ORTHOPAEDICS
for Physician Assistants

The second edition of *Orthopaedics for Physician Assistants* is dedicated to all my hard-working colleagues who strive to provide exceptional healthcare to their patients and to the following people who made this book possible:

Jennifer Hart for her perpetual loyalty to me and this book.

Alex Wix, who suddenly and serendipitously came into my family's life during the coronavirus school shut-down of 2020 and provided me time to focus amidst the chaos.

The contributing authors who devoted time they did not have and energy they could not waste to this project.

Dr. Bobby Chhabra for encouraging me to conceptualize and co-edit the first edition of *Orthopaedics for Physician Assistants* years ago, and who is still uplifting my career as a mentor.

I am deeply indebted to all my colleagues who I have worked with over the years in Virginia and Colorado. You have ALL made me a better PA.

And thank you to: my parents, who got me started off on this journey; my daughter, Asha, for understanding at such a young age that this project was important to me; and to my husband, Corey, for continuing to walk by my side— I love you all.—**SR**

This book is for my PA colleagues who work hard to deliver exceptional care to their patients every single day. This new update is thanks to the continued efforts of all of us who strive for success in this endeavor. I am thankful for the support of great supervising physicians, enthusiastic students, and supportive PA colleagues throughout the years. And I am forever thankful to my husband Joe and our family for supporting the years of training, work hours, and writing that is behind all of it. —**JAH**

ORTHOPAEDICS
for Physician Assistants

SECOND EDITION

SARA D. RYNDERS, MPAS, PA-C

Physician Assistant
Orthopaedic Surgery
University of Virginia
Charlottesville, Virginia

JENNIFER A. HART, MPAS, PA-C

Physician Assistant
Orthopaedic Surgery
University of Virginia
Charlottesville, Virginia

ELSEVIER

Elsevier
1600 John F. Kennedy Blvd.
Ste 1800
Philadelphia, PA 19103-2899

ORTHOPAEDICS FOR PHYSICIAN ASSISTANTS, SECOND EDITION   ISBN: 978-0-323-70984-2

Notice

Practitioners and researchers must always rely on their own experience and knowledge in evaluating and using any information, methods, compounds or experiments described herein. Because of rapid advances in the medical sciences, in particular, independent verification of diagnoses and drug dosages should be made. To the fullest extent of the law, no responsibility is assumed by Elsevier, authors, editors or contributors for any injury and/or damage to persons or property as a matter of products liability, negligence or otherwise, or from any use or operation of any methods, products, instructions, or ideas contained in the material herein.

Previous edition copyrighted 2013

Library of Congress Control Number: 2021946509

Senior Content Strategist: Lauren Wills
Senior Content Development Specialist: Angie Breckon
Content Development Manager: Meghan Andress
Publishing Services Manager: Shereen Jameel
Senior Project Manager: Karthikeyan Murthy
Design Direction: Renee Duenow

Printed in India

Last digit is the print number: 9   8   7   6   5   4   3

Deana Bhamidipati, PA-C, MPAS
Physician Assistant
Portland, Oregon

Nicholas Calabrese, BS, MPAS, PA-C
Physician Assistant
Orthopaedic Surgery
University of Virginia
Charlottesville, Virginia

Damond A. Cromer, BA, OTC
Orthopaedic Technologist Certified, II
Hand Center
University of Virginia
Charlottesville, Virginia

Jennifer A. Hart, MPAS, PA-C
Physician Assistant
Orthopaedic Surgery
University of Virginia
Charlottesville, Virginia

Michael Noordsy, PA-C, MPAS
Physician Assistant
Orthopaedics and Sports Medicine
Sanford/USD Medical Center
Sioux Falls, South Dakota

Michelle Post, PA-C
Sports Medicine PA
Orthopaedics
University of Virginia
Charlottesville, Virginia

Sara D. Rynders, MPAS, PA-C
Physician Assistant
Orthopaedic Surgery
University of Virginia
Charlottesville, Virginia

Christine Seeger, MAOT, CHT
Occupational Therapist
Austin Public School District
Austin, Minnesota

Rosemarie Tyger, PA-C
University of Virginia
Department of Orthopaedic Surgery
Division of Spine
Charlottesville, Virginia

Chad Wilson, MPAS, PA-C
Orthopaedic Surgery
UVA Health System
Charlottesville, Virginia

PREFACE

Orthopaedics for Physician Assistants is designed for those PAs who at some point find themselves alone in the vast world of musculoskeletal care and need a fast, reliable source to make it through the day. This text is the first of its kind. It is written for PAs by PAs or PA advocates. Its format is made for quick reading and referencing. Its small size is meant for storage in a pocket or at a clinic workstation. Its content and depth of knowledge are meant to appeal to the level of orthopaedic care provided by PAs working in the emergency department, primary care office, urgent care office, or orthopaedic clinic. This text is a reference and meant to be part of every PA student's library upon graduation.

The topics covered in this text are some of the most common orthopaedic conditions, organized by body location. Each chapter begins with an overview of anatomy with beautiful, detailed anatomic illustrations. The chapter is then subdivided into specific orthopaedic conditions. Each condition has an overview of the history and presentation, the pertinent physical examination findings, suggestions on what imaging or tests to order, and a treatment guide. Surgical indications and contraindications are also reviewed, and an overview of a common surgical treatment is outlined with pertinent surgical risks and expected recovery course. Also included is a beautifully photographed chapter that provides step-by-step guidance for splinting and casting. It really is a complete orthopaedic resource.

We sincerely thank all of our contributors, who range from physicians to residents, PAs, and cast technicians who are truly masters in their specialty areas. We appreciate your time and effort and support of PAs in medicine and orthopaedic surgery.

—*Sara D. Rynders*
—*Jennifer A. Hart*

CONTENTS

Spine

Rosemarie Tyger

ANATOMY

Bones: Fig. 1.1
- Cervical: Figs. 1.2 and 1.3

- Thoracic: Figs. 1.4 and 1.5
- Lumbar: Figs. 1.6 and 1.7

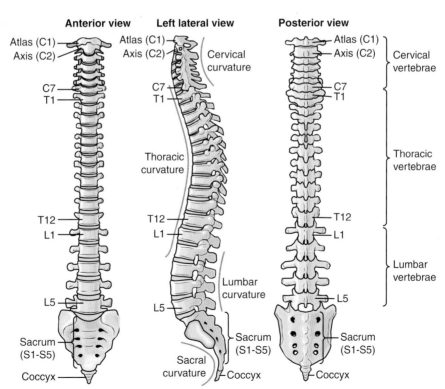

Fig. 1.1 The Bony Anatomy and Alignment of the Spine. (From Miller MD, Hart JA, MacKnight JM, editors: *Essential orthopaedics*, Philadelphia, 2010, Saunders, p 454.)

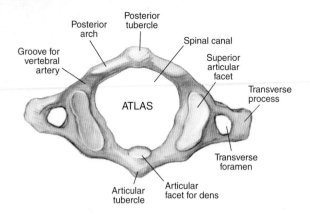

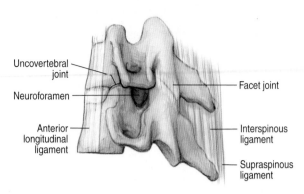

Fig. 1.3 **Anatomy of the Cervical Spine, Lateral View.** (From Miller MD, Chhabra AB, Hurwitz S, et al, editors: *Orthopaedic surgical approaches*, Philadelphia, 2008, Saunders, p 217.)

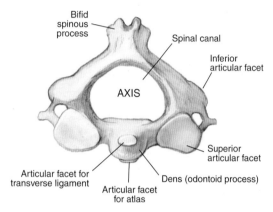

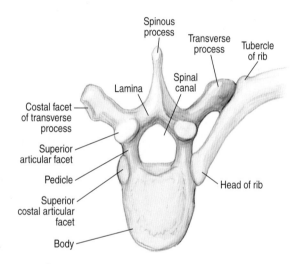

Fig. 1.4 **Bony Anatomy of a Thoracic Vertebra (Shown With Rib).** (From Miller MD, Chhabra AB, Hurwitz S, et al, editors: *Orthopaedic surgical approaches*, Philadelphia, 2008, Saunders, p 215.)

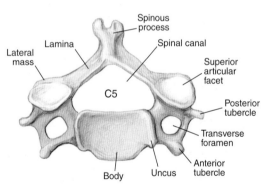

Fig. 1.2 **Bony Anatomy of the Cervical Vertebrae (C1, C2, and C5).** (From Miller MD, Chhabra AB, Hurwitz S, et al, editors: *Orthopaedic surgical approaches*, Philadelphia, 2008, Saunders, p 213.)

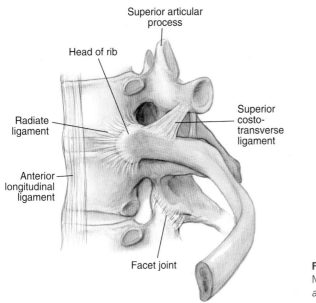

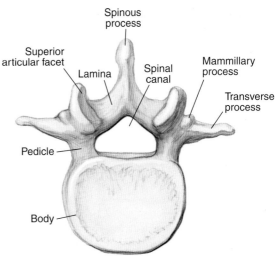

Fig. 1.6 Bony Anatomy of a Lumbar Vertebra. (From Miller MD, Chhabra AB, Hurwitz S, et al, editors: *Orthopaedic surgical approaches*, Philadelphia, 2008, Saunders, p 215.)

Fig. 1.5 Anatomy of the Thoracic Spine, Lateral View. (From Miller MD, Chhabra AB, Hurwitz S, et al, editors: *Orthopaedic surgical approaches*, Philadelphia, 2008, Saunders, p 218.)

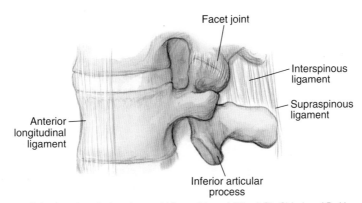

Fig. 1.7 Anatomy of the Lumbar Spine, Lateral View. (From Miller MD, Chhabra AB, Hurwitz S, et al, editors: *Orthopaedic surgical approaches*, Philadelphia, 2008, Saunders, p 218.)

Muscles and Soft Tissue: Figs. 1.8 through 1.11

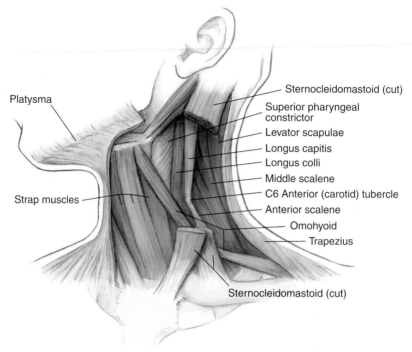

Fig. 1.8 Anterior Cervical Spine Muscles. (From Miller MD, Chhabra AB, Hurwitz S, et al, editors: *Orthopaedic surgical approaches*, Philadelphia, 2008, Saunders, p 219.)

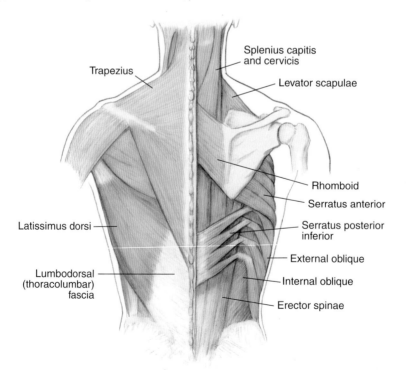

Fig. 1.9 Posterior View of the Spinal Musculature, Superficial and Intermediate Layers. (From Miller MD, Chhabra AB, Hurwitz S, et al, editors: *Orthopaedic surgical approaches*, Philadelphia, 2008, Saunders, p 222.)

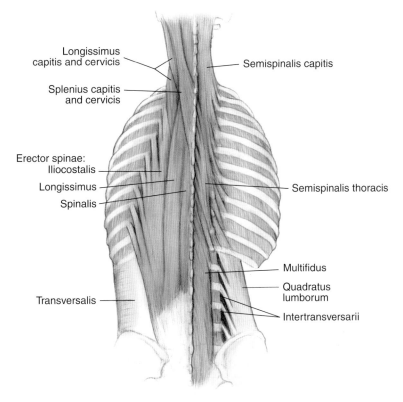

Longissimus capitis and cervicis

Semispinalis capitis

Splenius capitis and cervicis

Erector spinae:
  Iliocostalis
  Longissimus
  Spinalis

Semispinalis thoracis

Multifidus

Quadratus lumborum

Transversalis

Intertransversarii

Fig. 1.10 Posterior View of the Spinal Musculature, Deep View. (From Miller MD, Chhabra AB, Hurwitz S, et al, editors: *Orthopaedic surgical approaches*, Philadelphia, 2008, Saunders, p 223.)

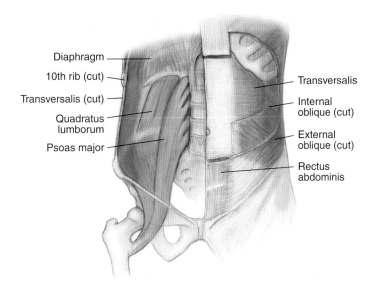

Diaphragm

10th rib (cut)

Transversalis (cut)

Quadratus lumborum

Psoas major

Transversalis

Internal oblique (cut)

External oblique (cut)

Rectus abdominis

Fig. 1.11 Anterior View of the Lumbar Spine Musculature. (From Miller MD, Chhabra AB, Hurwitz S, et al, editors: *Orthopaedic surgical approaches*, Philadelphia, 2008, Saunders, p 221.)

Nerves and Arteries: Figs. 1.12 through 1.14

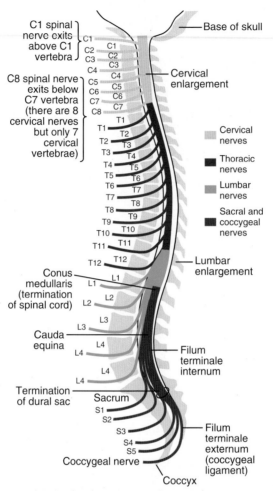

Fig. 1.12 The Spinal Cord and Nerve Root Orientation. (From Miller MD, Hart JA, MacKnight JM, editors: *Essential orthopaedics*, Philadelphia, 2010, Saunders, p 457.)

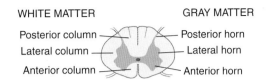

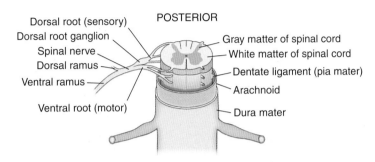

Fig. 1.13 The Cross-sectional Anatomy of the Spinal Cord. (From Miller MD, Chhabra AB, Hurwitz S, et al, editors: *Orthopaedic surgical approaches*, Philadelphia, 2008, Saunders, p 225.)

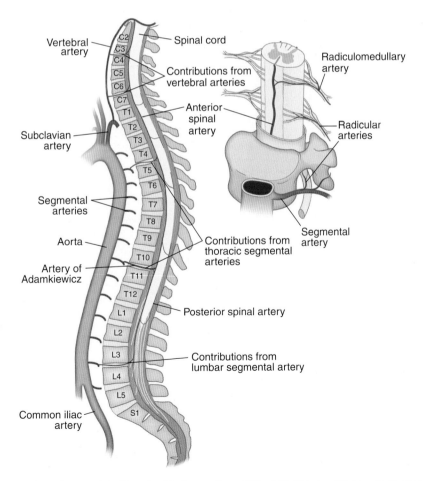

Fig. 1.14 The Vasculature of the Vertebral Column. (From Miller MD, Chhabra AB, Hurwitz S, et al, editors: *Orthopaedic surgical approaches*, Philadelphia, 2008, Saunders, p 227.)

Surface Anatomy: Fig. 1.15

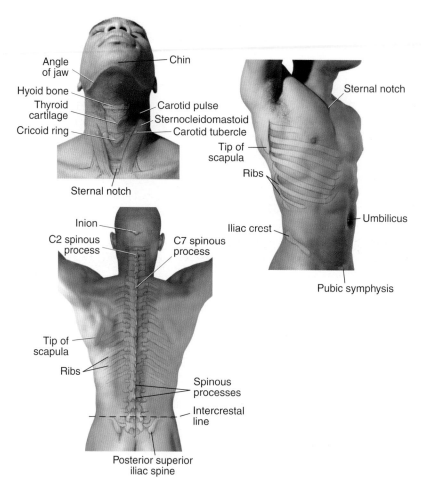

Fig. 1.15 The Surface Anatomy of the Spine. (From Miller MD, Chhabra AB, Hurwitz S, et al, editors: *Orthopaedic surgical approaches*, Philadelphia, 2008, Saunders, p 231.)

Normal X-Ray Appearance: Figs. 1.16 and 1.17

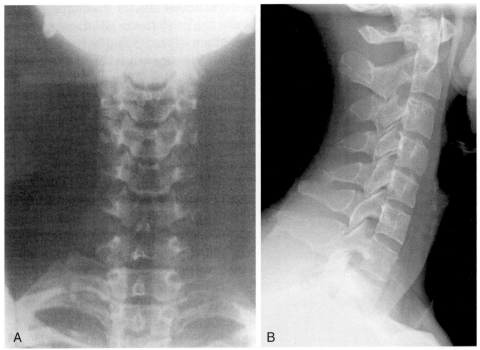

Fig. 1.16 Normal Cervical Spine X-ray Studies. **A,** Anteroposterior view. **B,** Lateral view. (**A,** From Schwartz AJ: Imaging of degenerative cervical disease, *Spine State Art Rev* 14:545–569, 2000; **B,** from Pretorious ES, Solomon JA, editors: *Radiology secrets,* ed 2, Philadelphia, 2006, Mosby.)

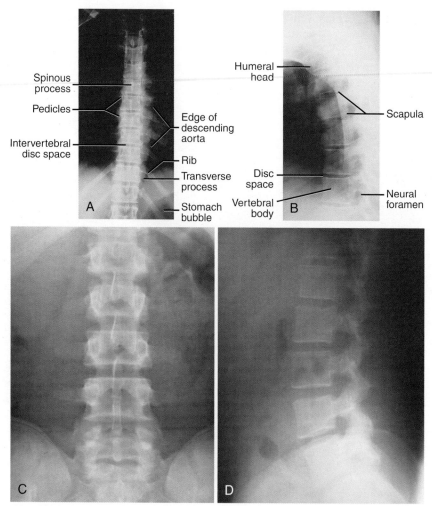

Fig. 1.17 Normal Spine X-ray Studies. **A,** Anteroposterior (AP) view of the thoracic spine. **B,** Lateral view of the thoracic spine. **C,** AP view of the lumbar spine. **D,** Lateral view of the lumbar spine. (**A** and **B,** From Mettler F: *Essentials of radiology,* ed 2, Philadelphia, 2005, Saunders; **C** and **D,** from Mercier L: *Practical orthopedics,* ed 6, Philadelphia, 2008, Mosby.)

PHYSICAL EXAMINATION

Inspect

- Skin for edema, rash, or discoloration
- Overall alignment in sagittal and coronal planes (evaluate for scoliosis or kyphosis)

Inspect gait for:

- Use of a cane, walker, or wheelchair
- Forward leaning posture (shopping cart sign): spinal stenosis
- Trendelenburg gait: hip disease
- Wide-based gait (antalgic): myelopathy

Palpate specific structures to evaluate complaint:

- Spinous processes
- Facet joints
- Musculature of trunk and spine
- Sacroiliac (SI) joints
- Greater trochanters

Percuss costovertebral angles (CVAs).

Normal range of motion (ROM): Table 1.1

Neurovascular examination: Fig. 1.18

- Cervical reflexes: include biceps (C5), triceps (C7), and brachioradial (C6).
- Lumbar reflexes: include patella (L4) and Achilles (S1).
- Pulses to be checked: include radial, dorsalis pedis, and posterior tibialis.
- Sensation of gross soft touch in the dermatomal pattern is assessed.
- Pinprick and point discrimination is tested as needed.

Special Tests

- **Hoffman reflex**: Hoffmann reflex most often reflects the presence of an upper motor neuron lesion from spinal cord compression. A **positive test** result is elicited by flicking either the volar or dorsal surfaces of the middle finger and observing the reflex contraction of the thumb and index finger to form an "OK" sign (Fig. 1.19).
- **Babinski reflex**: The Babinski reflex tests the integrity of the cortical spinal tract (CST). This is an abnormal reflex in adults and if it is present, represents an upper motor neuron lesion. A **positive test** is when there is involuntary dorsiflexion of the extensor hallucis longus (or big toe) and abduction of the lesser toes in response to forceful scratching of the plantar or lateral aspect of the foot (Fig. 1.20).
- **Clonus**: Involuntary repetitive dorsiflexion of ankle occurs in response to one-time forceful dorsiflexion of the ankle by the examiner (Fig. 1.21).
- **Bulbocavernosus reflex (BCR)**: This refers to anal sphincter contraction in response to squeezing the glans penis or clitoris, or by tugging on the Foley catheter tube carefully and involves the S2–S4 nerve roots. This is a spinal cord–mediated reflex. Following spinal cord trauma, the presence or absence of this reflex carries prognostic significance; in cases of cervical or thoracic spinal cord injury (SCI), absence of this reflex documents continuation of spinal shock or spinal injury at the level of the reflex arc. Return of the reflex signals the end of spinal shock. In lumbar injuries below the level of the spinal cord, absence of the reflex may reflect cauda equina injury.
- **Straight leg raise**: The test is performed by passively raising the leg while the patient is supine. **A positive test** result is indicated by reproduction of radicular symptoms on the involved side (Fig. 1.22).
- **Waddell signs**: These are a group of physical signs that test for nonorganic or psychological components to chronic low back pain:
  1. Tenderness test: superficial and diffuse tenderness and/or not anatomic
  2. Stimulation test: axial loading and pain of stimulated rotation (should not cause low back pain)
  3. Distraction test: positive test (such as a straight leg raise) that is rechecked when the patient's attention is distracted
  4. Regional disturbances: nonanatomic or breakaway weakness
  5. Overreaction (the most important Waddell sign): subjective signs regarding the patient's demeanor and reaction to testing

TABLE 1.1	Normal Range of Motion
Motion	**Range (Degrees)**
Cervical extension	60
Cervical flexion	75
Cervical lateral flexion	45
Cervical rotation	80
Thoracic flexion	50
Thoracic rotation	30
Lumbar extension	60
Lumbar flexion	25

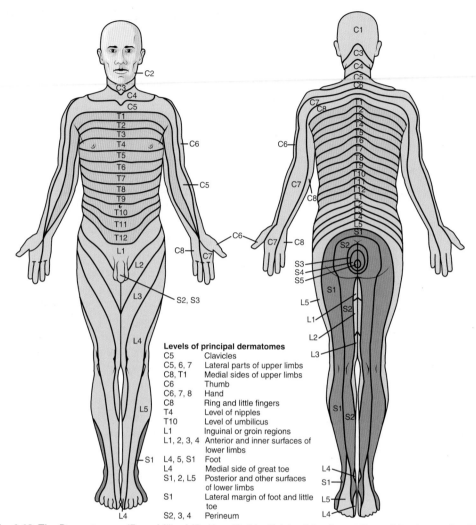

Levels of principal dermatomes

C5	Clavicles
C5, 6, 7	Lateral parts of upper limbs
C8, T1	Medial sides of upper limbs
C6	Thumb
C6, 7, 8	Hand
C8	Ring and little fingers
T4	Level of nipples
T10	Level of umbilicus
L1	Inguinal or groin regions
L1, 2, 3, 4	Anterior and inner surfaces of lower limbs
L4, 5, S1	Foot
L4	Medial side of great toe
S1, 2, L5	Posterior and other surfaces of lower limbs
S1	Lateral margin of foot and little toe
S2, 3, 4	Perineum

Fig. 1.18 The Dermatomes. (From Miller MD, Hart JA, MacKnight JM, editors: *Essential orthopaedics*, Philadelphia, 2010, Saunders, p 458.)

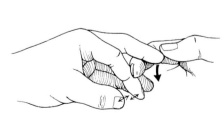

Fig. 1.19 Hoffman Reflex. (From Fong W, et al: Evaluation of cervical spine disorders. In Devlin VJ, editor: *Spine secrets plus*, ed 2, St. Louis, 2012, Mosby, p 38.)

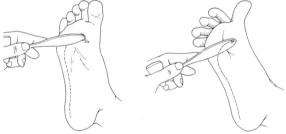

Fig. 1.20 Babinski Reflex. (From Fong W, et al: Evaluation of cervical spine disorders. In Devlin VJ, editor: *Spine secrets plus*, ed 2, St. Louis, 2012, Mosby, p 38.)

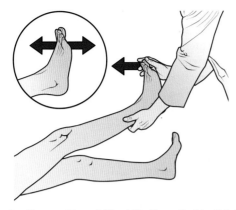

Fig. 1.21 Clonus. (From Miller MD, Hart JA, MacKnight JM, editors: *Essential orthopaedics*, Philadelphia, 2010, Saunders, p 460.)

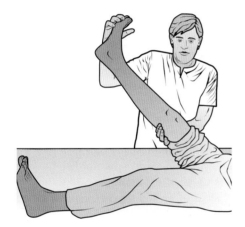

Fig. 1.22 Straight Leg Raise. (From Miller MD, Hart JA, MacKnight JM, editors: *Essential orthopaedics*, Philadelphia, 2010, Saunders, p 462.)

Board Review

1. Upward Babinski reflex is a physical examination finding suggestive of an upper motor neuron lesion.
2. A positive Babinski Reflex is characterized by an upward-going great toe (dorsiflexion) and abduction of the lesser toes.

SUGGESTED READINGS

Van Gijn J: The Babinski reflex, *Postgrad Med J* 71(841):645–648, 1995.

Differential Diagnosis

See Table 1.2

TABLE 1.2	**Differential Diagnosis**
Low back pain	Lumbar muscle pain
	Degenerative disc disease
	Lumbar facet disease
	Nephrolithiasis
	Lumbar compression fracture
	Osteomyelitis
	Malingering
	Ovarian cyst
Lumbar radiculopathy	Herniated disc
	Foraminal stenosis
	Spinal stenosis
	Neuropathy
Cervical or thoracic pain	Muscle strain
	Abdominal Aortic Aneurysm (AAA)
	Fracture
	Facet disease
	Degenerative disc disease
	Ankylosing spondylitis
Regional or dermatomal pain	Shingles
Deformity	Scoliosis
	Kyphosis

CERVICAL SPINE

CERVICAL DEGENERATIVE DISC DISEASE

Cervical degenerative disc disease (DDD), also known as cervical spondylosis, is chronic disc degeneration and associated facet arthropathy that can result in four clinical entities:

1. Discogenic neck pain (axial pain)
2. Radiculopathy (root compression)
3. Myelopathy (cord compression)
4. Myeloradiculopathy (root and cord compression)

DISCOGENIC NECK PAIN

Discogenic neck pain is secondary to intervertebral disc degeneration without other pathologic entities, such as spinal instability, fractures, dislocations or neural compression. This condition accounts for a large proportion of chronic neck pain and stiffness.

History

- Insidious onset of neck pain without neurologic signs or symptoms, exacerbated by vertebral motion
- Can also get occipital headaches

Physical Examination

- Typically benign; normal motor and sensory exam, normal reflexes

Imaging

- Cervical standing radiographs: anteroposterior (AP), lateral, flexion, and extension—typically normal without evidence of instability; may demonstrate disc space narrowing

Additional Imaging

- Magnetic resonance imaging (MRI): typically demonstrates intervertebral disc degeneration (dark disc) and facet arthropathy—decreased signal in the disc on T2-weighted imaging

Nonoperative Management

- **Patient Education.** Emphasizing the self-limiting nature of symptoms is important
- Nonoperative therapy: nonsteroidal antiinflammatory drugs (NSAIDs), physical therapy and symptomatic care

CERVICAL RADICULOPATHY

Cervical radiculopathy is caused by nerve root compression due to herniated disc, discosteophytic complex, facet arthropathy, thickened ligamentum flavum, or uncovertebral osteophyte. It can involve one or multiple nerve roots (polyradiculopathy). Cervical nerve roots exit above their corresponding vertebra so the caudal nerve root at a given level is usually affected (e.g., C5 exits at C4–5 neural foramen). It is also important to recognize that a disc herniation at C7–T1 involves the C8 nerve root.

History

- Neck pain and radicular symptoms
- Pain, numbness, paresthesia in a dermatomal distribution to upper extremity

Physical Examination

- Motor: weakness when present is associated with the myotome
- Sensory: pain, numbness or dysesthesias along dermatomal distribution is common
- Reflexes: typically normal or hyporeflexive
- Special tests
  - **Spurlings Test**: suggestive for nerve root pain when radicular symptoms occur with rotation and lateral bend of the neck, with vertical compression on the head
  - **Shoulder abduction sign**: relief of radicular pain with shoulder abduction (placing hand on top of patient's head)

Imaging

- Cervical standing radiographs: AP, lateral, flexion, and extension views—may see disc space narrowing

Additional Imaging

- **MRI (modality of choice):** on T2 weighted image look for herniated nucleus pulposus (HNP) causing nerve root compression
- Computed tomography (CT) or myelogram if previous instrumented spine surgery or if MRI contraindicated

Nonoperative Management

- Nonoperative management is always the first step in management of cervical radiculopathy.
- NSAIDs, physical therapy, gentle cervical traction, or gabapentin.
- Oral steroids should be used cautiously and may be reserved for severe acute radiculopathy rather than chronic symptom presentation.
- If noninvasive measures are not helpful to improve symptoms, then epidural spine injections can give good relief of symptoms, particularly for radicular pain.

Operative Management

ICD-10 codes:

  M54.12 Cervical radiculopathy

  M50.20 Cervical herniated disc

CPT codes:

  22551 to 22552 Anterior cervical discectomy and fusion (ACDF)

  22845 to 22846 Anterior instrumentation code

  63081 Cervical corpectomy

  22856 Cervical disc replacement

  63020, 63035 Cervical hemilaminectomy (laminotomy)

Indications

- Progressive motor weakness, persistent disabling pain despite conservative treatment.
- Surgical indications: progressive motor weakness, persistent disabling pain despite conservative treatment.

Informed consent and counseling

All anterior cervical spine surgery carries a risk of injury to the recurrent laryngeal nerve which can result in hoarseness or anterior neck edema and dysphagia. Frequently these complications are temporary, but there is a risk of permanent nerve injury.

Surgical Procedures
Anterior Cervical Discectomy Fusion (ACDF)

A left-sided approach is common to avoid the recurrent laryngeal nerve. Use a transverse incision from the anterior edge of the sternocleidomastoid muscle to near the midline through the fascia to the platysma. Deep dissection occurs carefully through the anterior neck structures. The herniated disc and associated ostephytes are removed and the disc space is filled with bone graft. The vertebral levels are then fused with anterior instrumentation.

Anterior Cervical Corpectomy and Fusion (ACCF)

This procedure is the same as ACDF except if neural compression is due to pathology behind the vertebral body then removal of the vertebral body (corpectomy) is preformed and replaced with a bone graft or cage.

Estimated Postoperative Recovery Course

- Postoperative 2 to 3 weeks:
  - Patient returns for wound check
  - Upright AP and lateral cervical x-rays are obtained
  - Cervical collar is discontinued, can start gentle ROM
  - Continue to have patient limit lifting <5–8 lbs until 6-week mark then patient can start physical therapy
- Postoperative 3 to 4 months:
  - Recheck x-rays (AP, lateral, flexion, and extension) and evaluate for fusion. Fusion site should be complete.
  - If patient is doing well and radiographs look good, can release back to normal activities.
- Postoperative 6 months:
  - Routine follow-up and recheck x-rays
- Postoperative 9 to 12 months:
  - Routine follow-up and recheck x-rays

Cervical Disc Replacement (CDR)

CDR uses the same anterior approach as ACDF to remove a herniated disc and replace it with an artificial device. This has been developed as an alternative to fusion with the possible benefit of preventing premature breakdown in adjacent levels of the spine. Only used in patients who have maintained normal lordotic cervical sagittal alignment.

Estimated Postoperative Recovery Course

- Postoperative 2 to 3 weeks:
  - Patient returns for wound check
  - Upright AP and lateral cervical x-rays are obtained
  - Continue to have patient limit lifting <5–8 lbs until 6-week mark then patient can start physical therapy
- Postoperative 3 to 4 months:
  - Recheck x-rays (AP, lateral, flexion, and extension) and make sure the cervical disc has good placement.
  - If patient is doing well and radiographs look good can release back to normal activities.
- Postoperative 6 to 9 months:
  - Routine follow-up and recheck x-rays

Posterior Keyhole Laminoforaminotomy

Posterior keyhole laminoforaminotomy is less commonly performed but it is an option for radiculopathy secondary to posterior compression from facet hypertrophy, osteophytes or lateral soft disc herniations. This procedure is used to remove the bone spur, part of the facet or a portion of the disc causing the compression therefore making more room for the nerve to pass through.

Estimated Postoperative Recovery Course

- Postoperative 2 to 3 weeks
  - Patient returns for wound check
  - Staples or sutures are removed if they were used
  - Upright AP and lateral cervical x-rays can be obtained, not always needed since there is no fusion to assess—*depends on surgeon preference*
  - Continue to have patient limit lifting <5–8 lbs until 6-week mark then patient can start physical therapy
- Postoperative 3 months:
  - Patient returns for routine follow-up, if doing well can release back to normal activities

CERVICAL MYELOPATHY

Cervical myelopathy is a progressive degenerative disease and is the most common cause of cervical spinal cord dysfunction.[1] Cervical myelopathy can be due to direct compression of the spinal cord, or surrounding blood vessels, resulting in varied clinical symptoms. Spondylosis has been shown as the most common etiology for cervical myelopathy in people aged 55 years or older.[2] The most common cause of compression is due to anterior degenerative changes, such as osteophytes and discosteophytic complexes. It can also be from trauma, tumor, or infection.

History

- Finger clumsiness, deterioration of handwriting, difficulty with fine motor control of hands
- Ataxia with wide-based gait, leg heaviness, and inability to perform tandem walk
- Urinary retention or incontinence
- Characterized by three presentations:
  1. Stepwise deterioration in symptomatology followed by a period of stability (most common, 65%–80%)[1]
  2. Slowly progressive decline (over months to years, 20%–25%)[1]
  3. Rapidly progressive decline (over days to weeks, 3%–5%)[1]

Physical Examination

- Upper motor neuron signs will be seen in myelopathy
  - Hyperreflexia, Hoffman's sign, clonus or Babinski
- Inverted radial reflex (ipsilateral finger flexion when eliciting brachioradialis reflex)

Imaging

- MRI (modality of choice)
  - May see myelomalacia, which is a hyperintense signal seen on T2-weighted images
- CT or myelogram if previous instrumented spine surgery or if MRI contraindicated
  - CT is also useful in looking for ossification of posterior longitudinal ligament (PLL) and surgical planning

Initial Management

- **Patient Education.** The Natural history of myelopathy is that it is typically progressive, therefore surgical decompression is frequently indicated.

Operative Management

ICD-10 codes:
  M48.02 Cervical stenosis
  G95.9 Cervical myelopathy

CPT codes:
  22551 to 22552 ACDF
  22845 to 22846 Anterior instrumentation code
  63081 Cervical corpectomy
  63001, 63015, 63045, 63048 Posterior cervical decompression codes
  22840, 22842, 22600 Posterior arthrodesis and instrumentation codes
  63051 Laminoplasty

Surgical Procedures

Posterior Cervical Decompression and Fusion

Posterior cervical decompression and fusion is procedure during which the posterior elements that are causing compression on the cervical spine are removed and the spine is stabilized with instrumentation.

Estimated Postoperative Recovery Course

- Postoperative 2 to 3 weeks:
  - Patient returns for wound check
  - Upright AP and lateral cervical x-rays are obtained
  - Suture or staples are removed
  - Cervical collar is discontinued
  - Continue to have patient limit lifting <5–8 lbs until 6-week mark then patient can start physical therapy
- Postoperative 3 to 4 months:
  - Recheck x-rays (AP, lateral, flexion, and extension) and evaluate for fusion. Fusion site should be complete.
  - If patient is doing well and radiographs look good can release back to normal activities.
- Postoperative 6 months:
  - Routine follow-up and recheck x-rays
- Postoperative 9 to 12 months:
  - Routine follow-up and recheck x-rays

Laminoplasty

Laminoplasty is a motion preserving procedure in which the lamina are hinged open laterally like a door, and secured in their new position with a metal plate to enlarge the spinal canal.

Estimated Postoperative Recovery Course

- Postoperative 2 to 3 weeks:
  - Patient returns for wound check
  - Upright AP and lateral cervical x-rays are obtained

- Suture or staples are removed
- Continue to have patient limit lifting <5–8 lbs until 6-week mark then patient can start physical therapy
- Postoperative 3 to 4 months:
  - Recheck x-rays (AP, lateral, flexion, and extension)
  - If patient is doing well and radiographs look good can release back to normal activities
- Postoperative 6 months:
  - Routine follow-up and recheck x-rays
- Postoperative 9 to 12 months:
  - Routine follow-up and recheck x-rays

Board Review

1. The modality of choice to look for cervical stenosis in a patient with suspected myelopathy is a cervical MRI.
2. A left-sided disc herniation at C5–6 will cause pain to radiate into the left arm in an anterior pattern down to the dorsoradial forearm and into the thumb and index finger. On physical examination look for weakness of the biceps muscle group and loss of brachioradialis reflex on that side.

SUGGESTED READINGS

Shen F, Samartiz D, Fessler R, editors: *Textbook of the cervical spine* (2). Elsevier/Saunders Maryland Heights, MI, 2015, pp 117–145(12-14).

REFERENCES

1. Singh A, Tetreault L, Casey A, Laing R, Statham P, Fehlings MG: A summary of assessment tools for patients suffering from cervical spondylotic myelopathy: a systematic review on validity, reliability and responsiveness, *Eur Spine J* 24(suppl 2):209–228, 2015.
2. Klineberg E: Cervical spondylotic myelopathy: a review of the evidence, *Orthop Clin North Am* 41:193–202, 2010.

LUMBAR SPINE

LUMBAR STRAIN

A lumbar strain is the most common cause of low back pain. The injury can be minor or mild and normally occurs due to overuse, improper use, or trauma. If it is classified as "acute" if it has been present for days to weeks. However, if the strain lasts longer than 3 months, it is referred to as "chronic."

History

- Bending, twisting, and lifting reproduce pain
- Pain in back occurs with movement, coughing, or sneezing
- Leg pain or weakness is lacking

Physical Examination

- Slow gait
- Tenderness to palpation over muscular structures
- Pain with flexion, extension, and/or rotation of the trunk
- Normal neurologic examination

Imaging

- Lumbar standing radiographs — AP or lateral views are obtained initially only if the mechanism warrants.

Differential Diagnosis

- Lumbar Compression fracture.
- Intra-abdominal or pelvic disease such as nephrolithiasis, pyelonephritis, abdominal aortic aneurysm, intraabdominal, intrapelvic, or spinal mass, or metastasis.
- SI joint instability or inflammation.
- Occult vertebral body fracture: bone scan or MRI will identify injury in cases of persistent pain.
- Malingering: secondary gain must be considered. Assess with Waddell signs.

Initial Management

- **Patient Education.** Back pain, one of the most common medical problems, affects 8 out of 10 people at some point during their lives. Most back pain goes away on its own, although it may take a while. However, staying in bed for more than 1 or 2 days can make it worse.

Nonoperative Management

- A short 1- to 2-day rest period for severe pain is prescribed.
- Heat and/or ice and over-the-counter NSAIDs or acetaminophen
- Skeletal muscle relaxants can be used sparingly.
- Physical therapy and "back school" can be beneficial for persistent pain.
- Advanced imaging is used only after 6 to 8 weeks of failed conservative treatment.
- Long-term prevention with core strengthening and ROM exercises is indicated.

ICD-10 Codes

M45.9 Back pain
M54.5 Lumbosacral pain
S39.012A Lumbar strain
Z76.5 Malingerer

LUMBAR DEGENERATIVE DISC DISEASE

Lumbar degenerative disc disease (also known as lumbar spondylosis) is a major cause of morbidity, with a financial impact in the United States. Low back pain affects approximately 60%–85% of adults during some point in their lives. Fortunately, for the large majority of individuals symptoms are mild and transient, with 90% subsiding within 6 weeks.[1] It has an array of symptoms that can result in several clinical entities such as discogenic back pain (axial pain), lumbar disc herniation (or HNP), lumbar spinal stenosis, and spondylolisthesis.

Discogenic Back Pain

Secondary to intervertebral disc degeneration without other pathologic entities, such as spinal instability, fractures, dislocations, or neural compression.

History

- Insidious onset of back pain without neurologic signs or symptoms, exacerbated by vertebral motion
- Back pain greater than leg pain
- No radiculopathy

Physical Examination

- Typically benign; normal motor and sensory examination, normal reflexes

Imaging

- Lumbar standing radiographs: AP, lateral, flexion, and extension views—typically normal without evidence of instability; may demonstrate disc space narrowing

Additional Imaging

- MRI: typically demonstrates decreased signal in the disc on T2-weighted imaging (dark disc), with or without annular tear or high intensity zone (HIZ).
- Discography: controversial study designed as a preoperative test to correlate MRI findings with a clinically significant pain generator.
  - Needle placed into the intervertebral disc space and contrast dye injected. To be considered reliably positive, the procedure should elicit pain after injection similar to that usually described by the patient.

Initial Management

- **Patient Education.** Counsel the patient that discogenic back pain is usually self-limited.
  - More than half of patients who seek treatment for low back pain recover in 1 week, and 90% recover within 1 to 3 months.[2]
  - Counsel patient on the importance of adhering to proper bending and lifting mechanics, back and core strengthening, weight control, and smoking cessation to prevent future episodes of pain.

Nonoperative Management

- NSAIDs, physical therapy, and conditioning

Operative Management

ICD-10 codes:

M51.26 Lumbar discogenic pain syndrome
M51.36 Lumbar degenerative disc disease

CPT codes:

22558, 22585 Anterior retroperitoneal or oblique lateral approach for interbody lumbar fusion
22857 Lumbar total disc arthroplasty

Indications

- Controversial: surgery should be avoided whenever possible for discogenic back pain
- Currently no good surgical option available that reliably reduces symptoms

Surgical Procedures

Anterior Lumbar Interbody Fusion (ALIF)

ALIF is accomplished through an anterior retroperitoneal approach, normally with the help of a vascular surgeon, to remove lumbar disc with excision of associated osteophytes followed by replacement of the disc with structural constructs (femoral ring allografts or cages) with or without anterior instrumentation.

Oblique Lateral Interbody Fusion (OLIF)

During an OLIF procedure the disc is accessed from an incision through the psoas muscle obliquely, removed and replaced with a cage.

Estimated Postoperative Recovery Course

- Postoperative 2 to 3 weeks:
  - Patient returns for wound check
  - Upright AP and lateral lumbar x-rays are obtained

- Suture or staples are removed
- Continue to have patient limit lifting <5–8 lbs and no bending or twisting until 6-week mark then patient can start physical therapy
- Postoperative 3 to 4 months:
  - Recheck x-rays (AP, lateral, flexion, and extension) and evaluate for fusion. Fusion site should be complete.
  - If patient is doing well and radiographs look good, can release back to normal activities.
- Postoperative 6 months:
  - Routine follow-up and recheck x-rays
- Postoperative 9 to 12 months:
  - Routine follow-up and recheck x-rays

LUMBAR HERNIATED NUCLEUS PULPOSUS

Nucleus pulposus herniation is the most common cause of sciatic pain and one of the most common indications for spine surgery worldwide. This condition presents as a displacement of the nucleus pulposus beyond the intervertebral disc space. The disc anatomy consists of two main structures, the *nucleus pulposus* (NP) and the *annulus fibrosus* (AF).[3] Most lumbar herniations are posterolateral (where the posterior longitudinal ligament is the weakest) and involve the lower nerve root at that level (e.g., S1 nerve at L5–S1). Herniations lateral to the neural foramen (also known as "far lateral" disc herniations) involve the upper nerve root (e.g., L4 nerve at the L4–5 level). Central herniations are often associated with back pain only; however, may precipitate a cauda equine compressive syndrome. **Cauda equina syndrome** is a rare disorder affecting the bundle of nerve roots (cauda equina) at the lower end of the spinal cord. It is considered a surgical emergency.

History

- Back pain and radicular symptoms that are worse with sitting and better with standing and lying down
- Pain or numbness radiating beyond the knee, typically in a dermatomal distribution
- **Cauda equina syndrome ("red flag" symptoms)**
  - Severe low back pain
  - Sciatica: often bilateral but sometimes absent
  - Loss of bowel or bladder control

- "Saddle anesthesia"—numbness and loss of sensation in the buttocks, perineum, and inner surfaces of the thighs

Physical Examination

- Motor: typically normal but weakness may be present, depending on nerve root involved
- Sensory: pain, numbness, or dysesthesias along dermatomal distribution is common
- Reflexes: typically normal or hyporeflexive
- Special tests
  - **Straight leg test:** while patient is supine, raise symptomatic leg with knee extended between 30 and 70 degrees. Positive test is when it reproduces and/or exaggerates symptoms radiating down the leg. Sensitive for L4, L5, and S1 nerve root irritation but not very specific.
  - **Contralateral straight leg test:** raising contralateral asymptomatic leg with knee straight results in pain radiating down the symptomatic leg. More specific for axillary disc herniation.
  - **Femoral tension sign:** patient is prone and on the symptomatic side. The knee is passively flexed while the hip is being extended. A positive test occurs when this maneuver reproduces and/or exaggerates symptoms radiating down anterior thigh. Sensitive for L2, L3, and L4 nerve root irritation but not very specific.
  - **Lasegue sign:** relief of radiating leg symptoms with knee flexion while hip is flexed.
  - **Digital rectal examination:** should be used for initial diagnosis of cauda equina syndrome.
  - Check for presence of rectal tone, perianal sensation, and volitional control/contraction. In particular, evaluation of perianal sensation is important for immediate diagnosis.

Imaging

- **Lumbar standing radiographs:** AP, lateral, flexion, and extension views—stimulate spinal alignment and help assess for spinal instability or deformity
  - May note sciatic scoliosis on radiograph, which is a lateral deformity of the trunks secondary to a HNP or sciatica

Additional Imaging

- **MRI (modality of choice):** use T2 weighted image to look for HNP and area of nerve root compression

- Urgent MRI is needed with suspected cases of cauda equina syndrome
- MRI with gadolinium is the best study for recurrent disc herniations
- CT or myelogram if previous instrumented spine surgery or if MRI contraindicated

Initial Management
Nonoperative Management
- NSAIDs, activity modification, Medrol dose pack and physical therapy are often effective in the first 6 weeks of symptom onset.
- If noninvasive conservative treatments are not helpful to improve symptoms, then epidural spine injections can give good relief of symptoms, particularly for radicular pain.

Operative Management
ICD-10 codes:
  M54.16 Lumbar radiculopathy
  M51.26 Lumbar herniated disc
  G83.4 Cauda equina compression
CPT codes:
  63030 Discectomy (open or with tubes)
  63042 Revision discectomy
  63056 Far lateral discectomy
  Indications
Progressive motor weakness, persistent disabling pain despite conservative treatment and predominately nerve root pain or cauda equina
- **Cauda equina syndrome**: timing of surgical decompression remains controversial, but decompression within the first 48 hours was reported to lead to the best outcomes

Surgical Procedure
Discectomy
A discectomy is a posterior procedure that can be performed open or with tubes (minimal invasive). A microscope may be utilized to remove the herniated part of the disc and decompress the affected nerve root. A far lateral discectomy can also be performed and will typically utilize an incision slightly off the midline on the affected side.

Estimated Postoperative Recovery Course
- Postoperative 2 to 3 weeks:
  - Patient returns for wound check

- Upright AP and lateral lumbar x-rays can be obtained, not necessarily needed since there is no fusion—*depends on surgeon preference*
- Continue to have patient limit lifting <5–8 lbs and no bending or twisting until 6-week mark then patient can start physical therapy
- Postoperative 3 months:
  - Patient returns for routine follow-up, if doing well can release back to normal activities

LUMBAR STENOSIS

Spinal stenosis is narrowing of the spinal canal or neural foramina, producing nerve root compression, root ischemia, and a variable syndrome of back and leg pain. Stenosis is not usually symptomatic until patients reach late middle age; men are affected somewhat more than women. Stenosis can be broken down into three main classifications: central stenosis (neurogenic claudication), lateral recess stenosis, and foraminal stenosis (Fig. 1.23)

Central Stenosis—Thecal Sac Compression
The *central canal* is defined as the space posterior to the posterior longitudinal ligament, anterior to the ligamentum flavum and laminae, and bordered laterally by the medical border of the superior articular process. The etiology of stenosis can be broken down into two categories: congenital versus acquired.
- Congenital (idiopathic or developmental in achondroplasia dwarfism), due to shortened pedicles
- Acquired (most common)
  - Degenerative secondary to enlargement of osteoarthritic facets
  - Degenerative secondary to spondylolisthesis
  - Posttraumatic
  - Iatrogenic (postsurgical)

History
- Insidious pain and paresthesia with ambulation and relieved with sitting or flexion of the spine (positive shopping cart sign)
- Patients commonly complain of lower extremity pain, usually in the buttock and thighs, with numbness or "giving away"
- Neurogenic claudication should be differentiated from vascular claudication. Neurogenic claudication is characterized by:
  - Differentiate from vascular claudication

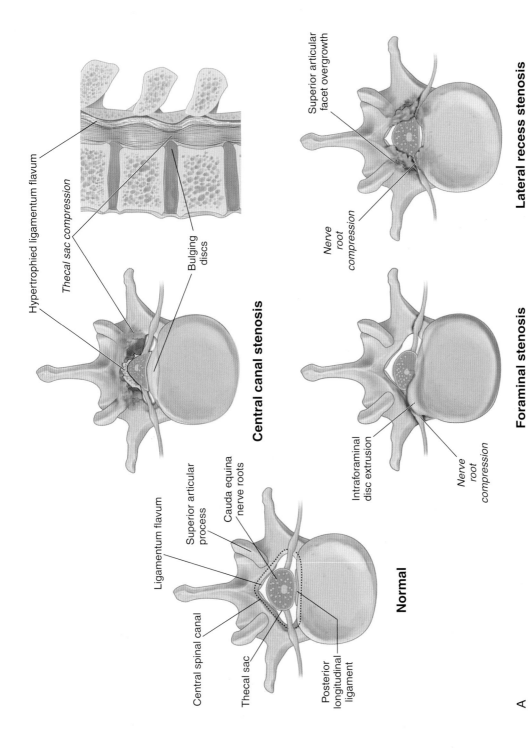

A

Fig. 1.23 Pathoanatomy of Spinal Stenosis. (From Shen FH: Spine. In Miller MD, Thompson SR, editors, *Miller's review of orthopedics* Philadelphia, Elsevier; 2016: p 671.)

Hypertrophied ligamentum flavum

Thecal sac compression

Bulging discs

Central canal stenosis

Superior articular facet overgrowth

Nerve root compression

Lateral recess stenosis

Intraforaminal disc extrusion

Nerve root compression

Foraminal stenosis

Ligamentum flavum

Superior articular process

Cauda equina nerve roots

Central spinal canal

Thecal sac

Posterior longitudinal ligament

Normal

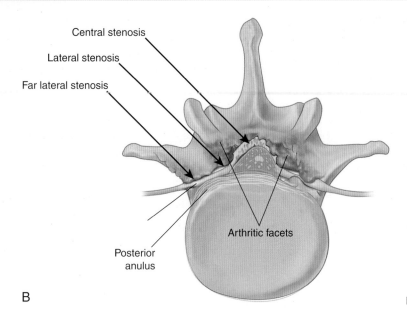

Central stenosis

Lateral stenosis

Far lateral stenosis

Arthritic facets

Posterior anulus

B

Fig. 1.23, cont'd

- Pain that starts proximal (buttocks) and extends distal
- Pain that is relieved only when sitting, not when standing
- Normal vascular examination

Physical Examination

- Primary finding is typically limited extension, which may exacerbate pain
- Motor: typically normal
- Sensory: normal
- Check for extremity perfusion and pulses
- Reflexes: typically normal or hyporeflexive

Imaging

- Lumbar standing radiographs: AP, lateral, flexion, and extension views
  - Interspace narrowing due to disc degeneration
  - Flattening of the lordotic curve
  - Degeneration of the facet joints

Additional Imaging and Testing

- MRI (test of choice)
  - Hypertrophy of the ligamentum flavum
  - Foraminal stenosis and nerve root entrapment
  - Evaluation for malignancy
- CT or myelogram if previous instrumented spine surgery or if MRI contraindicated

- Electromyography and Nerve Conduction Studies (EMG/NCS) may be used to help differentiate radiculopathy from peripheral neuropathy

Initial Management
Nonoperative Management

- Rest, Williams flexion exercises, NSAIDs, weight reduction
- If noninvasive conservative treatments are not helpful to improve symptoms, then epidural spine injections can give good short-term relief of symptoms

Operative Management

ICD-10 codes:
  M48.062 Lumbar stenosis with neurogenic claudication
  M48.062 Lumbar stenosis without neurogenic claudication
CPT codes:
  63047 Lumbar decompression
  63048 Additional level decompression
  Indications
- Progressive motor weakness and a persistently impaired quality of life

Surgical Procedure
Lumbar Decompression

A laminectomy is a posterior procedure that involves removing the lamina, ligamentum flavum, and part of the facets, which can usually be accomplished without destabilizing the spine, thus avoiding a fusion

Estimated Postoperative Recovery Course
- Postoperative 2 to 3 weeks:
  - Patient returns for wound check
  - Suture or staples are removed if they were used
  - Upright AP and lateral lumbar x-rays can be obtained, not necessarily needed since there is no fusion–*depends on surgeon preference*
  - Continue to have patient limit lifting <5–8 lbs and no bending or twisting until 6-week mark then patient can start some physical therapy
- Postoperative 3 months:
  - Patient returns for routine follow-up, if doing well can release back to normal activities

Lateral Recess Stenosis—Nerve Root Compression
Lateral recess stenosis is impingement of the nerve roots lateral to the thecal sac as they pass through the lateral recess and into the neural foramen. It is associated with facet joint arthropathy (superior articular process enlargement) and degenerative disc disease. The nerve root affected is the traversing (lower) nerve root (e.g., L5 root at L4–5).

History
- Back pain and radiculopathy that is worse with sitting and better with standing and lying down
- Pain or numbness radiating beyond the knee, typically in a dermatomal distribution

Physical Examination
- Motor: typically normal but may be present, depending on nerve root involved
- Sensory: pain, numbness, or dysesthesias along dermatomal distribution is common

Imaging
- Lumbar standing radiographs: AP, lateral, and flexion or extension views—dynamic views evaluate spinal alignment and help assess for spinal instability or deformity

Additional Imaging
- **MRI (modality of choice)**
- CT or myelogram if previous instrumented spine surgery or if MRI contraindicated

Initial Management
Nonoperative Management
- NSAIDs, activity modification, Medrol dose pack, and physical therapy are often effective in the first 6 weeks of symptom onset.
- If noninvasive conservative treatments are not helpful to improve symptoms, then epidural spine injections can give good relief of symptoms, particularly for radicular pain.

Operative Management
Indications
- Progressive motor weakness, persistent disabling pain despite conservative treatment and predominately nerve root pain

Surgical Procedures
Lumbar Decompression
Usually a full laminectomy is not needed and a smaller decompression is performed, such as **hemilaminectomy or hemilaminotomy.** This involves decompressing the hypertrophied lamina, ligamentum flavum, and part of the facet.

Estimated Postoperative Recovery Course
- Postoperative 2 to 3 weeks:
  - Patient returns for wound check
  - Upright AP and lateral lumbar x-rays can be obtained, not necessarily needed since there is no fusion—*depends on surgeon preference*
  - Continue to have patient limit lifting <5–8 lbs and no bending or twisting until 6 week mark then patient can start physical therapy
- Postoperative 3 months:
  - Patient returns for routine follow-up, if doing well can release back to normal activities

Foraminal Stenosis—Nerve Root Compression
Neural foraminal stenosis refers to the narrowing of the small openings between each vertebra in the spine, called foramen, through which nerve roots pass. This can be caused by intraforaminal disc protrusion, impingement of the tip of the superior facet, or degenerative changes that cause disc height collapse. The lower lumbar areas (L4–5 and L5–S1) are usually involved because the foramina decrease in size and the nerve root size increases at these levels. Foraminal stenosis affects the exiting nerve root (e.g., L4 root at L4–5)[4]

History

- Back pain and radicular symptoms that are worse with sitting and better with standing and lying down
- Pain or numbness radiating beyond the knee, typically in a dermatomal distribution

Physical Examination

- Motor: typically normal but may be present and depend on nerve root involved
- Sensory: pain, numbness, or dysesthesias along dermatomal distribution is common

Imaging

- Lumbar standing radiographs: AP, lateral, and flexion or extension views—stimulate spinal alignment and help assess for spinal instability or deformity

Additional Imaging

- **MRI (modality of choice)**
- CT or myelogram if previous instrumented spine surgery or if MRI contraindicated

Initial Management
Nonoperative Management

- NSAIDs, activity modification, Medrol dose pack, and physical therapy are often effective in the first 6 weeks of symptom onset.
- If noninvasive conservative treatments are not helpful to improve symptoms, then epidural spine injections can give good relief of symptoms, particularly for radicular pain.

Operative Management
Indications

- Progressive motor weakness, persistent disabling pain despite conservative treatment and predominately nerve root pain

Surgical Procedures
Lumbar Decompression

Nerve root compression can be managed with a smaller type of decompression called a **foraminotomy**. During this procedure the bone is removed from around the neural foramen, typically part of the medial facet is taken down, and part of the superior articular process is resected. In addition, a discectomy may also be needed to adequately decompress the nerve such as in the case of an intraforaminal disc herniation. Care should be taken to preserve greater than 50% of the facet joint and the pars intraarticularis to preserve stability.

Estimated Postoperative Recovery Course

- Postoperative 2 to 3 weeks:
  - Patient returns for wound check
  - Upright AP and lateral lumbar x-rays can be obtained, not necessarily needed since there is no fusion—*depends on surgeon preference*
  - Continue to have patient limit lifting <5–8 lbs and no bending or twisting until 6-week mark then patient can start physical therapy
- Postoperative 3 months:
  - Patient returns for routine follow-up, if doing well can release back to normal activities

Board Review

1. Pain radiating to one buttock helps differentiates a lumbar disk herniation from cauda equina syndrome.
2. The most appropriate initial step for a lumbar strain is antiinflammatory and muscle relaxant therapy.
3. Lumbar central stenosis with neurogenic claudication is associated with progressive difficulty with ambulating long distances secondary to leg pain and increasing leg heaviness. The leg pain is improved with forward flexion and sitting but aggravated with standing.
4. A far lateral disc herniated at L4–5 will cause radiating pain down the anterior aspect of the leg, weakness of the ankle dorsiflexion muscle, and loss of the knee jerk reflex.

SUGGESTED READINGS

Amin RM, Andrade NS, Neuman BJ: Lumbar Disc Herniation, *Curr Rev Musculoskelet Med* 10(4):507–516, 2017.

Jordan J, Konstantinou K, O'Dowd J: Herniated lumbar disc, *BMJ Clin Evid*1118, 2009.

Schoenfeld AJ, Weiner BK: Treatment of lumbar disc herniation: Evidence-based practice, *Int J Gen Med* 3:209–214, 2010.

REFERENCES

1. Middleton K, Fish DE: Lumbar spondylosis: clinical presentation and treatment approaches, *Curr Rev Musculoskelet Med* 2(2):94–104, 2009.
2. Atlas SJ, Deyo RA: Evaluating and managing acute low back pain in the primary care setting, *J Gen Intern Med* 16(2):120–131, 2001.

3. De Cicco FL, Camino Willhuber GO: *Nucleus Pulposus Herniation*, Treasure Island (FL), 2020, StatPearls Publishing. [Updated 2020 Mar 25]. In: StatPearls [Internet].
4. Miller MD, Thompson SR, editors: *Miller's review of orthopedics*, Philadelphia, 2016, Elsevier, p 673.

SPONDYLOLYSIS

Spondylolysis is a defect in the pars interarticularis and is one of the most common causes of low back pain in children and adolescents. It is a fatigue fracture from repetitive hyperextension stresses and most commonly seen in gymnasts and football lineman. There is also a probable hereditary predisposition.

History
- Axial back pain
- May or may not be associated with radicular symptoms and nerve root irritation

Physical Examination
- Pain is aggravated with extension and improves with flexion
- Motor: typically normal
- Sensory: usually normal

Imaging
- Lumbar standing radiographs: AP, lateral, oblique, and flexion or extension views—stimulate spinal alignment and help assess for spinal instability or deformity
  - 80% of these fractures can be seen on lateral radiographs
  - Another 15% are visible on oblique radiographs which show a defect in the neck of the "Scottie dog"

Additional Imaging
- CT, bone scanning and single emission computed tomography (SPECT) may be helpful in identifying subtle fractures
  - Increased uptake on SPECT is more compatible with acute lesions that have the potential to heal

Initial Management
Nonoperative Management
ICD-10 codes:

    M43.00 Spondylolysis

- Usually aimed at symptomatic relief rather that fracture healing in spondylolysis without spondylolisthesis
  - Activity restriction
  - Flexion exercises
  - Bracing
- If noninvasive conservative treatments are not helpful to improve symptoms, then pars injections can be used to provide relief of pain
  - **Prognosis**: unilateral defects rarely have progression of slippage

SPONDYLOLISTHESIS

Spondylolisthesis is a condition wherein there is anterior, posterior, or lateral shift of one vertebral body on an adjacent vertebral body. It can occur as a part of a degenerative or traumatic process. It can also be associated with spondylolisis wherein the fractured pars interarticularis separates, allowing the injured vertebra to shift or slip forward on the vertebra directly below it. In children and adolescents, this slippage most often occurs during periods of rapid growth—such as an adolescent growth spurt.

History
- Wide variety of symptoms based on type and severity of spondylolisthesis
- Low back pain with or without radiculopathy
- Possible neurogenic claudication

Physical Examination
- Motor: typically normal but weakness may be present depending on nerve root involved
  - Isthmic types: typically compress exiting nerve root, so L5–S1 slips have L5 radicular nerve pain
  - Degenerative types: typically compress trasversing nerve root, so L4–5 slips have L5 radicular pain
- Sensory: pain, numbness or dysesthesias along dermatomal distribution is common
- Reflexes: typically normal or hyporeflexive

Imaging
- Lumbar standing radiographs: AP, lateral, oblique, and flexion or extension views—stimulate spinal alignment and help assess for spinal instability or deformity
- MRI: helpful for looking for nerve root compression

- CT: useful for better defining bony anatomy, especially if surgery is being considered

Classification: six types

- Dysplastic: congenital dysplasia of S1 superior facet
- Isthmic: most common type, predisposition leading to elongation/fracture of pars (L5–S1)
- Degenerative: facet arthrosis leading to subluxation (L4–5)
- Traumatic: acute fracture other than pars
- Pathologic: incompetence of bony elements
- Postsurgical: excessive resection of neural arches/facets

Grading

Meyerding classification: five grades based on the amount or percentage of slip as compared with S1 width[1]:

- Grade I: 0%–25%
- Grade II: 25%–50%
- Grade III: 50%–75%
- Grade IV: greater than 75%
- Grade V: greater than 100% (spondyloptosis)

Initial Management
Nonoperative Management

- NSAIDs, hamstring stretching, core strengthening, lumbar flexion-extension based exercises.
- If noninvasive conservative treatments are not helpful to improve symptoms, then epidural steroid injection or selective nerve root injections can give good relief of pain from nerve root compression.

Operative Management

ICD-10 codes: M43.10 to M43.19 Spondylolisthesis codes

Q76.2 Congenital spondylolisthesis

CPT codes:

63047 Lumbar decompression

63048 Additional level decompression

22800 to 22819 Spinal fusion codes

22840 to 22855 Spinal instrumentation codes

Indications

- Persistent pain despite conservative treatments or progressive neurological symptoms or progression of the slip

- Prophylactic fusion is recommended in growing children with slippage of more than 50% (grade III–V)

Surgical Procedures

- Surgical techniques can vary depending on severity of slip, patient's age and surgeon preference, most common types are listed below

Lumbar Decompression and Posterior Fusion with Instrumentation and Interbody Cage

This is a posterior procedure that normally involves removing the lamina, ligamentum flavum, and part of the facets in order to decompress the nerves, then stabilization with pedicle screws and rods. Use of an interbody cage is done the help with realignment of spine and reduction of the slip. It should be noted that reduction of the spondylolisthesis is controversial in higher grade slips due to risk of nerve root injury.

ALIF with Posterior Fusion

As described on Page 18.

Estimated Postoperative Recovery Course

- Postoperative 2 to 3 weeks:
  - Patient returns for wound check
  - Upright AP and lateral lumbar x-rays are obtained
  - Suture or staples are removed
  - Continue to have patient limit lifting <5–8 lbs and no bending or twisting until 6-week mark then patient can start physical therapy
- Postoperative 3 to 4 months:
  - Recheck x-rays (AP, lateral, flexion, and extension) and evaluate for fusion. Fusion site should be complete.
  - If patient is doing well and radiographs look good, can release back to normal activities.
- Postoperative 6 months:
  - Routine follow-up and recheck x-rays
- Postoperative 9 to 12 months:
  - Routine follow-up and recheck x-rays

Board Review

1. The most common level for an isthmic spondylolisthesis is L5–S1.
2. The most common level for degenerative spondylolisthesis is L4–5 and typically compress traversing nerve root.

SUGGESTED READINGS

Kalichman L, Hunter DJ: Diagnosis and conservative management of degenerative lumbar spondylolisthesis, *Eur Spine J* 17(3):327–335, 2008.

Wang Y, Káplár Z, Deng M, Leung J: Lumbar degenerative spondylolisthesis epidemiology: A systematic review with a focus on gender-specific and age-specific prevalence, *J Orthopaed Transl* 11:39–52, 2016.

REFERENCES

1. Miller MD, Thompson SR, Hart J, editors: *Review of orthopedics*, Philadelphia, 2012, Elsevier, p 607.

ADULT SCOLIOSIS

Scoliosis is defined as a deviation of the normal vertical line of the spine, consisting of a lateral curvature with rotation of the vertebrae within the curve. Typically, for scoliosis to be considered, there should be at least 10 degrees of spinal angulation on the posterior-anterior radiograph associated with vertebral rotation.[1] It is usually defined in patients older than age 20. Curves may increase in size 0.5 to 2 degrees per year. Adolescent curves less than 30 degrees are unlikely to progress significantly into adulthood, while those over 50 degrees are likely to get bigger, which is why the curve should be monitored over time.[2]

History
- Backache or low back pain
- Fatigue
- Cosmetic deformity may be present—uneven appearance of shoulders, shoulder blades, hips, thoracic rib hump
- Cardiopulmonary problems (thoracic curves >60–65 degrees may alter pulmonary function test: curves >90 degrees may affect mortality)
- May have neurologic or radiculopathy signs in cases of impingement

Curve Progression
- Unlikely in curves of less than 30 degrees
- Right thoracic curves of more than 50 degrees are at the highest risk for progression (usually one degree a year), followed by lumbar curves

Physical Examination
- Progressive curve of the spine is noted
- Curve changes can be subtle and require consistent radiographic measurement over time
- Shoulder and pelvis height is often uneven
- Check for skin changes or hairy patches on the back, signs of neurofibromatosis
- Complete neuromuscular examination includes strength, Hoffman and Babinski reflexes, and clonus testing

Imaging
- Radiographs
  - Standing full-length spine plain film: AP and lateral views.
  - Lateral bending films while standing can be obtained to assess the flexibility of the curves or the primary and compensatory curves.
  - Check the Cobb angle, which is the angle between two lines, drawn perpendicular to the upper endplate of the uppermost involved vertebrae and the lower endplate of the lowest involved vertebrae. For patients with two curves, Cobb angles are followed for both curves (Fig. 1.24).

Additional Imaging
- CT myelogram or MRI is useful for evaluation of nerve root compression

Classification
- Idiopathic: progression of untreated adolescent scoliosis
  - more common in girls

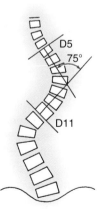

Fig. 1.24 Cobb Angle. (From Canale ST, Beaty JH, editors: *Campbell's operative orthopaedics*, ed 11, Philadelphia, 2008, Mosby, p 1934.)

- De novo
  - Neuromuscular: cerebral palsy, polio, tethered spinal cord, neurofibromatosis
  - Degenerative: secondary to degenerative disc disease or osteoporosis
  - Posttraumatic
  - Iatrogenic

Initial Management
Nonoperative Management

- Close follow up with radiographs is indicated to determine whether the curve is accelerating. An adult or skeletally mature patient can be monitored yearly. Progression of the curve is generally defined as a change of 5 degrees or more on consecutive x-ray studies.
- Symptomatic care is indicated for resulting pain or neural impingement if present: such as NSAIDs, weight reduction, physical therapy, muscle strengthening, facet joint injections, and orthoses (used with activity).

Operative Management
Indications

- Young adults (<30 years) with curves of greater than 50–60 degrees
- Older patients with refractory pain
- Sagittal plane imbalance
- Progressive curves
- Cardiopulmonary compromise with worsening pulmonary function tests (PFT's)
- Refractory spinal stenosis

Surgical Procedures

ICD-10 codes: M41.9 to M43.9 Curvature of spine
  M41.20 Scoliosis [and kyphoscoliosis], idiopathic
  M43.9 Curvature of spine associated with other conditions
CPT codes: 22800 to 22819 Spinal fusion codes
  22840 to 22855 Spinal instrumentation codes

- Numerous procedures may be performed, based on the type and severity of deformity and the surgeon's preference. In general, spinal fusion with instrumentation is the treatment of choice.
- Stabilization of the curve takes priority over correction. If correction is attempted, it may involve osteotomy (pedicle subtraction, Smith-Peterson, vertebrectomy) to correct sagittal or coronal deformity.

Long or short segment instrumented fusions are used to stabilize these corrections.
- Selective posterior instrumented fusions for flexible thoracic curves
- Combined anterior release and fusion in addition to posterior fusion and instrumentation may be beneficial for large (>70 degrees), more ridged curves (as determined on side-bending films) or curves in the lumbar spine
- Fusion to L5
  - Associated with development of L5–S1 degenerative disc disease
- Fusion to sacrum
  - Increases stability of long lumbar fusions
  - Increased incidence of pseudoarthrosis and potential for postoperative gait disturbances
- Fixation to ilium
  - Indicated in lumbosacral fusions involving more than three levels
- Anterior interbody fusion
  - Achieve anterior column support
  - Increases stability of long fusions including L5–S1
  - Helps maintain corrections of sagittal and coronal deformities
  - Increased fusion rates

Board Review

1. Right thoracic curves >50 degrees are at the highest risk for progression
2. At least 10 degrees of spinal angulation is needed for a diagnosis of scoliosis

SUGGESTED READINGS

Shen FH, Shaffrey CI: *Arthritis and arthroplasty: the spine*, 25. Philadelphia, 2010, Saunders, pp 195–200.
Spivak JM, Connolly PJ: *Orthopaedic knowledge update*, 46. Rosemont, IL, 2006, American Academy of Orthopaedic Surgeons, pp 443–455.

REFERENCES

1. Morrissy RT, Weinstein SL: *Lovell and Winter's pediatric orthopaedics*, Philadelphia, 2006, Lippincott Williams & Wilkins, pp 693–762.
2. Joseph A, Janicki MD, Alman, MD FRCSC Benjamin: Scoliosis: Review of diagnosis and treatment, *Paediatrics Child Health* 12(9):771–776, 2007.

KYPHOSIS

The thoracic spine should have a natural curve or kyphosis that is between 20 and 40 degrees. Postural or structural abnormalities can result in a curve that is outside this normal range and cause a sagittal plane deformity.

Etiology

- Idiopathic
  - **Scheuermann's disease:** developmental disorder of the spine that causes the abnormal growth of the thoracic vertebrae. The back of the vertebral body grows normally and the front grows more slowly or abnormally. This leads to a vertebra with a distinct wedge shape.
- Posttraumatic (missed posterior ligamentous complex injury)
- Ankylosing spondylitis
- Metabolic bone disease
  - Progressive kyphosis secondary to multiple osteoporotic compression fractures

History

- Mid back pain that is achy and constant in nature
- Fatigue
- Feeling "bent over" and unable to stand up straight

Physical Examination

- Normally a benign exam, can have pain to palpation over center of the curve

Imaging

- Thoracic standing radiographs: AP and lateral views
  - Look for fractures, wedging of anterior endplates
  - **Scheuermann's disease:** needs to meet a number of criteria (Sorensen classification)
    - thoracic spine kyphosis >40 degrees (normal 25–40 degrees) or
    - thoracolumbar spine kyphosis >30 degrees (normal ~zero degrees) and
    - at least three adjacent vertebrae demonstrating anterior wedging of >5 degrees[1]

Initial Management

Nonoperative Management

- Symptomatic care is indicated for resulting pain or neural impingement if present: NSAIDs, weight reduction, physical therapy, muscle strengthening, facet joint injections, and orthoses (used with activity)

Operative Management

ICD-10 codes: M40.0 to M40.209 Kyphosis codes

   M40.0 Kyphosis (acquired) (postural)

   M42.0 Scheuermann's disease

   M4.209 Kyphosis deformity of the spine

CPT codes: 22800 to 22819 Spinal fusion codes

   22840 to 22855 Spinal instrumentation codes

   22212-22216 Smith-Peterson osteotomy (SPO) codes: 5 to 10 degrees of sagittal plane correction

   22206-22207 Pedicle subtraction osteotomy (PSO) codes: 30 degrees of sagittal plane correction

Indications

- Deformity and pain is debilitating and all other conservative measures have been exhausted
- Numerous procedures may be performed, based on the type and severity of deformity and the surgeon's preference. In general, spinal fusion with instrumentation and osteotomies is the treatment of choice.

Board Review

1. In order to diagnose Scheuermann's disease on radiographs there needs to be at least three adjacent vertebrae demonstrating anterior wedging of more than 5 degrees.

SUGGESTED READINGS

Spivak JM, Connolly PJ: Orthopaedic knowledge update, *Rosemont, IL: Am Acad Orthopaedic Surg.* 47:465–468, 2006.

Thompson SR, Miller MD: Millers Review of Orthopaedics, 6. Philadelphia, PA, 2015, Elsevier, pp 300–301.

REFERENCES

1. Gokce E, Beyhan M: Radiological imaging findings of Scheuermann disease, *World J Radiol* 8(11):895–901, 2016.

VERTEBRAL COMPRESSION FRACTURE

Compression fractures of the spine generally occur from too much pressure on the vertebral body. This usually results from a combination of bending forward and downward pressure on the spine. The most

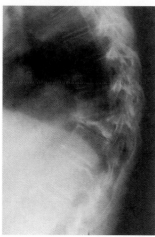

Fig. 1.25 Radiographic Appearance of **T11 Compression Fracture.** (From Barr JD, Barr MS, Lemley TJ, et al: Percutaneous vertebroplasty for pain relief and spinal stabilization *Spine* 25:923, 2000.)

common area for a compression fracture to occur in the spine is in the thoracic spine or at the thoracolumbar junction.

Causes
- Osteoporosis
- Low-velocity fall occurs in older adults; injury could be very minor in this population
- Higher-velocity injury may occur in younger patients
- Pathologic fracture—consider this in young patient with fracture and no history of trauma

History
- Patients complain of severe back pain with or without a known inciting event

Physical Examination
- Decreased ROM due to pain
- Pain with flexion, extension, and/or rotation of the trunk
- Tenderness to palpation over muscular structures
- Normal neurologic examination

Imaging
- Standing plain radiographs: AP and lateral—will show depressed or wedged end plates, Fig. 1.25
  - Look for other injuries such as spinous process fracture in higher-velocity injuries

Additional Imaging
- CT or MRI is useful to better assess extent of fracture and to look for edema, concurrent ligamentous injuries, and any spinal cord or nerve compression

Initial Management
Nonoperative Management
- **Patient Education.** important to explain the self-limiting nature of this injury and that most will heal around 8 to 10 weeks
- Short course of narcotics to help with initial pain
- Bracing for comfort and to promote healing
  - Cervical thoracic lumbar sacral orthosis (CTLSO): used for cervical or upper thoracic compression fractures to stabilize the cervicothoracic junction
  - Thoracic lumbar sacral orthosis (TLSO): used for thoracic or upper lumbar fractures in order to stabilize thoracolumbar junction
  - Lumbar sacral orthosis (LSO): used for lumbar fractures
- Follow in clinic and take x-rays to make sure fracture is healing

Operative Management
ICD-10 codes: S22.009A Closed fracture of dorsal thoracic vertebra without mention of spinal cord injury
S32.009A Closed fracture of lumbar vertebra without mention of spinal cord injury
CPT codes: 22510 Percutaneous vertebroplasty: cervicothoracic
22511 Percutaneous vertebroplasty: lumbosacral
22512 Each additional vertebral body treated during the same session
22513 Percutaneous vertebral augmentation, including cavity creation using mechanical device, one vertebral body; thoracic
22514 Percutaneous vertebral augmentation, including cavity creation using mechanical device, one vertebral body; lumbar
22515 Each additional thoracic or lumbar vertebral body
Indications
- Intractable pain despite conservative treatment for 8 to 10 weeks
  - Should get a new MRI to make sure there is still edema in the fracture site
- Pathologic fracture for palliative care

Surgical Procedures

- Vertebroplasty: approach depends on lesion location, with the classic approach being transpedicular, a trocar and cannula are introduced into the bone, one or two transpedicular needles are placed using fluoroscopy, and cement is introduced per the manufacturer's instructions.
- Kyphoplasty: same as vertebroplasty, except that first a balloon tamp is inserted and inflated to restore vertebral body height, then the balloon is removed, and cement is introduced.

Estimated Postoperative Recovery Course

- Postoperative 2 to 3 weeks:
  - Patient returns for routine follow-up
  - Upright AP and lateral x-rays are obtained

SUGGESTED READINGS

Robinson Y, Heyde CE, Försth P, et al.: Kyphoplasty in osteoporotic vertebral compression fractures—Guidelines and technical considerations, *J Orthop Surg Res* 6:43, 2011.

SPINAL TRAUMA AND SPINE FRACTURES

History

It is important to understand the mechanism of a patient's injury and perform a thorough trauma evaluation to determine the extent of a patient's injuries. Coordination with other medical and surgical services may be necessary in order to provide comprehensive care and reduce anesthetic exposure. Frequently, patients will have high-energy injuries such as a fall from a height or motor vehicle crash (MVC). However, low-velocity injury can result in severe injury in patients with underlying osteoporosis or tumor. Fractures of the thoracolumbar spine are four times more common in men.

Physical Examination

- Adherence to Advanced Trauma Life Support (ATLS) protocols remain imperative
  - Primary survey (ABCs, with D and E)
  - A – airway maintenance with cervical spine protection
  - B – Breathing and ventilation
  - C – Circulation with hemorrhage control
  - D – Disability and neurologic assessment
  - E – Exposure of patient

- Complete examination is critical for determining the injury extent and prognosis, especially in the case of a spine cord injury (SCI).
- In addition to standard examinations and reflexes discussed in the beginning of the chapter, perform a rectal examination for tone in all suspected cases of SCI.

Cervical Clearance

- An alert, asymptomatic patient without a distracting injury or neurologic deficit and who is able to complete a functional ROM examination may safely be cleared from cervical spine immobilization without radiographic evaluation.
- If cross-table x-ray studies of the cervical spine from the skull to T1 are negative and the patient has cervical spine tenderness, leave the collar in place until voluntary flexion and extension radiographs or MRI can be performed.
- An initial CT scan during trauma evaluation is ideal and may discover occult injuries, especially with high-velocity mechanisms.
- Cervical spine injuries in patients with altered mental status are more difficult to evaluate. Recommendations for evaluation include removal of the cervical collar after 24 hours in patients with normal radiographs; indefinite immobilization in a cervical collar; CT scan evaluation; and more recently cervical flexion-extension examinations using dynamic fluoroscopy. CT may be more beneficial in that it allows for examination of the skull and cervical spine during same examination.

Spinal Cord Injury Classification

- American Spinal Injury Association (ASIA) Examination and Classification: Fig. 1.26

Imaging

- During initial trauma evaluation, CT is becoming more common to evaluate a head injury. Cervical spine or other isolated cuts can be done with little risk to the patient but a high yield in the ability to clear spine injury.
- Cervical radiographs are used for cervical clearance as noted earlier (make sure it includes C7-T1 junction), as well as to evaluate possible bony injury in the thoracolumbar spine.
  - Assess radiographic lines for continuity

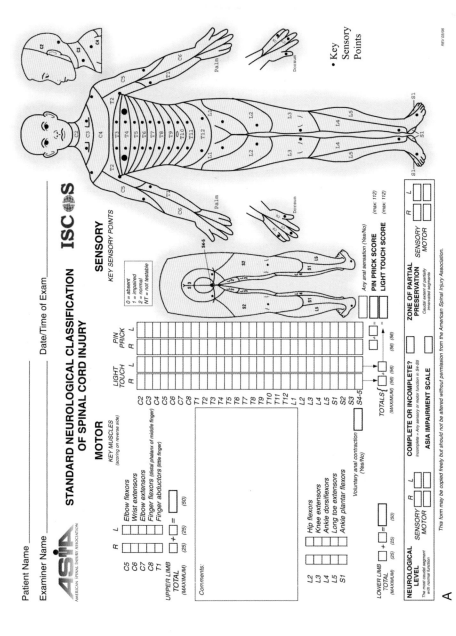

Fig. 1.26 A and **B,** Standard neurologic classification of spinal cord injury from the American Spinal Injury Association (ASIA). (From Canale ST, Beaty JH, editors: *Campbell's operative orthopaedics* Philadelphia, 2008, Mosby/Elsevier, Vol 2, Fig. 35-3, p 1765.)

STEPS IN CLASSIFICATION

The following order is recommended in determining the classification of individuals with SCI.

1. Determine sensory levels for right and left sides.

2. Determine motor levels for right and left sides.
   Note: in regions where there is no myotome to test, the motor level is presumed to be the same as the sensory level.

3. Determine the single neurological level.
   This is the lowest segment where motor and sensory function is normal on both sides, and is the most cephalad of the sensory and motor levels determined in steps 1 and 2.

4. Determine whether the injury is Complete or Incomplete (sacral sparing).
   *If voluntary and contraction = **No** AND all S4-5 sensory scores = **0** AND any anal sensation = **No**, then injury is COMPLETE. Otherwise injury is incomplete.*

5. Determine ASIA Impairment Scale (AIS) Grade:
   Is injury Complete? If **YES**, AIS=A Record ZPP
   (For ZPP record lowest dermatome or myotome on each side with some (non-zero score) preservation)

   NO

   Is injury motor incomplete? If **NO**, AIS=B
   (Yes=voluntary anal contraction OR motor function more than three levels below the motor level on a given side.)

   YES

   Are at least half of the key muscles below the (single) neurological level graded 3 or better?

   NO → AIS=C   YES → AIS=D

If sensation and motor function is normal in all segments, AIS=E
Note: AIS E is used in follow-up testing when an individual with a documented SCI has recovered normal function. If at initial testing no deficits are found, the individual is neurologically intact; the ASIA Impairment Scale does not apply.

ASIA IMPAIRMENT SCALE

☐ **A = Complete:** No motor or sensory function is preserved in the sacral segments S4-S5.

☐ **B = Incomplete:** Sensory but not motor function is preserved below the neurological level and includes the sacral segments S4-S5.

☐ **C = Incomplete:** Motor function is preserved below the neurological level, and more than half of key muscles below the neurological level have a muscle grade less than 3.

☐ **D = Incomplete:** Motor function is preserved below the neurological level, and at least half of key muscles below the neurological level have a muscle grade of 3 or more.

☐ **E = Normal:** Motor and sensory function are normal.

CLINICAL SYNDROMES (OPTIONAL)

☐ Central Cord
☐ Brown-Séquard
☐ Anterior Cord
☐ Conus Medullaris
☐ Cauda Equina

MUSCLE GRADING

0 Total paralysis

1 Palpable or visible contraction

2 Active movement, full range of motion, gravity eliminated

3 Active movement, full range of motion, against gravity

4 Active movement, full range of motion, against gravity and provides some resistance

5 Active movement, full range of motion, against gravity and provides normal resistance

5* Muscle able to exert, in examiner's judgment, sufficient resistance to be considered normal if identifiable inhibiting factors were not present

NT, [?] not testable. Patient unable to reliably exert effort or muscle unavailable for testing due to factors such as immobilization, pain on effort, or contracture.

Fig. 1.26, cont'd

B

- Anterior soft tissue shadows
  - At C2: 6 mm
  - At C6: 20 mm
  - Anterior spinal line
  - Posterior spinal line
  - Spinolaminar line
  - Spinous process line

Additional Imaging

- CT is useful for evaluation of fracture at all levels of the spine.
- MRI without contrast is used for evaluation of ligamentous structures, as well as for occult fracture of the spinal column.

Fracture Types

Cervical Fractures

Rule of 3s:
- The predentate space should be less than 3 mm
- The prevertebral soft tissue at C3 is usually 3 mm
- Anterior wedging of 3 mm or more suggests a fracture

Occipitocervical Dislocation (OCD)

- Head is disconnected from C1
- Usually fatal
- Children more commonly affected then adults
- Diagnosis is challenging on plain films (CT/MRI = 85% sensitive)
- **Treatment:** nonoperative treatments are not an option
  - **Operative Procedure:** posterior occipitocervical fusion (occiput to C2)

C1 Ring Fractures

- Neural arch Fractures: most common
  - Posterior arch fractures: axial loading and hyperextension
  - Isolated anterior arch fractures: axial loading and flexion
- Lateral mass fractures: axial loading with lateral bend
- **Burst fractures (Jefferson): axial load: Fig. 1.27**
  - Seen on an open-mouth (odontoid view) x-ray as a bilateral offset of C1–2
- **Treatment**: based predominantly on stability of transverse ligament
  - Combined lateral mass displacement of greater than 6.9 mm indicates transverse ligament rupture

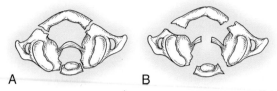

Fig. 1.27 **A** and **B**, Jefferson fracture. (From Canale ST, Beaty JH, editors: *Campbell's operative orthopaedics,* ed 11, Philadelphia, 2008, Mosby, p 1787.)

- Atlantodens interval (ADI)
  - If greater than 3.5 mm indicates transverse ligament is damaged
  - If greater than 5 mm indicates both the transverse and alar ligaments are damaged
- Operative procedures
  - Halo vest stabilization for 6 to 12 weeks for fractures with intact transverse ligament
  - Posterior spinal fusion (C1–2 or occiput-C2) if transverse ligament is incompetent

C2 Fracture (Hangman's)

- Traumatic spondylolisthesis of the axis: fracture through the pedicles of C2 with anterior slippage of C2 on C3
- Most common cervical spine fracture
- **Classification—Levine (Fig. 1.28)**
  - Type I: minimally displaced fracture of the pars secondary to hyperextension and axial loading (<3 mm displacement, no angulation)
  - Type IA: same as type I except fracture lines are asymmetric
  - Type II: displaced fracture (>3 mm) of the pars, with subsequent flexion after hyperextension and axial loading
  - Type IIA: flexion without displacement
  - Type III: bilateral pars fracture with bilateral facet dislocations then hyperextension mechanism
- **Treatment**
  - Type I: immobilization in rigid cervical orthosis
  - Type II: operative, typically C1–2 fixation or direct osteosynthesis
  - Type IIA: halo vest or surgery (no traction—which could worsen fracture)
  - Type III: usually operative, generally C2–3 fusion

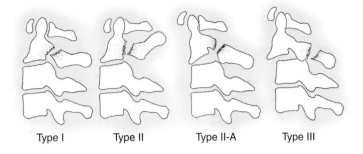

Type I   Type II   Type II-A   Type III

Fig. 1.28 Hangman's Fracture. (From Canale ST, Beaty JH, editors: *Campbell's operative orthopaedics*, ed 11, Philadelphia, 2008, Mosby, p 1796.)

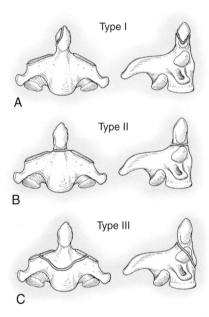

Type I

A

Type II

B

Type III

C

Fig. 1.29 A–C, The three types of odontoid fractures. (From Canale ST, Beaty JH, editors: *Campbell's operative orthopaedics*, ed 11, Philadelphia, 2008, Mosby, p 1791.)

Odontoid Fractures
- Hyperextension injury
- **Classification—Anderson-D'Alonso (Fig. 1.29)**
  - Type I: avulsion of alar ligament from the tip
  - Type II: fracture at the base of the odontoid
  - Type IIA: communicated fracture of the base of the odontoid
  - Type III: fractures that extend into the body of C2

- **Treatment**
  - Type I: immobilization in rigid cervical orthosis
  - Type II and IIA
    - Nondisplaced: immobilization in ridged cervical orthosis
    - Displaced: generally considered operative because of high rate on nonunion (C1–2 fusion or direct anterior osteosynthesis)
      - Nonreduced fractures are a contraindication to anterior odontoid screw
  - Type III: most will heal in rigid cervical orthosis, consider operative treatment if more than 5 mm displacement

Clay Shoveler's Fracture
- C6, C7, or T1 spinous process fracture
- Stable
- **Treatment**: managed with collar, nonoperative care

Thoracic and Lumbar Spine Injuries
- Upper thoracic spine (T1–T10) is stabilized by ribs, facet joint orientation, and sternum and may provide additional stability and is less susceptible to trauma
- Thoracolumbar junction is a transition zone from a relatively rigid thoracic spine to a relatively mobile lumbar spine
- Spinal cord ends and the cauda equina begins at L1–2, so lesions below L1 have a better prognosis because the cord is not affected
- **Column theory:** Fig. 1.30—described by Francis Denis to classify thoracolumbar spinal fractures

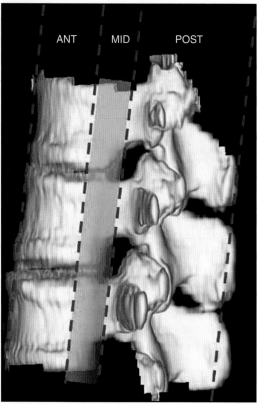

Fig. 1.30 Three column theory for spinal trauma as demonstrated on lateral 3D computed tomography reconstruction. (From Cianfoni A, Colosimo C: Imaging of spine trauma. In Law M et al, editors: *Problem solving in neuroradiology*, Philadelphia, 2011, Elsevier, p476.)

- **Anterior column**
  - anterior longitudinal ligament (ALL)
  - anterior two-thirds of the vertebral body
  - anterior two-thirds of the intervertebral disc (annulus fibrosus)
- **Middle column: if intact, the fracture is stable**
  - posterior one-third of the vertebral body
  - posterior one-third of the intervertebral disc (annulus fibrosus)
  - posterior longitudinal ligament (PLL)
- **Posterior column**
  - everything posterior to the PLL
    - pedicles
    - facet joints and articular processes
    - ligamentum flavum
    - neural arch and interconnecting ligaments

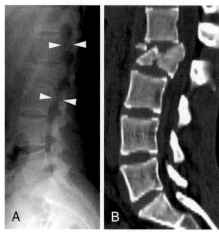

Fig. 1.31 Burst Fracture. **A**, X-ray appearance. **B**, Computed tomography appearance (note retropulsed fragment). (From Czervionke LF, Fenton DS: *Imaging painful spinal disorders*, Philadelphia, 2011, Saunders, p 97.)

Burst Fracture: Fig. 1.31
- Axial loading injury
- May be treated in a hyperextension orthosis if there is no neurologic deficit and PLC remains intact
- **Treatment**
  - Disruption of PLC – typically posterior fusion with instrumentation to reconstruct PLC. Traditionally three levels above and two level below
  - Presence of neurologic deficit – consider anterior approach for decompression of retropulsed middle column
  - Laminectomy alone is contraindicated due to high risk of progressive kyphosis

Flexion-Distraction (Chance) Fracture: Fig. 1.32
- Distraction and flexion mechanism of injury (seat-belt injury)
- Horizontal fracture through the vertebra, lamina, pedicles, or spinous process
- High rate of neurologic injury and associated intraabdominal injuries
- **Treatment**
  - **Bony flexion-distraction injury:** hyperextension external orthosis if neurologically and PLC intact
  - **Ligamentous flexion distraction injury:** has high rate of posttraumatic kyphosis due to incompetent PLC and will need a posterior spinal fusion.

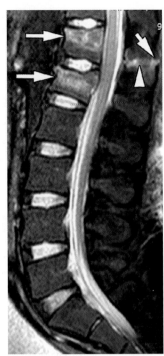

Fig. 1.32 Chance Fracture (flexion-distraction injury). The *arrows* indicate the fractures to the vertebral bodies and spinous process. (From Czervionke LF, Fenton DS: *Imaging painful spinal disorders*, Philadelphia, 2011, Saunders, p 100.)

Fracture-Dislocation: Fig. 1.33

- Rotation and shear mechanic of injury
- Frequently associated with neurologic injury
- **Treatment**
  - Most are unstable and require surgery with multiple points of fixation above and below the injury
  - May require anterior approach for decompression and/or to achieve anterior column support for additional stability

ICD-10 Codes

These are the codes for fracture of vertebral column without mention of spinal cord injury.
S12.9XXA Cervical vertebra fracture, closed
S12.9XXA, S1 Cervical vertebra fracture, open
S22.009A Dorsal (thoracic) vertebra fracture, closed
S22.009B Dorsal (thoracic) vertebra fracture, open

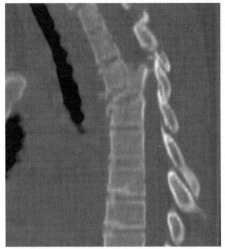

Fig. 1.33 Fracture-dislocation appearance on sagittal computed tomography reconstructions. (From Kim DH, Ludwig SC, Vaccaro AR, et al: *Atlas of spine trauma: adult and pediatric*, Philadelphia, 2008, Saunders, p 353.)

S32.009A Lumbar vertebra fracture, closed
S32.000B Lumbar vertebra fracture, open
S13.10 Cervical vertebra dislocation, closed
These are the codes for fracture of vertebral column *with* spinal cord injury.
S14.109A Cervical, closed
S12.9XXA Cervical, open
S24.109A Dorsal (thoracic), closed
S22.009B Dorsal (thoracic), open
S34.109A Lumbar, closed
S32.009A Lumbar, open

Surgical Procedures

CPT Codes
22035 Closed treatment of vertebral process fracture
22318 to 22328 Fracture-dislocation treatment codes
22532 to 22634 Arthrodesis codes
63001 to 63048 Posterior extradural laminotomy or laminectomy for exploration or decompression of neural elements or excision of herniated intervertebral discs

Surgical Procedures

- Anterior cervical discectomy and fusion
- Posterior instrumented decompression and fusion
- Lateral thoracolumbar decompression and fusion

Board Review

1. A Jefferson fracture is a burst fracture of C1.
2. The best way to see a Jefferson fracture on radiographic is with an odontoid view.
3. A Hangman's fracture is a fracture through the pedicles of C2 with anterior slippage of C2 on C3.
4. If a patient who was in a trauma complains of neck pain and cervical spine tenderness, leave the cervical collar in place until voluntary flexion and extension radiographs or MRI can be performed to rule out instability.

SUGGESTED READINGS

El-Faramawy A, El-Menyar A, Zarour A, et al.: Presentation and outcome of traumatic spinal fractures, *J Emerg Trauma Shock* 5(4):316–320, 2012.

Gupta MC, Bridwell KH, Anderson P: *Bridwell and DeWalds textbook of spinal surgery*, 129. Philadelphia, PA, 2020, Lippincott Williams & Wilkins, pp 1409–1419.

ACKNOWLEDGMENTS

The authors would like to acknowledge the contribution of the previous edition author, Ian Marks.

Shoulder and Humerus

Jennifer A. Hart

ANATOMY OF JOINT

Bones: Figs. 2.1 through 2.3

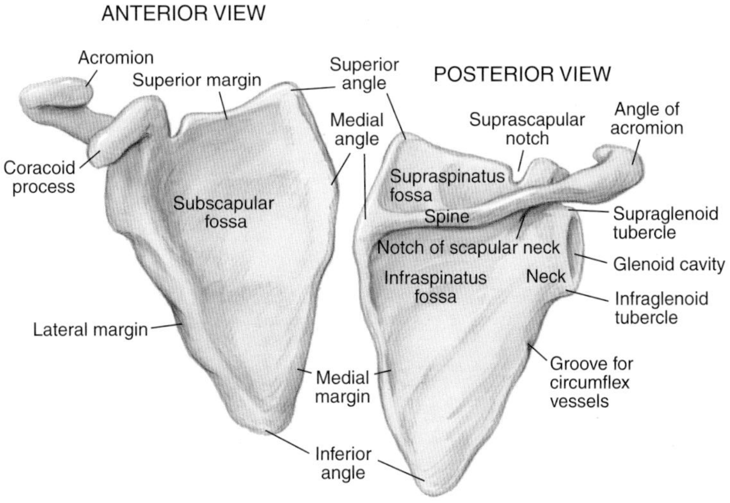

Fig. 2.1 The Scapula. (From Miller MD, Chhabra AB, Hurwitz SR, et al., editors: *Orthopaedic surgical approaches*, Philadelphia, 2008, Saunders, p 8.)

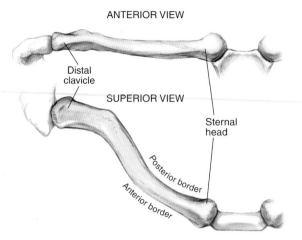

Fig. 2.2 The Clavicle. (From Miller MD, Chhabra AB, Hurwitz SR, et al., editors: *Orthopaedic surgical approaches,* Philadelphia, 2008, Saunders, p 9.)

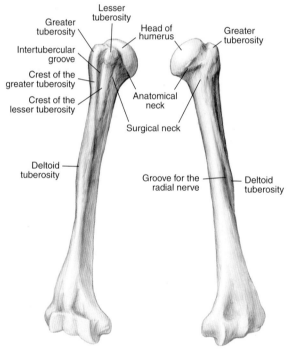

Fig. 2.3 The Humerus. (From Miller MD, Chhabra AB, Hurwitz SR, et al., editors: *Orthopaedic surgical approaches,* Philadelphia, 2008, Saunders, p 11.)

Ligaments: Figs. 2.4 and 2.5

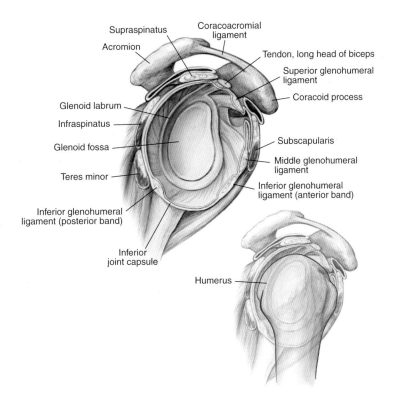

Fig. 2.4 The Glenohumeral Joint. (From Miller MD, Chhabra AB, Hurwitz SR, et al., editors: *Orthopaedic surgical approaches,* Philadelphia, 2008, Saunders, p 13.)

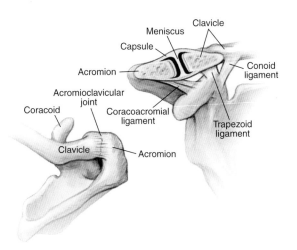

Fig. 2.5 The Acromioclavicular (AC) Joint. (From Miller MD, Chhabra AB, Hurwitz SR, et al., editors: *Orthopaedic surgical approaches,* Philadelphia, 2008, Saunders, p 13.)

Muscles and Tendons: Fig. 2.6

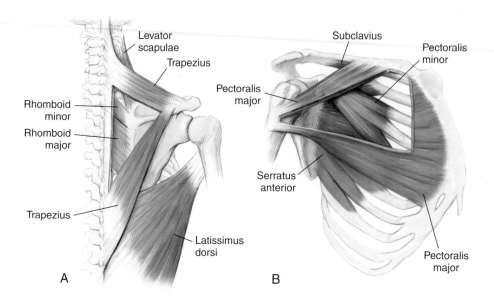

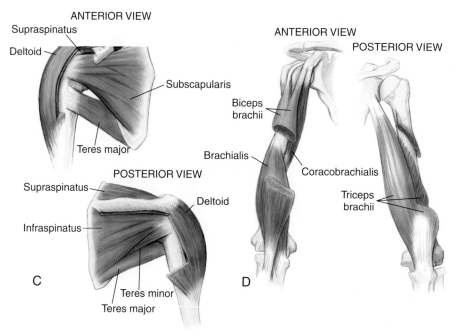

Fig. 2.6 A–D, The Muscles of the Shoulder and Upper Arm. (From Miller MD, Chhabra AB, Hurwitz SR, et al., editors: *Orthopaedic surgical approaches*, Philadelphia, 2008, Saunders, p 15.)

Nerves and Arteries: Figs. 2.7 through 2.9

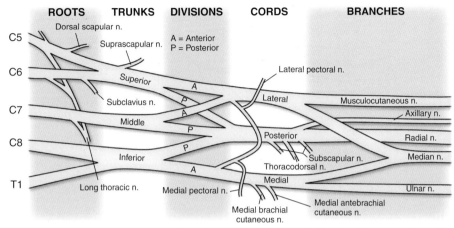

Fig. 2.7 The Brachial Plexus. *n.,* Nerve. (From Miller MD, Chhabra AB, Hurwitz SR, et al., editors: *Orthopaedic surgical approaches,* Philadelphia, 2008, Saunders, p 16.)

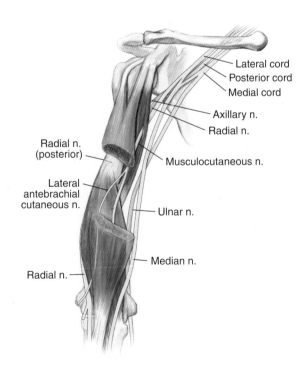

Fig. 2.8 Major Branches of the Brachial Plexus in the Upper Arm. *n.,* Nerve. (From Miller MD, Chhabra AB, Hurwitz SR, et al., editors: *Orthopaedic surgical approaches,* Philadelphia, 2008, Saunders, p 17.)

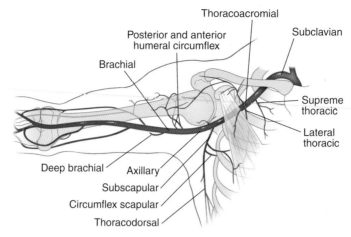

Fig. 2.9 Arteries of the Shoulder and Upper Arm. (From Miller MD, Chhabra AB, Hurwitz SR, et al., editors: *Orthopaedic surgical approaches,* Philadelphia, 2008, Saunders, p 18.)

Surface Anatomy: Fig. 2.10

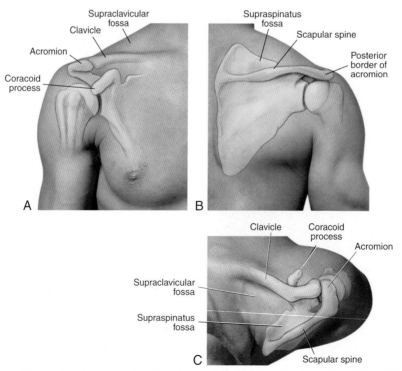

Fig. 2.10 A–C, Surface Landmarks and Underlying Anatomy of the Shoulder. (From Miller MD, Chhabra AB, Hurwitz SR, et al., editors: *Orthopaedic surgical approaches,* Philadelphia, 2008, Saunders, p 20.)

Normal Radiographic Appearance: Fig. 2.11 A–C

PHYSICAL EXAMINATION

Inspect for deformity, muscle atrophy, skin changes (ecchymosis, rash, erythema), asymmetry of the axillary fold or acromioclavicular (AC) joint.

Palpate the specific structures to evaluate for deformity or tenderness:

- AC joint
- Glenohumeral joint
- Scapula body
- Coracoid process
- Biceps tendon/bicipital groove

Normal range of motion (ROM):
Table 2.1

Special Tests
Neer Impingement Sign

- Tests for shoulder impingement

TABLE 2.1	Normal Shoulder Range of Motion
Forward Flexion	180 degrees
Abduction	180 degrees
External Rotation	90 degrees
Internal Rotation	90 degrees

- Performed by putting the shoulder in full passive forward flexion
- Positive test indicated by pain in this position

Hawkins Impingement Sign

- Tests for shoulder impingement
- Performed by passively forward flexing the shoulder and the elbow to 90 degrees and internally rotating the arm
- Positive test indicated by pain in this position

Cross-Body Adduction Test

- Tests for AC joint dysfunction (e.g., osteolysis, shoulder separation, arthritis)

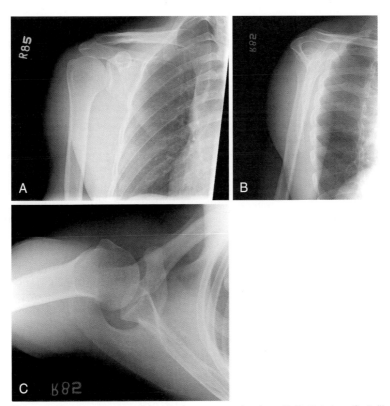

Fig. 2.11 Normal Shoulder Radiographs. **A,** Anteroposterior view. **B,** Outlet view. **C,** Axillary view.

- Performed by passively moving the arm into maximum adduction across the body
- Positive test indicated by pain over the AC joint in this position

Supraspinatus Stress Test
- Tests for rotator cuff abnormality (e.g., impingement or tear)
- Performed by having the patient hold the arm in 90 degrees of abduction and the thumb pointed down to the floor while holding against downward resistance by the examiner
- Positive test indicated by weakness and/or pain

Drop Arm Sign
- Tests for rotator cuff tear, usually massive
- Performed by having the patient hold the arms with the shoulder abducted to 90 degrees with the thumbs down
- Positive test indicated by an inability to hold the arm in this position

External Rotation Strength
- Tests for rotator cuff tear (infraspinatus)
- Performed by asking the patient to hold the arm against the side with the elbow in 90 degrees of flexion and externally rotating against resistance from the examiner
- Positive test indicated by weakness

Lift-Off Test
- Tests for rotator cuff tear (subscapularis)
- Performed by asking the patient to internally rotate the arm to allow the dorsum of the hand to rest just off the back and then to hold that position against resistance by the examiner
- Positive test indicated by weakness

Belly Press Test
- Tests for rotator cuff tear (subscapularis); alternative to lift-off test for patients unable to position their arm behind their back
- Performed by asking the patient to use the heel of the hand and press it into his or her abdomen while holding the elbow forward
- Positive test indicated by an inability to hold the elbow forward, thus allowing it to drift back to the side

Sulcus Sign
- Tests for general shoulder laxity

- Performed by applying downward force on the humerus
- Positive test indicated by the appearance of a "gap" between the humeral head and the acromion

Apprehension Test
- Tests for shoulder instability (anterior)
- Performed by asking the patient to lie supine while the examiner passively moves the shoulder into an abducted and externally rotated position
- Positive test indicated by "apprehension" on the part of the patient as he or she feels the shoulder slide anteriorly

Relocation Test
- Tests for shoulder instability
- Performed by first doing an apprehension test and, after obtaining a positive response, applying a posterior force to the humeral head with the examiner's other hand
- Positive test indicated by relief of the "apprehension"

Jerk Test
- Tests for posterior shoulder instability
- Performed by abducting the arm to 90 degrees, internally rotating it, and applying an axial load to the shoulder while adducting the arm
- Positive test indicated by a sudden jerk as the humeral head slides over the edge of the glenoid

O'Brien Test
- Tests for superior labrum anterior to posterior (SLAP) tear
- Performed by having the patient hold the arm in 90 degrees of forward flexion and 10 to 20 degrees of adduction with the thumb down then resisting a downward force to the arm applied by the examiner; test repeated with the thumb up
- Positive test indicated by pain, which should be worse with the "thumb down" position; if pain present also in the "thumb up" position, may indicate an AC joint problem

Differential Diagnosis: Table 2.2

SHOULDER IMPINGEMENT
History
- Overuse, repetitive activity.

TABLE 2.2	Differential Diagnosis
Anterior shoulder pain	Shoulder impingement Biceps tendinitis Arthritis Rotator cuff tear Instability Labral tear
Posterior shoulder pain	Periscapular muscle pain Posterior instability Cervical radiculopathy Posterior labral tear Subscapular bursitis Scapula fracture
Superior shoulder pain	Acromioclavicular (AC) joint osteolysis AC joint arthritis Clavicle fracture Shoulder (AC) separation Superior labral tear
Arm pain	Humerus fracture Rotator cuff tear Shoulder impingement Cervical radiculopathy

- Shoulder pain, worse with over-head lifting or reaching, can radiate to lateral upper arm (deltoid area).

Physical Examination
- May be tender anteriorly.
- ROM typically normal but may be painful.
- Positive Hawkins and/or Neer impingement signs.
- May have weakness secondary to pain with abduction (supraspinatus) strength testing.

Imaging
- Anteroposterior (AP), axillary, outlet commonly used standard radiographic views.

Radiographic Image: Fig. 2.12A and B

Differential Diagnoses
- Rotator cuff tear
- Labral tear
- Cervical radiculopathy

Initial Management
- **Patient Education.** Shoulder impingement is part of the spectrum of rotator cuff injury. Generally, this involves inflammation (bursitis and rotator cuff tendinitis) without actual tearing of the tendon. Partial tears can develop over time and can progress to a full-thickness tear. If symptoms do not improve with early treatment, call the office because a magnetic resonance imaging (MRI) scan may be necessary to evaluate for a rotator cuff tear.
- Begin general antiinflammatory measures including nonsteroidal antiinflammatory drugs (NSAIDs), ice, and activity modification.
- Perform subacromial steroid injection.
- Begin physical therapy that emphasizes rotator cuff strengthening exercises.
- If symptoms persist despite injection and physical therapy, consider ordering an MRI scan with or without an arthrogram of the shoulder to evaluate the integrity of the rotator cuff.
- Use of a sling is generally discouraged because this can lead to shoulder stiffness and adhesive capsulitis.

Nonoperative Management
Indications
- Nonoperative management is indicated if the patient has pain without evidence of a full-thickness rotator cuff tear (night pain, weakness on examination, history of recent shoulder dislocation in patient over the age of 40 years).
- Treatment generally begins with the addition of NSAIDs and/or subacromial steroid injection.
- Physical therapy and/or a home program with Thera-Bands should be started to focus on rotator cuff strengthening.
- Work restrictions may be necessary if the patient has a job that involves repetitive activity or overhead reaching with the affected arm, to prevent repeat aggravation.
- Prognosis for shoulder impingement is good with these nonsurgical treatment options.
- Generally, the patient should be reevaluated in 6 weeks to check ROM and strength.
- Failure to improve at that point may warrant further evaluation of rotator cuff integrity with an MRI.
- Generally, failure to improve with one to two subacromial injections and a minimum of 6 weeks of physical therapy should prompt referral to a surgeon to consider surgical options for shoulder impingement.

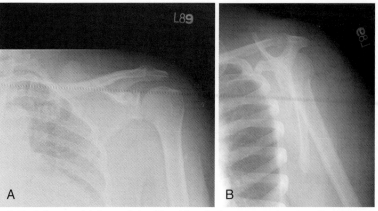

Fig. 2.12 Subacromial Spur of the Shoulder. A, Anteroposterior view. B, Outlet view.

Operative Management: Subacromial Decompression

Codes

ICD-10 code: M75.40 Shoulder impingement

CPT codes: 29826 Arthroscopic acromioplasty (shoulder arthroscopic decompression of the subacromial space with partial acromioplasty, with or without coracoacromial release)

> 23130 Open acromioplasty (acromioplasty or acromionectomy, partial with or without coracoacromial ligament release)

Indications

- Shoulder pain that has failed to improve with nonoperative treatment including subacromial injection and physical therapy and which interferes with patient activity.
- Absence of other potential causes of shoulder pain such as cervical radiculopathy.

Informed consent and counseling

- Routine surgical risks should be discussed with the patient (infection, bleeding, bruising, surgical pain, continued symptoms, and anesthesia complications).
- If your institution routinely uses nerve blocks as part of postoperative pain management, the expected duration of action of these blocks should be discussed.
- Generally, the patient is expected to be in a sling for up to 2 weeks, and use of the sling is discontinued based on patient comfort.
- Physical therapy is generally expected after surgery for approximately 6 weeks.
- Informed consent should include the possibility of rotator cuff repair if an unexpected tear is discovered at the time of surgery because this could lead to a longer recovery time (6 weeks in a sling and an average of 12 weeks of physical therapy).

Anesthesia

- General anesthesia with or without nerve block.

Patient positioning

- Beach chair or lateral decubitus (surgeon preference).

Surgical Procedures

- Arthroscopic acromioplasty
- Open acromioplasty (less common but may be necessary for posttraumatic deformity or large osteophytes)

Arthroscopic Acromioplasty

- The posterior portal is first created as the primary viewing portal for the arthroscope, followed by the anterior portal (working portal) for instruments.
- Diagnostic arthroscopy should be performed before the initiation of any procedure, with careful evaluation of the glenohumeral joint, labrum, biceps tendon, rotator cuff, and joint capsule.
- Placing the camera in the posterior portal and directing it superiorly allows visualization of the subacromial space.
- A lateral portal can be made to pass instruments for the acromioplasty.
- Electrocautery or radiofrequency devices may be superior to routine arthroscopic shavers because they help to control bleeding as the highly vascular bursa is débrided.
- After the bursa is adequately débrided, the coracoacromial ligament is cut, and an arthroscopic bur is used to remove impinging bone from the inferior surface of the acromion.

- Adequate bony resection should be confirmed before removing the arthroscope and closing the portals.

Estimated Postoperative Course

- Initial postoperative visit (7 to 14 days)
  - Suture removal
  - Physical therapy orders
  - Discussion of current pain control and plan for transitioning to nonnarcotic pain medications/modalities if applicable
  - Discontinuation of sling as tolerated
  - Review of work status, light duty desk work generally for 6 weeks
- 6-week postoperative visit
  - Evaluate wound healing, ROM, and strength
  - Determine the need for additional physical therapy
  - Review the return-to-work plan
- 12-week postoperative visit (optional)
  - Generally, only if pain is persistent, motion is limited, or reevaluation of work status is needed

SUGGESTED READINGS

Mazzocca AD, Alberta FG, Cole BJ, et al.: Shoulder: patient positioning, portal placement, and normal arthroscopic anatomy. In Miller MD, Cole BJ, editors: *Textbook of arthroscopy*, Philadelphia, 2004, Saunders.

Miller MD, Hart JA, MacKnight JM, editors: *Essential orthopaedics*, Philadelphia, 2010, Saunders.

Willenborg MD, Miller MD, Safran MR: Shoulder arthroscopy. In Miller MD, Chhabra AB, Safran MR, editors: *Primer of arthroscopy*, Philadelphia, 2010, Saunders.

ROTATOR CUFF TEARS

History

- Pain is located in the anterior and lateral shoulder.
- Pain frequently radiates to the deltoid area, but not usually below elbow.
- Tears are generally atraumatic, with progression of pain and weakness over time.
- They may be related to an acute trauma (e.g., fall on the outstretched hand).
- Waking at night is one of the frequently described symptoms.
- The patient may or may not complain of weakness in that arm.

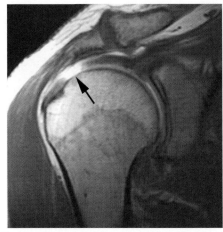

Fig. 2.13 Complete tear of the supraspinatus tendon *(arrow).* (From Miller MD, Sanders TG, editors: *Presentation, imaging, and treatment of common musculoskeletal conditions: MRI-arthroscopy correlation*, Philadelphia, 2012, Saunders, p 41.)

Physical Examination

- Active ROM may be limited, but passive ROM is generally full.
- Hawkins and Neer impingement signs may or may not be present.
- The drop arm sign (inability to hold the arm in an abducted position against gravity) indicates a likely massive rotator cuff tear.
- The supraspinatus stress test (weak with resisted abduction) is positive.
- Weakness with resisted external rotation indicates involvement of the infraspinatus.
- A positive lift-off or belly press sign indicates involvement of the subscapularis.
- A positive O'Brien sign indicates involvement of the biceps tendon.

Imaging

- Plain radiography should include AP, axillary, and outlet views.
- An MRI scan with or without arthrogram (often dictated by local protocol) is the "gold standard" for diagnosing and evaluating the extent of rotator cuff disease, although ultrasound evaluations are increasing in popularity due to the lower cost associated with them (Fig. 2.13).
- A computed tomography (CT) arthrogram may be necessary for patients who are unable to undergo MRI (e.g., patients with a pacemaker).

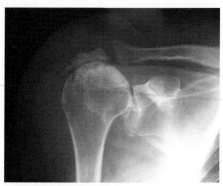

Fig. 2.14 Radiologic Appearance of Rotator Cuff Arthropathy. Note superior migration of the humeral head.

Classification System

- Rotator cuff tears are typically described by the number of tendons involved, the size of the tear, the amount of tendon retraction, and the degree of fatty atrophy of the rotator cuff muscles.
- Partial tears are commonly seen in patients who are more than 40 years old and may or may not be symptomatic. It is helpful to determine the percentage of involved tendon with MRI to determine treatment.
- Complete rotator cuff tears should be described by the number of involved tendons and the amount of retraction.
- Massive tears are generally defined as those involving two or more tendons and retracted more than 5 cm.
- Rotator cuff arthropathy denotes massive, retracted, chronic rotator cuff tears that are generally considered irreparable.
  - These patients are significantly weak on examination and may demonstrate a drop arm sign.
  - Diagnosis can be made by plain radiographs when proximal migration of the humeral head relative to the glenoid is seen (Fig. 2.14).
- At the time of arthroscopy, rotator cuff tears can further be described by the shape of the tear (e.g., U-shaped tear).

Differential Diagnoses

- Shoulder impingement
- Labral tear
- Cervical radiculopathy

Initial Management

- Initial treatment is determined by the size of the rotator cuff tear.
- Partial rotator cuff tears involving less than 50% of the total tendon area may respond well to conservative treatment including NSAIDs, subacromial steroid injections, and physical therapy.
- High-grade partial rotator cuff tears (involving >50% of the total tendon area) may be treated conservatively but may require surgical repair. This decision is determined by the degree of the patient's pain and dysfunction and the severity of the tear (for a 60% tear, an attempt at conservative treatment is more likely, whereas a 90% tear may suggest the need for earlier operative intervention).
- Complete rotator cuff repairs usually require surgical repair.
- **Patient Education.** Rotator cuff tears occur as a spectrum of injury ranging from tendinitis to partial tearing to complete tear to irreparable tear.
- Complete tears of the rotator cuff require surgery to repair the tendon in most cases to restore normal shoulder function.
- Patients should use the shoulder normally to maintain ROM but avoid repetitive overhead activities and heavy lifting.
- Complete rotator cuff tears should be referred to a shoulder surgeon.
- Although surgical treatment is not urgent, ideally surgery occurs in the first 1 to 3 months of diagnosis because of the risk of tendon retraction with longer delays.
- The use of a sling should be avoided because this can lead to the development of adhesive capsulitis.

Nonoperative Management

- Nonoperative management typically is reserved for partial, low-grade rotator cuff tears.
- NSAIDs, subacromial steroid injections, and physical therapy effective in managing pain and improving function.
- Patients should be instructed to follow up for a new evaluation if conservative treatment does not improve symptoms in 6 to 8 weeks.
- MRI (with or without arthrogram), if not already performed, may be necessary at that point to evaluate for a full-thickness rotator cuff tear.

Operative Management: Rotator Cuff Repair

Codes
ICD-10 code: M75.100 Complete rupture of the rotator cuff

CPT code: 29827 Arthroscopy, shoulder, with rotator cuff repair

Indications
- Complete tear of the rotator cuff.
- High-grade partial tear of the rotator cuff.
- Partial rotator cuff tear that has failed to improve with conservative treatment.

Informed consent and counseling
- Routine surgical risks should be discussed with the patient (infection, bleeding, bruising, surgical pain, continued symptoms, and anesthesia complications).
- If your institution routinely uses nerve blocks as part of the postoperative pain management, the expected duration of action of these blocks should be discussed.
- Generally, the patient is expected to be in a sling for approximately 6 weeks postoperatively.
- Physical therapy is generally started after the first postoperative appointment and continued for 12 weeks or until motion and strength goals are obtained.
- Return to full function can take 6 to 12 months.

Anesthesia
- General, often with accompanying nerve block

Patient positioning
- Beach chair or lateral decubitus (surgeon's preference)

Surgical Procedures
- Arthroscopic rotator cuff repair
- Open rotator cuff repair (may be used based on the surgeon's experience or because of massive tears in which adequate repair cannot be obtained arthroscopically)

Rotator Cuff Repair
- For arthroscopic repair, the posterior portal is first created as the primary viewing portal for the arthroscope, followed by the anterior portal (working portal) for instruments.
- Diagnostic arthroscopy should be performed before the initiation of any procedure, with careful evaluation of the glenohumeral joint, labrum, biceps tendon, rotator cuff, and joint capsule.

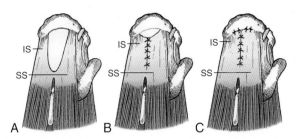

Fig. 2.15 A–C, Margin convergence technique. *IS,* Infraspinatus; *SS,* supraspinatus. (From Miller MD, Cole BJ: *Textbook of arthroscopy*, Philadelphia, 2004, Saunders.)

- For open repair, an incision is made in the anterior aspect of the shoulder lateral to the acromion along the Langer lines; access to the joint capsule is gained through the deltoid either by splitting the fibers (traditional open approach) or detaching it from the acromion (mini-open approach).
- Acromioplasty is typically performed as described earlier.
- The rotator cuff is evaluated to determine the degree of tear, the shape of the tear, and retraction.
- Partial-thickness tears of less than 50% can be débrided with the shaver rather than repaired.
- Full-thickness tears and high-grade partial tears must be mobilized and repaired.
- Arthroscopic repair is performed by passing sutures through the cuff tissue and directly repairing it to the bone by suture anchors.
- Margin convergence may be necessary before direct repair of tendon back to bone in the case of L-shaped or U-shaped tears (Fig. 2.15).
- Sutures are then passed either in antegrade or retrograde fashion and are secured to suture anchors placed in the footprint (single row, double row, suture bridge technique, as preferred by the surgeon).
- In open repair, direct suture repair to bone is performed by passing sutures through bone tunnels and then tying knots.
- Sutures are tensioned, and the repair is examined before irrigation and closure of the portals and/or incision.

Estimated Postoperative Course
- Initial postoperative visit (7 to 14 days)
  - Suture removal
  - Physical therapy orders given to focus on passive ROM of the shoulder only

- Pain control should be reviewed and plan made to transition to nonnarcotic pain medications/modalities if applicable
- Continued use of sling removing only for pendulum exercises and elbow motion
- Review of work status; light duty desk work begun as tolerated by patient, with no use of surgical arm
- 6-week postoperative visit
  - Evaluation of wound healing, ROM, and strength
  - New physical therapy orders to begin active-assisted ROM, active motion, and gentle early rotator cuff strengthening exercises
  - Removal of sling
  - Light duty work continued for a minimum of 6 additional weeks
- 12-week postoperative visit
  - Evaluate the progression of ROM and strength
  - Determine the need for additional physical therapy
  - Discuss the return-to-work plan

Board Review

Rotator cuff tears can be traumatic from a fall but often occur from overuse and are most common in patients over 40 years of age.

SUGGESTED READINGS

Amoo-Achampong K, Krill MK, Acheampong D, Nwachukwu BU, McCormick F: Evaluating strategies and outcomes following rotator cuff tears, *Shoulder Elbow* 11:4–18, 2019.

Jancuska J, Matthews J, Miller T, Kluczynski MA, Bisson LJ: A systematic summary of systematic reviews on the topic of the rotator cuff, *Orthop J Sports Med* 60(6), 2018.

Miller MD, Hart JA, MacKnight JM, editors: *Essential orthopaedics*, Philadelphia, 2010, Saunders.

Willenborg MD, Miller MD, Safran MR: Shoulder arthroscopy. In Miller MD, Chhabra AB, Safran MR, editors: *Primer of arthroscopy*, Philadelphia, 2010, Saunders.

Wolf BR, Dunn WR, Wright RW: Clinical sports medicine update: indications for repair of full-thickness rotator cuff tears, *Am J Sports Med* 35:1007–1016, 2007.

SHOULDER INSTABILITY

History

- Shoulder instability may be traumatic or atraumatic.
- Traumatic shoulder dislocations most commonly occur with the shoulder in an abducted and externally rotated position causing immediate pain, shoulder deformity, and loss of motion.
- Patients may report a "dead" arm syndrome resulting from transient traction on the brachial plexus or the axillary nerve.
- Atraumatic shoulder instability may be vaguer, with pain or subluxation events during activity such as overhead throwing or swimming.
- It is important to differentiate dislocation from subluxation during the history, as well as the number of episodes (acute, recurrent).
- Other causes of shoulder dislocation include seizure disorders and electric shock (posterior dislocation).
- Hyperligamentous laxity can predispose to instability, as can a history of such conditions as Ehlers-Danlos syndrome or Marfan syndrome.

Physical Examination

- Acute dislocations produce deformity and loss of motion.
- Decreased sensation occurs over the "deltoid patch" initially and resolves with time.
- Apprehension and relocation tests are positive.
- A positive sulcus sign with inferior instability, often bilateral, indicates multidirectional instability.
- A positive supraspinatus stress test may indicate an associated rotator cuff tear in patients who are more than 40 years old.

Imaging: Figs. 2.16 and 2.17

- AP and axillary views are indicated at a minimum (the **axillary view** is important to confirm reduction).
- Stryker notch and West Point views can be helpful for chronic, recurrent instability:
  - Stryker notch: Hill Sachs lesion
  - West Point view: bony Bankart lesion
- MRI arthrogram is used to evaluate labral tear (patients <40 years old) or rotator cuff tear (patient >40 years old) with shoulder dislocation or instability.
- CT scan may be helpful in recurrent shoulder instability to evaluate the glenoid for bone loss (important to determine the need for a concomitant bony procedure).

Classification System

- Direction of instability (anterior, posterior, multidirectional).

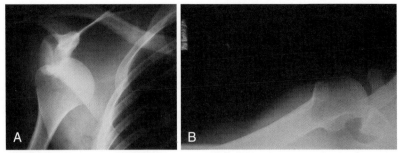

Fig. 2.16 A, Anteroposterior view of anterior shoulder dislocation. B, Axillary view; note the large Hill Sachs lesion.

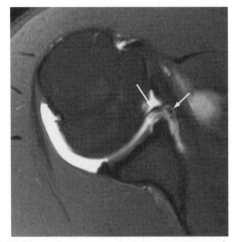

Fig. 2.17 Magnetic resonance imaging appearance of anterior labral tear (cartilaginous Bankart lesion; *arrows*). (From Miller MD, Sanders TG, editors: *Presentation, imaging, and treatment of common musculoskeletal conditions: MRI-arthroscopy correlation*, Philadelphia, 2012, Saunders, p 56.)

- Chronicity (acute or chronic, first-time dislocation, recurrent).
- By anatomic description of injury:
  - Glenoid labrum articular disruption (GLAD)
  - Anterior labral periosteal sleeve avulsion (ALPSA)
  - Humeral avulsion of the glenoid labrum (HAGL)

Initial Management

- **Patient Education.** Shoulder dislocations should be reduced as soon as possible, usually in an emergency department. Pain improves rapidly after the shoulder is reduced and can usually be controlled with antiinflammatory medications and ice. Typically, the shoulder remains sore for several weeks after an acute dislocation. Shoulder strengthening with physical therapy is helpful after acute shoulder dislocation. The rate of recurrence is highest in younger patients.

- Acute dislocation should be treated with reduction, although this may need to be done in the emergency department because sedation may be required.
- A sling is useful for patient comfort initially.
- Antiinflammatory medication may be provided for early postinjury pain.
- Follow up in the clinic 1 to 2 weeks after acute dislocation should be set up to reevaluate motion and strength.

Nonoperative Management

- Nonoperative management is indicated for most first-time shoulder dislocations and cases of multidirectional instability.
- Narcotic pain medications should be used only for initial very severe postinjury pain and discontinued as soon as the patient is comfortable. NSAIDs may be used at that point if necessary.
- A sling can be used initially and discontinued based on patient comfort.
- Physical therapy can be helpful to decrease pain, restore normal ROM, and improve rotator cuff and scapula stabilizer strength.
- Recurrent episodes of instability or failure to improve with this nonoperative treatment plan may necessitate MRI with arthrogram to evaluate the labrum.
- Clinicians should have a high index of suspicion for rotator cuff tear in patients more than 40 years old who have shoulder dislocation.

Operative Management: Arthroscopic Bankart Repair and Capsulorrhaphy

Codes
ICD-10 codes: M25.319 Shoulder instability
    M24.419 Recurrent shoulder dislocation
    S43.006A Shoulder dislocation

CPT codes: 29806 Arthroscopy, shoulder, surgical; capsulorrhaphy

Indications

- Recurrent shoulder dislocation.
- Symptomatic shoulder instability after failure of conservative treatment.
- Multidirectional instability with failure of appropriate course of conservative treatment.

Informed consent and counseling

- Routine surgical risks should be discussed with the patient (infection, bleeding, bruising, surgical pain, continued symptoms, and anesthesia complications).
- If your institution routinely uses nerve blocks as part of the postoperative pain management, the expected duration of action of these blocks should be discussed.
- Generally, the patient is expected to be in a sling for approximately 6 weeks postoperatively.
- Physical therapy is generally started after the first postoperative appointment and continued for 12 weeks.
- Return to sport should be restricted until 6 months postoperatively.

Anesthesia

- General with or without nerve block

Patient positioning

- Beach chair or lateral decubitus (surgeon preference)

Surgical Procedures

- Arthroscopic Bankart repair (with or without capsulorrhaphy)
- Open Bankart repair (with or without capsulorrhaphy)
- Latarjet procedure
- Open glenoid bone grafting

Arthroscopic Bankart Repair

- Routine diagnostic arthroscopy is performed.
- Examination under anesthesia with arthroscopic visualization can identify engaging Hill Sachs lesions.
- Labral tears should be identified and may require mobilization and elevation up onto the face of the glenoid if the tissue has scarred down medially.
- The "bumper pad" effect of the labrum is restored by passing suture secured to anchors placed on the glenoid rim.

Estimated Postoperative Course

- Initial postoperative visit (7 to 14 days)
  - Suture removal
  - Physical therapy orders given to focus on passive ROM, with avoidance of extreme abduction and external rotation
  - Pain medication refill, if necessary
  - Continued use of the sling, removed only for pendulum exercises and elbow motion
  - Review of work or sports status; light duty desk work begun as tolerated by the patient, with no use of surgical arm or athletics
- 6-week postoperative visit
  - Evaluation of wound healing, ROM, and strength
  - New physical therapy orders to advance ROM and begin strengthening exercises
  - Removal of sling
- 12-week postoperative visit
  - Evaluate the progression of ROM and strength
  - Determine the need for additional physical therapy
  - Discuss the return-to-work and sports plan (usually no collision or throwing sports until 6 months postoperatively)

Board Review

First-time acute shoulder dislocations can often be managed conservatively with physical therapy and activity modification while recurrent instability often requires surgical stabilization.

SUGGESTED READINGS

Camp C: An age-based approach to anterior shoulder instability in patients under 40 years old: Analysis of a US population, *Am J Sports Med* 48(1):56–62, 2020.

Best MJ, Tanaka MJ: Multidirectional instability of the shoulder: treatment options and considerations, *Sports Med Arthrosc Rev* 26(3):113–119, 2018.

Leland DP, Bernard CD, Keyt LK, Provencher MT, Bhatia S, Ghodadra NS, et al.: Recurrent shoulder instability: current concepts for evaluation and management of glenoid bone loss, *J Bone Joint Surg Am* 92(Suppl 2):133–151, 2010.

Young AA, Maia R, Berhouet J, et al.: Open Latarjet procedure for management of bone loss in anterior instability of the glenohumeral joint, *J Shoulder Elbow Surg* 20(2):S61–S69, 2011.

SUPERIOR LABRAL TEARS AND BICEPS TENDON DISORDERS

History

- These injuries are common in overhead throwing athletes from repetitive stress on the biceps anchor.
- They may be traumatic, most commonly from a fall on the outstretched hand or a traction injury (e.g., catching oneself from a fall by grabbing something overhead).
- Patients typically report pain anterior and deep in the shoulder that is worse with overhead reaching and the throwing motion.
- They can be associated with mechanical catching.

Physical Examination

- Several special tests have been described to identify SLAP tears such as the O'Brien (active compression) test.
- Glenohumeral internal rotation deficit (GIRD) should be documented because this is a common finding with internal impingement in throwing athletes.
- Otherwise, ROM and strength are generally normal.

Imaging

- Standard AP, outlet, and axillary radiographs (usually normal).
- MRI with arthrogram (the preferred imaging modality).

Magnetic Resonance Imaging: Fig. 2.18

Classification System: Fig. 2.19

- The original Snyder classification system of SLAP tears included types I to IV, but types V to VII were added later:
  - Type I: degenerative tearing of the superior labrum with intact biceps anchor
  - Type II: detachment of the superior labrum and biceps anchor (most common)
  - Type III: bucket handle tear of the superior labrum but intact biceps anchor
  - Type IV: tearing of the superior labrum that extends up into the biceps tendon
  - Type V: superior labral tear in addition to anterior or posterior labral tear
  - Type VI: flap tear of the superior labrum
  - Type VII: superior labral tear with extension to the capsule

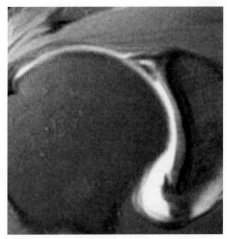

Fig. 2.18 Magnetic resonance imaging appearance of superior labrum anterior to posterior (SLAP) tear. (From Miller MD, Sanders TG, editors: *Presentation, imaging, and treatment of common musculoskeletal conditions: MRI-arthroscopy correlation*, Philadelphia, 2012, Saunders, p 69.)

- Classification of proximal biceps disease is typically descriptive (tendinopathy, partial tear, complete rupture).

Differential Diagnoses

- Rotator cuff tear
- Labral tear
- Distal biceps tendon injury

Initial Management

- **Patient Education.** Although tears of the biceps tendon attachment in the shoulder can result from an injury, they more commonly occur from repetitive activity that stresses this area. Injections may provide some temporary relief, but these conditions often require surgery for correction.
- Any loss of motion should first be corrected with physical therapy (sleeper stretch may be necessary for GIRD to stretch the posterior capsule).
- NSAIDs may be helpful if the patient is in pain and has pain-related difficulty doing exercises.
- Glenohumeral injections may temporarily relieve pain and can be diagnostic if the patient has other symptoms that confuse the clinical picture (e.g., cervical radiculopathy).

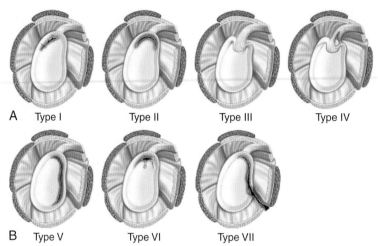

Fig. 2.19 Classification of Superior Labrum Anterior to Posterior (SLAP) Tears. (From Miller MD, Thompson S, Hart JA, editors: *Review of orthopaedics,* ed 6, Philadelphia, 2012, Saunders. Adapted from Kepler CL, Nho SJ, Sherman SL, et al: Superior labral tear. In: Reider B, Terry M, Provencher MT, editors: *Operative techniques: sports medicine surgery,* Philadelphia, 2009, Saunders.)

Nonoperative Management

- Nonoperative management can be initiated early with NSAIDs, activity modification, glenohumeral injection, biceps tendon sheath injection, and/or physical therapy.
- MRI with arthrogram should be performed when conservative treatment fails or when symptoms severely limit normal levels of activity.
- If surgery is considered, tenotomy versus tenodesis should be discussed because the best procedure is still debated in the literature.
- Complete ruptures of the proximal biceps tendon are treated conservatively with reassurance, ice, NSAIDs, and rest.

Operative Management

Codes
ICD-10 codes: S43.439A Superior glenoid labrum lesion (SLAP tear)

    S46.119A Biceps rupture, proximal

    M75.20 Biceps tendinitis

    M67.929 Biceps tendinopathy

CPT codes: 29807 Arthroscopy, shoulder, surgical; repair of SLAP lesion

    29822 Arthroscopy, shoulder, débridement, limited (biceps tenotomy)

    29828 Arthroscopy, shoulder, biceps tenodesis

    23430 Tenodesis of long tendon of biceps, open

Indications
- Symptomatic SLAP tears.

- Biceps tendinopathy that has failed to improve with conservative treatment.
- Symptomatic biceps tendon subluxation.

Informed consent and counseling
- Routine surgical risks (infection, bleeding, bruising, surgical pain, continued symptoms, and anesthesia complications) should be discussed, as well as expectations of nerve blocks if these blocks are used at your institution.
- For patients considered for biceps tenotomy or tenodesis, the difference between these two procedures should be discussed (e.g., "popeye" deformity for tenotomy, longer sling for tenodesis).
- Generally, the patient is expected to be in a sling for approximately 6 weeks postoperatively for SLAP repairs and biceps tenodesis and only to comfort (about 2 weeks) for tenotomy.
- Physical therapy is generally started after the first postoperative appointment and is continued for 12 weeks.
- Return to sport should be restricted until 6 months postoperatively.

Anesthesia
- General, with or without a nerve block

Patient positioning
- Beach chair or lateral decubitus (surgeon preference)

Surgical Procedures
- Arthroscopic débridement

- Arthroscopic superior labral repair
- Biceps tenotomy
- Biceps tenodesis

Arthroscopic Labral Débridement or Repair

- Diagnostic arthroscopy is initially performed according to routine protocol.
- Repair of the superior labrum, if indicated, is performed by placing anchors on either side of the biceps tendon and passing or tying sutures.

Arthroscopic Biceps Tenotomy or Tenodesis

- Diagnostic arthroscopy is initially performed according to routine protocol.
- The biceps tendon should be visually inspected by using a probe to pull the proximal tendon into the joint.
- Biceps tenotomy is performed by simply releasing the proximal biceps and débriding the stump.
- Biceps tenodesis is performed by first releasing the tendon and then reattaching it by suturing it to the rotator cuff or securing it to the proximal humerus through a bone tunnel.
- The tenodesis is secured by anchors or a screw.

Estimated Postoperative Course

- Initial postoperative visit (7 to 14 days)
  - Suture removal
  - Physical therapy orders given to focus on passive ROM, with avoidance of resisted elbow flexion (biceps tenotomy can progress strengthening immediately)
  - Pain medication refill, if necessary
  - Continued use of sling, with removal only for pendulum exercises and elbow motion (biceps tenotomy, can remove as comfortable)
  - Review of work or sports status, light duty desk work begun as tolerated by the patient, with no use of surgical arm or athletics
- 6-week postoperative visit
  - Evaluation of wound healing, ROM, and strength
  - New physical therapy orders to advance ROM and begin strengthening exercises
  - Removal of sling
- 12-week postoperative visit
  - Evaluate the progression of ROM and strength
  - Determine the need for additional physical therapy
  - Discuss the return-to-work and sports plan (usually no collision or throwing sports until 6 months postoperatively)

SUGGESTED READINGS

Chen RE, Voloshin I: Long head of biceps injury: treatment options and decision making, *Sports Med Arthrosc Rev* 26(3):139–144, 2018.

Crum RJ, Lin A, Lesniak BP: Labral repair versus biceps tenodesis for primary surgical management of type II superior labrum anterior to posterior tears: a systematic review, *Arthroscopy* 35(6):1927–1938, 2019.

De Sa D, Arakgi ME, Lian J, et al.: Current concepts in the evaluation and management of type II superior labral lesions of the shoulder, *Open Orthop J* 12:331–341, 2018.

Hassan S, Patel V: Biceps tenodesis versus biceps tenotomy for biceps tendinitis without rotator cuff tears, *J Clin Orthop Trauma* 10(2):248–256, 2019.

Rainey R, Miller MD, Anderson M, et al.: Superior labral injuries. In Miller MD, Sanders TG, editors: *Presentation, imaging, and treatment of common musculoskeletal conditions: MRI-arthroscopy correlation*, Philadelphia, 2012, Saunders, pp 65–69.

GLENOHUMERAL OSTEOARTHRITIS

History

- Most commonly a progressive degenerative condition.
- May be posttraumatic.
- May be secondary to chronic rotator cuff tear (rotator cuff arthropathy).
- Often seen in patients with a history of shoulder instability and a remote history of surgical treatment of that instability (e.g., Putti-Platt or Magnuson procedure).
- Complaints of pain, crepitus, and progressive loss of motion.

Physical Examination

- Active and passive ROM is often limited.
- Crepitus is frequently noted during motion testing.
- Strength is typically not affected, except in cases of associated rotator cuff disease (e.g., rotator cuff arthropathy).

Imaging

- AP and axillary radiographs are usually sufficient to make the diagnosis.
- The most common findings are an inferior humeral osteophyte and glenohumeral joint space narrowing.

Radiographic Image: Fig. 2.20

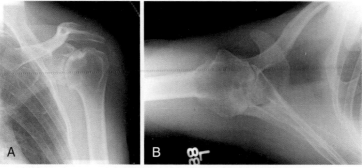

Fig. 2.20 **A** and **B,** Radiographic appearance of glenohumeral osteoarthritis. Note inferior humeral osteophyte and joint space narrowing.

Classification

- Mild, moderate, or severe, based on the amount of glenohumeral joint space narrowing and associated bony deformity.

Differential Diagnoses

- Rotator cuff tear
- Adhesive capsulitis
- Cervical radiculopathy

Initial Management

Patient Education. Glenohumeral osteoarthritis refers to progressive "wear and tear" changes to the ball and socket joint in the shoulder. Although this can occur from an old injury, it more commonly develops with increasing age from use. Arthritis has no definitive cure, so treatment is based on modifying activities and trying various treatments to control the pain that range from antiinflammatory medications to injections to shoulder replacement.

- Ice, NSAIDs, rest, activity modification.
- Glenohumeral steroid injections, usually done under fluoroscopic or ultrasound guidance for improved accuracy.
- Physical therapy to improve ROM and rotator cuff strength.

Nonoperative Management

- Ice, NSAIDs, rest, activity modification.
- Glenohumeral steroid injections, usually done under fluoroscopic guidance for improved accuracy.
- Physical therapy to improve ROM and rotator cuff strengthening.

Operative Management

Codes

ICD-10 codes: M19.019 Osteoarthritis shoulder
M19.119 Posttraumatic osteoarthritis of the shoulder
M12.819 Rotator cuff arthropathy
CPT codes: 29823 Shoulder arthroscopy, débridement, extensive
23472 Total shoulder replacement

Indications

- Shoulder osteoarthritis that has failed to respond to nonoperative treatment.
- Pain secondary to shoulder osteoarthritis that affects activities of daily living.

Informed consent and counseling

- Standard surgical risks should be discussed in detail (e.g., bleeding, infection, failure, anesthesia risks).
- Shoulder arthroscopy can be useful in relieving some mechanical catching and locking related to osteoarthritis, but it rarely relieves all the symptoms.
- Total shoulder replacements are effective at treating pain from osteoarthritis but they do not usually restore normal function and ROM (some stiffness should be expected postoperatively).
- Reverse total shoulder implants may be preferred for cases of a chronically torn rotator cuff or some cases of posttraumatic arthritis.

Anesthesia

- General, likely with nerve block

Patient positioning

- Beach chair or lateral decubitus (arthroscopy)
- Modified beach chair (total shoulder replacement)

Surgical Procedures

- Arthroscopic débridement
- Total shoulder arthroplasty

Total Shoulder Arthroplasty
- A standard deltopectoral approach is used to access the glenohumeral joint.
- The biceps tendon is released within the bicipital groove.
- Osteotomy of the lesser tuberosity is performed, and the subscapularis is taken down to allow dislocation of the joint for access.
- The humeral canal is reamed, and a humeral head cutting jig is used for the humeral head osteotomy.
- The glenoid is exposed, the labral tissue is excised, and the glenoid bone is reamed in preparation for the implant.
- The appropriately sized implants are cemented into place, and the shoulder is reduced; the final position is confirmed with imaging.
- After copious irrigation, the wound is closed in layers according to routine protocol.

Estimated Postoperative Course
- Initial postoperative visit (7 to 14 days)
  - Suture or staple removal
  - Physical therapy orders given to focus on ROM in the early period
  - Pain medication refill, if necessary
  - Sling used for 6 weeks postoperatively
- 6-week postoperative visit
  - Evaluation of wound healing, ROM, and strength
  - New physical therapy orders to advance ROM and begin strengthening exercises
- 12-week postoperative visit
  - Evaluate the progression of ROM and strength
  - Determine the need for additional physical therapy
  - Counsel the patient that ROM and strength improvements continue over upcoming months

SUGGESTED READINGS

Ansok CB, Muh SJ: Optimal management of glenohumeral osteoarthritis, *Orthop Res Rev* 10:9–18, 2018.

Saltzman BM, Leroux TS, Verma NN, Romeo AA: Glenohumeral osteoarthritis in the young patient, *J Am Acad Orthop Surg* 26(17):e361-370, 2018.

Takamura KM, Chen JB, Petrigliano FA: Nonarthroplasty options for the athlete or active individual with shoulder osteoarthritis, *Clin Sports Med* 37(4):517–526, 2018.

Tashjian RZ, Chalmers PN: Future frontiers in shoulder arthroplasty and the management of shoulder osteoarthritis, *Clin Sports Med* 37(4):609–630, 2018.

ADHESIVE CAPSULITIS

History
- The patient has progressive loss of motion.
- Pain is worse at the end ROM in all planes.
- The origin of adhesive capsulitis not well understood, but the condition is believed to be an inflammatory process and is often seen in patients with a history of an autoimmune disorder, especially diabetes mellitus.
- Other related factors may include history of trauma, thyroid disease, period of immobilization, associated cervical disease, and multiple medical comorbidities, but often occurs in the absence of all these conditions.

Physical Examination
- Both passive ROM and active ROM are restricted.
- The patient exhibits increased pain at the end ROM during the examination.
- Often supine ROM measurements are more accurate with this condition.
- Careful documentation is important to assess improvement after treatment.

Imaging
- Standard AP, axillary, and outlet radiographs are usually normal but are important to evaluate for other conditions that can affect ROM, such as shoulder osteoarthritis.

Differential Diagnoses
- Rotator cuff tear
- Shoulder osteoarthritis
- Cervical radiculopathy

Initial Management
Patient Education. Adhesive capsulitis is better known as "frozen shoulder." It is caused by scarring of the joint capsule that causes pain and stiffness in the shoulder joint. It is more common in diabetic patients but can also be seen in completely healthy patients with no history of shoulder problems. Generally, frozen shoulder is self-limiting, but the process can be long and can take more than a year or two to resolve without appropriate treatment steps.
- Ice and antiinflammatory medications are generally used to help control pain.

- The use of a sling should be avoided in cases when it is not absolutely necessary (e.g., fracture) because this can increase joint stiffness.
- Glenohumeral joint steroid injections, generally done under fluoroscopic or ultrasound guidance for improved accuracy, are extremely helpful initially.
- Physical therapy is the key to the nonoperative management, with the focus on both passive and active ROM. It is often best in conjunction with steroid injection.
- Patients should be encouraged to work on passive ROM exercises on their own at home in addition to formal physical therapy sessions.

Nonoperative Management

- Ice and antiinflammatory medications are generally used to help control pain.
- The use of a sling should be avoided because this can increase joint stiffness
- Glenohumeral joint steroid injections, generally done under fluoroscopic guidance for improved accuracy, are extremely helpful initially.
- Physical therapy is the key to the nonoperative management, with the focus on both passive and active ROM.
- Patients should be encouraged to work on passive ROM exercises on their own at home in addition to formal physical therapy sessions.

Operative Management: Arthroscopic Lysis of Adhesion and Manipulation under Anesthesia

Codes

ICD-10 codes: M75.00 Adhesive capsulitis, shoulder
CPT codes: 29825 Arthroscopic lysis of adhesions and manipulation under anesthesia

Indications

- Adhesive capsulitis that has been refractory to conservative treatment (often two glenohumeral injections and 6 to 12 weeks of physical therapy)

Informed consent and counseling

- Standard surgical risks should be discussed in detail (e.g., bleeding, infection, failure, anesthesia risks).
- Physical therapy should be set up before surgery to begin in the immediate postoperative period (postoperative day 1 or 2).
- Recurrence of this condition is common even with surgical treatment.

Anesthesia

- General, with or without a block
- Consideration of leaving a catheter in place for continuous block infusion for severe refractory cases, to allow early aggressive physical therapy

Patient positioning

- Beach chair or lateral decubitus (surgeon preference)

Surgical Procedures

Arthroscopic Lysis of Adhesions and Manipulation under Anesthesia

- Examination under anesthesia should be done before beginning the surgical procedure and preoperative ROM recorded.
- Standard arthroscopic portals are made, and diagnostic arthroscopy is performed as described earlier.
- A shaver is used to débride the rotator interval, and the middle glenohumeral ligament is released along with the capsular tissue, with caution used to avoid the rotator cuff tendon.
- After changing portals, the posterior joint is similarly débrided, and tight posterior capsular tissue is released.
- Postoperative ROM should be measured and recorded to ensure that adequate release was performed before portal closure.

Estimated Postoperative Course

- Early postoperative period (days 0 to 6)
  - Physical therapy to emphasize ROM should start as early as 1 to 2 days after surgery
  - Use of a sling should be avoided, and home ROM exercises should be encouraged immediately
- Initial postoperative visit (7 to 14 days)
  - Suture or staple removal
  - Physical therapy orders given to focus on ROM in the early period
  - Pain medication refill, if necessary
  - Sling used for comfort and discontinued as tolerated by the patient
- 6-week postoperative visit
  - Evaluation of wound healing, ROM, and strength
  - New physical therapy orders to advance ROM and begin strengthening exercises
- 12-week postoperative visit
  - Evaluate the progression of ROM and strength
  - Determine the need for additional physical therapy

- Counsel the patient that ROM and strength improvements continue over upcoming months
- Additional fluoroscopically guided glenohumeral injections may be necessary for patients with persistent symptoms postoperatively, but these injections are typically delayed for at least 6 weeks after surgery

Board Review

Adhesive capsulitis is primarily diagnosed by a physical examination that shows a loss of *passive* ROM.

SUGGESTED READINGS

Hannafin JA, Chiaia TA: Adhesive capsulitis: a treatment approach, *Clin Orthop Relat Res* 372:95–109, 2000.

MacKnight JM: Adhesive capsulitis (frozen shoulder). In Miller MD, Hart JA, MacKnight JM, editors: *Essential orthopaedics*, Philadelphia, 2010, Saunders, pp 172–174.

Neviaser AS, Neviaser RJ: Adhesive capsulitis of the shoulder, *Am Acad Orthop Surg* 19(9):536–542, 2011.

Xiao RC, DeAngelis JP, Smith CC, Ramappa AJ: Evaluating nonoperative treatments for adhesive capsulitis, *J Surg Orthop Adv* 26(4):193–199, 2017.

ACROMIOCLAVICULAR JOINT INJURIES AND DISORDERS

History

- AC separations
  - Trauma with most likely reported mechanism a fall onto the lateral point of the shoulder
  - Common in collision sports (e.g., football) from a direct hit to the shoulder
  - Pain localized over the AC joint
  - Often a "lump" or deformity reported over the AC joint
- AC joint osteolysis and osteoarthritis
  - Usually more insidious onset of pain, although old trauma possibly reported
  - Pain again localized over the AC joint
  - Pain worse when reaching across the body (adduction)
  - Possible history of weight lifting or other repetitive activity

Physical Examination

- Possible deformity over the AC joint in acute or chronic separations.
- Focal tenderness over the AC joint.

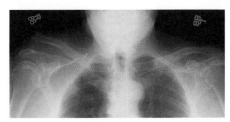

Fig. 2.21 Radiographic appearance of acromioclavicular separation. Note bilateral radiographs for comparison of coracoclavicular distance.

- Palpation of the entire clavicle and also the sternoclavicular joint in cases of trauma.
- Cross-body adduction pain.

Imaging

- Plain radiographs of the shoulder include a bilateral AP view of the AC joint (comparison), as well as an axillary view of the affected shoulder (type IV AC separation; see later).
- The Zanca view may be helpful to visualize the AC joint for osteolysis or osteoarthritis.

Radiographic Image: Fig. 2.21

Classification System

- AC separation (Fig. 2.22)
  - Type I: AC sprain only, possible widening of the AC joint but no elevation of the distal clavicle
  - Type II: complete tear of the AC ligament but intact coracoclavicular (CC) ligament
  - Type III: AC and CC ligament rupture, elevation of distal clavicle up to 100% of the contralateral side
  - Type IV: *posterior* displacement of the distal clavicle through the trapezius (need axillary view to diagnose)
  - Type V: AC and CC ligament injury with elevation greater than 100% of the contralateral side (twice the other CC distance)
  - Type VI: inferior displacement of the distal clavicle below the coracoid (rare)
- AC osteolysis and osteoarthritis
  - Mild, moderate, severe

Differential Diagnoses

- Clavicle fracture
- Shoulder contusion
- Cervical radiculopathy

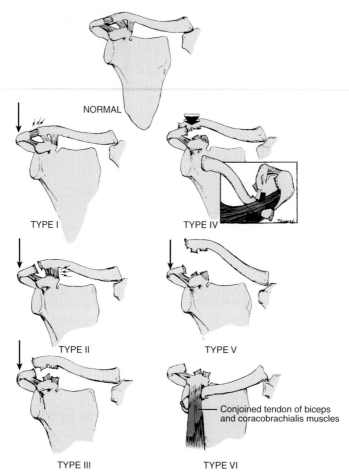

Fig. 2.22 Classification of Acromioclavicular (AC) Separations. Type I: AC sprain. Type II: Complete AC tear, intact coracoacromial (CC) ligament. Type III: AC and CC ligament tear, displacement up to 100% of contralateral side. Type IV: Posterior displacement of clavicle through trapezius muscle; requires axillary view for diagnosis. Type V: Displacement of more than 100% of the contralateral side. Type VI: (Rare) inferior displacement of clavicle below coracoids. (From Rockwood CA Jr, Young DC: Disorders of the acromioclavicular joint. In Rockwood CA Jr, Matsen III FA, editors: *The shoulder,* ed 2, Philadelphia, 1998, Saunders.)

Initial Management

- **Patient Education.** AC separation
  - AC separations are very painful in the first few weeks of injury, and treatment is based on the degree of separation. More minor separations begin to improve rapidly after that time, and symptoms generally resolve within 6 to 8 weeks. More severe separations may require surgery to repair the damaged structures.
- **Patient Education.** AC osteolysis and osteoarthritis
  - These conditions occur secondary to repetitive stresses across this small joint and can affect people of all ages. Generally, treatment is

conservative with antiinflammatory medications (pills or injections) and avoidance of activities that aggravate the pain. If symptoms persist, surgery to remove the affected bone end surfaces is an option.
- Treatment of AC separations begins with identifying the severity of the injury (radiographs)
  - Types I and II AC separations are treated conservatively with rest, activity modification, and antiinflammatory medications.
  - Type III separations are most commonly treated conservatively initially, and surgery is considered only for patients with persistent symptoms.

- Types IV, V, and VI separations require surgery to restore the AC joint.
- Treatment of AC joint osteolysis and osteoarthritis should begin with ice, rest, activity modification, and antiinflammatory medications.

Nonoperative Management

- Conservative treatment for AC joint injuries (types I, II, and most type III), as well as osteolysis or osteoarthritis, should begin with resting the shoulder and avoiding activities that aggravate the pain.
- Antiinflammatory medications are useful.
- AC joint injections are very effective in controlling pain and are also useful to localize symptoms in cases of more generalized pain.
- Activities can progress as pain improves.
- AC joint padding should be used for collision athletes (e.g., football players) as they return to play.

Operative Management: Acromioclavicular Joint Reconstruction and Distal Clavicle Excision

Codes

ICD-10 codes:

M19.019 Acromioclavicular joint arthritis

S43.109A AC separation

CPT codes: 29824 Shoulder arthroscopic distal claviculectomy

23120 Open distal claviculectomy

23550 Open treatment of acromioclavicular dislocation

23552 Open treatment of acromioclavicular dislocation, with graft

Indications

- Types IV, V, and VI AC separations
- Type III AC separations that are persistently symptomatic despite adequate conservative treatment
- AC joint osteolysis, AC joint degenerative disease, very distal clavicle fractures (distal clavicle excision)

Informed consent and counseling

- Standard surgical risks should be discussed in detail (e.g., bleeding, infection, failure, anesthesia risks).
- The use of a sling will be necessary for a minimum of 6 weeks postoperative (AC joint reconstruction).
- No heavy lifting, reaching, or repetitive activity with this shoulder is permitted for 3 to 6 months.

- Recurrence is a relatively common complication of AC joint reconstruction procedures.

Anesthesia

- General anesthesia, with or without nerve block

Patient positioning

- Beach chair or lateral decubitus (arthroscopic distal clavicle excision)
- Beach chair or modified beach chair (AC reconstruction)

Surgical Procedures

Arthroscopic Distal Clavicle Excision

- Standard arthroscopic portals are made, and diagnostic arthroscopy performed as previously described.
- The coracoacromial ligament is incised, with care taken to limit the dissection medially to avoid vascular injury.
- An arthroscopic bur is used to remove 1 to 1.5 cm of bone from the distal clavicle, with careful evaluation to ensure that adequate bony resection is performed before closure.

Acromioclavicular Joint Reconstruction (Modified Weaver-Dunn Procedure)

- An incision is made starting approximately 2 to 3 cm posterior to the AC joint and extending to the tip of the coracoid.
- The approach is carried down to expose the lateral clavicle and the AC joint.
- The distal clavicle (1 to 1.5 cm) is resected, and then the coracoid is exposed.
- Reconstruction is performed using surgical tape, braided suture, or tendon graft (allograft or autograft) according to the preference of the surgeon.
- This tape, suture, or graft is passed either through drill holes through the coracoid and distal clavicle or looped around the bone and secured after appropriate reduction of the AC joint is obtained.
- Reduction should be confirmed and maintained through passive ROM of the shoulder before irrigating and closing the wound in layers according to routine protocol.

Estimated Postoperative Course

- Early postoperative period (days 0 to 6)
  - Sling at all times, with removal only for elbow motion (AC joint reconstruction)
  - Sling for comfort only (AC joint resection)

- Initial postoperative visit (7 to 14 days)
  - Suture or staple removal
  - Physical therapy generally delayed until the 2- to 6-week point (surgeon's preference) for reconstructions but may begin immediately for distal clavicle excision
  - Pain medication refill, if necessary
  - Sling continued for AC joint reconstruction but weaned as tolerated by the patient after simple AC joint resection
- 6-week postoperative visit
  - Evaluate wound healing and distal clavicle deformity.
  - Radiographs of AC joint should be obtained.
  - Begin physical therapy to start gentle ROM exercises.
- 12-week postoperative visit
  - Evaluate the progression of ROM and strength.
  - Obtain new radiographs of the AC joint.
  - Assess job status and consider continued light duty for next 2 to 3 months.

SUGGESTED READINGS

Deans CF, Gentile JM, Tao MA: Acromioclavicular joint injuries in overhead athletes: a concise review of injury mechanisms, 12(2):80–86, 2019.

Phadke A, Bakti N, Bawale R, Singh B: Current concepts in management of ACJ injuries, *J Clin Orthop Trauma* 10(3):480–485, 2019.

Simpson M, Howard MS: Acromioclavicular degenerative joint disease. In Miller MD, Hart JA, MacKnight JM, editors: *Essential orthopaedics*, Philadelphia, 2010, Saunders, pp 178–181.

FRACTURES OF THE SHOULDER

History

- The patient usually has a history of a fall or other trauma.
- Pain is the most common symptom.
- Deformity may be present at the site of injury.
- Numbness or tingling into the hand or discoloration distal to the shoulder should prompt neurovascular evaluation.

Physical Examination

- Inspect for laceration or skin defects (possible open fracture), ecchymosis, and deformity.

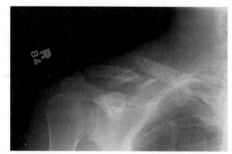

Fig. 2.23 Radiographic Appearance of Midshaft Clavicle Fracture.

- Skin tenting is common with displaced clavicle fractures, and the integrity of skin overlying fracture fragment is important in determining possible surgical treatment.
- ROM should be evaluated, with acute loss concerning for fracture-dislocation.
- Tenderness and crepitus are noted over the fracture site.
- A thorough neurovascular examination of the extremity should be performed.

Imaging

- Radiographs
  - AP and axillary radiographs are indicated at a minimum.
  - AP and tangential views of the clavicle should be added for suspected clavicle fracture.
  - Scapula views are useful for posterior pain and suspicion of scapula fracture.
- CT scan may be necessary for displaced proximal humerus fractures and scapula fractures.

Radiographic Image: Figs. 2.23 and 2.24

Classification System
Clavicle Fractures

- Described by displacement and location (middle third, medial third, lateral third).
- Distal clavicle fractures are further classified based on involvement of the CC ligaments:
  - Type I: intact CC ligaments, nondisplaced fracture
  - Type II: displaced fracture, medial to CC ligaments
    - Type IIA: CC ligaments attached to fracture fragment (Fig. 2.25)
    - Type IIB: fracture between the CC ligaments
  - Type III: intraarticular fracture (involves AC joint)

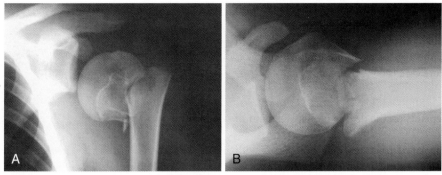

Fig. 2.24 Radiographic Appearance of Proximal Humerus Fracture. **A,** Anteroposterior view. **B,** Axillary view.

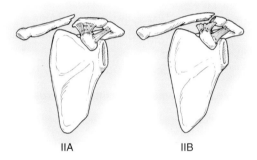

IIA   IIB

Fig. 2.25 Neer Type II Clavicle Fractures. (From Canale ST, Beaty JH, editors: *Campbell's operative orthopaedics,* ed 11, Philadelphia, 2008, Mosby, p 3372.)

Proximal Humerus Fractures

- Neer classification (Fig. 2.26)

Initial Management

Patient Education. Fractures around the shoulder joint commonly occur from falls and motor vehicle accidents. These injuries can be very painful, and a sling is helpful to limit shoulder motion and reduce pain. Many shoulder fractures can be treated without surgery, but others may require a surgical procedure to align the bone ends more accurately for improved outcome. Radiographs and/or CT scan will be necessary to make the best treatment decision.

- Treatment depends on the degree of displacement of the fracture.

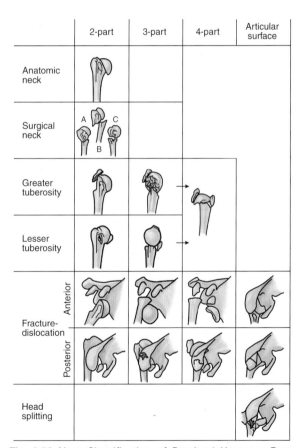

Fig. 2.26 Neer Classification of Proximal Humerus Fractures. (From Miller MD, Hart JA, MacKnight JM, editors: *Essential orthopaedics,* Philadelphia, 2010, Saunders, p 201.)

- Minimally displaced fractures may be treated with the application of a sling or shoulder immobilizer.
- Adequate pain control may require narcotic pain medications; the use of antiinflammatory medications in fracture care is controversial.

Nonoperative Management

- Treatment depends on the degree of displacement of the fracture.
- Minimally displaced fractures may be treated with the application of a sling or shoulder immobilizer.
- Adequate pain control may require narcotic pain medications; the use of antiinflammatory medications in fracture care is controversial.

Operative Management: Open Reduction and Internal Fixation of Clavicle Fractures

Codes

ICD-10 code: S42.009A Fracture of clavicle
CPT code: 23515 Clavicle open reduction, internal fixation

Indications

- Still controversial: traditionally, most clavicle fractures treated nonoperatively, but more of these fractures currently managed surgically for improved shoulder mechanics.
- Open fracture or skin compromise (severe skin tenting from fracture fragment).
- More than 2 cm of clavicle shortening, 100% displacement, or severe comminution.

Informed consent and counseling

- Standard surgical risks should be discussed in detail (e.g., bleeding, infection, failure, anesthesia risks).
- Hardware failure and nonunion are known complications of fracture treatment.
- A minimum of 6 to 8 weeks in a sling is usually required following surgery.

Anesthesia

- General anesthesia, with or without nerve block

Patient positioning

- Beach chair or modified beach chair

Surgical Procedure: Clavicle Open Reduction, Internal Fixation: Fig. 2.27

- A 5- to 8-cm longitudinal incision is made in line with the clavicle.
- The deltotrapezius fascia is stripped off the clavicle.

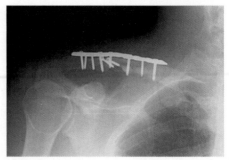

Fig. 2.27 Open Reduction, Internal Fixation of a Clavicle Fracture.

- The fracture fragments may be reduced by Steinmann pins and the reduction verified with fluoroscopy.
- A four- to five-hole low-profile clavicle plate should be fitted to the contour of the clavicle.
- Screws are placed carefully with an instrument placed along the inferior clavicle border to protect the subclavian vessels.
- Closure is in layers according to routine protocol.

Operative Management: Proximal Humerus Fractures

Codes

ICD-10 code: S42.209A Proximal humerus fracture
CPT codes: 23615 Open treatment of proximal humerus fracture, with internal fixation

23470 Arthroplasty glenohumeral joint, hemiarthroplasty

Indications

- Displaced two-part surgical neck fractures.
- Displaced three- and four-part fractures in relatively young, healthy patients.
- Greater tuberosity fractures with more than 5 mm displacement (also require surgical open reduction, internal fixation [ORIF]).

Informed consent and counseling

- Standard surgical risks should be discussed in detail (e.g., bleeding, infection, failure, anesthesia risks).
- Hardware failure and nonunion are known complications of fracture treatment.
- A minimum of 6 to 8 weeks in a sling is usually required following surgery.

Anesthesia

- General anesthesia, with or without nerve block

Patient positioning

- Beach chair or modified beach chair

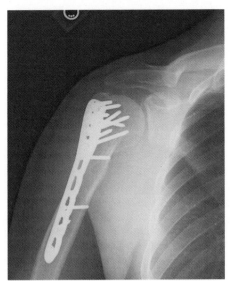

Fig. 2.28 Open Reduction, Internal Fixation of a Proximal Humerus Fracture.

Surgical Procedure: Open Reduction, Internal Fixation of Proximal Humerus Fracture: Fig. 2.28

- An anterior shoulder incision is made for a standard deltopectoral approach to the shoulder.
- The fracture is exposed by releasing the deltoid, and the fracture fragments are reduced using a Cobb elevator or threaded pin.
- Kirschner wires (K-wires) are used to hold the reduction in place, as confirmed with fluoroscopy.
- A proximal humerus plate is placed on the lateral aspect of the bone posterior to the biceps tendon and is secured with locking screws in the humeral head and nonlocking screws in the shaft.
- The rotator cuff is sutured to the proximal plate, and the wound is closed in layers according to routine protocol.

Estimated Postoperative Course
- Early postoperative period (days 0 to 6)
  - A sling should be used at all times, except for elbow motion
- Initial postoperative visit (7 to 14 days)
  - Sutures should be removed, and the wound should be inspected
  - Refill pain medications
  - Address the patient's work status
  - Check AP and tangential views of the clavicle or AP and axillary views of the shoulder for proximal humerus fracture

- 6-week postoperative visit
  - Repeat radiographs
  - Consider physical therapy for early gentle passive ROM
  - Continue light duty work status with limited to no use of the affected arm
- 12-week postoperative visit
  - Repeat radiographs (last time if united)
  - Advance physical therapy to include active ROM and strengthening
  - Determine the need for additional follow-up visits

SUGGESTED READINGS

Crenshaw Jr AH, Perez EA: Fractures of the shoulder, arm, and forearm. In ed 11, Canale ST, Beaty JH, editors: *Campbell's operative orthopaedics*, vol 3. Philadelphia, 2008, Mosby, pp 3371–3460.
Johnston PS, Bushnell BD, Taft TN: Proximal humerus fractures. In Miller MD, Hart JA, MacKnight JM, editors: *Essential orthopaedics*, Philadelphia, 2010, Saunders, pp 199–203.
Rubright JH, Bushnell BD, Taft TN: Clavicle fractures. In Miller MD, Hart JA, MacKnight JM, editors: *Essential orthopaedics*, Philadelphia, 2010, Saunders, pp 212–216.

ORTHOPAEDIC PROCEDURES (SHOULDER)

Subacromial Injection
CPT code: 20610
Indications
- Shoulder impingement
- Partial rotator cuff tear
- Rotator cuff arthropathy
- Shoulder pain (diagnostic)
Contraindications
- Shoulder infection
- Local skin rash or active skin lesion over the injection site
- Allergy to injection material

Equipment Needed
- Ethyl chloride
- Topical cleansing agent (e.g., povidone-iodine [Betadine])
- Sterile gloves
- Syringe with a 21-gauge, 1½-inch or longer needle
- Steroid (e.g., triamcinolone [Kenalog], 40 mg/mL)
- Anesthetic (e.g., lidocaine, 1% without epinephrine)
- Sterile dressing and tape or self-adhesive bandage

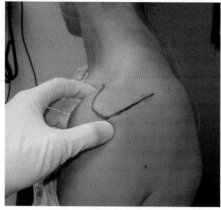

Fig. 2.29 Identify the inferior edge of the acromion as the site for the injection. (From Miller MD, Hart JA, MacKnight JM, editors: *Essential orthopaedics*, Philadelphia, 2010, Saunders, p 226.)

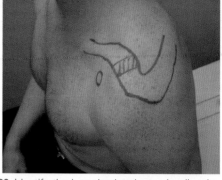

Fig. 2.30 Identify the bony landmarks to visualize the area of the injection just lateral to the end of the clavicle (*hashed line*). (From Miller MD, Hart JA, MacKnight JM, editors: *Essential orthopaedics*, Philadelphia, 2010, Saunders, p 229.)

Procedure

1. Palpate and locate the injection site (Fig. 2.29).
2. Apply ethyl chloride to the area before injection (not sterile).
3. Prepare the area with a cleaning agent such as povidone-iodine (Betadine) and include the skin well beyond the injection site.
4. Insert the needle just below the inferior border of the acromion.
5. As you insert the needle past the acromion, angle the need tip up into the subacromial space.
6. Inject the steroid or anesthesia medication.
7. Withdraw the needle, remove any residual cleansing agent from the skin, and apply a dressing.

Aftercare Instructions

1. Apply ice to the area if local pain is present that day.
2. Expect the anesthetic to wear off later that same day, but know that the steroid does not take effect for an average of 3 to 5 days.
3. Call the office with any local erythema, increased pain, fever, or chills.
4. Call the office if symptoms fail to improve or if pain returns within 2 to 3 weeks of injection because this may indicate the need for additional imaging to evaluate the rotator cuff.

Acromioclavicular Joint Injection
CPT code: 20605
Indications
- AC joint osteoarthritis

- AC joint osteolysis
- AC joint pain
Contraindications
- Shoulder infection
- Local skin rash or active skin lesion over the injection site
- Allergy to injection material

Equipment Needed
- Ethyl chloride
- Topical cleansing agent (e.g., povidone-iodine [Betadine])
- Sterile gloves
- Syringe with a 21-gauge, 1.5-inch or longer needle
- Steroid (e.g., triamcinolone [Kenalog], 40 mg/mL)
- Anesthetic (e.g., lidocaine, 1% without epinephrine)
- Sterile dressing and tape or self-adhesive bandage

Procedure
- Palpate and locate the injection site at the lateral tip of the clavicle (Fig. 2.30).
- Apply ethyl chloride to the area before injection (not sterile).
- Prepare the area with cleaning agent such as povidone-iodine (Betadine) and include the skin well beyond the injection site.
- Hold the syringe vertically, and insert the needle with a slight medial angle until it passes between the acromion and clavicle and a small "pop" is felt when the joint capsule is penetrated (Fig. 2.31).

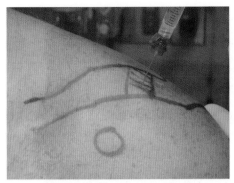

Fig. 2.31 Injection just lateral to the end of the clavicle (*hashed line*). (From Miller MD, Hart JA, MacKnight JM, editors: *Essential orthopaedics*, Philadelphia, 2010, Saunders, p 230.)

- Inject the steroid or anesthesia medication.
- Withdraw the needle, remove any residual cleansing agent from skin, and apply a dressing.

Aftercare Instructions

1. Apply ice to the area if local pain is present that day.
2. Expect the anesthetic to wear off later that same day, but know that the steroid does not take effect for an average of 3 to 5 days.
3. Call the office with any local erythema, increased pain, fever, or chills.

Shoulder Reduction

CPT code: 23650 Closed treatment with manipulation of shoulder dislocation not requiring anesthesia
23655 Closed treatment with manipulation of shoulder dislocation requiring anesthesia

Indications
- Shoulder dislocation, anterior

Contraindications
- Multitrauma in which medical status is unstable
- Displaced, unstable fracture

Anesthesia
- Intraarticular lidocaine or
- Conscious sedation

Equipment Needed
- Minimal equipment necessary; traction/counter-traction method requiring the use of weights or intravenous bags

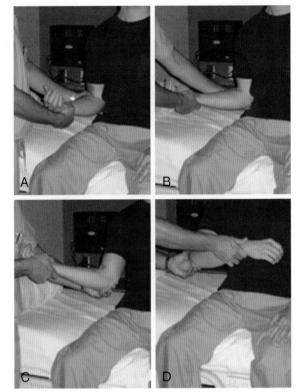

Fig. 2.32 Kocher Method of Shoulder Reduction. **A,** Start with adduction at the shoulder and elbow flexion. **B,** Externally rotate the arm at the shoulder. **C,** Flex the arm forward at the shoulder until resistance is felt. **D,** Internally rotate the arm at the shoulder. (From Miller MD, Hart JA, MacKnight JM, editors: *Essential orthopaedics,* Philadelphia, 2010, Saunders, p 218.)

Procedure

Traction/countertraction technique (Stimson method)

1. The patient is placed prone on the table, with his or her arm hanging down vertically off the side.
2. Weights are added to the arm, beginning with 5 to 10 pounds, or manual pressure is applied to the arm to provide gentle traction (the table provides counter-traction).
3. This may take time (15 to 20 minutes typically) as the muscles fatigue.
4. Scapula manipulation may be helpful to facilitate reduction.

   Kocher method. *Fig. 2.32*

1. With the patient's arm adducted and the elbow flexed to 90 degrees, externally rotate the arm.

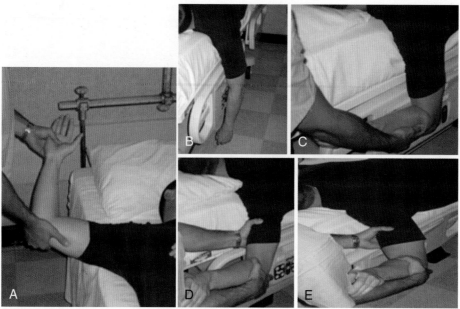

Fig. 2.33 Milch Method of Shoulder Reduction. **A,** Supine. **B–E,** Prone. (From Miller MD, Hart JA, MacKnight JM, editors: *Essential orthopaedics,* Philadelphia, 2010, Saunders, pp 218–219.)

2. At the point of resistance, maximally forward flex the shoulder then internally rotate it until reduction is felt.

Milch method. Fig. 2.33

1. The patient is placed either supine or prone, and the patient's arm is placed in an abducted position with the elbow flexed to 90 degrees.
2. The arm is passively abducted and externally rotated while the examiner's other hand gently pushes the humeral head back into proper position.

Aftercare Instructions

1. The arm is placed in a sling for patient comfort, with instructions to remove the sling for pendulum exercises and elbow motion, to prevent stiffness.
2. External rotation slings are increasingly popular after shoulder reduction because some literature suggests improved healing in this position.
3. Follow-up evaluation should be set for 1 to 2 weeks after to assess motion and rotator cuff strength.

Elbow and Forearm

Sara D. Rynders

ANATOMY

Bones: Fig. 3.1

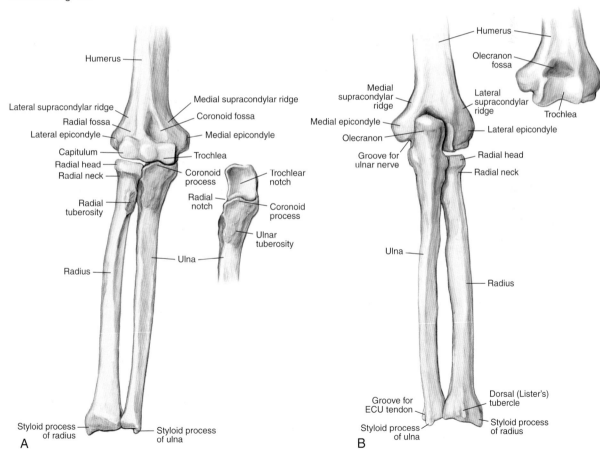

Fig. 3.1 **A,** Anterior view of the elbow and forearm bony anatomy. **B,** Posterior view of the elbow and forearm bony anatomy. *ECU,* Extensor carpi ulnaris. (From Chhabra AB: Elbow and forearm. In: Miller MD, Chhabra AB, Hurwitz S, et al., editors, *Orthopaedic surgical approaches,* Philadelphia, 2008, Saunders, pp 63, 64.)

Ligaments: Fig. 3.2

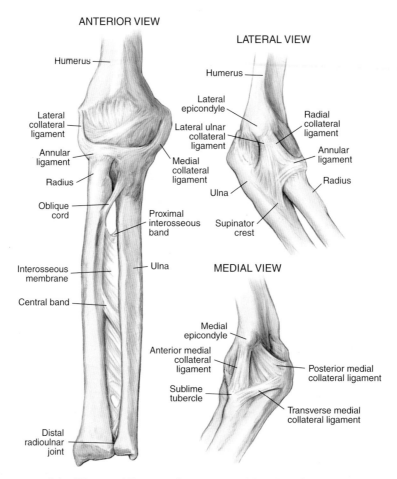

ANTERIOR VIEW

Humerus

Lateral collateral ligament

Annular ligament

Radius

Oblique cord

Interosseous membrane

Central band

Distal radioulnar joint

Proximal interosseous band

Ulna

LATERAL VIEW

Humerus

Lateral epicondyle

Lateral ulnar collateral ligament

Medial collateral ligament

Ulna

Radial collateral ligament

Annular ligament

Radius

Supinator crest

MEDIAL VIEW

Medial epicondyle

Anterior medial collateral ligament

Sublime tubercle

Posterior medial collateral ligament

Transverse medial collateral ligament

Fig. 3.2 Ligaments of the Elbow and Forearm. Components of the elbow ligaments—ulnar collateral ligament: anterior band, posterior band, and transverse band; lateral collateral ligament: annular ligament, radial collateral ligament, accessory collateral ligament, and lateral ulnar collateral ligament. (From Chhabra AB: Elbow and forearm. In: Miller MD, Chhabra AB, Hurwitz S, et al., editors, *Orthopaedic surgical approaches,* Philadelphia, 2008, Saunders, p 67.)

Muscles and Tendons: Fig. 3.3

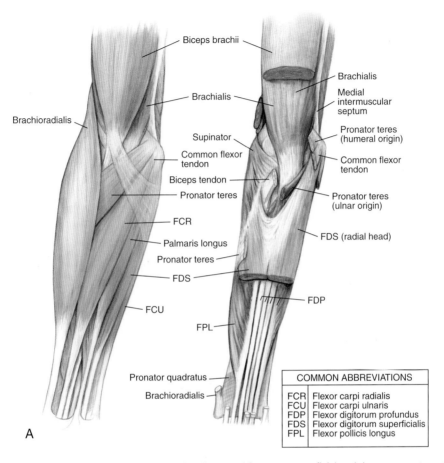

A

COMMON ABBREVIATIONS	
FCR	Flexor carpi radialis
FCU	Flexor carpi ulnaris
FDP	Flexor digitorum profundus
FDS	Flexor digitorum superficialis
FPL	Flexor pollicis longus

Fig. 3.3 A, Muscles and tendons of the anterior elbow and forearm: superficial and deep compartments. B, Muscles and tendons of the posterior elbow and forearm: superficial and deep compartments. (From Chhabra AB: Elbow and forearm. In: Miller MD, Chhabra AB, Hurwitz S, et al., editors, *Orthopaedic surgical approaches*, Philadelphia, 2008, Saunders, pp 68, 69.)

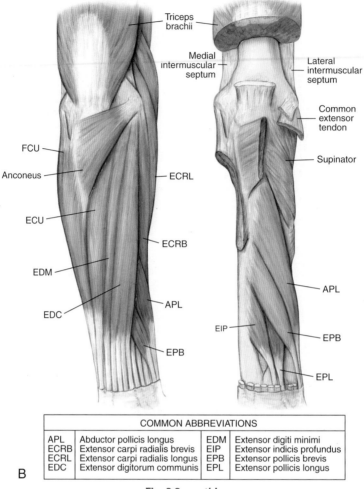

COMMON ABBREVIATIONS			
APL	Abductor pollicis longus	EDM	Extensor digiti minimi
ECRB	Extensor carpi radialis brevis	EIP	Extensor indicis profundus
ECRL	Extensor carpi radialis longus	EPB	Extensor pollicis brevis
EDC	Extensor digitorum communis	EPL	Extensor pollicis longus

B

Fig. 3.3, cont'd

Nerves and Arteries: Fig. 3.4 and Table 3.1

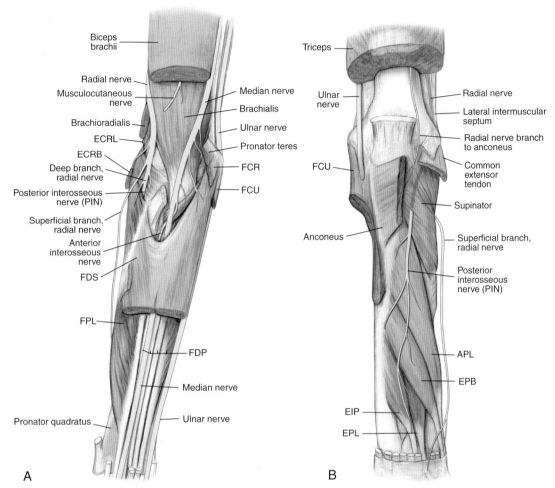

Fig. 3.4 A, Anterior view of the nerves of the elbow and forearm. **B,** Posterior view of the nerves of the elbow and forearm. **C,** Arteries of the elbow and forearm. *APL,* Abductor pollicis longus; ECRB, extensor carpi radialis brevis; *ECRL,* extensor carpi radialis longus; *EIP,* extensor indicis profundus; *EPB,* extensor pollicis brevis; *EPL,* extensor pollicis longus; *FCR,* flexor carpi radialis; *FCU,* flexor carpi ulnaris; *FDP,* flexor digitorum profundus; *FDS,* flexor digitorum superficialis; *FPL,* flexor pollicis longus; *PT,* pronator teres. (From Chhabra AB: Elbow and forearm. In: Miller MD, Chhabra AB, Hurwitz S, et al, editors, *Orthopaedic surgical approaches,* Philadelphia, 2008, Saunders, pp 74, 75, 81.)

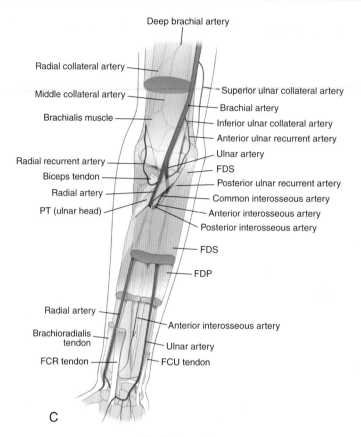

Deep brachial artery

Radial collateral artery

Middle collateral artery

Brachialis muscle

Radial recurrent artery

Biceps tendon

Radial artery

PT (ulnar head)

Superior ulnar collateral artery

Brachial artery

Inferior ulnar collateral artery

Anterior ulnar recurrent artery

Ulnar artery

FDS

Posterior ulnar recurrent artery

Common interosseous artery

Anterior interosseous artery

Posterior interosseous artery

FDS

FDP

Radial artery

Brachioradialis tendon

FCR tendon

Anterior interosseous artery

Ulnar artery

FCU tendon

C

Fig. 3.4, cont'd

TABLE 3.1	**Muscle Innervation and Testing**			
Nerve	**Branch**	**Motor**	**Test**	**Sensory**
Musculocutaneous	Proper	Biceps brachii, brachialis	Elbow flexion, forearm supination	
	Lateral antebrachial cutaneous			To lateral elbow and forearm
Medial cord	Medial antebrachial cutaneous			To anterior antebrachium and medial forearm
Radial	Proper	Triceps, anconeus, brachioradialis	Elbow extension, elbow flexion	
	Superficial sensory radial nerve (SSRN)			To dorsal aspect of radial wrist and thumb, dorsal hand
	Posterior interosseous nerve (PIN)	ECRB, EDM, ECRL, APL, ECU, EPB, supinator, EPL, EIP	Wrist extension, thumb extension, finger extension	

TABLE 3.1 Muscle Innervation and Testing—cont'd

Nerve	Branch	Motor	Test	Sensory
Median	Proper	Pronator teres, FCR, FDS, palmaris longus, index and middle finger lumbricals	Radial wrist flexion, finger flexion, pronation	Thumb, index finger, middle finger, and radial half of ring finger
	Recurrent motor branch	Thenar muscles: APB	Thumb abduction	
	Anterior interosseous nerve (AIN)	FDP to index finger, FPL, pronator quadratus	Index finger DIP joint flexion, thumb IP joint flexion, pronation	
	Superficial sensory palmar branch			Sensation to palm
Ulnar	Proper	FDP to ring and small fingers, FCU	Flexion of ring and small fingers, ulnar wrist flexion	
	Superficial sensory branch			Sensation to volar fifth finger and ulnar half of ring finger
	Deep motor branch	Adductor pollicis, hypothenar muscle, interosseous muscle, ring and small finger lumbricals, deep branch of FPB	Finger abduction and adduction, thumb adduction	
	Dorsal sensory branch			Dorsal sensation to small finger and ulnar half of ring finger

APB, Abductor pollicis brevis; *APL*, abductor pollicis longus; *DIP*, distal interphalangeal; *ECRB*, extensor carpi radialis brevis; *ECRL*, extensor carpi radialis longus; *ECU*, extensor carpi ulnaris; *EDM*, extensor digiti minimi; *EIP*, extensor indicis proprius; *EPB*, extensor pollicis brevis; *EPL*, extensor pollicis longus; *FCR*, flexor carpi radialis; *FCU*, flexor carpi ulnaris; *FDP*, flexor digitorum profundus; *FDS*, flexor digitorum superficialis; *FPB*, flexor pollicis brevis; *FPL*, flexor pollicis longus; *IP* interphalangeal.

Surface Anatomy: Fig. 3.5

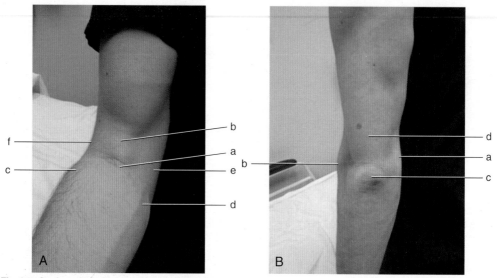

Fig. 3.5 Surface Anatomy of the Anterior and Posterior Elbow and Forearm. **A,** Anterior labels: (a) antebrachial fossa, (b) biceps tendon, (c) common extensor tendons, (d) common flexor tendons, (e) medial epicondyle, (f) lateral epicondyle. **B,** Posterior labels: (a) medial epicondyle, (b) lateral epicondyle, (c) olecranon process, (d) triceps tendon.

Normal Radiographic Appearance: Figs. 3.6 and 3.7

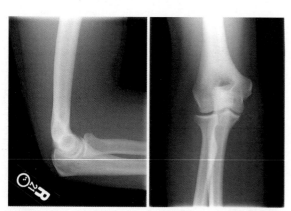

Fig. 3.6 Normal Radiographs of the Elbow. Anteroposterior *(right)* and lateral *(left)* views. (From Hart JA: Overview of the elbow. In: Miller MD, Hart JA, MacKnight JM, editors, *Essential orthopaedics,* Philadelphia, 2010, Saunders, 2010, p 239.)

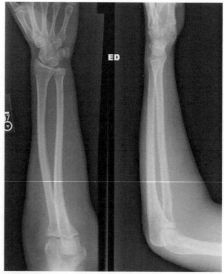

Fig. 3.7 Normal Radiographs of the Forearm. Anteroposterior *(left)* and lateral *(right)* views.

PHYSICAL EXAMINATION

(Tables 3.2 through 3.4)

Inspect for edema, deformity, ecchymosis, biceps muscle.

Palpate:
- Medial epicondyle
- Ulnar nerve in cubital tunnel
- Lateral epicondyle
- Radial head
- Distal biceps tendon
- Brachial artery
- Common extensor muscles (also known as "mobile wad")
- Olecranon and olecranon bursa

LATERAL EPICONDYLITIS

Lateral epicondylitis, commonly known as "tennis elbow," is a condition of tendinopathy of the common extensor tendon origin at its insertion site at the lateral epicondyle of the humerus. Although initially thought to be a condition of inflammation, histopathologic studies have now determined that tennis elbow is actually a condition of tendinosis, or degeneration, as few inflammatory cells are actually present at the affected tendon insertion site.[1] It is characterized by lateral-sided elbow pain that may arise from injury, overuse, or poor ergonomics. Treatment is largely nonoperative and focused on symptom control and avoidance of aggravating activity. Frequently this condition will "burn itself out" over time, though the length of time is variable over months to years, and patients may experience recurrence that interfere with activities and work.

History
- Lateral-sided elbow pain
- Possible reported history of injury or repetitive trauma
- Pain worse with lifting and gripping
- Pain also possible at night when the elbow is moved from a resting position

Physical Examination
- Possible mild edema over lateral epicondyle.
- Point tenderness to palpation over lateral epicondyle.
- Pain with resisted wrist extension.

TABLE 3.2	Normal Elbow and Forearm Range of Motion
Extension	0 degrees
Flexion	135 degrees
Supination	90 degrees
Pronation	90 degrees

TABLE 3.3	Neurovascular Examination	
Nerve	**Location of Test**	**Tests**
Ulnar nerve	Cubital tunnel at elbow	Tinel sign, look for subluxation over medial epicondyle; distally, check Froment and Wartenburg sign (see cubital tunnel syndrome on p. 83)
Median nerve	Wrist and hand	Radial-sided wrist flexion and finger flexion checked distally
Radial nerve	Triceps	Resisted elbow extension
Posterior interosseous nerve	Test strength distally at wrist and hand	Resisted wrist extension, finger extension, thumb extension
Brachial artery; radial and ulnar artery	At medial brachium; at volar wrist	

- Pain at the lateral epicondyle caused by grip strength testing with a dynamometer; pain worse when test performed with the elbow extended rather than flexed.

Imaging: Fig. 3.8
- Not always necessary for diagnosis; considered if history of injury.
- X-ray elbow: anteroposterior (AP), lateral, oblique views. X-rays will be negative for abnormality.

Additional Imaging
- Not always necessary. Magnetic resonance imaging (MRI) can help differentiate causes of lateral-sided

TABLE 3.4	Differential Diagnosis of Elbow Pain
Medial-sided elbow pain	Medial epicondylitis
	Ulnar collateral ligament injury
	Arthritis
	Cubital tunnel syndrome
Lateral-sided elbow pain	Lateral epicondylitis
	Radial head fracture
	Lateral collateral ligament injury
Anterior elbow pain	Biceps tendinitis or biceps tendon rupture
Posterior elbow pain	Olecranon bursitis
	Triceps tendinitis
Forearm pain	Radial tunnel syndrome
	Muscle strain

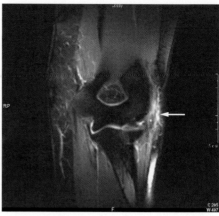

Fig. 3.8 Magnetic Resonance Image of Lateral Epicondylitis. Edema and high-grade partial tearing of the common extensor tendon origin are visible *(arrow)*.

elbow pain in patients who fail to respond to treatment for lateral epicondylitis. Diagnosis of lateral epicondylitis can be confirmed by MRI. Lateral epicondylitis may be described on an MRI as "high-grade partial tearing of the common extensor tendon origin."

Differential Diagnosis

- Lateral collateral ligament (LCL) sprain
- Radial tunnel syndrome (compression of the posterior interosseous nerve [PIN] in the supinator)
- Distal humerus fracture

Initial Management

- **Patient education** and activity modification are paramount to successful treatment. Ergonomic work evaluation may be indicated and patient should be counseled on proper lifting techniques that utilize the elbow flexors (biceps brachii and brachialis). Patients should understand at the time of diagnosis that the condition is usually treated nonoperatively and is self-limited but that recurrences may happen over a period of years. Treatment should focus on reducing pain and dysfunction by way of modifying activities, utilizing multimodal antiinflammatory techniques, and patient education for self-management when symptoms occur.
- Initial management includes avoidance of aggravating activities and repetitive lifting and gripping, correction of improper lifting or gripping techniques, a nonsteroidal antiinflammatory drug (NSAID)

regimen if tolerated, possible use of transdermal anesthetic patches, heat and ice modalities with stretching, and occupational therapy referral.
- Some advocate for use of a wrist brace to limit wrist extension during activities.

Nonoperative Management

- Lateral epicondylitis is usually a self-limited condition, causing pain and dysfunction for 12 to 18 months, with or without intervention.[2]
- In addition to initial treatments listed earlier, several injectable treatment modalities may be considered. Traditionally, cortisone injections have been a treatment of choice (see p. 105 for lateral epicondyle injection). But newer methods such as autologous blood injection or platelet rich plasma injection are becoming more widely used. Currently, no one modality has been proven superior over another for long-term management of lateral epicondylitis and all may be considered as part of a nonoperative armament.[3]
- Avoid multiple repeat cortisone injections over a short time because they can result in local tissue destruction and possible tendon or ligament rupture.
- Advise the patient on a period of rest and activity modification after injection.
- Occupational therapy referral for elbow stretching, gradual protected strengthening, counseling on lifting techniques, and use of local modalities such as iontophoresis for inflammation.

- If the patient notes no improvement or diminishing improvement in symptoms with injections, consider an MRI scan to evaluate for any other causes of lateral elbow pain such as an LCL injury.

Operative Management

ICD-10 code: M77.0 Lateral epicondylitis
CPT code: 24359 Débridement of soft tissue and/or bone at lateral epicondyle
Additional surgical techniques for treatment of lateral epicondylitis also include percutaneous release and arthroscopic débridement.

Indications

- Conservative management for at least 1 year has failed.
- Indications and techniques vary, and more studies are necessary for an evidence-based approach.

Informed consent and counseling

- Surgical treatment, regardless of technique, has been found to provide 80% good to excellent results.[4]
- The surgical procedure is not likely to be successful if the patient fails to modify activities or cease repetitive trauma postoperatively.
- The patient will require a 2- to 3-month recovery period with monitored progressive occupational therapy.

Anesthesia

- Regional block with sedation, or general anesthesia

Patient positioning

- Supine with the arm on an arm board, with the shoulder internally rotated and the elbow flexed
- Nonsterile tourniquet high on the brachium

Surgical Procedures

Lateral Epicondyle Débridement

An oblique incision is made just anterior to the lateral epicondyle and common extensor tendon origin. Care is taken to avoid injury to the lateral antebrachial cutaneous nerve. The lateral epicondyle is identified, and a split is made in the common extensor tendon origin parallel to the fibers. The tissue is divided in layers until the underlying joint capsule is identified. A rongeur or curette is used to débride the dysvascular tissue and to stimulate bleeding. Avoid injury to the underlying LCL. Sometimes, a Kirschner wire (K-wire) is used to puncture the lateral epicondyle several times and stimulate bleeding at the origin of the tendon. Once débridement has concluded, the common extensor tendon is repaired in layers using suture. The fascia is also closed followed by the subcutaneous tissues and the skin. Most surgeons immobilize the patient in a long-arm posterior splint for 10 to 14 days.

Estimated Postoperative Course

Postoperative days 10 to 14:

- Perform a wound check and suture removal.
- *Therapy*: Start therapy for gentle elbow range of motion (ROM). The patient should avoid lifting with the operative extremity.

Postoperative 6 weeks:

- Perform a motion check. Evaluate and document whether the patient has tenderness to palpation at the lateral epicondyle.
- *Therapy*: Start a graduated strengthening program.

Postoperative 3 months:

- Perform a motion and strength check. Evaluate and document whether the patient has tenderness at the lateral epicondyle, and test for pain with resisted wrist extension.
- If the patient is asymptomatic, release him or her to regular activities.

Board Review

Lateral-sided elbow pain worse with lifting, gripping, and repetitive activity may indicate tennis elbow, or lateral epicondylitis.

SUGGESTED READINGS

Calfee RP, Patel A, DaSilva MF, Akelman E: Management of lateral epicondylitis: current concepts, *J Am Acad Orthop Surg* 16:19–29, 2008.

Faro F, Wolf JM. Lateral epicondylitis: review and current concepts, *J Hand Surg Am.* 32:1271, 2007.

Nirschl RP, Ashman ES: Elbow tendinopathy: tennis elbow, *Clin Sports Med* 22:813–836, 2003.

Rineer CA, Ruch DS: Elbow tendinopathy and tendon ruptures: epicondylitis, biceps and triceps ruptures, *J Hand Surg Am* 34(3):566–576, 2009.

REFERENCES

1. Duran A, Gresham GA, Rushton N, Watson C: Tennis elbow: a clinicopathologic study of 22 cases followed for 2 years, *Acta Orthop Scand* 61(6):535–538, 1990.
2. Sims SE, Miller K, Elfar JC, Hammert WC: Non-surgical treatment of lateral epicondylitis: a systemic review of randomized controlled trials, *Hand (N.Y.)* 9(4):419–446, 2014.

3. Tang S, Wang X, Wu P, et al.: Platelet-rich-plasma vs. autologous blood vs. corticosteroid injections in treatment of lateral epicondylitis: a systemic review, pairwise and network meta-analysis of randomized controlled trials, *PM R* 12(4):397–409, 2020.

4. Lo MY, Satran MR: Surgical treatment of lateral epicondylitis: a systemic review, *Clin Orthop Rel Res* 463:98–106, 2007.

MEDIAL EPICONDYLITIS

Medial epicondylitis, also known as "golfer's elbow," is a condition of tendinopathy that occurs on the medial aspect of the elbow where the common flexor tendon origin inserts on the medial epicondyle of the humerus. It can be caused by injury, overuse, or poor ergonomics. Occasionally it is associated with a concurrent irritation of the ulnar nerve, or cubital tunnel syndrome. The condition is usually self-limited and nonoperative management should be maximized in order to relieve pain and dysfunction and prevent recurrence.

History
- Medial-sided elbow pain
- Possible reported history of injury or repetitive trauma
- Possible patient-reported associated paresthesias in the fourth and fifth fingers (possible simultaneous cubital tunnel syndrome resulting from inflammation)

Physical Examination
- Possible mild edema over medial epicondyle.
- Point tenderness to palpation over medial epicondyle.
- Pain with resisted wrist flexion.
- Elbow stable to stress testing of the ulnar collateral ligament (UCL).
- Evaluation of the ulnar nerve at the cubital tunnel for subluxation or neuritis (see p. 83 for cubital tunnel syndrome).

Imaging: Fig. 3.9
- Not necessary for diagnosis but possibly warranted if history of recent trauma or examiner suspects arthritis.
- X-rays: elbow AP, lateral, and oblique views. X-rays will be negative for abnormality.

Additional Imaging
- MRI of the elbow can aid in diagnosis and evaluation for other causes of medial-sided elbow pain.

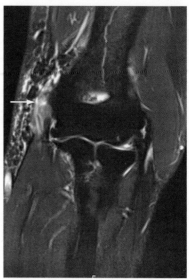

Fig. 3.9 Magnetic Resonance Image of Medial Epicondylitis. Edema and high-grade partial tearing of the common flexor tendon origin are visible *(arrow)*.

Differential Diagnosis
- UCL sprain
- Cubital tunnel syndrome
- Distal humerus fracture

Initial Management
- **Patient education** and activity modification are paramount to successful treatment.
- Advise patient to avoid aggravating activities and repetitive tasks. Biomechanical or ergonomic education is important.
- NSAID regimen if tolerated, heat and ice modalities with stretching, and occupational therapy referral.
- Some advocate use of a wrist brace to limit wrist flexion during activities.
- If fourth and fifth finger paresthesias are present, consider obtaining an electromyography and nerve conduction study (EMG/NCS) to evaluate for concomitant cubital tunnel syndrome (see p. 83 for treatment recommendations).

Nonoperative Management
Indications
- Conservative management is reserved for patients with no previous treatment or whose previous treatment was successful but the problem recurred after several months or years.

CHAPTER 3 Elbow and Forearm

- In addition to initial treatments listed earlier, a cortisone injection may be performed (see p. 106 for medial epicondyle injection). Additional therapies such as platelet-rich-plasma injection or autologous blood injection may also be an option.
- Avoid multiple repeat cortisone injections over a short time because this can result in local tissue destruction and possible tendon or ligament rupture.
- A relative contraindication to injection is a subluxating ulnar nerve.
- Advise the patient on a period of rest and activity modification after injection.
- If referring the patient to occupational therapy, the referral should include instructions to provide elbow stretching, gradual protected flexor-pronator strengthening, and use of local modalities for inflammation.
- If the patient notes no improvement or diminishing improvement in symptoms with injections, consider an MRI scan to evaluate for any other causes of medial elbow pain such as a UCL injury.

Operative Management

ICD-10 code: M77.0 Medial epicondylitis

CPT code: 24359 Débridement of soft tissue and/or bone at medial epicondyle

Indications

- Conservative management for at least 1 year has failed.
- Indications and techniques vary, and more studies are necessary for an evidence-based approach.

Informed consent and counseling

- The surgical procedure is not likely to be successful if the patient fails to modify activities or cease repetitive trauma postoperatively.
- The patient will require a 2- to 3-month recovery period with monitored progressive occupational therapy.

Anesthesia

- Regional block with sedation, or general anesthesia

Patient positioning

- Supine with the arm on an arm board, with the shoulder externally rotated and the elbow flexed
- Nonsterile tourniquet placed high on the brachium

Surgical Procedures

- The medial approach is used for tendon débridement
- If cubital tunnel syndrome is present, an ulnar nerve transposition can be performed simultaneously with this procedure (see next section for cubital tunnel syndrome)

Medial Epicondyle Débridement

An oblique incision is made just anterior to the medial epicondyle. Care is taken to avoid injury to the medial antebrachial cutaneous nerve and ulnar nerve in the cubital tunnel. The medial epicondyle is identified, and a split is made in the common flexor tendon origin parallel to the fibers. The tissue is divided in layers until the underlying joint capsule is identified. A rongeur or curette is used to débride the dysvascular tissue and to stimulate bleeding. Avoid injury to the underlying UCL. Sometimes, a K-wire is used to puncture the medial epicondyle several times to stimulate bleeding at the origin of the tendon. The common flexor tendon is then repaired in layers using a suture. The fascia is also closed followed by the subcutaneous tissues and the skin. Most surgeons immobilize the patient in a long-arm posterior splint for 10 to 14 days.

Estimated Postoperative Course

Postoperative days 10 to 14:

- Perform a wound check and suture removal.
- *Therapy*: Start gentle elbow ROM. The patient is to avoid lifting with the operative extremity.

Postoperative 6 weeks:

- Perform a motion check. Evaluate and document whether the patient has tenderness to palpation at the medial epicondyle.
- *Therapy*: Start a graduated strengthening program.

Postoperative 3 months:

- Perform a motion and strength check. Evaluate and document whether the patient has tenderness to palpation at the medial epicondyle, and test for pain with resisted wrist flexion.
- If the patient is asymptomatic, release him or her to regular activities.

SUGGESTED READINGS

Ciccotti MG, Ramani MN: Medial epicondylitis, *Tech Hand Up Extrem Surg* 7:190–196, 2003.

Jobe FW, Ciccotti MG: Lateral and medial epicondylitis of the elbow, *J Am Acad Orthop Surg* 2:18, 1994.

CUBITAL TUNNEL SYNDROME

Cubital tunnel syndrome is a compression neuropathy of the ulnar nerve as it courses posteromedially at the elbow within the cubital tunnel. The nerve is known to the layman as the "funny bone" at this level. Symptoms of cubital tunnel syndrome are numbness, tingling, and sometimes pain in the fourth and fifth digit and can lead to irreversible weakness in the hand. In severe cases of nerve compression and atrophy, a claw-hand can develop. Treatment can range from postural adjustments, splints, and therapy to surgery for nerve decompression or transposition.

History

- Medial-sided elbow pain
- Numbness and tingling in the fourth and fifth fingers
- Achy pain radiating down the ulnar side of the forearm to the wrist and hand
- Worse when the elbow is flexed or while leaning on the elbow; possibly while sleeping
- Hand weakness (late finding)

Physical Examination

- Palpate for tenderness over the ulnar nerve at the cubital tunnel.
- Perform a Tinel sign over the ulnar nerve at the cubital tunnel. A positive test reproduces numbness and tingling into the fourth and fifth fingers distally.
- Evaluate for subluxation of the ulnar nerve. Place the elbow through flexion and extension and palpate the ulnar nerve. Observe if it remains posterior to the medial epicondyle or subluxes over the medial epicondyle.
- Evaluate and record sensory changes using two-point discrimination on the ulnar border of the fourth finger and the entire fifth finger. Abnormal two-point discrimination occurs at 7 mm or more.
- Inspect the hand for intrinsic muscle atrophy or claw deformity (late finding).

Wartenburg Test: Fig. 3.10

- This test evaluates for weakness of the adductor digiti minimi, which is the earliest sign of muscle weakness.
- Ask the patient to adduct all fingers together.
- A positive test result is when the fifth finger remains in an abducted position.

Froment Sign: Fig. 3.11

- This test evaluates for weakness of the adductor pollicis muscle caused by ulnar nerve injury.

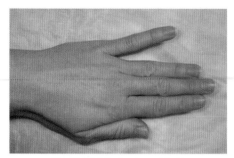

Fig. 3.10 Wartenburg Test.

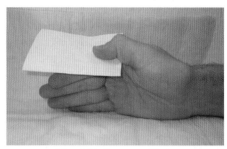

Fig. 3.11 Froment Sign.

- Ask the patient to hold a piece of paper between the thumb and index finger while the fingers are extended. The examiner then tries to remove paper from the patient's grip.
- A positive sign is when the patient flexes the thumb interphalangeal joint and thereby activates the flexor pollicis longus (a median nerve innervated muscle) to hold the paper, instead of using the adductor pollicis.

Imaging

- Not necessary for diagnosis; considered only if symptoms are trauma-related.

Additional Tests

Electromyography and Nerve Conduction Study

EMG/NCS can identify ulnar nerve compression at the cubital tunnel and can determine severity of compression. Ask the electromyographer to evaluate for the differential diagnosis, which includes carpal tunnel syndrome, ulnar nerve compression at Guyon's canal, cervical radiculopathy, and peripheral neuropathy. Sometimes an "inching study" is performed across the elbow to identify a specific area of compression.

Differential Diagnosis

- Medial epicondylitis
- Cervical radiculopathy
- Peripheral neuropathy
- Ulnar tunnel syndrome: compression of the ulnar nerve at the hand at Guyon's canal
- Carpal tunnel syndrome
- Snapping triceps tendon

Initial Management

- Educate the patient how to avoid leaning on the elbow and flexing it for long periods of time.
- Discuss activity modifications.
- Suggest that the patient obtain an elbow pad to protect the nerve and possibly refer the patient to an occupational therapist to have a night-time splint made.

Nonoperative Management

- Conservative management is reserved for patients with no evidence of muscle wasting on EMG/NCS or physical examination and for those without any previous treatment.
- Patient education is key. Discuss in detail how the patient should avoid leaning on the elbow and flexing the elbow repetitively or for extended periods of time. Discuss appropriate sleep posture.
- NSAIDs can help with pain.
- Attempt nonoperative management for at least 6 weeks.

Rehabilitation

- Refer the patient to an occupational therapist for ulnar nerve gliding exercises, night splinting with the elbow in 45 degrees of flexion, and discussion of activity modifications.

Operative Management

ICD-10 code: G56.20 Lesion of ulnar nerve
CPT code: 64718 Ulnar nerve neuroplasty and/or transposition at elbow

Indications

- Nonoperative management has failed.
- Patient has evidence of severe ulnar nerve compression and/or muscle denervation on EMG/NCS.
- Surgical treatment may be appropriate for patients with evidence of intrinsic wasting on physical examination, to prevent further progression.

- There are several different surgical procedures including in-situ decompression, decompression and transposition, and medial epicondylectomy. No one procedure has currently been proven superior.[1]

Informed consent and counseling

- Care will be taken to avoid injury to the cutaneous nerves at the elbow, but some residual numbness occasionally occurs near the incision site at the elbow.
- The purpose of the surgical procedure is to relieve the sites of compression, and the goal is to prevent progression of nerve damage; if the patient has advanced disease, the operation may not restore normal sensation to the fingers, and strength may never return.
- If symptoms fail to improve or worsen over time, a revision surgery may be indicated.
- The patient can expect to have limited use of the arm for about 6 to 8 weeks.

Anesthesia

- Regional upper extremity block with sedation, or general anesthesia

Patient positioning

- Supine, with the shoulder abducted and externally rotated and the arm on the hand table
- Nonsterile tourniquet high on the brachium

Surgical Procedure

- Medial approach over the ulnar nerve at the elbow
- In-situ ulnar nerve decompression, or decompression and transposition of the ulnar nerve
- The ulnar nerve can be transposed subcutaneously or submuscular
- Endoscopic ulnar nerve decompression is also an option

Ulnar Nerve Transposition (Subcutaneous or Submuscular): Fig. 3.12

A longitudinal incision is made over the medial elbow. Take care to identify and protect the medial antebrachial cutaneous nerve. Elevate the subcutaneous flaps off the fascia overlying the flexor-pronator mass. Identify the medial epicondyle. Just posteriorly, identify the ulnar nerve within the cubital tunnel. With tenotomy scissors and smooth forceps, the ulnar nerve is carefully decompressed. Minimal traction and manipulation of the nerve are ideal, and a vessel loop can be used to retract and control the nerve gently while operating. All sites of ulnar nerve compression at the elbow are addressed: arcade of Struthers, medial intramuscular septum of

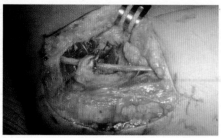

Fig. 3.12 Intraoperative Photograph of a Transposed Ulnar Nerve. The nerve now lies anterior to the medial epicondyle and is held in place by lengthened flexor-pronator fascia.

the triceps, Osborne ligament, the flexor carpi ulnaris (FCU) fascia, and the heads of the FCU. If transposing subcutaneously, a sling is created within the medial subcutaneous flap. The nerve is transposed, and then a suture is used to tack the subcutaneous tissue back down to the flexor pronator fascia, thus securing the nerve anterior to the medial epicondyle.

If transposing submuscularly, the flexor-pronator fascia may be lengthened using a steplike incision. A trough may also be created in the musculature and the nerve transposed anterior to the medial epicondyle. The fascia is then sutured back together over the nerve but in a lengthened position.

Once the nerve has been transposed, the elbow is placed through ROM to ensure that the nerve no longer subluxes with flexion, has no areas of compression, and is not under tension. The wound is then irrigated and the skin closed. A soft dressing or a splint may be applied based on preference and surgical procedure. A long-arm posterior splint with the elbow at 90 degrees and the forearm in neutral is appropriate.

Estimated Postoperative Course
Postoperative days 3 to 5:
- Some clinicians advocate for an early therapy session for gentle elbow ROM and edema control to prevent stiffness. A removable thermoplastic long-arm posterior splint may be fabricated to support the arm between therapy sessions.

Postoperative days 10 to 14:
- Sutures are removed, and ROM is assessed.
- Inquire about and document changes in preoperative paresthesias.
- Perform and document Froment and Wartenburg signs.

Postoperative 6 weeks:
- Reassess ROM.
- Perform a wound check, and evaluate for hypersensitivity.
- Inquire about and document changes in preoperative paresthesias.
- Perform and document Froment and Wartenburg signs.
- The patient can start strengthening exercises between 6 and 8 weeks and gradually return to everyday activities without restrictions.

SUGGESTED READINGS

Boone S, Gelberman RH, Calfee R: The management of cubital tunnel syndrome, *J Hand Surg Am* 40(9):1897–1904, 2015.

Cobb TK: Endoscopic cubital tunnel release, *J Hand Surg* 35:1690–1697, 2010.

Palmer BA, Hughes TB: Cubital tunnel syndrome, *J Hand Surg Am* 35:153–163, 2010.

Staples JR, Calfee R: Cubital tunnel syndrome: current concepts, *J Am Acad Orthop Surg* 25(10):e215–e224, 2007.

Szabo RM, Kwak C: Natural history and conservative management of cubital tunnel syndrome, *Hand Clin* 23:311–318, 2007.

REFERENCES

1. Calliandro P, LaTorre G, Padua R, Giannini F, Padua L: Treatment for ulnar neuropathy at the elbow, *Cochrane Database Syst Rev* 7:Cd006839, 2012.

OLECRANON BURSITIS

The olecranon bursa is a fluid-filled sac that overlies the bony olecranon process on the posterior aspect of the elbow. Under normal conditions, the fluid is minimal and the sac is flat. But the bursa can become enlarged and swollen, a condition called olecranon bursitis. The key to understanding and managing this disorder is to accurately diagnose the bursitis as a condition of inflammation or infection, as both conditions have similar presentation. Anecdotally, there are nuanced physical examination findings particular to each type of bursitis. A thorough history and physical examination combined with a keen sense of clinical judgment and a few objective data can help to guide treatment. Please refer to Table 3.5 for common similarities and differences to aid in diagnosis.

TABLE 3.5 Comparison of Inflammatory vs. Infectious Olecranon Bursitis

Inflammatory Olecranon Bursitis	Infectious Olecranon Bursitis
Gradual onset	Acute onset
Warmth present	Warmth present
Less erythema, localized to bursa	More erythema, deeper red
Less tenderness to palpation	Very tender to palpation
ROM not reduced, or reduced very little	ROM reduced and painful
No surrounding cellulitis	Likely surrounding cellulitis
Afebrile	Probably afebrile, but fever possible
Normal ESR, CRP, WBC	ESR, CRP may be elevated
	WBC may be elevated or normal

CRP, C-reactive protein; *ESR*, erythrocyte sedimentation rate; *ROM*, range of motion; *WBC*, white blood cell.

Aspiration of the bursa should be reserved for severe inflammatory cases, cases that fail conservative treatment, or if the aspirate is needed to confirm a diagnosis of infection and obtain cultures. Aspiration of a chronic, noninflamed bursa can result in a persistent draining sinus or introduction of bacteria into a previously aseptic bursa.

History
- Possible history of elbow trauma, repetitive activity, or abrasion
- Patient-reported edema and sometimes pain over the posterior elbow
- Possible erythema and warmth
- Possible pain with ROM

Physical Examination
- Observe enlargement of the bursa at the posterior elbow.
- Note the presence of any erythema and whether it is localized to the bursa or extends to the surrounding tissues in a cellulitic pattern.
- Warmth will be present in both inflammatory and infectious bursitis.
- Palpation of the bursa reveals bogginess and mild tenderness. Severe tenderness could indicate infection.
- Evaluate ROM and assess whether it is painful. Severe, painful, and limited ROM could suggest deeper joint infection.

Imaging
- X-rays: elbow AP and lateral views. Occasionally a posterior osteophyte is observed on the olecranon process at the triceps insertion.
- X-rays are generally not necessary for diagnosis and are indicated only to evaluate for any underlying elbow joint injury or if a septic joint is suspected.

Classification
Classification System: Inflammatory versus Infectious Table 3.5

Differential Diagnosis
- Rheumatoid nodules
- Elbow joint effusion
- Cellulitis
- Gouty arthritis or gouty tophi
- Pigmented villonodular synovitis

Initial Management
- Determine whether bursitis is inflammatory or infectious.
- Consider obtaining a baseline complete blood count (CBC), erythrocyte sedimentation rate (ESR), and c-reactive protein (CRP).
- The distinction between inflammatory and infectious bursitis may be made by a nuanced history and physical examination and a trial of tailored treatment, or an aspirate may be necessary to identify a pathogen, if present.
- If possible, avoid aspiration and treat conservatively.
- **Patient Education.** Treatment success takes time and is highly associated with patient compliance. Fluid reaccumulation in the bursa is possible and may require repeat treatment. Aspiration, while frequently requested by patients, should be avoided and reserved for refractive cases and to confirm the presence of infection, as it can cause iatrogenic infection. After the bursitis has resolved, the skin overlying the bursa can remain remarkably sensitive or tender and produce a "rug burn" type pain with even light touch. This eventually resolves over weeks to months.

Nonoperative Management
- When deciding on a treatment algorithm, always consider the host and base clinical decision-making on the patient, predicted compliance with recommendations and follow up, and coexisting medical conditions.

- **For mild inflammatory bursitis**: Suggest ice, NSAIDs, an elbow pad or elastic (Ace) wrap for compression, and avoidance of leaning on the elbow. An elbow splint can be used short-term to reduce acute inflammation. The patient should be educated that these treatments may take several weeks to be successful. Aspiration of the inflamed bursa may not be necessary for successful treatment.[1] Corticosteroid injection is generally not recommended due to the increased incidence of infection and skin atrophy.[2]

- **For severe or refractive inflammatory bursitis**: Consider aspiration in addition to the foregoing treatments. Use of a compression wrap over the decompressed bursa is key to prevent recurrence. The patient may need to apply constant compression for 7 to 10 days. Repeat aspirations may be necessary, but treatment is usually successful. If the aspirated fluid is cloudy or purulent, suspect infection, send cultures, and start antibiotics.

- **For mild infectious bursitis with cellulitis**: Obtain baseline lab values for CBC, ESR, and CPR. Draw demarcation lines near cellulitis to evaluate effectiveness of treatment at the subsequent appointment. Initiate rest, ice, compression with an Ace wrap, and elevation. High-dose NSAIDs (if appropriate) can reduce pain and inflammation, and a well-padded elbow splint in 90 degrees of elbow flexion should be worn at all times. Select an appropriate antibiotic and counsel the patient to start it immediately. Reevaluate the patient's condition in 24 hours to monitor response to treatment.

- **For refractive or severe infectious bursitis**: Aspirate bursa and send fluid for Gram stain, aerobic and anaerobic culture with sensitivities, white blood cell (WBC) count, crystals, and fluid glucose. A WBC count greater than 10,000 is considered diagnostic for septic bursitis. A fluid glucose to serum glucose ratio less than 50% is also indicative of septic bursitis. Consider empiric oral antibiotic treatment in addition to ice, rest, and a compression wrap because most infections are caused by *Staphylococcus aureus* or other gram-positive bacteria. Intravenous antibiotics can also be used. Once the susceptibility of the pathogen is known, a 2-week course of oral antibiotics is indicated (see Olecranon Bursa Aspiration, p. 107).

- **Incision and drainage with wound packing** is reserved for cases of infectious olecranon bursitis that does not resolve after treatment with antibiotics. An incision is made just lateral to the olecranon process (an incision directly over the process can lead to delayed wound healing, a chronic open wound, and pain over the posterior elbow). A wick can be placed into the bursa and changed frequently. Avoid overpacking the wound, and use less packing with each dressing change, to encourage healing and wound closure.

Operative Management

ICD-10 code: M70.2 Olecranon Bursitis

CPT code: 24105 Excision of olecranon bursa

Indications

- Surgical excision of the bursa should be reserved for chronic or severe infections and for failure of multiple aspirations.

Informed consent and counseling

- The risk of wound breakdown over the olecranon is high. The skin over the olecranon may become painful or hypersensitive.

Anesthesia

- General anesthesia or a regional anesthetic with sedation

Patient positioning

- Supine, with the operative arm extended on the arm table, the shoulder internally rotated, and the elbow flexed so that the lateral aspect of the elbow is easily exposed
- Nonsterile tourniquet placed high on the brachium

Surgical Procedure

Olecranon Bursectomy

An oblique incision is made just lateral to the olecranon. Take care to avoid injury to the lateral antebrachial cutaneous nerve. The inflamed or infected bursa is usually easily identified and completely excised. Consider sending the bursa for pathologic examination and for cultures. Care should be taken to avoid injury to the insertion of the triceps tendon. The wound is then copiously irrigated, and the skin is closed using suture. Most surgeons advocate for a 2-week period of postoperative splinting in a long-arm posterior elbow splint with the elbow at 90 degrees and neutral forearm rotation, to reduce the risk of hematoma formation.

Estimated Postoperative Course

Postoperative days 10 to 14:

- Return to the clinic for a wound check and for splint and suture removal.

- A therapy referral may be necessary to encourage elbow ROM and strengthening.

Postoperative 6 weeks:

- A wound and motion check is performed.
- If the injury is healed, return to all activities as tolerated.

SUGGESTED READINGS

Aaron DL, Patel A, Kayiaros S, et al.: Four common types of bursitis: diagnosis and management, *J Am Acad Orthop Surg* 19:359–367, 2011.

Blackwell JR, Hay BA, Bolt AM, Hay SM: Olecranon bursitis: a systemic overview, *Shoulder Elbow* 6(3):182–190, 2014.

REFERENCES

1. Deal Jr JB, Vaslow AS, Bickley RJ, Verwiebe EG, Ryan PM: Empirical treatment of uncomplicated septic olecranon bursitis without aspiration, *J Hand Surg Am* 45(1):20–25, 2020.
2. Soderquist B, Hedstrom SA: Predisposing factors, bacteriology and antibiotic therapy in 35 cases of septic bursitis, *Scand J Infect Dis* 18(4):305–311, 1986.

DISTAL BICEPS TENDON RUPTURE

A rupture of the distal biceps tendon from its insertion on the radial tuberosity is an injury that can result in pain, weakness, and disability of the affected arm. This condition usually affects men between 30 and 50 years of age and occurs when a sudden extension load is placed on the arm. When a rupture occurs, it is a time-sensitive injury that requires treatment ideally within 3 weeks of injury for ease of surgical procedure and optimal outcome. Reconstruction of the tendon can be performed for ruptures that are identified late or have delayed treatment.

History

- Generally, patients are men 30 to 50 years old
- Patients may have prior history of some biceps tendinitis
- Patients report a "pop" while lifting or using the arm with an extension load
- Patients may report pain and a "popeye deformity" of the biceps muscle
- A chronic tear may manifest with arm weakness as the primary complaint

Physical Examination

- Observe for prominence of the biceps muscle belly ("popeye deformity"), and compare it with the contralateral side.
- The distal biceps tendon insertion site is tender to palpation just distal to the antecubital fossa.
- Pain or weakness is noted with resisted forearm supination and flexion. (Remember: The brachialis muscle is the primary elbow flexor; the biceps brachii is a primary forearm supinator when the elbow is flexed.)
- **Hook test.** The examiner attempts to hook the distal biceps tendon in the antecubital fossa with the index finger while the patient's elbow is flexed and the forearm is supinated. When a rupture has occurred, the tendon is nonpalpable or flaccid and the hook cannot be performed.
- Palpate for bogginess or bulk proximal to the antecubital fossa which can indicate proximal retraction of the ruptured end of the tendon.

Imaging

- Radiographs of the elbow should be obtained: AP, lateral, and oblique views. The images are usually normal, however.

Additional Imaging
Magnetic Resonance Imaging

- Usually, this diagnosis is made clinically. MRI may be indicated if the diagnosis is unclear, if a partial tear is suspected, or if the surgeon requires additional studies for operative planning.

Classification

- Complete or partial
- Acute (<4 weeks old)
- Chronic (>4 weeks old)

Initial Management

- Splint the elbow in a posterior splint with the elbow at 90 degrees, and provide a sling for comfort.
- It is important to repair the tendon within 2 to 3 weeks of injury. The patient should be seen by an orthopaedic surgeon as soon as possible and within 2 weeks of injury so that surgery can be performed within the first 21 days.
- Repair is usually recommended to limit weakness of elbow flexion and supination, but in some situations

(patient is low demand, is of advanced age, or has significant medical comorbidities), an argument can be made against repair.

- If the injury is left unrepaired, the patient can expect a loss of about 30% of flexion strength and up to 40% of supination strength.[1]
- **Patient Education.** After tendon repair, a significant amount of rehabilitation is necessary, and full strength is not usually recovered until 6 months postoperatively.

Nonoperative Management

- Conservative management is indicated for partial ruptures of less than 50% of the tendon insertion, or if patient is low demand, is older, or has significant medical comorbidities.
- If nonoperative management is indicated, splint the elbow for no more than 3 weeks to allow pain and edema to subside.
- Use a hinged elbow brace with low-grade partial tears, and gradually increase the arc of motion over several weeks. Strengthening can begin at 3 months.
- For nonoperative complete tears, start early elbow ROM with a skilled occupational therapist. Later, the patient can start strengthening ancillary elbow muscles to minimize loss of strength.

Operative Management

ICD-10 code: 840.8 Rupture of the distal biceps tendon
CPT code: 24342 Reinsertion of distal biceps tendon

Indications

- Acute rupture of the distal biceps tendon.
- Partial ruptures of more than 50% of the tendinous insertion.

Informed consent and counseling

- Recovery time is 6 months until return to full strength.
- Success of surgery depends on the patient's compliance with the postoperative therapy program.
- There is a risk of development of heterotopic ossification (HO), which could limit motion and result in the need for additional procedures. Compliance with therapy is crucial.
- A small (5%) risk of injury to the PIN exists, but usually this injury is transient neurapraxia.

Anesthesia

- Regional upper extremity block with general anesthesia

Patient positioning

- The patient is supine, with the arm extended on the arm table
- A nonsterile tourniquet is placed high on the brachium
- A sterile towel roll or upside-down basin may be used under the forearm to place the elbow in flexion once the repair is complete; this limits tension on the repair

Surgical Procedures

- Multiple approaches and techniques for repair have been described. These include:
  - Single incision extended Henry Approach (S-type or horizontal incision at the antecubital fossa)
  - Dual incision technique incorporating the S-type antecubital incision with a dorsal forearm incision that splits the extensor carpi ulnaris (ECU)
  - Tendon repair can be accomplished using bone tunnels, suture anchor technique, interference screw fixation, or suspensory cortical button but no one technique or fixation method has currently been proven superior to another[2]

Distal Biceps Tendon Repair: Fig. 3.13

An incision is made over the distal biceps tendon insertion. This may be a lazy-S incision made over the antecubital fossa, or a horizontal or longitudinal incision distal to the antecubital fossa. Avoid injury to the **lateral antebrachial cutaneous nerve**, which lies just lateral to the biceps tendon in the antecubital fossa. The radial artery and the basilic vein and its tributaries are also protected during this procedure. The proximal stump of the biceps tendon is identified, and a hematoma is frequently

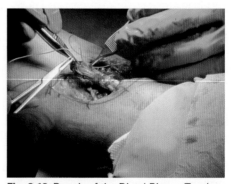

Fig. 3.13 Repair of the Distal Biceps Tendon.

encountered. The lacertus fibrosis (also known as the bicipital aponeurosis) often prevents the tendon from retracting. The stump of the tendon is mobilized and freed of adhesions. An interval is developed between the brachioradialis and the pronator teres. The forearm is placed in supination to avoid injury to the PIN, and blunt dissection is used to identify the radial tuberosity.

The radial tuberosity is prepared by débridement with a rongeur. If suture anchors, unicortical, or bicortical buttons are used for repair, these are then placed at the radial tuberosity. If a bone tunnel is used, a second incision is made posteriorly through the ECU tendon. The forearm is maintained in pronation during this portion of the surgical procedure. The radius is identified posteriorly, and a burr is used to create the tunnel at the radial tuberosity. A 2-mm drill bit is used to create two or three holes about 1 cm apart on the lateral side of the radius.

The biceps tendon is then prepared with a double-limbed running locking suture, also known as a Krackow suture technique. The suture limbs are then pulled down into the bone tunnel or to the suture anchor and are tied in place. The elbow must be flexed to approximate the tendon stump with the repair site, and must remain flexed and supinated for the remainder of the procedure, wound closure, and splint application.

After irrigation and closure of the wound, a posterior elbow splint is applied with the elbow flexed to 90 degrees and the forearm in neutral.

Estimated Postoperative Course
Postoperative days 10 to 14:
- A wound check and suture removal are performed.
- The elbow is continuously maintained in 90 degrees of flexion during examination.
- Occupational therapy is initiated for edema control, wrist and finger ROM, and shoulder pendulum exercises with the elbow in a splint. A splint is fabricated, or a hinged elbow brace is provided and locked at 90 degrees.

Postoperative 3 weeks:
- Therapy starts to increase dynamic elbow flexion. Elbow extension is incrementally increased from weeks 3 to 6 while in the hinged brace. The patient can perform active extension in the brace, but no active flexion. The patient also begins gentle active forearm pronation with the elbow at 90 degrees.

Postoperative 6 weeks:
- The patient returns for a clinic visit for a wound and motion check.
- The patient continues with therapy for progressive extension.

Postoperative 8 weeks:
- The patient can start gentle active elbow flexion.

Postoperative 12 weeks through 6 months:
- The patient returns for a clinic visit at 3 and 6 months postoperatively for a motion check.
- The patient continues with therapy for ROM and can start strengthening.

SUGGESTED READINGS

Bain GI, Johnson LJ, Turner PC: Treatment of partial distal biceps tendon tears, *Sports Med Arthrosc Rev* 16:154–161, 2008.

Cohen MS: Complications of distal biceps tendon repairs, *Sports Med Arthrosc Rev* 16:148–153, 2008.

Sutton KM, Dodds SD, Ahmad CS, et al.: Surgical treatment of distal biceps rupture, *J Am Acad Orthop Surg* 18:139–148, 2010.

REFERENCES

1. Morrcy BF, Askew NL, An KN, et al.: Rupture of the distal tendon of the biceps brachii: a biomechanical study, *J Bone Joint Surg Am* 67(3):418–421, 1985.
2. Srinivasan RC, Pedersen WC, Morrey BF: Distal biceps tendon repair and reconstruction, *J Hand Surg Am* 45(1):48–56, 2020.

ELBOW SPRAIN

A sprain of the elbow refers to a medial or lateral ligamentous injury that can result from an acute injury, such as a fall on an outstretched hand, or chronic stress, such as pitching a baseball. The key to identifying and managing this injury is knowledge of the anatomic structures that provide stability to the elbow and a good physical examination.

History
- Fall onto an outstretched hand
- Possible report of a "pop" at the time of injury
- Elbow pain, stiffness, and edema after a fall
- Overhead throwing athletes prone to UCL sprains or chronic instability

- Overhead throwing athlete with report of medial-sided elbow pain worse during late cocking and acceleration phases of throwing, decreased velocity, and loss of control

Physical Examination

- Observe edema, ecchymosis, and position of the elbow.
- Observe active elbow ROM including supination and pronation.
- Palpate for tenderness to palpation at the following areas:
  - Medial epicondyle and the UCL complex just anterior to the medial epicondyle
  - Lateral epicondyle and the LCL complex just anterior to the lateral epicondyle
  - Radial head
- Palpate the ulnar nerve in the cubital tunnel, and document a thorough neurovascular examination.

Evaluation of the Ulnar Collateral Ligament Complex

Valgus stress test. *Fig. 3.14*
The examiner places one hand on the lateral aspect of the patient's brachium and the other hand on the patient's forearm. The examiner stabilizes the brachium and places the elbow in about 30 degrees of flexion to "unlock" the olecranon and then applies valgus stress on the UCL. A positive test result is characterized by pain, apprehension, or instability of the ligament. The test is 66% sensitive and 60% specific for injury to the anterior band of the ulnar collateral ligament.[1]

Milking maneuver. *Fig. 3.15*
The patient lies supine on the examining table. The shoulder is abducted to 90 degrees, and the elbow is flexed to 90 degrees, with the thumb pointing toward the floor. The examiner grabs the patient's thumb and pulls downward toward the floor (hence, "milking maneuver"). This maneuver places stress over the UCL. A positive test result is characterized by pain, apprehension, or frank instability.

Evaluation of the Lateral Collateral Ligament Complex

Varus stress test. This test is similar to the valgus stress test. The examiner places one hand on the medial side of the patient's elbow and holds the medial and lateral epicondyles. With the other hand, the examiner places the patient's elbow in about 30 degrees of flexion

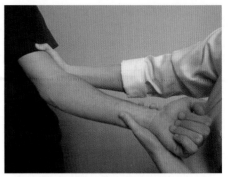

Fig. 3.14 Valgus Stress Test.

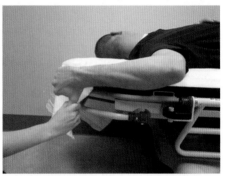

Fig. 3.15 Milking Maneuver.

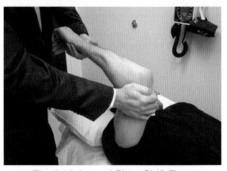

Fig. 3.16 Lateral Pivot Shift Test.

to "unlock" the olecranon and then applies varus stress across the LCL complex. A positive test result is characterized by pain, apprehension, or instability.

Lateral pivot shift test. *Fig. 3.16*
This tests the lateral-UCL (LUCL) for posterolateral rotatory instability (PLRI). The patient lies supine on the examining table. The shoulder is extended over the patient's head. The examiner stands at the head of the bed. The examiner places a hand on the

posterolateral aspect of the patient's elbow and grasps the medial and lateral epicondyles. The maneuver starts with the elbow in an extended position. The examiner applies axial force to the elbow joint and simultaneously flexes and supinates the forearm. A positive test result is characterized by pain, apprehension, a "clunk," or frank dislocation. This test has been found to be 100% sensitive for detecting PLRI but only in anesthetized patients. In awake patients, the test is only 38% sensitive likely due to patient muscle guarding.[2]

The push-up test and stand-up test (or chair push-up test). These two tests are designed to test for PLRI and when combined are more sensitive for detecting instability than the lateral pivot shift test. The push up test is performed by asking the patient to perform a push up on the floor. The elbows are at 90 degrees and the affected elbow is supinated. The patient attempts a push up in this position. A positive test is pain, instability, or inability to perform a push up. The stand-up test (or chair push up test) is performed by having the patient push themselves up out of a chair with their arms. The patient's hands are placed on bilateral arm rests and the elbows are placed in 90 degrees of flexion and supination. A positive test occurs when the patient has pain, instability, or inability to push up out of the chair. These tests are 87.5% sensitive when performed individually and 100% sensitive when performed together.[2]

Imaging

- Elbow AP, lateral, and oblique views.
- Varus or valgus stress views.
- Observation for unilateral widening of the joint or avulsion fractures.
- Radiographs often normal in simple dislocations.
- MRI with arthrogram helpful in the diagnosis of a partial or complete tear (Fig. 3.17).

Initial Management

- Confirm that the elbow joint is reduced on a radiograph.
- Place the elbow in a long-arm posterior splint.
- Refer the patient to be seen in follow-up clinic in 10 to 14 days.
- **Patient Education.** Most simple elbow sprains heal with nonoperative treatment. The patient may experience elbow stiffness as a result of this injury.

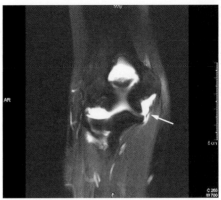

Fig. 3.17 Elbow Magnetic Resonance Imaging with Arthrogram with a Partial Ulnar Collateral Ligament Tear. A small strand of ligament is still attached to the ulna *(arrow).*

Nonoperative Management

Indications

- Reserved for sprained but intact ligaments and/or stable reduced joints.
- Remove the initial splint, and assess ROM.
- Place the patient in a hinged elbow brace, and allow gentle elbow ROM in the brace.
- Refer the patient to an occupational therapist to help guide protected elbow ROM.
- The patient is to be non–weight bearing for 6 to 8 weeks.
- Retest elbow ROM, and assess stability after about 2 months of treatment. If the joint is stable and there is no pain, the patient can return to all regular activities (overhead throwing athletes can return to a graduated throwing program at about 3 months).
- If the patient has continued pain or instability, obtain an MRI with an arthrogram of the elbow to evaluate the location and degree of tear.

Operative Management
ICD-10 codes:

S53.43 Sprain of elbow radial (lateral) collateral ligament

S53.44 Sprain of elbow ulnar (medial) collateral ligament

S53.4 Sprain of elbow or forearm unspecified site

CPT codes:

24344 Reconstruction of radial (lateral) collateral ligament with tendon graft

24346 Reconstruction of ulnar (medial) collateral ligament with tendon graft

Indications

- UCL injury
  - Complete tear with significant elbow instability
  - A partial tear with no improvement after 2 to 3 months of conservative management
  - High-level overhead throwing athlete in whom 6 weeks of splinting and rehabilitation fail
- LCL injury
  - The presence of PLRI

Informed consent and counseling

- A significant amount of postoperative therapy is required for a successful outcome.
- The medial antebrachial cutaneous nerve and the ulnar nerve are at risk for injury during UCL surgery.
- This procedure carries a risk of elbow stiffness.
- Overhead throwing athletes will not be back to baseline for at least 1 year and may not be able to achieve preinjury level of performance.

Anesthesia

- Regional block with general anesthesia

Patient positioning

- The patient is supine, with the arm extended on an arm table. The elbow is flexed.
- A nonsterile tourniquet is placed high on the brachium.

Surgical Procedures

Ulnar Collateral Ligament Reconstruction or Lateral Collateral Ligament Reconstruction

- Direct ligament repair is performed on acute injuries usually associated with elbow dislocation or an acute avulsion from the humerus (see p. 95 for elbow dislocation).

Ulnar Collateral Ligament Reconstruction (Also Known as Tommy John Surgery): Fig. 3.18

- An incision is made just anterior to the medial epicondyle. Blunt dissection is used in the subcutaneous tissue so that the medial antebrachial cutaneous nerve can be identified and protected. The underlying medial epicondyle and common flexor tendon origin are identified. Note whether the tendon origin has been injured because this is a secondary stabilizer of the elbow.
- A longitudinal incision is made through the common flexor tendon origin running parallel to the muscle fibers. A plane is developed between the tendon origin and the underlying joint capsule and UCL. At

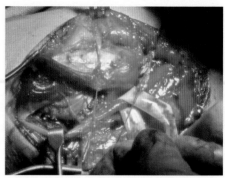

Fig. 3.18 Reconstruction of the ulnar collateral ligament with a palmaris longus tendon graft (also known as Tommy John surgery).

this point, it may be pertinent to dissect, identify, and protect the ulnar nerve in the cubital tunnel for the remainder of the procedure. The UCL is identified, and injuries are noted, most of which occur in the midsubstance of the anterior bundle.

- Bone tunnels are created next with a 3.5-mm or similar drill bit. **Extreme care should be taken to protect the ulnar nerve while drilling.** Two converging holes are made in the humerus at the origination point of the UCL.
- Next, a single tunnel is created in the ulna at the insertion point of the UCL. An autologous tendon graft is harvested (usually the palmaris longus tendon, or a strip of the Achilles or hamstring). With the elbow in 45 degrees of flexion, the graft is woven through the bone tunnels in a figure-8 fashion and is sutured together.
- The elbow is placed through ROM, and the graft is stressed to ensure stability and appropriate tightening. At this point, the surgeon may choose to transpose the ulnar nerve. The joint capsule is then closed, and the common flexor tendon origin is repaired as indicated. Some surgeons use a temporary drain. The patient is placed in a long-arm posterior splint with the elbow in 90 degrees of flexion and the forearm in neutral.

Lateral Collateral Ligament Reconstruction

- A posterior midline approach or Kocher approach is used. The common extensor tendon origin is identified, and an interval is created through the ECU and anconeus to expose the underlying LCL and joint capsule. The elbow is placed under varus stress, and the ligamentous injury is identified.

- Anteriorly converging bone tunnels are then created on the posterior surface of the lateral epicondyle with a 3.5-mm or similar drill bit. A single tunnel is created on the ulna from the supinator tubercle to the ulnar attachment of the annular ligament.
- An autologous tendon graft is harvested (usually the Palmaris longus, or a strip of the Achilles or hamstring). The graft is then woven through the bone tunnels in a figure of 8 or similar fashion.
- The elbow is placed through ROM and varus stress to ensure proper stability and graft tension.
- The joint capsule is closed, and the common extensor tendon origin is repaired as needed. The wound is closed in layers. A long-arm posterior splint is applied with the elbow in 90 degrees of flexion and the forearm in neutral.

Estimated Postoperative Course

Ulnar collateral and lateral collateral ligament reconstruction
Postoperative day 7:
- Remove the postoperative dressing for a wound check.
- UCL: Start gentle elbow ROM under the guidance of an occupational therapist or athletic trainer. For protection, a hinged elbow brace may be prescribed with full ROM.
- LCL: Provide a hinged elbow brace locked at 30 degrees of extension and gradually extend the elbow at 10-degree increments over a 6-week period. Initiate gentle elbow ROM in the brace as guided by an occupational therapist.
- The patient is non–weight bearing for 6 to 8 weeks.
Postoperative 2 weeks:
- Return for suture removal.
Postoperative 4 weeks:
- Start strengthening of the wrist and forearm.
Postoperative 6 weeks:
- Start gradual strengthening of the elbow.
Postoperative 3 months:
- Most patients return to activities as tolerated.
- A graduated throwing program may be initiated for the overhead throwing athlete.
Postoperative 9 to 18 months:
- Overhead throwing athletes can usually return to play at preinjury level.

SUGGESTED READINGS

Cain Jr EL, Dugas JR, Wolf RS, et al.: Elbow injuries in throwing athletes: a current concepts review, *Am J Sports Med* 31:621–635, 2003.

Chen FS, Rokito AS, Jobe FW: Medial elbow problems in the overhead throwing athlete, *J Am Acad Orthop Surg* 9:99–113, 2001.

Hausman MR, Lang P: Examination of the elbow: current concepts, *J Hand Surg Am* 39(12):2534–2541, 2014.

Mehta JA, Bain GI: Posterolateral rotatory instability of the elbow, *J Am Acad Orthop Surg* 12:405–415, 2004.

REFERENCES

1. Hariri S, Safran MR: Ulnar collateral ligament injury in overhead athlete, *Clin Sports Med* 29(4):619–644, 2010.
2. Regan W, Lapner PC: Prospective evaluation of two diagnostic apprehension signs for posterolateral rotatory instability of the elbow, *J Shoulder Elbow Surg* 15(3):344–346, 2006.

ACUTE ELBOW DISLOCATIONS

An acute dislocation of the elbow joint usually results from a high-energy mechanism or fall. The injury usually results in a posterior or posterolateral dislocation. Early reduction is necessary and repeat physical examination to reassess elbow stability is important.

History
- Fall onto an outstretched arm
- High-energy trauma or fall from a height

Physical Examination
- Inspect for evidence of elbow deformity, and identify open injuries.
- Inspect skin integrity, and identify abrasions.
- Palpate known landmarks: lateral epicondyle, medial epicondyle, olecranon process, and radial head.
- Assess neurovascular function and, in particular, the distal motor and sensory function of the median, ulnar, and radial nerves, the brachial artery, and the radial and ulnar arteries distally. Document findings before and after reduction.
- Neurovascular injury is rare and usually transient. The brachial and radial pulse may be diminished initially but should return to normal once the joint is reduced. The ulnar or median nerve may incur

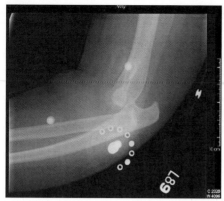

Fig. 3.19 Radiograph of a Posterior Elbow Dislocation.

stretch neurapraxia while the joint is dislocated, and this should resolve once the injury is reduced.

Imaging: Fig. 3.19

- Radiographs of the elbow: AP, lateral, and oblique views

Ligaments

see Fig. 3.2

Classification

- Of dislocations, 90% are posterior or posterolateral (radius and ulna dislocate posterior to humerus).[1]

Simple Instability

- Injury to the UCL or the LCL (specifically the LUCL)
- General pattern of simple dislocation has been described by O'Driscoll, et al.[2]: stage 1, disruption of the LUCL; stage 2, disruption of the remainder of the LCL in addition to the anterior and posterior capsules; stage 3, partial (posterior band only) or complete UCL disruption

Complex Instability: Ligamentous and Osseous Injury

- Radial head fracture with dislocation
- Coronoid fracture with dislocation
- Monteggia fracture-dislocation
- Transolecranon fracture-dislocation
- Terrible triad: a constellation of elbow dislocation, radial head fracture, and coronoid fracture

Primary Stabilizers of the Elbow

- LCL complex

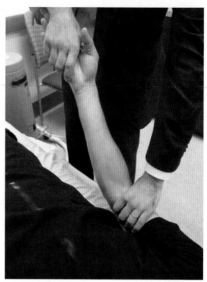

Fig. 3.20 Closed Reduction of a Dislocated Elbow.

- UCL complex
- Ulnohumeral joint

Secondary Stabilizers of the Elbow

- Radial head
- Common flexor and extensor tendon origins
- Elbow joint capsule

Initial Management

Elbow Joint Closed Reduction: Fig. 3.20

CPT code: 24605 Closed reduction with anesthesia

Procedure

1. Obtain adequate pain control, and use conscious sedation to provide muscle relaxation and to ease reduction.
2. Perform and document prereduction and postreduction neurovascular examinations.
3. For posterior dislocations, the patient is supine on a stretcher. An assistant is used to apply traction at the brachium. Apply traction at the forearm with one hand. With the other hand, apply pressure to the posterior aspect of the olecranon by pushing it anteriorly into the trochlea. Varus or valgus stress may also be applied to reduce the joint. The elbow can be flexed during this maneuver to aid in reducing the ulnohumeral joint. An audible "clunk" usually accompanies successful reduction.

4. Once reduced, move the elbow through passive ROM to ensure reduction and stability. Occasionally, the elbow redislocates in extension. When this occurs, the elbow should be reduced again, and an extension blocking splint should be applied to maintain the reduction.

5. Postreduction radiographs are taken: AP and true lateral views of the elbow. Evaluate for adequate reduction and a congruent joint.

6. Document a postreduction neurovascular examination of the median, ulnar, and radial nerves, as well as the radial and ulnar arteries.

7. Place the patient in a sugar tong splint with the elbow flexed to 90 degrees and the forearm in neutral rotation, and advise the patient not to remove the splint.

8. The patient should return to the clinic in 10 to 14 days for repeat radiographs to ensure that the joint has stayed reduced.

Nonoperative Management

Indications
- Most acute simple dislocations can be treated with reduction followed by a brief period of immobilization and do not require surgery.
- The elbow is considered stable after reduction if the joint can be ranged through 50 to 60 degrees of flexion
- **Patient Education.** Most simple dislocations do not require surgical intervention. Some loss of elbow ROM, especially in terminal extension, and residual elbow pain can result after an elbow dislocation. Chronic elbow instability after a simple dislocation is unusual. HO can occur after a dislocation but rarely limits function.[3] Recovery and rehabilitation can take 6 to 8 weeks.

Postreduction procedures and therapy
- The postreduction splint can be removed within 7 to 14 days of injury and replaced with a hinged elbow brace or sling.
- Gentle ROM is initiated when pain and swelling allow, and before 3 weeks postinjury. The extremity is non–weight bearing. The patient may require supervised therapy visits for ROM.
- If the elbow feels unstable in extension, an extension block should be applied to the hinged elbow brace and gradually increased over 3 to 6 weeks.
- The patient should return to the clinic in 6 to 8 weeks. If the elbow is stable on repeat examination, the

patient can be released to gradual weight bearing at 6 to 8 weeks.

Operative Management
ICD-10 codes: S53 Closed dislocation of the elbow

CPT codes: 24615 Open treatment of acute or chronic elbow dislocation

    24586 Open treatment of elbow periarticular fracture and/or dislocation

    24343 Repair of radial (lateral) collateral ligament

    24345 Repair of ulnar (medial) collateral ligament

Indications
- An unreducible joint.
- Acute dislocations that require more than 50 to 60 degrees of flexion to maintain reduction.
- Elbow dislocation with an associated unstable periarticular fracture.

Informed consent and counseling
- Significant stiffness may occur after an elbow fracture-dislocation; therefore, extensive therapy is needed postoperatively.
- Posttraumatic stiffness may need to be addressed later with anterior or posterior capsulotomies. Functional ROM of the elbow is 30 to 130 degrees.

Anesthesia
- Regional upper extremity block with general anesthesia

Patient positioning
- Supine on the operating table, with the arm extended on an arm board
- Sterile or nonsterile tourniquet applied high on the brachium

Surgical Procedures
- Repair of collateral ligaments
- External fixation (rigid or dynamic): for persistent instability after ligament repair
- Other:
  - Open reduction, internal fixation (ORIF) is indicated for fractures (radial head, coronoid) with repair of collateral ligaments as needed. External fixators can be applied during this procedure
  - Occasionally, implants such as a radial head implant are used

Collateral Ligament Repair
- Hardware includes suture anchors and intraoperative fluoroscopy equipment.

- The medial collateral ligament and LCL are approached through two separate incisions. On the medial side of the elbow, an incision is made over the medial epicondyle. Care is taken to avoid injury to the ulnar nerve, which is identified in the cubital tunnel and is protected. The flexor-pronator mass is identified, as is the injured UCL. Often, the entire flexor pronator mass is disrupted from the medial epicondyle in addition to the UCL. The ligament and flexor pronator mass can be repaired back to their origins either with suture through bone tunnels or with suture anchors.
- Next, an incision is made over the lateral aspect of the elbow by using a posterior midline or Kocher approach. The lateral epicondyle and the common extensor tendon origin are identified. Often, the common extensor tendon insertion is disrupted, and the underlying ruptured LCL is easily identified. The ligament and common extensor tendon origin can be repaired back to their origins either with suture through bone tunnels or with suture anchors. The elbow is then placed through ROM, and intraoperative fluoroscopy is used to confirm joint reduction through ROM.
- It may be necessary to apply an external fixator if the joint is unstable. The fixator is applied with two pins in the humerus and two pins in the ulna. Care should be taken when placing the humeral pins to avoid injury to the axillary nerve, which lies 4 to 7 cm distal to the acromion, and the radial nerve in the spiral groove, which is found 9 cm from the acromion and 10 cm from the lateral epicondyle. Pins are placed through small incisions under direct visualization. A drill guide firmly seated on bone is used to avoid soft tissue injury. The fixator is usually left in place for 3 to 4 weeks to allow the ligaments to heal.

Estimated Postoperative Course

Postoperative days 10 to 14:
- Remove sutures, and perform a wound check.
- Document a neurovascular examination.
- Obtain radiographs of the elbow: AP and lateral.
- Therapy for stable elbows after ligament repair: Some clinicians advocate for early protected motion. The patient is taken out of the postoperative splint and placed into a hinged elbow brace, and protected motion is started.
- For elbows in external fixators: Provide pin site care education.

Postoperative 4 weeks:
- For stable elbows after ligament repair: Obtain radiographs to check joint reduction after initiation of therapy.
- For elbows in an external fixator: The fixator can be removed in the clinic. Provide a hinged elbow brace, and start gentle protected motion now or in 2 more weeks, depending on strength of repair and the severity of injury.

Postoperative 8 weeks:
- Perform a motion check.
- Obtain radiographs to confirm joint reduction.
- Therapy: Progress ROM and start a gradual strengthening program.

Postoperative 3 months:
- Perform a final check for ROM and strengthening.
- Continue to follow the patient if ROM is not yet functional (30 to 130 degrees).

SUGGESTED READINGS

Cohen MS, Hastings 2nd H: Acute elbow dislocation: evaluation and management, *J Am Acad Orthop Surg* 6:15–23, 1998.

Ebrahimzadeh MH, Amadzadeh-Chabock H, Ring D: Traumatic elbow instability, *J Hand Surg* 35:1220–1225, 2010.

Morrey BF: Current concepts in the management of complex elbow trauma, *Surgeon* 7:151–161, 2009.

Robinson PM, Griffiths E, Watts AC: Simple elbow dislocation, *Shoulder Elbow* 9(3):195–204, 2017.

REFERENCES

1. Josefsson PO, Nilsson BE: Incidence of elbow dislocation, *Acta Orthop Scand* 57(6):537–538, 1986.
2. O'Driscoll SW, Morrey BF, Korinek S, An KN: Elbow subluxation and dislocation: a spectrum of instability, *Clin Orthop Relat Res* 280:186–197, 1992.
3. Anakwe RE, Middleton SD, Jenkins PJ, McQueen MM, Court-Brown CM: Patient reported outcomes after simple dislocation of the elbow, *J Bone Joint Surg Am* 93(13):1220–1226, 2011.

FOREARM (RADIUS AND ULNA) FRACTURES AND DISLOCATIONS

A fracture that occurs in the forearm usually results from a trauma or high-energy impact. These injuries may result

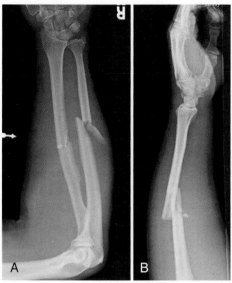

Fig. 3.21 (A) Anteroposterior and (B) lateral radiographs of a comminuted displaced both bone forearm fracture.

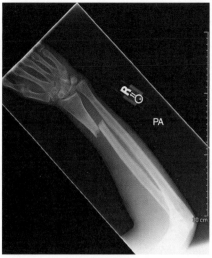

Fig. 3.22 Galeazzi fracture-dislocation: distal third radius fracture with dislocation of the ulna at the distal radioulnar joint. *PA*, Posteroanterior. (From Dacus AR: Radial and ulnar shaft fractures. In: Miller MD, Hart JA, MacKnight JM, editors, *Essential orthopaedics*, Philadelphia, 2010, Saunders, 2010, p 280.)

in an ulnar shaft fracture (night-stick fracture), radial shaft fracture, both bone forearm fracture (Fig. 3.21), or a fracture-dislocation affecting the wrist or elbow. A Galeazzi fracture-dislocation is a distal third radius fracture with dislocation of the distal ulna (Fig. 3.22). A Monteggia fracture-dislocation is a proximal third ulna fracture with dislocation of the proximal radius (Fig. 3.23).

History

- Usually, high-energy trauma such as motor vehicle crash (MVC) or a fall from a height
- Pain and deformity in the forearm and/or elbow

Physical Examination

- Look for evidence of open injury, inspect skin integrity, and identify abrasions.
- Edema and deformity may be present.
- Palpate for instability of the forearm bones and crepitus, and palpate for concomitant wrist injury.
- Assess compartments for compartment syndrome.
- Assess distal motor function for finger and wrist flexor and extensors.
- Assess the neurovascular examination, especially function of the PIN, and document it.

Imaging: Figs. 3.21 through 3.23

- Obtain routine elbow, forearm, and wrist films as indicated.

Classification System: Monteggia Fractures

Type I (most common): Anterior dislocation of the radial head and ulnar diaphysis fracture

Type II: Posterior or posterolateral dislocation of the radial head and ulnar diaphysis fracture

Type III: Lateral or anterolateral dislocation of the radial head and fracture through the ulnar metaphysis

Type IV (rare): Anterior dislocation of radial head and fracture of both forearm bones

Initial Management

- All patients with open injuries should be taken to the operating room urgently.
- Reduce closed fractures by using traction and manipulation, if necessary.
- Splint the forearm in a sugar tong splint or a long-arm posterior splint with the elbow at 90 degrees and the forearm in neutral pronation.
- **Patient Education.** Both bone forearm fractures, Monteggia fractures, and Galeazzi fractures should be treated with ORIF unless medical status prohibits. Elbow or wrist stiffness may occur postoperatively. The recovery period is 6 to 8 weeks, depending on bone healing.

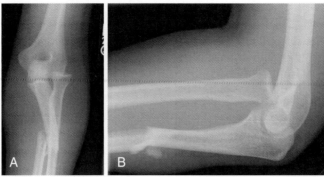

Fig. 3.23 Type I Monteggia Fracture-Dislocation: Proximal Third Ulna Fracture with Dislocation of the Radial Head. **A,** Anteroposterior view; **B,** lateral view.

Nonoperative Management

Both bone forearm fractures
- Nonoperative treatment generally not recommended.

Ulnar shaft fractures and radial shaft fractures
- Nonoperative management is indicated if the patient has less than 10 degrees of angulation and at least 50% cortical contact.
- A sugar tong splint is used for 1 to 2 weeks.
- Apply a short arm cast or a Muenster cast for an additional 4 weeks.
- Place a functional splint for 2 weeks, and start elbow and therapy referral for forearm ROM.
- Monitor fractures with radiographs at each visit to evaluate for displacement.

Galeazzi fracture-dislocation
- Nonoperative treatment generally not recommended.

Monteggia fracture-dislocation
- Nonoperative treatment generally not recommended.

Operative Management
ICD-10 codes:
> S52.27 Monteggia fracture of the ulna
> S52.37 Galeazzi fracture of the radius
> S52.60 closed, S52.61 open
> Both Bone forearm fracture
- **CPT codes**: 25515 ORIF radial shaft fracture
  25525 ORIF radial shaft fracture and closed treatment of DRUJ (distal radioulnar joint) dislocation
  25526 ORIF radial shaft fracture and open treatment DRUJ dislocation
  24635 ORIF Monteggia fracture
  25545 ORIF ulnar shaft fracture
  25575 ORIF radius and ulna shaft fractures
  +20690 Application of uniplanar external fixator

Indications
- All open injuries
- Both bone forearm fractures
- Galeazzi fractures
- Monteggia fractures
- Radial or ulnar shaft fractures with more than 10 degrees of angulation or a more than 50% loss of cortical contact

Informed consent and counseling
- Treatment of open injuries has a higher risk of infection and nonunion.
- Significant elbow stiffness can result from these injuries, and aggressive postoperative therapy is the key to a good functional outcome.
- A risk of PIN injury or palsy related to exposure of the proximal and middle radius exists.

Anesthesia
- Regional upper extremity block with sedation or general anesthesia

Patient positioning
- The patient is supine on the operating table, with the arm extended on an arm board
- A nonsterile tourniquet is placed high on the brachium
- Intraoperative fluoroscopy is used

Surgical Procedures

Open Reduction, Internal Fixation of the Radius and Ulna Shaft: Fig. 3.24
- Two approaches are needed: the approach to the ulnar shaft and the Thompson approach to the dorsal forearm.

Open Reduction, Internal Fixation of Both Bone Forearm Fractures
- Equipment: 3.5-mm dynamic compression plate, intraoperative fluoroscopy, and mini–C-arm

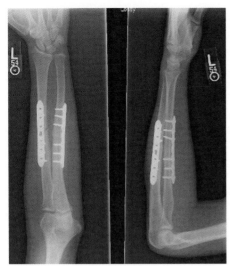

Fig. 3.24 Radiographs of a both bone forearm fracture treated with open reduction, internal fixation. *Left,* Anteroposterior view; *right,* lateral view.

Approach to the Ulna Shaft

Make a longitudinal incision directly over the midulnar shaft at the interval between the ECU and FCU muscle bellies. Use a periosteal elevator to lift the ECU and FCU from their attachments on the ulna. Identify the fracture site, and débride any hematoma. Reduce the fracture with the aid of retractors or towel clips. Apply an appropriate plate, and use lag screws across the fracture site as necessary. Use intraoperative fluoroscopy to confirm the placement of hardware and fracture reduction. Once fixation is in place, the wound is irrigated, and the fascia is closed using suture. The skin is closed in layers.

Thompson (Dorsal) Approach to the Radius

The forearm is pronated, and a longitudinal incision is made between the extensor carpi radialis brevis (ECRB) and extensor digitorum communis (EDC) muscle bellies. The interval lies just anterior to the lateral epicondyle and travels distally toward the Lister tubercle on the dorsal radius. The ECRB and EDC muscles are retracted at this interval to expose the underlying supinator and abductor pollicis longus (APL). Extreme care should be taken to identify the **PIN** as it runs through and exits the supinator. The radius is identified between the supinator and the APL, and a periosteal incision is made down its shaft. The periosteum can be elevated down the length of the radius as needed. The APL and extensor pollicis brevis are retracted to expose more distal fractures. An appropriate plate is selected, and lag screws are used as indicated. Intraoperative fluoroscopy is used to confirm hardware placement and fracture reduction. Once the fracture is fixed, the wound is irrigated, and the fascia is closed. The skin is closed in layers.

Henry Approach (Volar Approach) to the Forearm (for Galeazzi Fractures)

A longitudinal incision is made directly over the FCR tendon. Sharp dissection is carried down through the skin and subcutaneous tissues, the FCR tendon sheath is divided, and the tendon is mobilized. The interval of this approach is between the FCR and the brachioradialis. The FCR and the underlying flexor pollicis longus are retracted. The flexor compartment with the **median nerve** is retracted ulnarly as a unit and is protected. Care is taken to protect the **radial artery** and the **superficial sensory radial nerve** on the radial aspect of the surgical field. If operating on the distal aspect of the radius, the pronator quadratus is visible once the tendons have been retracted. If operating on the radial shaft, the interval of exposure lies between the flexor digitorum superficialis and the pronator teres. The periosteum of the radius is sharply incised and elevated from the bone at the fracture site. Usually, the distal radioulnar joint (DRUJ) will reduce once the radius fracture has been stabilized.

A sugar tong or long-arm posterior splint is applied. It is important to assess the patient's PIN postoperatively during exposures of the proximal forearm if a nerve block was not used.

Estimated Postoperative Course

Postoperative days 10 to 14:

- Wound check and suture removal.
- Radiographs are obtained as follows: for shaft fractures, forearm posteroanterior (PA) and lateral views; for Monteggia fracture, elbow AP and lateral views; for Galeazzi fracture, wrist PA and lateral views.
- If fixation is stable, the patient can wear a removable custom forearm splint and start therapy for gentle hand, wrist, forearm, and elbow ROM. The patient is non–weight bearing on the extremity.
- For severely comminuted fractures, a long-arm or Muenster cast may be necessary for several weeks. In addition, consider casting in patients who need to bear weight on the forearm such as with a platform attachment on a walker.

Postoperative 6 weeks:
- Radiographs are obtained as described earlier.
- If healing is evident, start strengthening and gradual weight bearing.
- If no healing is present, continue the current program.

Postoperative 3 months:
- Radiographs are obtained as described earlier.
- If healing is evident, release the patient to all regular activities.
- If no healing is present, consider supplying the patient with a bone stimulator. Consider reasons for nonunion including infection. It may be beneficial to order appropriate laboratory tests.

Board Review

- A Galeazzi fracture-dislocation is a distal third radius fracture with dislocation of the distal ulna at the wrist.
- A Monteggia fracture-dislocation is a proximal third ulna fracture with dislocation of the proximal radius at the elbow.

SUGGESTED READINGS

Chhabra AB: Elbow and forearm. In Miller MD, Chhabra AB, Hurwitz S, et al.: *Orthopaedic surgical approaches,* Philadelphia, 2008, Saunders, pp 61–144.

Eathiraju S, Mudgal CS, Jupiter JB: Monteggia fracture-dislocations, *Hand Clin* 23:165–177, 2007.

Giannoulis FS, Sotereanos DG: Galeazzi fractures and dislocations, *Hand Clin* 23:153–163, 2007.

Moss JP, Bynum DK: Diaphyseal fractures of the radius and ulna in adults, *Hand Clin* 23:143–151, 2007.

Sauder DJ, Athwal GS: Management of isolated ulnar shaft fractures, *Hand Clin* 23:179–184, 2007.

Sebastin SJ, Chung KC: A historical report on Riccardo Galeazzi and the management of Galeazzi fractures, *J Hand Surg* 35:1870–1877, 2010.

RADIAL HEAD FRACTURES

A fracture of the radial head can result in a wide range of symptom presentation. A minor nondisplaced fracture may produce little in the way of pain and loss of motion, while a large fracture fragment may cause severe elbow dysfunction, pain, locking, or even instability. Appropriate radiographic fracture assessment will help guide treatment.

History
- Fall on an outstretched hand
- Lateral elbow pain, edema, and stiffness

Physical Examination
- Possible elbow edema.
- Possible limited and/or painful ROM.
- Tenderness to palpation at the radial head and pain and possible crepitus with forearm rotation.

Imaging: Figs. 3.25 and 3.26
- AP, lateral, and oblique radiographic views, and possibly a "radial head view," of the elbow are obtained.
- A radial head view or Greenspan view is a modified lateral view with the beam angled 45 degrees toward the radial head.

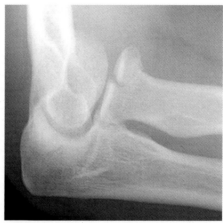

Fig. 3.25 Radial Head View or Greenspan View of a Type I Radial Head Fracture.

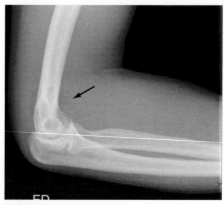

Fig. 3.26 Radiograph of an occult radial head fracture with a "sail sign" *(arrow).*

- Look for the "sail sign" on the radiograph. This is a shadow created by the anterior fat pad when elbow effusion is present. This sign may indicate intraarticular injury even if radiographic findings are negative.
- A computed tomography (CT) scan may be helpful to characterize comminuted fracture fragments further.

Mason Classification System (as Modified by Hotchkiss)

Fig. 3.27 and Table 3.6

Initial Management

- Evaluate ROM. If a significant block to supination or pronation is noted, attempt hematoma aspiration and/or intraarticular injection of 1% plain lidocaine. If block remains, a CT scan may be necessary to evaluate for a displaced, intraarticular fracture.
- Splint the elbow in a long-arm posterior splint.
- **Patient Education.** Elbow stiffness can develop after this fracture; the patient may require occupational therapy during healing. Intraarticular fractures are associated with an increased risk of posttraumatic arthritis. Follow up with an orthopedic specialist is recommended.

Nonoperative Management

- Nonoperative management is indicated for a nondisplaced or minimally displaced (1-mm intraarticular step-off or less) fracture without block to motion.
- Maintain in a posterior splint for 7 to 14 days, and no longer than 21 days, to prevent permanent elbow stiffness.

- Obtain a repeat radiograph of the elbow at the first follow-up visit to evaluate for displacement.
- If reduction is maintained, transition the patient to a hinged elbow brace, and start gentle elbow ROM. Based on the patient's level of discomfort, the brace may need to have a limited arc of motion initially, with graduated progression to full ROM.
- Monitor more severe fractures with weekly radiographs to ensure maintenance of reduction.
- The patient will require 6 to 8 weeks of protected ROM and is non–weight bearing during this time.
- If the patient is asymptomatic and radiographs show evidence of healing at 6 to 8 weeks, release the patient to regular activities.

Operative Management

ICD-10 code: S52.12 Closed fracture of head of radius

CPT codes: 24665 ORIF radial head or neck fracture (includes radial head excision)

24666 With radial head prosthetic replacement

Indications
- Displaced and or comminuted fracture or evidence of bony block to motion

Informed consent and counseling
- A risk of permanent elbow stiffness exists.
- The patient will require weeks of therapy to regain elbow ROM.
- A risk of injury or neurapraxia of the PIN exists.
- A risk of the development of HO exists.
- If the fracture is severe, the patient should be counseled on the possibility of converting an ORIF procedure to a radial head replacement.

Anesthesia
- Regional block with sedation or general anesthesia

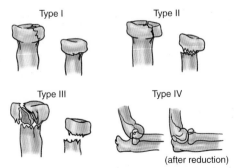

Fig. 3.27 Classification of Radial Head Fractures. (From Dacus AR: Radial head or neck fractures. In: Miller MD, Hart JA, MacKnight JM, editors, *Essential orthopaedics,* Philadelphia, 2010, Saunders, 2010, p 274.)

TABLE 3.6 **Mason Classification System (as Modified by Hotchkiss)**	
Type I	Minimally displaced radial head fracture (<2 mm intraarticular step-off) with no block to motion
Type II	Radial head fracture displaced >2 mm or angulated
Type III	Comminuted fracture of the radial head with block to motion
Type IV	Radial head fracture with elbow dislocation

Patient positioning

- The patient is supine, with the arm on a hand table, the elbow flexed, and the forearm pronated
- A sterile or nonsterile tourniquet is used high on the brachium
- Intraoperative fluoroscopy is used

Surgical Procedures

- ORIF with screws is used for most fractures.
- Radial head prosthetic replacement is used for severely comminuted fractures.
- ORIF with radial head plate is used for fractures that extend into the radial neck.
- Radial head excision is falling out of favor with more advanced technology. It is associated with proximal migration of the radius resulting in an Essex-Lopresti lesion and wrist pain.

Open Reduction, Internal Fixation of a Radial Head Fracture

- A Kocher approach to the elbow is used to gain access to the radial head. A lateral incision is made from the lateral epicondyle to the ECU. The muscle fascia over the common extensor tendon and ECU insertions is identified and divided at the interval between the ECU and anconeus. A plane is developed between the muscles and the underlying joint capsule and LCL.
- It is important to keep the forearm in pronation during the procedure to protect the **PIN** in the supinator.
- The joint capsule is incised anterior to the LUCL from the lateral epicondyle to the annular ligament. The annular ligament can be incised and later repaired to gain access to the radial neck. With the radiocapitellar joint now exposed, the fracture is débrided, and individual pieces are aligned. K-wires are used for provisional fixation of the fracture fragments.
- Then, mini-fragment screws are used for definitive fixation. Alternatively, a plating system can also be used, especially if there is involvement of the radial neck, or a radial head replacement in an older patient with a severely comminuted fracture.
- Once fracture reduction and hardware placement are confirmed by intraoperative fluoroscopy, the wound is irrigated and closed in layers to avoid development of a synovial sinus tract. A long-arm posterior splint is applied with the elbow in 90 degrees of flexion and the forearm in neutral rotation.

Estimated Postoperative Course

Postoperative days 10 to 14:

- Return to the clinic for a wound check and suture removal.
- Some clinicians advocate for early protected elbow ROM if fixation is good and comminution is minimal.
- Radiography: Obtain routine postoperative radiographs: AP, lateral, and oblique views of the elbow.
- Therapy: Provide a hinged elbow brace and start gentle, protected ROM with no weight bearing. The brace may need to be placed in an extension block, depending on the patient's motion, elbow stability, or fracture severity.

Postoperative 4 weeks:

- Return to the clinic for a wound and motion check.
- Radiography: Obtain routine radiographs to evaluate for healing.
- Therapy: Progress ROM.

Postoperative 6 to 8 weeks:

- Return to the clinic for a motion check.
- Radiography: Obtain routine radiographs to evaluate for healing.
- Therapy: Start aggressive ROM and weight bearing.

Postoperative 3 months:

- Return for a motion check.
- Obtain radiographs if concerned for healing.
- Release to regular activities without restrictions.

SUGGESTED READINGS

Dacus AR: Radial head or neck fractures. In Miller MD, Hart JA, MacKnight JM, editors: *Essential orthopaedics,* Philadelphia, 2010, Saunders, pp 273–275.

Pike JM, Athwal GS, Faber KJ, et al.: Radial head fractures: an update, *J Hand Surg* 34:557–565, 2009.

Tejwani NC, Mehta H: Fractures of the radial head and neck: current concepts in management, *J Am Acad Orthop Surg* 15:380–387, 2007.

ORTHOPAEDIC PROCEDURES

Intraarticular Elbow Injection and Aspiration

Code

CPT code: 20605

Indications
- Elbow arthritis
- Intraarticular block for fracture reduction
- Diagnostic injection
- Elbow aspiration

Contraindications
- Steroid injections contraindicated if infection suspected
- Skin abrasions over lateral elbow

Equipment Needed: Fig. 3.28
- Gloves
- Iodine and alcohol swabs or another antiseptic of choice
- Injection: 5-mL syringe and 25-gauge needle
- Injectate: 3 mL of 1% plain lidocaine mixed with 1 mL of 40 mg/mL triamcinolone (Kenalog) or other corticosteroid
- Aspiration: 20-mL empty syringe and 18-gauge needle
- Adhesive bandage

Procedure: Fig. 3.29
1. Position the patient's elbow in 90 degrees of flexion with the arm internally rotated so that the lateral aspect of the elbow is exposed.
2. Identify the lateral epicondyle, radial head, and olecranon process. Triangulate the area among these three structures, and identify the "soft spot" that is the location for the intraarticular injection. Mark the injection site.
3. Prepare the skin with iodine and alcohol swabs or antiseptic of choice.
4. Ethyl chloride spray may be used for patient comfort.
5. Place the needle directly into the "soft spot," and inject the medication or aspirate synovial fluid.
6. Withdraw the needle, and apply an adhesive bandage.

Aftercare Instructions
1. The elbow joint may be sore and even mildly edematous for the 24-hour period following the injection.
2. A risk of subcutaneous fat atrophy, skin depigmentation, and damage to surrounding structures exists when cortisone is used as a treatment modality.
3. Apply ice and take acetaminophen (Tylenol) or NSAIDs if pain is intolerable.

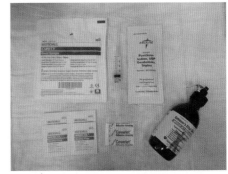

Fig. 3.28 Equipment needed for intraarticular elbow injection and aspiration. Manufacturers and supplies may vary.

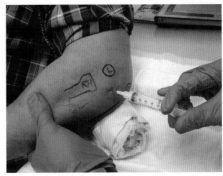

Fig. 3.29 Intraarticular Elbow Injection and Aspiration.

4. The injection may take several weeks to exert maximum effect.
5. The injection may provide temporary relief; return to the clinic if symptoms recur.

Lateral Epicondyle Injection
Code
CPT code: 20551

Indications
- Lateral epicondylitis that has failed to respond to therapeutic exercise, rest, and NSAIDs.

Contraindications
- Injection is contraindicated if the integrity of the skin over the lateral epicondyle has been compromised, such as from an abrasion or from subcutaneous fat atrophy from previous treatment.
- Multiple repeated injections are a relative contraindication, and length between injections should be considered before administration.

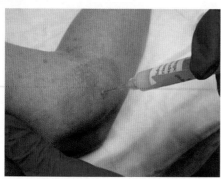

Fig. 3.30 Injection for Lateral Epicondylitis.

Equipment Needed
- Gloves
- Iodine and alcohol swabs or topical antiseptic of choice
- Ethyl chloride spray considered for patient comfort
- 5-mL syringe and 25-gauge needle
- Injectate: 3 mL of 1% plain lidocaine mixed with 1 mL of 40 mg/mL triamcinolone (Kenalog) or other corticosteroid
- Adhesive bandage

Procedure: Fig. 3.30
1. Position the patient's elbow in 90 degrees of flexion with the arm in internal rotation so that the lateral epicondyle is exposed.
2. Palpate the lateral epicondyle and mark the area for the injection directly over the bony prominence of the epicondyle. Administration of the injection too far distal, posterior, and anterior could result in damage to surrounding structures such as the LCL or the PIN.
3. Prepare the skin directly over the lateral epicondyle with the iodine and alcohol swabs or antiseptic of choice.
4. Ethyl chloride may be used before injection for patient comfort.
5. Administer the injection directly over the lateral epicondyle into the common extensor tendon origin. Manipulate the needle during the injection so that the injectate is distributed evenly over the fanlike insertion of the tendons. However, do not administer the injection distal to the epicondyle.
6. Withdraw the needle, and place an adhesive bandage over the injection site.

Aftercare Instructions
1. The injection site may be sore and even mildly edematous for the 24-hour period following the injection.
2. A risk of subcutaneous fat atrophy, skin depigmentation, and damage to surrounding structures is present when cortisone is used as a treatment modality.
3. Apply ice and take acetaminophen (Tylenol) or NSAIDs if pain is intolerable.
4. The injection may take several weeks to exert maximum effect.
5. Avoid lifting heavy objects or returning to repetitive activity in the period following the injection, and ease back into such tasks gradually.
6. The injection may provide temporary relief; return to the clinic if symptoms recur.

Medial Epicondyle Injection
Code
CPT code: 20551

Indications
- Medial epicondylitis that has failed to respond to therapeutic exercise, rest, and NSAIDs.

Contraindications
- A subluxating ulnar nerve or previous ulnar nerve transposition is a relative contraindication, and the injection should be performed with extreme caution in this situation.
- Injection is contraindicated if the integrity of the skin over the medial epicondyle has been compromised such as from an abrasion or from subcutaneous fat trophy from previous treatment.
- Multiple repeated injections are a relative contraindication, and length between injections should be considered before administration.

Equipment Needed
- Gloves
- Iodine and alcohol swabs or topical antiseptic of choice
- Ethyl chloride spray considered for patient comfort
- 5-mL syringe and 25-gauge needle
- Injectate: 3 mL of 1% plain lidocaine mixed with 1 mL of 40 mg/mL triamcinolone (Kenalog) or other corticosteroid
- Adhesive bandage

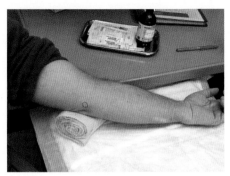

Fig. 3.31 Elbow and Arm Positioning for Medial Epicondyle Injection.

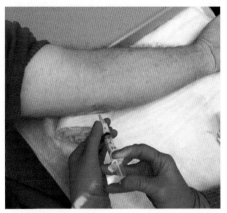

Fig. 3.32 Injection for Medial Epicondylitis.

Procedure: Fig. 3.31

1. Position the patient's elbow in full extension, and externally rotate the arm so that the medial epicondyle is exposed. The ulnar nerve should remain behind the medial epicondyle in the cubital tunnel when the elbow is extended.
2. Palpate the medial epicondyle and then ulnar nerve posteriorly to confirm its position. While palpating the medial epicondyle, ask the patient to confirm that he or she does not feel any distal paresthesias.
3. Mark the area for the injection directly over the medial epicondyle.
4. Prepare the skin directly over the medial epicondyle with the iodine and alcohol swabs or antiseptic of choice.
5. Ethyl chloride may be used before injection for patient comfort.
6. Administer the injection directly over the medial epicondyle and into the common flexor tendon origin with the elbow in extension. Discontinue injection if the patient reports paresthesias in the ulnar nerve. Minimal manipulation of the needle is ideal so that the injectate is distributed evenly over the tendon insertion but does not penetrate posteriorly into the cubital tunnel or anteriorly into the UCL (Fig. 3.32).
7. Withdraw the needle, and place an adhesive bandage over the injection site.

Aftercare Instructions

1. The injection site may be sore and even mildly edematous for the 24-hour period following the injection.
2. A risk of subcutaneous fat atrophy, skin depigmentation, and damage to surrounding structures exists when cortisone is used as a treatment modality.

3. Apply ice and take acetaminophen (Tylenol) or NSAIDs if pain is intolerable.
4. The injection may take several weeks to exert maximum effect.
5. Avoid lifting heavy objects or returning to repetitive activity in the period following the injection, and ease back into such tasks gradually.
6. The injection may provide temporary relief; return to the clinic if symptoms recur.

Olecranon Bursa Aspiration
Code
CPT code: 20605

Indications
- Symptomatic inflammatory bursitis
- Diagnostic aspiration of potential septic bursitis
- Treatment of septic bursitis

Contraindications
- Aspiration should be avoided in minimally symptomatic bursitis, to reduce the potential for iatrogenic infection.

Equipment Needed: Fig. 3.33
- Gloves
- Iodine and alcohol swabs or other antiseptic of choice
- 30-mL syringe
- 21-gauge needle
- Adhesive bandage
- Compression wrap

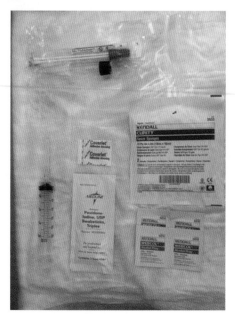

Fig. 3.33 Equipment needed for olecranon bursa aspiration. Manufacturers and supplies may vary.

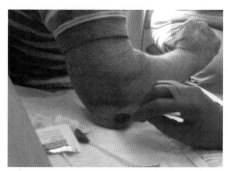

Fig. 3.34 The elbow is positioned, and the skin is prepared.

- Culture swabs and specimen tube for aerobic or anaerobic culture with Gram stain

Procedure

1. Position the patient's elbow in 90 degrees of flexion with the lateral surface of the bursa exposed.
2. Identify area on the lateral side of bursa for aspiration site (avoid punctures directly posterior, because of sensitivity and increased risk for fistula formation, and in the ulnar direction, to avoid injury to the ulnar nerve).
3. Prepare the skin with antiseptic (Fig. 3.34).

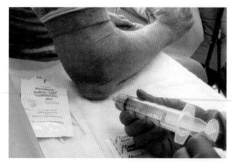

Fig. 3.35 Olecranon Bursa Aspiration.

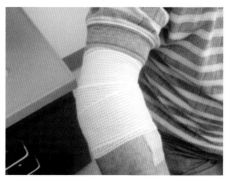

Fig. 3.36 The arm has been wrapped firmly with a compression wrap. An arm tourniquet should not be created.

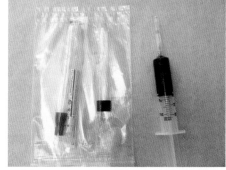

Fig. 3.37 Cultures should be taken for suspected infection or if fluid looks cloudy or purulent.

4. Puncture the skin and bursa, and begin to aspirate fluid. Manual compression of the bursa may be necessary to extract all the fluid. No need exists to move the needle around in the bursa because it is one continuous space (Fig. 3.35).
5. Once the bursa is decompressed, apply an adhesive bandage.

6. Wrap the arm firmly with a compression wrap (but avoid creating an arm tourniquet) (Fig. 3.36).
7. Send cultures if fluid looks cloudy or purulent or if infection is suspected (Fig. 3.37).
8. Consider starting empiric antibiotics if infection is suspected.

Aftercare Instructions

1. Instruct the patient to leave the wrap on for at least 24 hours, then remove wrap only for bathing and replace it immediately. The wrap will be necessary for 7 to 10 days.
2. If the bursa recurs, the patient should return either for repeat aspiration or a discussion of surgical management.
3. If erythema, pain, or edema worsens, the patient is to return to the clinic.

4

Wrist and Hand

Sara D. Rynders

ANATOMY

Bones: Fig. 4.1

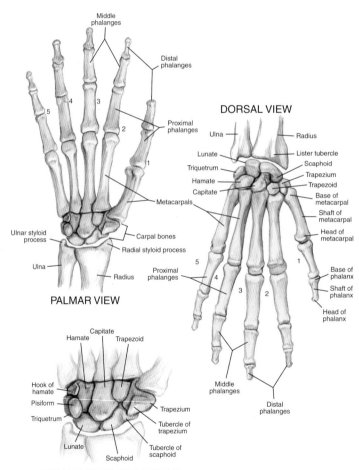

Fig. 4.1 Bones of the Hand and Wrist. (From Chhabra AB: Wrist and hand. In: Miller MD, Chhabra AB, Hurwitz S, et al., editors, *Orthopaedic surgical approaches,* Philadelphia, 2008, Saunders, p 148.)

Ligaments: Fig. 4.2

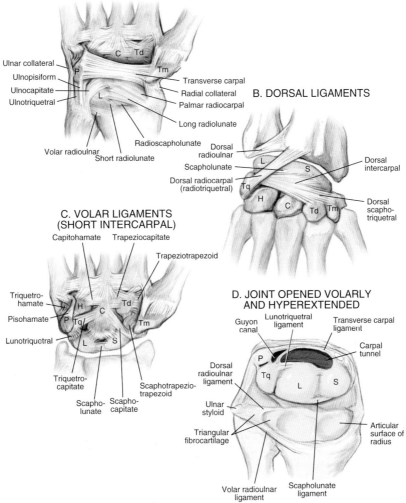

Fig. 4.2 A–D, Ligaments of the wrist. *Ca,* Capitate; *H,* hamate; *L,* lunate; *P,* pisiform; *S,* scaphoid; *Td,* trapezoid; *Tm,* trapezium; *Tq,* triquetrum. (From Chhabra AB: Wrist and hand. In: Miller MD, Chhabra AB, Hurwitz S, et al., editors, *Orthopaedic surgical approaches*, Philadelphia, 2008, Saunders, p 150.)

Muscles and Tendons: Figs. 4.3 through 4.7

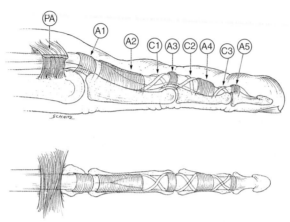

Fig. 4.3 Flexor Tendon Pulley System. *A1 to A5,* Annular pulleys; *C1 to C3,* cruciate pulleys; *PA,* palmar aponeurosis. (From Strickland JW: Flexor tendons: acute injuries. In: Green DP, editor, *Operative hand surgery,* ed 4, New York, 1999, Churchill Livingstone, p 1853.)

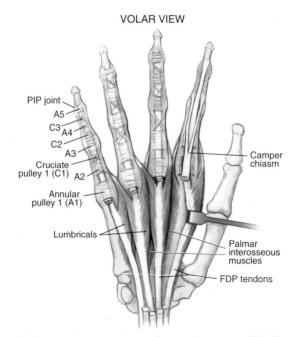

Fig. 4.4 Volar Muscles of the Hand: Lumbricals and Palmar Interossei. *FDP,* Flexor digitorum profundus; *PIP,* proximal interphalangeal. (From Chhabra AB: Wrist and hand. In: Miller MD, Chhabra AB, Hurwitz S, et al., editors, *Orthopaedic surgical approaches, Philadelphia,* 2008, Saunders, p 154.)

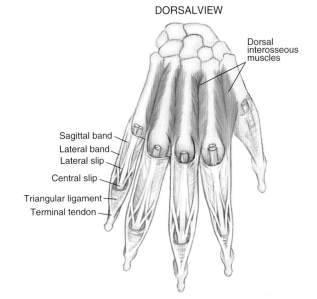

DORSAL VIEW

Dorsal interosseous muscles

Sagittal band
Lateral band
Lateral slip
Central slip
Triangular ligament
Terminal tendon

Fig. 4.5 Dorsal Muscles of the Hand: Dorsal Interossei and Extensor Mechanism of the Finger. (From Chhabra AB: Wrist and hand. In: Miller MD, Chhabra AB, Hurwitz S, et al., editors, *Orthopaedic surgical approaches*, Philadelphia, 2008, Saunders, p 155.)

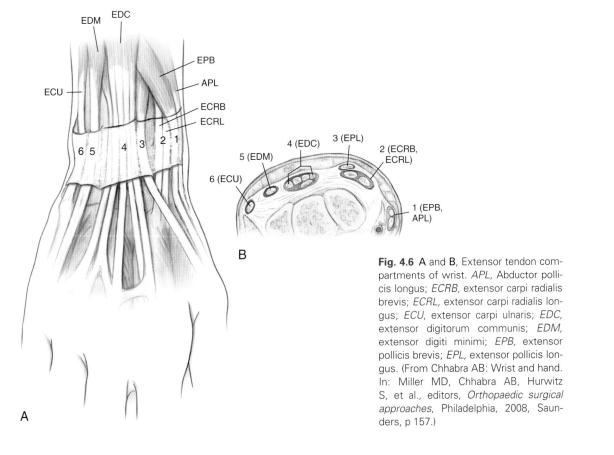

EDM   EDC
ECU
EPB
APL
ECRB
ECRL
6 5   4 3   2 1

5 (EDM)
6 (ECU)
4 (EDC)   3 (EPL)   2 (ECRB, ECRL)
1 (EPB, APL)

A

B

Fig. 4.6 A and B, Extensor tendon compartments of wrist. *APL,* Abductor pollicis longus; *ECRB,* extensor carpi radialis brevis; *ECRL,* extensor carpi radialis longus; *ECU,* extensor carpi ulnaris; *EDC,* extensor digitorum communis; *EDM,* extensor digiti minimi; *EPB,* extensor pollicis brevis; *EPL,* extensor pollicis longus. (From Chhabra AB: Wrist and hand. In: Miller MD, Chhabra AB, Hurwitz S, et al., editors, *Orthopaedic surgical approaches*, Philadelphia, 2008, Saunders, p 157.)

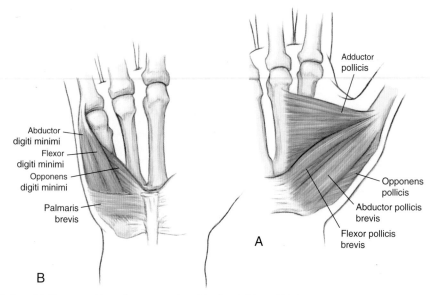

Fig. 4.7 **A** and **B,** Thenar and hypothenar muscles of the hand. (From Chhabra AB: Wrist and hand. In: Miller MD, Chhabra AB, Hurwitz S, et al., editors, *Orthopaedic surgical approaches,* Philadelphia, 2008, Saunders, p 156.)

Nerves and Arteries: Figs. 4.8 through 4.10 and Table 4.1

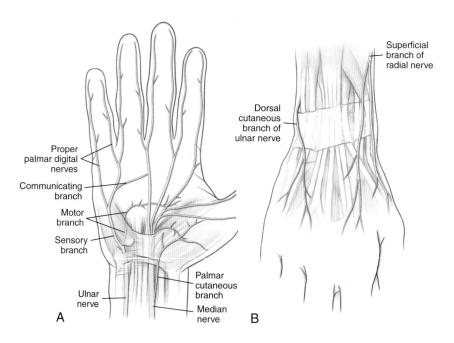

Fig. 4.8 **A** and **B,** Nerves of the hand and wrist. (From Chhabra AB: Wrist and hand. In: Miller MD, Chhabra AB, Hurwitz S, et al., editors, *Orthopaedic surgical approaches,* Philadelphia, 2008, Saunders, p 159.)

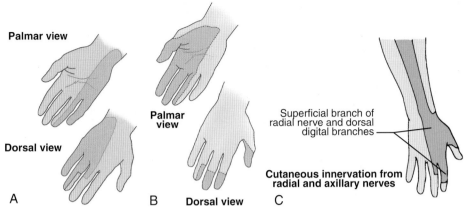

Fig. 4.9 Sensory patterns of the **(A)** ulnar, **(B)** median, and **(C)** radial nerves. (From Hart JA: Overview of the wrist and hand. In: Miller MD, Hart JA, MacKnight JM, editors, *Essential orthopaedics*, Philadelphia, 2010, Saunders, p 297.)

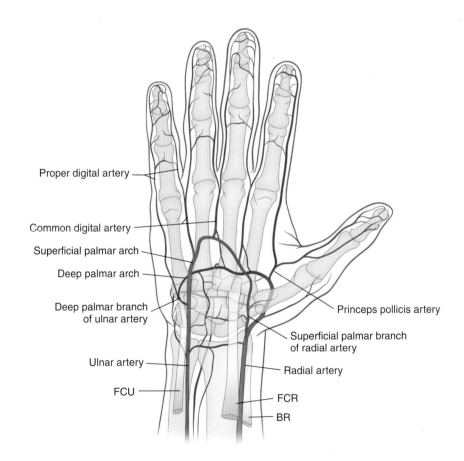

Fig. 4.10 Arteries of the Hand and Wrist. *BR,* Brachioradialis; *FCR,* flexor carpi radialis; *FCU,* flexor carpi ulnaris. (From Chhabra AB: Wrist and hand. In: Miller MD, Chhabra AB, Hurwitz S, et al., editors, *Orthopaedic surgical approaches*, Philadelphia, 2008, Saunders, p 161.)

TABLE 4.1   Nerves and Their Functional Testing

Nerve	Branch	Motor	Test	Sensory
Radial	Superficial sensory radial nerve			To dorsal aspect of radial wrist and thumb, dorsal hand
	PIN	ECRB EDM ECRL APL ECU EPB Supinator EPL EIP	Wrist extension Thumb extension Finger extension	
Median	Proper	Pronator teres FCR FDS Palmaris longus Index and middle finger lumbricals	Radial wrist flexion Finger flexion Pronation	Thumb, index finger, middle finger, and radial half of ring finger
	Recurrent motor branch	Thenar muscles: APB	Thumb abduction	
	AIN	FDP to index finger FPL Pronator quadratus	Index finger DIP joint flexion Thumb IP joint flexion Pronation	
	Superficial sensory palmar branch			Sensation to palm
Ulnar	Proper	FDP to 4 and 5 FCU	Flexion of ring and small fingers Ulnar wrist flexion	
	Deep motor branch	Adductor pollicis Hypothenar muscle Interosseous muscle Ring and small finger lumbricals Deep branch of FPB	Finger abduction and adduction Thumb adduction	
	Dorsal sensory branch			Palmar and dorsal sensation to small finger and ulnar half of ring finger

APB, Abductor pollicis brevis; *APL*, abductor pollicis longus; *AIN*, anterior interosseous nerve; *DIP*, distal interphalangeal; *ECRB*, extensor carpi radialis brevis; *ECRL*, extensor carpi radialis longus; *ECU*, extensor carpi ulnaris; *EDM*, extensor digiti minimi; *EIP*, extensor indicis proprius; *EPB*, extensor pollicis brevis; *EPL*, extensor pollicis longus; *FCU*, flexor carpi ulnaris; *FCR*, flexor carpi radialis; *FDP*, flexor digitorum profundus; *FDS*, flexor digitorum superficialis; *FPB*, flexor pollicis brevis; *FPL*, flexor pollicis longus; *IP*, interphalangeal; *PIN*, posterior interosseous nerve.

Surface Anatomy: Fig. 4.11

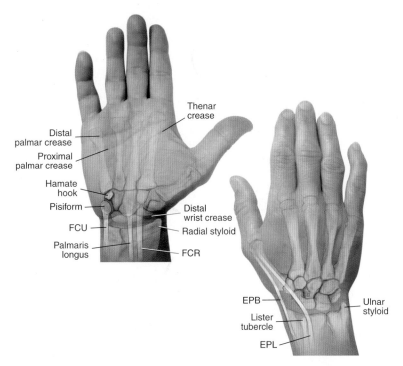

Fig. 4.11 Surface Anatomy of the Hand and Wrist. *EPB,* Extensor pollicis brevis; *EPL,* extensor pollicis longus; *FCR,* flexor carpi radialis; *FCU,* flexor carpi ulnaris. (From Chhabra AB: Wrist and hand. In: Miller MD, Chhabra AB, Hurwitz S, et al., editors, *Orthopaedic surgical approaches*, Philadelphia, 2008, Saunders, p 163.)

Normal Radiographic Appearance: Figs. 4.12 through 4.14

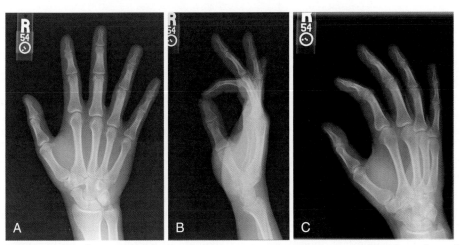

Fig. 4.12 Normal Radiographs of the Hand. (**A**) Anteroposterior, (**B**) lateral, and (**C**) oblique views of the hand. (From Hart JA: Overview of the wrist and hand. In: Miller MD, Hart JA, MacKnight JM, editors, *Essential orthopaedics*, Philadelphia, 2010, Saunders, p 303.)

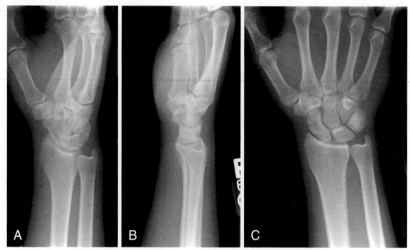

Fig. 4.13 Normal Radiographs of the Wrist. (A) Anteroposterior, (B) oblique, and (C) lateral views of the wrist.

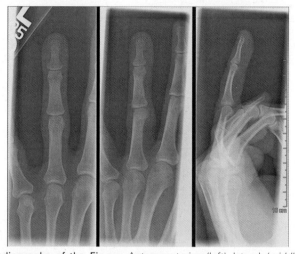

Fig. 4.14 Normal Radiographs of the Finger. Anteroposterior *(left)*, lateral *(middle)*, and oblique *(right)* views of the finger.

HISTORY

- Always obtain HAND DOMINANCE and OCCU-PATION.
- Inquire about TIMING OF SYMPTOMS and MECHANISM OF INJURY.
  - Was onset sudden or gradual? Was there a fall on an outstretched hand?
- Ask about the LOCATION OF THE PAIN and CHARACTERIZE if it is constant, intermittent, or only occurs with certain activities.
- Inquire if there is NUMBNESS AND TINGLING in the hand and if so, where?

- It may prove valuable to ask the patient to point to the area of most significant pain using one finger, as this can quickly help the evaluator narrow down the differential diagnosis.

PHYSICAL EXAMINATION

Inspect and document lacerations, abrasions, muscle atrophy, edema, erythema, or deformity.

Palpate structures specific to the complaint, as well as one joint above and below the zone of injury. There are many anatomic structures concentrated within a small area in the wrist and hand. Approach the physical examination with diligence and specificity. Note if tenderness is present and over which anatomic structures the tenderness is located. Common areas of bony tenderness include:

- Distal radius
- Anatomic snuffbox and scaphoid tubercle
- Scapholunate (SL) interval
- First carpometacarpal (CMC) joint
- A1 pulley of the flexor tendon
- Proximal interphalangeal (PIP) joint of the finger

Normal wrist range of motion (ROM): Table 4.2
Neurovascular examination of the wrist and hand: Table 4.3

Special Tests: Table 4.4

TABLE 4.2 Normal Wrist Range of Motion	
Extension	80 degrees
Flexion	70 degrees
Supination	90 degrees
Pronation	90 degrees
Ulnar deviation	30 degrees
Radial deviation	20 degrees

TABLE 4.3 Neurovascular Examination of the Wrist and Hand		
Nerve	**Location of Test**	**Tests**
Median nerve	Carpal tunnel	Tinel, Phalen, Durkan test (see page 147) Sensation testing on the volar thumb, index, middle, and radial side of the ring fingers
Ulnar nerve	Guyon canal/ medial epicondyle	Tinel test directly over nerve Froment's test Wartenburg's test Resisted finger abduction
Superficial sensory radial nerve	At radial styloid	Tinel test
Radial and ulnar artery	At volar wrist	Palpation of pulse Capillary refill in digits Allen test for dominance or perfusion

Differential Diagnosis of Wrist Pain: Table 4.5

Differential Diagnosis of Finger Pain: Table 4.6

SUGGESTED READINGS

Kenney RJ, Hammert WC: Physical examination of the hand, *J Hand Surg Am* 39:2324–2334, 2014.
Miller MD, Hart JA, MacKnight JM, editors: *Essential orthopaedics*, Philadelphia, 2010, Saunders.
Wolfe Hotchkiss, Pedersen Kozin, editors: *Greens operative hand surgery*, ed 6, Philadelphia, 2011, Elsevier.

SCAPHOID FRACTURE

Scaphoid fractures are the most commonly encountered carpal bone fracture, accounting for 70% of all carpal fractures.[1] The hallmark physical examination finding is tenderness at the anatomic snuffbox. Fractures of the scaphoid may not be visible on initial x-rays; therefore, a high level of suspicion and close follow up are necessary in order to avoid missing this injury. The scaphoid bone has a very tenuous blood supply in which the artery enters the bone in a retrograde fashion from the distal pole to the proximal pole. It is important to properly identify and treat scaphoid fractures in order to avoid fracture nonunion, avascular necrosis, and ultimately debilitating wrist arthritis. Information on the work-up and treatment of chronic scaphoid fractures, scaphoid nonunions, and advanced wrist arthritis can be found in the suggested readings.

History

- Fall on an outstretched hand
- Patient reports anatomic snuffbox pain, pain with wrist motion and weight bearing
- Patient may say they think they just "sprained" their wrist

Physical Examination

- Tenderness to palpation at anatomic snuffbox is hallmark finding for this condition (Fig. 4.15). Tenderness may also be present at the scaphoid tubercle on the volar wrist.
- Radial-sided wrist edema and/or ecchymosis may be present.
- Limitation and pain with all wrist motion, especially radial deviation and extension.

TABLE 4.4 Special Tests

Test	Associated Condition	Description of Positive Test
Anatomic snuffbox tenderness	Scaphoid fracture	Tenderness to palpation at the radial side of the wrist, base of the thumb, in the triangular recess formed by the first and third extensor compartments.
Finkelstein's test	DeQuervain's tenosynovitis	Pain with passive radial deviation of the wrist while the thumb is flexed into the palm.
Tinel's sign	Carpal tunnel syndrome Cubital tunnel syndrome Peripheral nerve lesion	Distal paresthesias produced by percussing over the affected nerve with one finger.
Phalen's test	Carpal tunnel syndrome	Flexing the wrists to 90 degrees and holding for 60 seconds produced paresthesias into the thumb, index, middle, and radial side of the ring finger.
Froment's sign	Ulnar neuropathy	The practitioner places a piece of paper in the first webspace and asks the patient to perform key pinch. A positive test is one in which the patient flexes the thumb IP joint, thereby activating the median-nerve innervated FPL, instead of performing pinch grasp using the adductor pollicis. A positive test indicates weakness of the adductor pollicis, an ulnar-innervated hand muscle.
Wartenburg's sign	Ulnar neuropathy	The 5th finger is observed to remain in an abducted position when the patient is asked to actively adduct their digits together. A positive test indicates weakness of the hand intrinsic muscles, particularly the 5th finger adductor.
Allen's test	Radial or ulnar artery injury, thrombosis, or dominance	Using both thumbs, the examiner applies pressure over BOTH the radial and ulnar arteries at the wrist. The patient open and closes the fist to exsanguinate the venous system while the arteries are occluded. Then the practitioner releases the radial artery and observes for reperfusion of the palm. The test is repeated, this time releasing the ulnar artery and observing for reperfusion. This test can indicate if an occlusion is present and/or if a patient has a dominant arterial blood flow pattern to the hand.
Watson's scaphoid shift test	Scapholunate ligament injury or instability	The examiner places his or her thumb firmly on the patient's volar wrist over the scaphoid tubercle and applies pressure. With the other hand, the examiner moves the patient's wrist from ulnar to radial deviation. A positive test occurs when there is a palpable and painful "clunk." The presence of a clunk alone is not a positive test result. The "clunk" occurs when the scaphoid has dissociated from the lunate because of an SLL tear and hits against the dorsal lip of the radius during the maneuver.
Piano key test	DRUJ instability	The examiner places one hand on the patient's radius and then applies dorsal pressure over the ulnar head with the opposite hand. Compare with contralateral side. Increased motion or pain with motion on injured side is a positive test result.
TFCC grind test	TFCC tear	The examiner extends, axially loads, and ulnarly deviates wrist; a positive test result is pain with this motion.
Elson's test	Extensor tendon central slip rupture or laceration	Rest the patient's hand on a table with the affected finger flexed at the PIP joint over the edge of the table. Hold the PIP joint fixed at 90 degrees as the patient attempts to extend at the PIP joint. If the DIP joint is supple during active extension, the central slip is intact. If the DIP joint is rigid during active extension, the central slip is likely completely ruptured. This occurs because the patient will inadvertently try to extend the finger by using the intact lateral bands and terminal extensor tendon that inserts onto the distal phalanx, thereby making the DIP joint rigid.

DRUJ, Distal radioulnar joint; *FPL,* flexor pollicis longus; *IP,* interphalangeal; *PIP,* proximal interphalangeal; *TFCC,* triangular fibrocartilage complex; *SLL,* scapholunate ligament.

TABLE 4.5	**Differential Diagnosis of Wrist Pain**
Radial-sided wrist pain	Distal radius fracture
	SLL tear
	Arthritis
	Scaphoid fracture
	Extensor tendinitis de Quervain's tenosynovitis
Ulnar-sided wrist pain	TFCC tear
	DRUJ instability
	FCU tendinitis
	Ulnar artery thrombosis
	Cubital tunnel syndrome
	Pisotriquetral arthritis
	ECU tendinitis
	ECU subluxation
	Distal ulnar fracture
	Lunotriquetral tear
	Hook hamate fracture
Dorsal wrist pain	Extensor tendinitis
	Arthritis
	SLL tear
	Scaphoid fracture
	Ganglion cyst
Volar wrist pain	FCU or FCR tendinitis
	Carpal tunnel syndrome
	First CMC joint arthritis

DRUJ, Distal radioulnar joint; *CMC,* carpometacarpal; *ECU,* extensor carpi ulnaris; *FCU,* flexor carpi ulnaris; *FCR,* flexor carpi radialis; *SLL,* scapholunate ligament; *TFCC,* triangular fibrocartilage complex.

TABLE 4.6	**Differential Diagnosis of Finger Pain**
Dorsal finger pain	Joint arthritis
	Extensor tendinitis
	Joint sprain
	Phalanx fracture
Volar finger pain	Trigger finger
	Joint arthritis
	Phalanx fracture

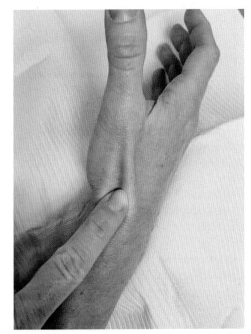

Fig. 4.15 Location of Anatomic Snuffbox. (Original Image.)

Imaging: Fig. 4.16

- Order standard wrist radiographs: posteroanterior (PA), lateral, oblique, AND a scaphoid view (also known as "navicular view" or "ulnar deviation PA view").
- Up to 25% of scaphoid fractures are not visible on initial x-rays.[1]

Additional Imaging

- A magnetic resonance imaging (MRI) scan without contrast is a good way to diagnose an occult scaphoid fracture early. Consider this imaging modality if two or more x-ray series at least 2 weeks apart cannot identify a fracture and the patient has persistent pain and anatomic snuffbox tenderness. An MRI scan can be useful before 3 weeks in high-level athletes or in patients for whom remaining out of work for 2 to 3 weeks while in a splint would be financially detrimental.

- Current literature suggests that MRI scan is 98% sensitive, 99% specific, and 96% accurate for detecting scaphoid fractures.[2]
- An MRI scan with *and* without contrast may be utilized months or years after an injury to assess for the presence of avascular necrosis of the scaphoid.
- A computed topography (CT) scan may be helpful to further characterize a fracture for surgical planning, or to assess for healing when plain x-rays are inconclusive.

Classification

- The majority of scaphoid fractures occur at the scaphoid waist, or middle of the bone. Less often, fractures occur at the proximal pole or distal pole.

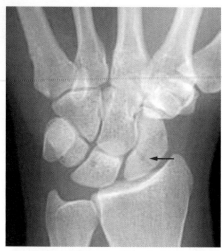

Fig. 4.16 Nondisplaced Scaphoid Fracture.

- Scaphoid fractures are further described as displaced or nondisplaced and by their orientation to the long axis of the scaphoid: transverse, oblique, or vertical oblique.
- Nonunion and avascular necrosis can be a problem with scaphoid fractures. Nondisplaced distal-third scaphoid fractures have the highest likelihood of healing; fractures of the proximal-third of the scaphoid have the highest likelihood of nonunion and avascular necrosis. This is due to the retrograde blood supply to the scaphoid bone which occurs from distal to proximal.

Differential Diagnosis

- Scapholunate ligament (SLL) injury (see p. 132)
- De Quervain's tenosynovitis
- First CMC joint arthritis
- Occult scaphoid fracture: If there is high level of suspicion for a scaphoid fracture but the initial radiographic findings are negative, place the patient into a thumb spica splint and obtain radiographs again 2 weeks after injury. If follow-up radiographic findings are negative but patient is still symptomatic, order MRI scan to evaluate for occult scaphoid fracture or SLL tear.

Initial Management

- Apply a thumb spica splint (Chapter 11, p. 388). Instruct patient to wear at all times.
- Refer the patient to an orthopaedic surgeon for evaluation within 7 to 10 days from injury.

Nonoperative Management

Indications

- Nondisplaced scaphoid waist fractures.
- Nondisplaced distal pole (distal third) scaphoid fractures.
- Nondisplaced scaphoid waist fractures may be treated with thumb spica cast immobilization for 8 to 12 weeks and have an 80% to 90% healing rate if treated within 3 weeks of injury.[1]
- Nondisplaced distal pole scaphoid fractures require thumb spica cast immobilization for 6 to 8 weeks and have a 95% chance of healing.[1]
- Counsel the patient that there is a 5% to 10% risk of nonunion for all scaphoid fractures treated nonoperatively. Encourage smoking cessation.
- See the patient in follow-up clinic at 3- or 4-week intervals to change the cast and obtain repeat radiographs of the fracture to assess healing. Document the presence or absence of tenderness at the anatomic snuffbox at each visit.
- A CT scan may be necessary to confirm healing after 8 to 12 weeks if plain x-rays are inconclusive.
- The fracture is considered healed if there is radiographic evidence of healing AND the patient is nontender to palpation at the anatomic snuffbox and scaphoid tubercle, *or* if a CT scan confirms healing.
- **Rehabilitation.** Once the fracture is healed, the patient can start active wrist ROM. An off-the-shelf wrist support may be used to transition from the cast.
- **Restrictions:** Non–weight bearing is indicated until the fracture is healed and patient is pain free.

> **! CLINICAL ALERT**
>
> Don't miss this injury! If a scaphoid fracture is left undiagnosed or untreated, the patient will develop wrist arthritis within 10 to 15 years after the injury.
> - This pattern of posttraumatic arthritis is called scaphoid nonunion advanced collapse (SNAC) and is similar to the pattern of arthritis associated with an untreated scapholunate ligament tear (see p. 132)
> - If arthritis is present, proceed as if treating the underlying arthritis and not the scaphoid nonunion. Treatment would include a wrist support, activity modification, nonsteroidal antiinflammatory drugs, and possible intraarticular steroid injection.

Operative Management

ICD-10 code: S62.0 Fracture of scaphoid/navicular bone of wrist

CPT codes: 25628 Open reduction, internal fixation (ORIF) scaphoid fracture

Indications
- Displaced fractures of the scaphoid waist and distal pole.
- Proximal pole scaphoid fractures.
- Nondisplaced fractures in patients who are high level athletes or who will benefit from early return to work.

Informed consent and counseling
- There is a risk of scaphoid nonunion even with timely treatment and good surgical fixation. Proximal pole scaphoid fractures have the highest incidence of nonunion.
- Smoking cessation is imperative for fracture healing.
- The patient can expect to be immobilized for approximately 6 weeks, although the type of immobilization depends on the surgeon's preference and on fracture fixation.
- The patient will require approximately 2 months of outpatient hand therapy to restore motion and strength.

Anesthesia
- Regional anesthetic such as a brachial plexus block with sedation or general anesthesia

Patient positioning
- Supine with the arm extended on a hand table
- Nonsterile tourniquet on the brachium

Surgical Procedure
- Hardware: cannulated headless compression screw

Open Reduction, Internal Fixation
The scaphoid bone may be approached over the volar or dorsal wrist depending on the location of the fracture. Approach a proximal pole scaphoid fracture from the dorsal wrist. A longitudinal incision is made over the midline of the wrist joint. The soft tissues and extensor tendons are retracted to protect the **dorsal branches of the superficial sensory radial nerve (SSRN).** The wrist is often flexed to improve visualization of the scaphoid during this procedure.

Distal pole and scaphoid waist fractures are approached from the volar wrist. A small incision is made over the scaphoid tubercle. The wrist is placed into and held in extension to deliver the scaphoid closer to the working surface. The soft tissues are retracted and care is taken to protect the **radial artery** during this approach.

Once the scaphoid is properly exposed and reduced with either approach, a guidewire is placed into the central long axis of the scaphoid bone using fluoroscopic

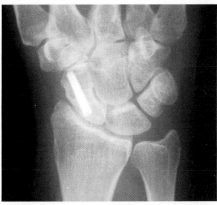

Fig. 4.17 Percutaneous Screw Fixation of a Scaphoid Fracture. (From Knoll VD, Tumble TE: Scaphoid fractures and nonunion. In: Trumble T, Budoff J, Cornwall R, editors, *Hand, elbow, and shoulder: core knowledge in orthopaedics.* Philadelphia, 2006, Mosby, p 123.)

guidance. Screw length is measured with a guide on the wire. A cannulated drill is placed over the wire, followed by an appropriate length cannulated screw. Fluoroscopic images confirm screw length, appropriate placement, and adequate fracture reduction and compression. The wrist capsule is closed with suture and the skin may be closed with 4.0 suture of choice. The patient's wrist is immobilized in a thumb spica splint.

Percutaneous Internal Fixation: Fig. 4.17
Nondisplaced scaphoid fractures that do not require reduction may be treated with a percutaneous screw technique. The scaphoid can be accessed percutaneously from a volar or dorsal approach and the procedure is accomplished in an identical manner to the open compression screw technique.

Estimated Postoperative Course
Postoperative days 10 to 14:
- Sutures are removed and a wound check is performed.
- Radiographs consist of wrist PA, lateral, oblique, and scaphoid views.
- Immobilization: The patient is placed into a removable thumb spica splint.
- *Therapy referral:* Start edema control and gentle finger and wrist ROM only. Non–weight bearing on the operative extremity.
- Note: Some surgeons prefer cast immobilization in a thumb spica cast during the initial postoperative period, especially if the fracture was difficult to reduce or particularly comminuted.

Postoperative 6 weeks:
- The patient returns for a motion check.
- Radiographs consist of wrist PA, lateral, and scaphoid views.
- *Therapy:* If healing is present, progress therapy to more aggressive wrist ROM, wean from the splint, and start gradual weight bearing.
- If no healing is noted, continue gentle ROM and have the patient wear the brace at all times until healing is evident on radiographs.

Postoperative 3 months:
- The patient returns for a motion check.
- Assess for tenderness at the anatomic snuffbox and scaphoid tubercle.
- Radiographs consist of wrist PA, lateral, and scaphoid views.
- If the injury is healed and no pain is noted on examination, release the patient to regular activities without restrictions.
- If no evidence of healing is seen on radiographs, consider use of a bone stimulator and possibly obtain a CT scan to evaluate for healing.
- Nonunion occurs if there has been no healing by 6 months postoperatively.

Board Review

Anatomic snuffbox tenderness is indicative of a scaphoid fracture.

SUGGESTED READINGS

Kawamura K, Chung C: Treatment of scaphoid fractures and non-unions, *J Hand Surg Am* 33(6):988–997, 2008.

Mack GR, Bosse MH, Gelberman RH, et al.: The natural history of scaphoid non-union, *J Bone Joint Surg Am* 66:504–509, 1984.

Pinder RM, Brkljac M, Rix L, Muir L, Brewster M: Treatment of scaphoid nonunion: a systemic review of the existing evidence, *J Hand Surg Am* 40:1797–1805, 2015.

REFERENCES

1. Geissler WB, Slade JF: Fractures of the carpal bones. In Wolfe SW, Hotchkiss RN, Pedersen WC, Kozin SH, editors: *Green's operative hand surgery*, ed 6, Philadelphia, 2011, Elsevier.
2. Ring D, Lozano-Calderon S: Imaging for suspected scaphoid fractures, *J Hand Surg Am* 33A:954–957, 2008.

DISTAL RADIUS FRACTURES

Fractures of the distal radius are one of the most commonly encountered fractures in the upper extremity and frequently occur from a fall on an outstretched hand (FOOSH). The term distal radius fracture refers to all fractures involving the distal aspect of the radius and is an umbrella term of fractures that are dorsally angulated (Colles fracture), volarly angulated (Smiths fracture), involve the radial styloid, or any other portion of the distal end of the radius bone.

History

- FOOSH, fall from height, fall backwards onto hands
- Patient reports generalized wrist pain, pain with motion and weight bearing, swelling, bruising, and possibly wrist deformity

Physical Examination

- Observe generalized wrist edema and/or ecchymosis. A silver fork wrist deformity may be present in which the forearm and wrist have a curve, similar to the back of a fork.
- Pain is present at rest and with all motion, especially wrist extension and flexion.
- There is tenderness to palpation over the distal radius and the radial aspect of the wrist.
- Evaluate sensation in the median and ulnar nerve distributions of the hand.

Imaging: Fig. 4.18

- Order wrist radiographs: PA, lateral, and oblique views.
- MRI or bone scan may be used in rare cases when a fracture is suspected by physical examination but plain radiographs are negative.
- CT scan may be helpful to qualify the severity of fracture comminution and for surgical planning.

Classification

Describe the fracture in terms of displacement, comminution, radial length, surface tilt, and intraarticular step-off (Table 4.7, page 126.). Named fracture patterns are:

- Colles fracture: a distal radius fracture with dorsal comminution and dorsal angulation
- Smith fracture: a distal radius fracture with volar angulation
- Barton fracture: a distal radius fracture with subsequent volar displacement, translation, or subluxation of the carpus with the displaced fragment

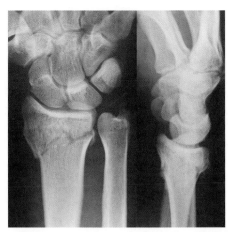

Fig. 4.18 Displaced Distal Radius Fracture. (From Wolf SW, Fernandez DL: Distal radius fractures. In: Green DP, Hotchkiss RN, Pederson WC, Kozin SH, editors, *Green's Operative Hand Surgery*, Ed 5, Philadelphia, 2005, Churchill Livingstone, p 660.)

Differential Diagnosis

- SLL injury
- Scaphoid fracture
- Wrist sprain
- First extensor compartment tendinitis

Initial Management

- Immediate closed reduction is indicated if the fracture is displaced (to be done in a setting where adequate pain control, muscular relaxation, and traction may be provided, such as an emergency department.) Note pre- and postreduction neurovascular examination and order postreduction wrist x-rays.
- Apply a sugar tong splint.
- Refer to an orthopaedic surgeon for evaluation within 7 days from injury.

Nonoperative Management
Indications
- Nondisplaced fractures.
- Stable, reduced fractures.
- Low-demand patients or patients too ill for surgery.
- Nondisplaced fractures require casting for 6 to 8 weeks in a short-arm cast.
- Stable, reduced fractures require 3 weeks in a sugar tong splint with *weekly radiographs* in the splint to ensure that fracture alignment is maintained. If the reduction is lost, surgery is recommended. If fracture reduction is maintained for 3 weeks, transition the patient to a short-arm cast.

- A fracture is considered healed if there is radiographic evidence of healing and the patient is nontender over the fracture site. This usually occurs in approximately 2 to 3 months, depending on the severity of the original injury.
- **Rehabilitation.** Once the fracture is healed, the patient can start active wrist motion and frequently require formal hand therapy. An off-the-shelf wrist brace may be used to transition from the cast.
- **Restrictions:** Non–weight bearing until the fracture is healed and pain free. Typically, this is around 6 to 8 weeks after injury.

Operative Management
ICD-10 code: S52.5 Fracture of lower end of radius
CPT codes: 25607 Open treatment of distal radial extraarticular fracture with internal fixation
25608 Open treatment of distal radial intraarticular fracture with internal fixation of two fragments
25609 Open treatment of distal radial intraarticular fracture with internal fixation of three or more fragments
Indications
- Displaced and/or unstable fractures of the distal radius (see Table 4.7).[1]
Informed consent and counseling
- Smoking cessation is important for fracture healing.
- The patient can expect to be immobilized for approximately 6 weeks, but the type of immobilization (cast vs. splint) will depend on the surgeon's preference and on fracture fixation.
- The patient may require several sessions of outpatient hand therapy to restore motion and strength.
Anesthesia
- Regional anesthetic such as a brachial plexus block with sedation or general anesthesia
Patient positioning
- Supine with the arm extended on a hand table
- Nonsterile tourniquet on the brachium

Surgical Procedure
ORIF of the Distal Radius
The most commonly encountered surgical procedure for fractures of the distal radius is ORIF (Fig. 4.19). Variations of this procedures are vast and sometimes internal fixation is augmented with dorsal approaches for fracture reduction, additional plates, or percutaneous pins. Generally, a volar longitudinal incision is made directly superficial to the flexor carpi radialis (FCR) tendon. An interval is developed between the FCR and the radial artery. Care is taken to identify and protect the **radial artery and**

TABLE 4.7   Classification of Distal Radius Fractures

Radiographic Anatomy	View To Assess	How To Measure	Normal	Acceptable
Radial inclination:	AP or PA view	Angle BC formed by the following two lines: • Line drawn perpendicular to the longitudinal axis of the radius (B) • Line drawn from the tip of the radial styloid process to the ulnar corner of the radius (C)	21–23 degrees	16–28 degrees (can accept 5-degree change either way)

How to Determine Whether a Distal Radius Fracture Meets Operative Criteria. A, Radial inclination. B, Volar tilt. C, Radial height. (Adapted from Baratz ME, Larsen CF: Wrist and hand measurements and classification schemes. In: Gilula LA, Yin Y, editors. *Imaging of the wrist and hand,* Philadelphia, Saunders, 1996.)

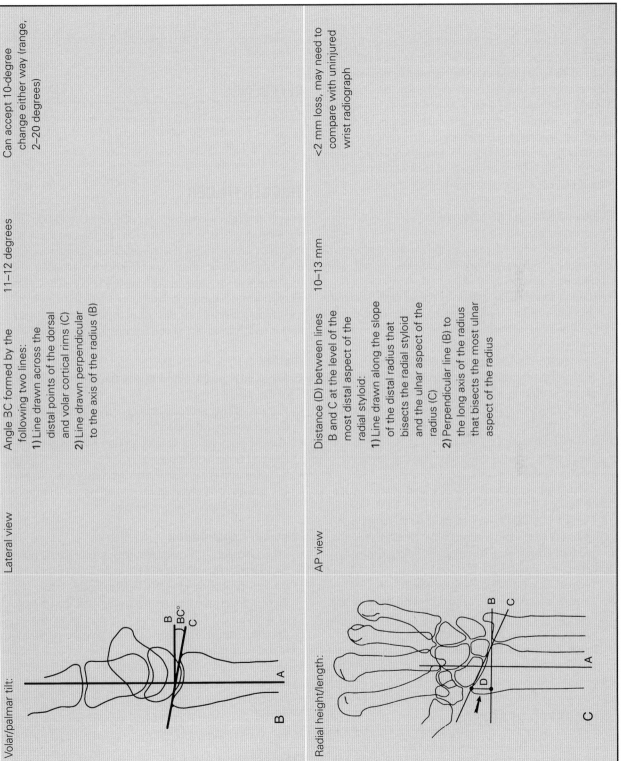

Volar/palmar tilt:	Lateral view	Angle BC formed by the following two lines: 1) Line drawn across the distal points of the dorsal and volar cortical rims (C) 2) Line drawn perpendicular to the axis of the radius (B)	11–12 degrees	Can accept 10-degree change either way (range, 2–20 degrees)
Radial height/length:	AP view	Distance (D) between lines B and C at the level of the most distal aspect of the radial styloid: 1) Line drawn along the slope of the distal radius that bisects the radial styloid and the ulnar aspect of the radius (C) 2) Perpendicular line (B) to the long axis of the radius that bisects the most ulnar aspect of the radius	10–13 mm	<2 mm loss, may need to compare with uninjured wrist radiograph

AP, Anteroposterior; PA, posteroanterior.

median nerve. Blunt deep dissection is carried down to the pronator quadratus muscle, which is sharply incised on its radial border and elevated off the periosteum of the radius to expose the fracture. Sometimes the brachioradialis tendon insertion must be released to decrease the deforming forces on the fracture. The fracture is provisionally reduced and a volar plate and screws are used to hold the reduction. Intraoperative fluoroscopy confirms reduction and hardware placement. The pronator quadratus is frequently closed with suture followed by closure of the skin with a 4.0 suture of choice. The patient is placed in a volar short-arm splint postoperatively.

Estimated Postoperative Course

Postoperative days 10 to 14:
- Sutures are removed, and a wound check is performed.
- Possible radiographs include wrist PA, lateral, and oblique views.
- Immobilization: The patient is placed into a removable spica splint. Some surgeons prefer cast immobilization in a short-arm cast during the initial postoperative period, especially if the fracture was difficult to reduce or especially comminuted.
- *Therapy referral*: Initiated if patient is in a splint. Start edema control and gentle finger and wrist motion. Some clinicians start therapy as soon as 3 to 5 days postoperatively.

Postoperative 6 weeks:
- The patient returns for either cast removal or a motion check.
- Radiographs consist of wrist PA, lateral, and navicular views.
- *Therapy:* If healing is present, progress therapy to more aggressive wrist motion, wean the patient from the splint, and start gradual weight bearing and strengthening.

Postoperative 3 months:
- The patient returns for a motion check.
- Assess for tenderness to palpation at the fracture site.
- Radiographs consist of wrist PA, lateral, and oblique views.
- If the fracture is healed and no pain is noted on examination, release the patient to regular activities without restrictions.

SUGGESTED READINGS

Alluri RK, Hill JR, Ghiassi A: Distal radius fractures: approaches, indications, and techniques, *J Hand Surg Am* 41:845–854, 2016.

Wolfe SW: Distal radius fractures. In Wolfe SW, Hotchkiss RN, Pedersen WC, Kozin SH, editors: *Green's operative hand surgery*, ed 6, Philadelphia, 2011, Elsevier, pp 561–638.

REFERENCE

1. Nesbitt KS, Failla JM, Clifford L: Assessment of instability factors in adult distal radius fractures, *J Hand Surg Am* 29:1128–1138, 2004.

TRIGGER FINGER

Trigger finger is a commonly encountered condition of the hand. It affects about 2.6% of the population and 4% to 10% of patients with diabetes mellitus.[1] Trigger finger is an inflammatory condition of the flexor tendon sheath that occurs in the palm at the level of the A1 pulley. The tenosynovium becomes inflamed, irritated, and enlarged and causes a mechanical clicking or locking during finger flexion and extension. The condition is frequently painful.

History
- Reported pain and tenderness in the palm at the base of the affected digit
- Painful locking and/or catching of the digit, but painless locking can also occur
- May be related to a specific period of overuse, but also can occur insidiously
- Symptoms may be worse after a period of inactivity such as on awakening in the morning and improve throughout the day, or be constant

Physical Examination
- There is tenderness to palpation directly over the A1 pulley, located at the volar base of the finger just proximal to the metacarpophalangeal (MCP) joint flexion crease.
- Place a finger over the A1 pulley and ask the patient to flex and extend the digit in an attempt to reproduce the triggering. Passive flexion may be required to feel the catching.
- There may be a palpable nodularity on the flexor tendon at the level of the A1 pulley.

Imaging
- Not necessary for diagnosis.

Classification: Fig. 4.20
- Grade 1: painful tenderness at the A1 pulley

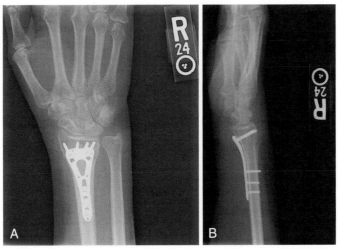

Fig. 4.19 Surgical fixation of a displaced distal radius fracture with a volar locking plate. Posteroanterior (**A**) and lateral (**B**) views.

- Grade 2: uneven finger movements, triggering, unlocks by self
- Grade 3: locking, triggering finger, unlocks by outside force
- Grade 4: fixed, irreducible flexion at the PIP joint

Differential Diagnosis

- Arthritis of the MCP or PIP joint
- Extensor tendon sagittal band injury or snapping
- Dupuytren's disease
- Infectious flexor tenosynovitis—Clinical Alert

> **! CLINICAL ALERT**
>
> Infectious flexor tenosynovitis is a condition that all practitioners should be aware of as urgent treatment is necessary. Infectious flexor tenosynovitis is an infection of the flexor tendon sheath and is distinguishable from trigger finger by the history and physical examination findings. Please see p. 132 for more information on infectious flexor tenosynovitis. If infectious flexor tenosynovitis is suspected, an urgent referral to a surgeon for intravenous antibiotics and incision and drainage is indicated.

Initial Management

- If symptoms are mild, intermittent, AND have been present for less than 2 to 3 weeks, consider a period of activity modification, ice or heat, and use of nonsteroidal antiinflammatory medication, if appropriate.

- **Patient Education.** Trigger finger is a condition caused by inflammation of the lining of the flexor tendon. It can affect any digit and may occur in multiple. Treatment involves use of cortisone injections into the flexor tendon sheath or surgery.

Nonoperative Management

Corticosteroid injection into the tendon sheath (see p. 177)

- A cortisone injection into the flexor tendon sheath is considered a good first line of management option to reduce inflammation and eliminate painful locking and triggering.
- It may take several days to weeks for symptoms to completely resolve after injection. Long-term success rate after one cortisone injection has been reported as 45% and may be higher during the first 1 to 2 years after injection based on previous studies.[2]
- If a trigger finger recurs after injection, the decision to administer additional cortisone injections should be based on the length of time that has passed since the previous injection, the degree of relief the patient experienced, as well as the patient's social situation or medical comorbidities that could preclude surgery. Occasionally, a second "booster" cortisone injection may be indicated if symptoms are improved but not completely resolved within 3 to 6 weeks of the first injection.
- 50% of patients who require and receive repeat cortisone injections have a year or more of symptom relief.[3]
- Trigger finger is more common in patients with diabetes mellitus. A cortisone injection may cause a

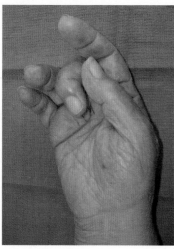

Fig. 4.20 Locked Trigger Finger. (From Wood MM, Ingari J: Trigger finger. In: Miller MD, Hart JA, MacKnight JM, editors, *Essential orthopaedics*, Philadelphia, 2010, Saunders, p 350.)

transient increase in blood glucose in patients with diabetes mellitus. Thoughtful patient selection and close glucose monitoring is recommended.

- Surgery is considered highly successful and is indicated if the patient has failed one or more cortisone injections.
- Splinting is generally contraindicated because it has been proven not effective and may lead to finger stiffness.

Operative Management

Codes

ICD-10 code: M65.3 Trigger finger

CPT code: 26055 Tendon sheath incision (A1 pulley release)

Indications

- Persistent painful triggering despite conservative measures (including cortisone injections)
- Grade 4 trigger finger

Informed consent and counseling

- Pertinent risks include finger stiffness, wound sensitivity, and infection. Postoperative finger motion (with or without guidance from a hand therapist), scar massage when appropriate, and proper wound care is paramount.
- Total recovery time is about 2 to 3 weeks to account for a period of wound healing and reduction in postoperative discomfort and wound sensitivity.

Anesthesia

- Local, or regional anesthetic with sedation for multiple digits

Patient positioning

- Supine with the arm extended on a hand table
- Nonsterile tourniquet on the brachium

Surgical Procedure

Open A1 Pulley Release

A local field anesthetic is administered prior the procedure, or a regional block may be provided by an anesthesiologist based on surgeon preference or involvement of multiple digits. Once anesthetized, a small approximately 1-cm incision is made in the palm overlying the A1 pulley. The soft tissues are retracted and the adjacent digital nerves and arteries are protected to expose underlying the flexor tendon sheath. The A1 pulley is identified and sharply incised in its entirety. Distally, the A2 pulley should be preserved to prevent bowstringing. After release of the pulley the finger is actively or passively placed through ROM to ensure no additional areas of triggering. The wound is closed with a 4.0 suture of choice and a light dressing that allows for finger motion is applied.

Percutaneous A1 pulley release is an additional surgical technique in which the A1 pulley is similarly sharply incised percutaneously using a large needle such as a tapered 18 g.

Estimated Postoperative Course

Postoperative days 10 to 14:

- Sutures are removed and a wound check is performed.
- A therapy referral may be indicated in some patients who present with postoperative edema or stiffness. Prescribe edema control, finger and wrist stretching and motion, and scar massage, as needed.

Postoperative week 4:

- The patient may return for final motion and wound check.

SUGGESTED READINGS

Sato ES, Gomes Dos Santos JB, Belloti JC, et al.: Treatment of trigger finger: randomized clinical trial comparing the methods of corticosteroid injection, percutaneous release and open surgery, *Rheumatology* 51(1):93–99, 2012.

REFERENCES

1. Griggs SM, Weiss AP, Lane LB, Schwenker C, Akelman E, Sachar K: Treatment of trigger finger in patients with diabetes mellitus, *J Hand Surg Am* 20(5):787–789, 1995.

2. Wojahn RD, Foeger MC, Gelberman RH, Calfee RP: Long-term outcomes following a single corticosteroid injection for trigger finger, *J Bone Joint Surg Am* 96:1849–1854, 2014.
3. Dardas AZ, VandenBerg J, Shen T, Gleberman RH, Calfee RP: Long-term effectiveness of repeat corticosteroid injections for trigger finger, *J Hand Surg Am* 42:227–235, 2017.

PYOGENIC FLEXOR TENOSYNOVITIS

Pyogenic flexor tenosynovitis, which is an infection of the flexor tendon sheath (and also known as infectious flexor tenosynovitis), is an orthopaedic emergency. This condition can be difficult to diagnose clinically but should always be suspected in a patient presenting with severe and rapid-onset finger pain isolated to one digit. Physical examination is paramount for diagnosis and advanced imaging should be reserved for cases of equivocal presentation. Infectious flexor tenosynovitis does not respond to oral antibiotics and usually requires both administration of IV antibiotics and surgical drainage. If missed or treated inappropriately, flexor tenosynovitis can lead to permanent necrosis of the flexor tendon and even loss of the digit. The most common causative organism is *Staphylococcus aureus*.

History
- Extreme finger pain that develops over hours to days.
- Usually involves only one digit with pain and tenderness in the palm at the base of the digit.
- Frequently the patient will have had a previous history of some type of laceration, surgical incision, or penetrating injury prior to symptom onset; occasionally an infection can seed from a secondary site or develop insidiously.
- Patient reports severe, constant pain in the digit that is worse with motion or palpation.

Physical Examination
- Evaluate the affected hand for nearby wounds, lacerations, abscesses, or abrasions.
- **Kanavel's signs:** There are four hallmark physical examination findings that are diagnostic for infection within the flexor tendon sheathe. The specificity and sensitivity of these signs have not been validated to date, but are widely considered to be the most useful clinical tool for diagnosis.[1] All four signs must be present to be conclusive of the diagnosis:
  1. Finger is held in a flexed posture
  2. Intense pain with passive extension
  3. Fusiform swelling involving entire finger
  4. Tenderness along the course of the flexor tendon sheath proximally in the palm and distally along the finger
- Always palpate the radial and ulnar aspects of the MCP joint, PIP joint, and distal interphalangeal (DIP) joint to evaluate for tenderness that could indicate a concurrent septic joint.

> **! CLINICAL ALERT**
>
> Finger pain and swelling alone does not portend to a diagnosis of an infection in the flexor tendon sheath. An examiner MUST perform all four Kanavel tests for diagnosis.

Imaging
- Not always necessary for diagnosis if Kanavel's signs are present
- An urgent nonvascular ultrasound or MRI of the finger can help to identify increased fluid within the flexor tendon sheath or can evaluate for cellulitis, septic arthritis, or localized abscess that can be confused with a flexor tendon sheath infection.

Differential Diagnosis
- Abscess
- Cellulitis
- Septic arthritis
- Trigger finger
- Inflammatory flexor tenosynovitis. Similar in presentation to trigger finger but without locking or catching. Can be observed in patients with autoimmune disease such as rheumatoid arthritis. Generally has a less severe and more gradual onset than infectious flexor tenosynovitis.

Initial Management
- Once the diagnosis of infectious flexor tenosynovitis is suspected or confirmed, apply a resting hand splint and refer the patient for immediate surgical evaluation by an orthopedist or hand surgery specialist.
- Check patient's vital signs. Order a complete blood count, erythrocyte sedimentation rate, and C-reactive protein if possible. Immediate surgical evaluation is prudent and obtaining laboratory work should not delay referral. Laboratory results are not necessary for diagnosis but baseline values can serve as markers for improvement postoperatively.

Operative Management

ICD-10 code: M65.04 Abscess of tendon sheath, hand, or M65.14 Other infective tenosynovitis, hand

CPT Code: 26020 Incision and drainage of flexor tendon sheath

Indications

Confirmed or suspected flexor tendon sheath infection

Informed consent and counseling

- An infection of the flexor tendon sheath is a surgical emergency that requires immediate care.
- Hospital admission is frequently necessary for administration of IV antibiotics over 24 hours.
- This condition can result in significant postoperative finger stiffness. A referral for hand therapy is almost always necessary.

Anesthesia

- Local anesthetic, or general anesthesia

Patient positioning

- Supine with the affected hand extended onto a hand table

Surgical Procedure

Incision and Drainage of Flexor Tendon Sheath

Consider withholding preoperative antibiotics to obtain accurate intraoperative cultures. Access to the flexor tendon sheath can be accomplished in a minimally invasive manner using a two-incision technique. This is only possible if no additional areas of abscess are present that require more thorough incision and drainage. Once anesthetized, an incision is made in the volar palm overlying the affected finger A1 pulley. A second incision is made over the volar distal phalanx at the distal end of the flexor tendon sheath. Obtain cultures if indicated and administer a broad-spectrum IV antibiotic. A pediatric feeding tube or angiocath may be inserted into the flexor tendon sheath at the proximal incision. Copious irrigation with saline is performed until fluids are clear. Incisions may be left open with gauze packing to allow for additional drainage and can be removed 1 or 2 days postoperatively. Apply a bulky dressing and a resting hand splint.

Estimated Postoperative Recovery Course

Postoperative day 1:

- Reevaluate patient to ensure subjective improvement in pain and check the wound to ensure objective improvement in redness and edema. Document findings and neurovascular status.
- Consider rechecking labwork to compare to baseline levels if they were obtained.

Postoperative day 2:

- Recheck patient as above to ensure improvement.
- Remove drains and provide wound care. Change dressings and reapply splint.
- Check cultures and labwork; adjust IV medication if organism is known and consider transitioning to oral medication. Infectious disease specialists can assist in this matter.

Postoperative day 3–5:

- Recheck patient to ensure improvement.
- Refer to hand therapy for early motion and wound care.
- Consider discontinuing splint or starting part-time use.

Postoperative week 1–2:

- Recheck patient as needed to ensure improvement.
- Remove sutures, if present, provide care, and check motion.

Postoperative week 3–4:

- Continue therapy until motion is improved and determine need for any ongoing treatment.

Postoperative 1–2 months:

- Therapy may be necessary for 1 to 2 months after an infection, depending on its severity. Monitor patient as needed.

SUGGESTED READINGS

McDonald LS, Bavaro MF, Hofmeister EP, Kroonen LT: Hand infections, *J Hand Surg Am* 30(8):1403–1412, 2011.

Neviaser JR: Closed tendon sheath irrigation for pyogenic flexor tenosynovitis, *J Hand Surg Am* 3(5):462–466, 1978.

Gialdi AM, Malay S, Chung KC: Management of acute pyogenic flexor tenosynovitis: literature review and current trends, *J Hand Surg Eur* 40(7):720–728, 2015.

REFERENCE

1. Kennedy CD, Huang JI, Hanel DP: Kanavel's signs and pyogenic flexor tenosynovitis, *Clin Orthop Relat Res* 474:280–284, 2016.

SCAPHOLUNATE LIGAMENT INJURY

The SLL is a very important stabilizing structure within the wrist. If it is injured, the carpal bones are subjected to abnormal motion and patterns of wear. Injury to the SLL is one of the most difficult conditions to identify and treat in the wrist. Nevertheless, if the injury is missed or inappropriately managed, the consequences to the patient can be devastating. Progressive loss of wrist motion, chronic pain, edema, and wrist arthritis will develop if this condition is not treated. A healthcare provider should have a high level of suspicion for this injury when a patient presents with a "wrist sprain."

History

- FOOSH or impact with wrist in extension.
- The patient reports dorsal wrist pain and pain with weight bearing with the wrist in extension (push-up position).
- The patient may report wrist weakness with lifting or grip.
- In later stages, the patient may report a remote injury and development of wrist stiffness.

Physical Examination

- Affected wrist may appear normal or may have dorsal wrist edema.
- Tenderness to palpation at the scapholunate (SL) interval. This interval is located in the soft spot on the dorsal wrist 1 cm distal to Lister's tubercle in the space between the third and fourth extensor compartments (Fig. 4.21).
- Positive Watson's scaphoid shift test (Fig. 4.22).

- **Watson's Scaphoid Shift Test.** This special test evaluates for SLL instability. The examiner places their thumb firmly on the patient's volar wrist over the scaphoid tubercle and applies pressure. With the other hand, the examiner moves the patient's wrist from ulnar to radial deviation. A positive test occurs when there is a palpable and painful "clunk." The presence of a clunk alone is not a positive test result. The "clunk" occurs when the scaphoid has dissociated from the lunate because of an SLL tear and hits against the dorsal lip of the radius during the maneuver.
- Watson's scaphoid shift test has a sensitivity of 48% and a specificity of 67% for detecting SL injuries. This test should be compared to the uninjured side.[1]

Imaging

- Order wrist radiographs: PA, lateral, and obliques and bilateral clenched fist views.
- The clenched fist view is obtained by the patient actively clenching the fist while taking the x-ray image. This causes force across the radiocarpal joint and drives the capitate into the SL interval. If the SLL is torn, the force created by the capitate with cause a visible gap between the scaphoid and the lunate bone. A wide SL interval occurs when there is a gap of more than 3 to 4 mm; this must be compared with the contralateral side as normally wide physiologic variants can exist (Fig. 4.23).
- The lateral view may show an SL angle greater than 60 degrees (an increased SL angle is also known as dorsal

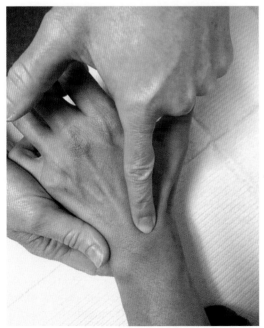

Fig. 4.21 Surface anatomy of the scapholunate interval, located between the third and fourth extensor compartments at the level of the radiocarpal joint. (Original image.)

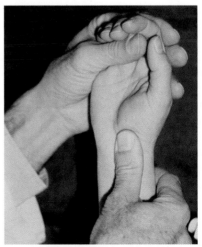

Fig. 4.22 Watson Maneuver. (From Hastings H: Arthrodesis, partial and complete. In: Green DP, Hotchkiss RN, Pederson WC, Kozin SH, editors, *Green's operative hand surgery*, Ed 5, Philadelphia, 2005, Churchill Livingstone, p 493.)

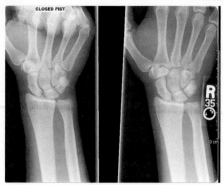

Fig. 4.23 Clenched fist view with widening of the scapholunate (SL) interval *(left)* and nonstress posteroanterior view with a normal SL interval *(right)*. (From Rynders SD, Chhabra AB: Scapholunate ligament injury. In: Miller MD, Hart JA, MacKnight JM, editors, *Essential orthopaedics*, Philadelphia, 2010, Saunders, p 306.)

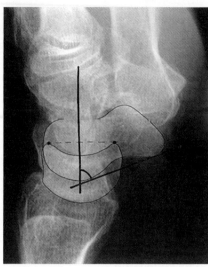

Fig. 4.24 Radiograph Showing an Abnormal Scapholunate Angle. (From Garcia-Elias M, Geissler WB: Carpal instability. In: Green DP, Hotchkiss RN, Pederson WC, Kozin SH, editors, *Green's operative hand surgery*, Ed 5, Philadelphia, 2005, Churchill Livingstone, p 558.)

intercalated segment instability or DISI deformity). A normal SL angle is 30 to 60 degrees (Fig. 4.24).
- The PA view may reveal a scaphoid ring sign (Fig. 4.25).

Additional Imaging
- MRI can help to identify SL injuries, but sensitivity and specificity vary depending on the quality of MRI and the expertise and experience of the radiologist. Recent studies have noted a 71% sensitivity, 88% specificity, and 84% accuracy.[2] CT arthrography can also be helpful with a slightly higher sensitivity (95%) and a similar specificity (86%).[3]
- The gold standard diagnostic tool to identify a SLL tear is wrist arthroscopy.

Classification
- The SLL has three bands: volar, interosseous, and dorsal. The thickest and most supportive portion is the dorsal band.
- Patterns of Instability Resulting from Scapholunate Ligament Injury

Predynamic Instability	Partial SL tear (detected by MRI or wrist arthroscopy) Normal stress x-rays
Dynamic Instability	Partial or complete SL tear Wide SL interval on stress x-rays ONLY
Static Instability	Complete SL tear SL interval greater than 3 mm on nonstress views SL angle >60° on lateral view

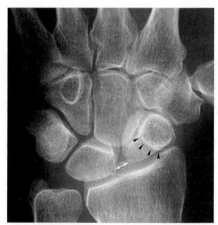

Fig. 4.25 Scaphoid ring sign *(arrowheads). Double arrow,* SL interval. (From Garcia-Elias M, Geissler WB: Carpal instability. In: Green DP, Hotchkiss RN, Pederson WC, Kozin SH, editors, *Green's operative hand surgery*, Ed 5, Philadelphia, 2005, Churchill Livingstone, p 558.)

- Scapholunate Advanced Collapse (SLAC) (Fig. 4.26): This term refers to a predictable pattern of osteoarthritis (OA) of the wrist that results from a chronic untreated SL tear. The radioscaphoid joint is first affected, followed by the lunatocapitate joint (Fig. 4.27):

> **! CLINICAL ALERT**
>
> If a scapholunate ligament tear is left undiagnosed or untreated, the patient will develop wrist arthritis within 10 to 15 years after the injury.

Stage 1: radial styloid arthritis and radial styloid beaking
Stage 2: radiocarpal joint arthritis
Stage 3: capitolunate interface arthritis
Stage 4: pan-carpal arthritis

Differential Diagnosis

- Kienbock disease
- Acute fracture of scaphoid
- de Quervain's tenosynovitis
- Gout or pseudogout
- Wrist tendinitis (flexor or extensor)

Initial Management

- Immobilize in a volar short-arm splint.
- Referral to an orthopaedic surgeon to be seen within 7 to 10 days from injury.
- **Patient Education.** A tear of the SLL creates instability within the wrist joint. If left undiagnosed or untreated, it can result in a predictable pattern of early-onset wrist arthritis.

Nonoperative Management

Indications

- Conservative management is reserved for patients with partial tears or chronic complete tears with evidence of static instability, arthritis, or patients too ill for surgery.
- Partial tears: Cast immobilization for 4 to 6 weeks is indicated. If immobilization does not provide relief, consider radiocarpal wrist injection.
- Chronic injuries (>6 months) respond poorly to surgical repair. Consider symptom control with splinting and radiocarpal cortisone injections as needed. Patients should be counseled that arthritic changes and loss of motion will be expected.
- Salvage procedures for symptomatic injuries that are identified late (chronic injuries) include proximal row carpectomy and limited or total wrist

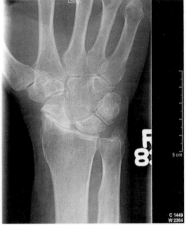

Fig. 4.26 Scapholunate Advanced Collapse. (From Rynders SD, Chhabra AB: Scapho-lunate ligament injury. In: Miller MD, Hart JA, MacKnight JM, editors, *Essential orthopaedics*, Philadelphia, 2010, Saunders, p 307.)

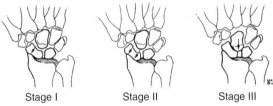

Stage I	Stage II	Stage III

Fig. 4.27 Stages of scapholunate advanced collapse *(arrows)*. Note with advancing stage, capitate migrates proximally. (From Shin AY, Moran SL: Carpal instability including dislocation. In: Trumble T, Budoff J, Cornwall R, editors, *Hand, elbow, and shoulder: core knowledge in orthopaedics*, Philadelphia, 2006, Mosby, p 151.)

fusion (for stages 3 and 4). Surgery should be suggested only after conservative treatment has failed.

Operative Management

ICD-10 code: S63.5 Sprain of carpal ligament
CPT codes: 29840 Diagnostic wrist arthroscopy
29846 Wrist arthroscopy with SLL débridement
25320 Capsulorrhaphy or reconstruction, wrist, any method (e.g., capsulodesis or ligament repair for carpal instability)

Indications

- Acute/subacute SLL tear

Informed consent and counseling

- Surgery will result in decreased wrist ROM but it will prevent arthritis and pain.

- The patient can expect to be immobilized for approximately 3 months.
- Approximately 1 to 2 months of outpatient hand therapy will be needed to restore motion and strength after immobilization.
  ### Anesthesia
- Regional anesthetic such as a brachial plexus block with sedation, or general anesthesia
  ### Patient positioning
- Supine with the arm extended on a hand table
- Nonsterile tourniquet on the brachium

Surgical Procedures

Surgical treatment techniques are numerous and ever-evolving. Treatment options are frequently determined by the degree of SL tear, type of instability present, and length of time since injury. Initial surgery may involve a diagnostic wrist arthroscopy with débridement of the SLL in order to directly visualize the ligament, qualify the degree tearing, and identify any cartilage loss. Treatment options for a known SL tear may include pinning of the SL interval, direct repair of the SLL, and ligament reconstruction techniques with tendon grafts or implants with or without a dorsal capsulodesis (a portion of dorsal wrist capsule is used to tether the scaphoid and prevent it from subluxing).

Estimated Postoperative Recovery Course

- The postoperative course depends on the type and extent of the procedure.
- If the SL is pinned, the patient is usually casted, and the pins are removed 6 to 8 weeks postoperatively.
- All procedures require postoperative rehabilitation with a hand therapist.

SUGGESTED READINGS

Shin AY, Moran SL: Carpal instability including dislocation. In Trumble TE, Budoff JE, Cornwall R, editors: *Hand, elbow, and shoulder: core knowledge in orthopaedics*, Philadelphia, 2006, Mosby, pp 139–176.

Walsh J, Berger R, Cooney W: Current status of scapholunate interosseous ligament injuries, *J Am Acad Orthop Surg* 10(1):32–42, 2002.

Watson HK, Ballet FL: The SLAC wrist: scapholunate advanced collapse pattern of degenerative arthritis, *J Hand Surg Am* 9(3):358–365, 1984.

REFERENCES

1. Ruston J, Konan E, Sorene E: Diagnostic accuracy of clinical examination and magnetic resonance imaging for common articular wrist pathology, *Acta Orthop Belg* 79(4):375–380, 2013.
2. Kuo CE, Wolfe SW: Scapholunate instability: current concepts in diagnosis and management, *J Hand Surg Am* 33:998–1013, 2008.
3. Bille B, Harley B, Cohen H: A comparison of CT arthrography of the wrist to findings during wrist arthroscopy, *J Hand Surg Am* 32:834–841, 2007.

KIENBOCK DISEASE

Kienbock disease is a condition of avascular necrosis of the lunate bone in the wrist. It is more common in men than in women and usually affects patients 20 to 40 years old. The etiology of Kienbock's disease is generally unknown but thought to be related to increased stress loading across the lunate, possibly in the setting of interosseous vascular abnormalities. One predisposing factor is thought to be the presence of ulnar negative variance in which the distal radius is anatomically longer than the distal ulna, thereby creating more loading across the radiolunate joint. Kienbock's disease generally presents as a painful, progressive, and unilateral loss of wrist motion and can be difficult to diagnose in early stages on plain radiographs. Treatment is based on symptoms and stage of the disease and prognosis is very difficult to predict.

History

- Pain over the dorsum of the wrist
- Possible swelling in the wrist
- Weakness in grip
- Pain with motion, eventual pain at rest
- Wrist stiffness

Physical Examination

- Tenderness to palpation directly over the lunate
- Decreased motion with advancing disease
- Possible reduction in grip strength

Imaging: Fig. 4.28

- Order wrist radiographs: PA, lateral, and oblique views.
- Evaluate for negative ulnar variance (defined as the distal ulna being shorter than the distal radius).

Additional Imaging

- Consider MRI if the diagnosis unclear on radiographs and to assist in staging the disease.

Classification

The Lichtman Classification System has long been used to stage disease and offer assistance in determining appropriate treatment options (Table 4.8). More recently, Bain and Begg have developed a classification and treatment algorithm that utilizes wrist arthroscopy to characterize the integrity of the cartilage joint surfaces in order to offer treatment recommendations

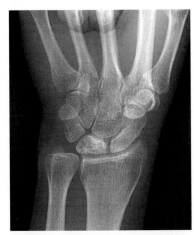

Fig. 4.28 Radiograph of Stage IIIa Kienbock Disease. The lunate shows increased sclerosis and collapse. (From Thaller JB: Kienbock's disease. In: Miller MD, Hart JA, MacKnight JM, editors, *Essential orthopaedics*, Philadelphia, 2010, Saunders, p 318.)

(Fig. 4.29). Currently both systems are valid and can be used simultaneously to assist with Kienbock disease staging and treatment recommendations.[1]

Differential Diagnosis

- Ulnocarpal impaction syndrome (ulna abuts the lunate and causes pain and degenerative changes over time)
- Avascular necrosis of the scaphoid (Preiser's disease)
- SLL injury
- Lunate fracture
- Ganglion cyst

Initial Management

- Provide the patient with an off-the-shelf wrist splint to wear for support and refer to an orthopaedic hand specialist. Nonsteroidal antiinflammatory drugs (NSAIDs) may be used for pain relief.

Nonoperative Management

Indications

May be considered in stage 1 disease but progression is common.

Operative Management

ICD-10 Code: M93.1
CPT Codes: 29840 Diagnostic wrist arthroscopy
29845 Wrist arthroscopy with complete synovectomy
25215 Proximal row carpectomy
25350 Radial shortening osteotomy
25800 Total wrist arthrodesis
25820 Limited wrist arthrodesis

TABLE 4.8	Lichtman Osseous Classification of Kienböck Disease		
Disease Stage	**X-Ray Findings**	**MRI Findings**	**Treatment**
I	Normal	T1 Signal: decreased T2 Signal: variable	Immobilization
II	Lunate sclerosis	T1 Signal: decreased T2 Signal: variable	Ulnar shortening (negative ulnar variance) Capitate shortening (positive ulnar variance)
IIIA	Lunate collapse	T1 Signal: decreased T2 Signal: variable	Same as stage II, and/or revascularization with dorsal pedicle
IIIB	Lunate and carpal collapse Scaphoid rotation (RS angle >60 degrees)	T1 Signal: decreased T2 Signal: usually decreased	Reconstructive procedure STT or SC fusion ± lunate excision (if fragmented), or PRC
IV	Pancarpal arthritis KDAC	T1 Signal: decreased T2 Signal: decreased	Salvage procedure (TWF, TWA, or PRC)

KDAC, Kienböck disease advanced collapse; *PRC*, proximal row carpectomy; *RS*, radioscaphoid; *SC*, scaphocapitate; STT, scaphotrapezio-trapezoid; *TWA*, total wrist arthroplasty; *TWF*, total wrist fusion.
From Lichtman DM, Pientka WF, Bain GI: Kienbock disease: moving forward. *J Hand Surg Am*, 41:630–638, 2016.

Grade	Description	Recommendation
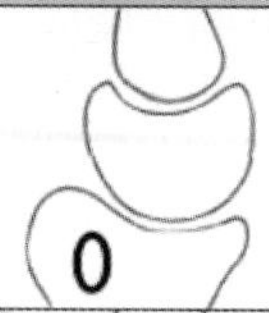 0	**Grade 0** 0 Nonfunctional surface	Joint levelling procedure Forage ± bone graft Vascularized bone graft
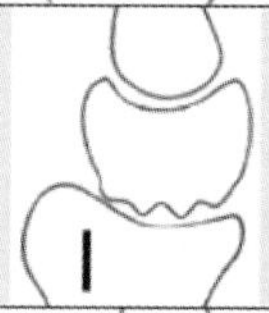 1	**Grade 1** 1 Nonfunctional surface - Proximal lunate	RSL fusion PRC Osteochondral grafting
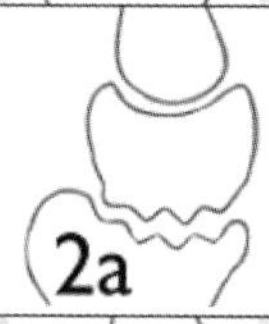 2a	**Grade 2a** 2 Nonfunctional surfaces - Proximal lunate and lunate facet of radius	RSL fusion
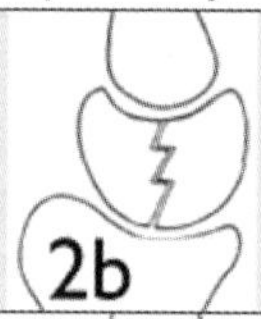 2b	**Grade 2b** 2 Nonfunctional surfaces - Proximal and distal lunate	PRC Lunate replacement Capitate Lengthening
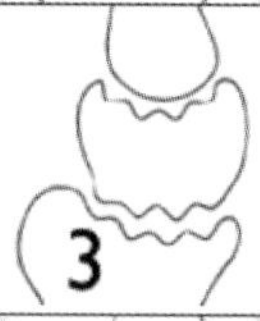 3	**Grade 3** 3 Nonfunctional surfaces - Capitate surface usually preserved	Hemiarthroplasty (SC fusion if radial column intact)
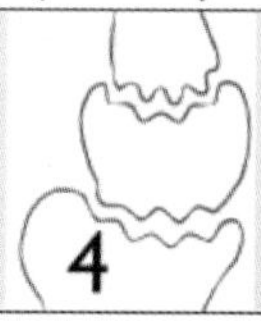 4	**Grade 4** All 4 articular surfaces are nonfunctional	Total wrist fusion Total wrist arthroplasty (SC fusion if radial column intact)

Synovectomy is performed in all patients.

PRC, proximal row carpectomy; RSL fusion, radioscapholunate fusion; SC fusion, scaphocapitate fusion; can be considered if the central column is nonfunctional, but the radial column is intact.

Fig. 4.29 Articular-Based Approach to Kienbock's Disease from Bain and Begg. (Modified from Bain GI, Begg M: Arthroscopic assessment and classification of Kienbock's disease, *Tech Hand Up Extrem Surg* 10(1):8–13, 2009.)

Indications: Table 4.8

Informed consent and counseling

- Even with appropriate treatment and good surgical technique Kienbock disease that is initially managed with bone shortening procedures or vascularized bone grafting may progress and require additional definitive surgical treatment such as proximal row carpectomy or limited or total wrist fusion.
- Smoking cessation is imperative for healing.

Anesthesia

- Regional anesthetic such as a brachial plexus block with sedation or general anesthesia

Patient positioning

- Supine with the arm extended on a hand table
- Nonsterile tourniquet on the brachium

Surgical Procedures

Multiple surgical procedures are used with varying indications. These include joint leveling procedures, vascularized bone grafting, proximal row carpectomy, and partial or total wrist fusions. Surgical techniques and indications are still evolving. The type of surgery indicated will depend upon factors such as disease severity, patient age, and occupation or activity level.

SUGGESTED READINGS

Allan CH, Joshi A, Lichtman DM: Kienbock's disease: diagnosis and treatment, *J Am Acad Orthop Surg* 9:128–136, 2001.

Geissler WB, Slade JF: Fractures of the carpal bones. In Wolfe SW, Hotchkiss RN, Pedersen WC, Kozin SH, editors: *Green's operative hand surgery*, ed 6, Philadelphia, 2011, Elsevier.

Innes L, Strauch RJ: Systematic review of the treatment of Kienbock's disease in its early and late stages, *J Hand Surg Am* 35(5):713–717, 2010.

Lichtman DM, Pientka WF, Bain GI: Kienbock disease: moving forward, *J Hand Surg Am* 41:630–638, 2016.

REFERENCE

1. Lichtman DM, Pientka WF, Bain GI: Kienbock disease: moving forward, *J Hand Surg Am* 41:630–638, 2016.

TRIANGULAR FIBROCARTILAGE COMPLEX TEAR

The triangular fibrocartilage complex (TFCC) is a group of structures located on the ulnar side of the wrist between the distal ulna and carpus. The TFCC is made up of a fibrocartilage disc, the volar and dorsal distal radioulnar ligaments, a meniscus homologue, volar ulnocarpal ligaments, and the floor of the extensor carpi ulnaris tendon subsheath (Fig. 4.30). The TFCC serves two main purposes: it acts as a stabilizer of the distal radioulnar joint (DRUJ) and bears about 20% of the load across the ulnocarpal joint. When the TFCC is injured, the patient is susceptible to ulnar-sided wrist pain, mechanical symptoms, and/or wrist instability.

TFCC tears may be traumatic or chronic/degenerative and may occur in the peripheral or central portion of the complex. It is important to note the blood supply of the TFCC in order to determine the healing potential of a tear. The peripheral portion of the TFCC is vascularized, whereas the central portion is largely avascular. Therefore, tears that occur in the periphery are frequently repaired, whereas tears that occur in the central portion are usually débrided.

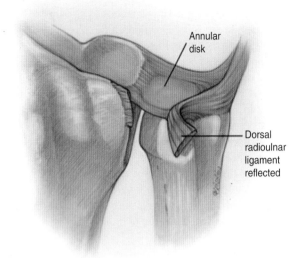

Fig. 4.30 Anatomy of the TFCC. (From Adams BD: Distal radioulnar joint instability. In: Wolfe, Hotchkiss, Pedersen, Kozin, editors, *Greens operative hand surgery*, ed 6, Philadelphia, 2011, Elsevier, Figure 16.1, p 524)

A condition of ulnar positive variance (where the distal ulna is >4 mm longer than the distal radius) may predispose a patient to a TFCC tear. When the ulna is slightly longer than the radius the forces across the ulnocarpal joint are increased and the ulna may repetitively impact the TFCC and lunate. This condition may be asymptomatic, but may also cause painful ulnocarpal impaction syndrome subsequent to TFCC tearing and lunate chondromalacia.

History

- Insidious onset, or related to a fall, twist, or sudden impact
- The patient reports ulnar-sided wrist pain, pain with rotational movements, ulnar deviation or loading in extension
- Patient may report clicking or popping in the wrist
- The patient may report weakness or sense of instability at the wrist
- The patient may have a history of distal radius malunion with ulnar positive variance

Physical Examination

- Wrist may appear normal or with ulnar-sided edema.
- The ulnar styloid may look prominent in the presence of DRUJ instability.

- Grip strength is reduced.
- **Positive fovea sign:** This sign consists of palpable tenderness in the soft depression on the ulnar side of the wrist located distal to the ulnar styloid and proximal to triquetrum and between the flexor carpi ulnaris (FCU) and extensor carpi ulnaris (ECU) tendons (Fig. 4.31).
- **Positive ulnar grind test:** The examiner extends, axially loads, and ulnarly deviates the wrist; a positive test result is pain with this motion (Fig. 4.32).
- **Piano key test** for stability of the DRUJ: The examiner places one hand on the patient's radius and then applies dorsal pressure over the ulnar head with the opposite hand. Compare with contralateral side. Increased motion or pain with motion on injured side is a positive test result (Fig. 4.33).

Imaging

- Order wrist radiographs: PA neutral, lateral, and oblique views, and a contralateral PA neutral view for comparison. A PA neutral view is obtained by abduction the patient's shoulder to 90 degrees and flexing the elbow to 90 degrees, creating a neutral condition across the radiocarpal joint.
- Frequently, x-rays are normal.
- Assess for ulnar positive variance on the PA neutral view. Measure the length of the distal ulnar relative to the distal radius. Ulnar positive variance is present when the ulna is more than 4 mm longer than the radius.
- Evaluate the ulnar aspect of the lunate for sclerosis or lytic lesions that could indicate the presence of ulnocarpal impaction syndrome (Fig. 4.34).
- Assess the DRUJ for widening compared to the uninjured wrist on the PA neutral view.

Additional Imaging

- MRI with arthrogram (or MRA) is recommended for evaluating TFCC injuries. This is considered a superior study to traditional MRI for identifying tears.[1] The quality of scans and the radiologist's experience

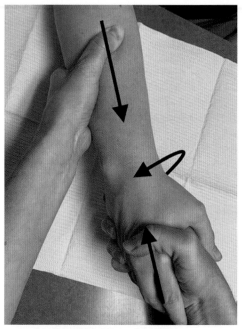

Fig. 4.32 Ulnar Grind Test.

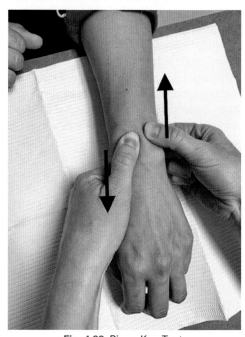

Fig. 4.33 Piano Key Test.

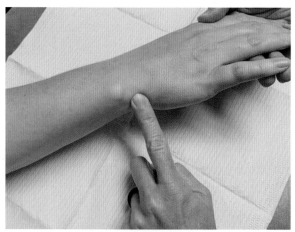

Fig. 4.31 Fovea Sign.

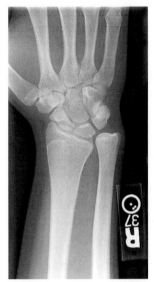

Fig. 4.34 Measuring Ulnar Positive Variance. Radiograph shows ulnar positive variance. (From Rynders SD, Chhabra AB: Triangular fibrocartilage complex injuries. In: Miller MD, Hart JA, MacKnight JM, editors, *Essential orthopaedics*, Philadelphia, 2010, Saunders, p 323.)

play a role in accurately diagnosing a tear. The gold standard for diagnosis of a TFCC tear remains wrist arthroscopy (Fig. 4.35).

Classification

The Palmar classification system was developed to categorize tears by location and provide corresponding treatment recommendations. Tears are divided into traumatic class 1 tears and degenerative class 2 tears.[2] Although this tool is extremely useful to classify a tear, it is generally sufficient to characterize TFCC tears as traumatic or degenerative, note their location as peripheral or central, and to identify concurrent conditions such as ulnocarpal impaction syndrome or DRUJ instability.

Differential Diagnosis

- Extensor or flexor tendinitis
- Pisotriquetral arthritis
- DRUJ arthritis
- Cubital tunnel syndrome
- Ulnar nerve compression at Guyon canal
- Ulnar artery thrombosis
- Hook hamate fracture
- Lunotriquetral ligament (LTL) tear
- SLL tear

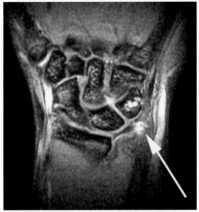

Fig. 4.35 Triangular fibrocartilage complex tear *(arrow)* as seen on magnetic resonance imaging. (From Rynders SD, Chhabra AB: Triangular fibrocartilage complex injuries. In: Miller MD, Hart JA, MacKnight JM, editors, *Essential orthopaedics*, Philadelphia, 2010, Saunders, p 324.)

- Calcium pyrophosphate dihydrate (CPPD) disease, also known as pseudogout

Initial Management

- Immobilize the wrist in a splint and refer for orthopaedic evaluation within 7 to 10 days of injury.
- **Patient Education.** The type and location of tear will guide treatment. Often degenerative central tears can be initially managed with splinting and/or injection whereas peripheral tears frequently require surgical repair. A wrist arthroscopy may be necessary to diagnose and treat the tear if conservative measures fail.

Nonoperative Management

Indications

- Degenerative tears or traumatic tears without gross DRUJ instability.
- Degenerative tears may respond well to use of an off-the-shelf wrist splint and activity modification and NSAIDs for 4 to 6 weeks. If the patient remains symptomatic, an ulnocarpal cortisone injection with additional immobilization and therapy may be indicated.
- Acute, stable tears may initially be managed with immobilization in a short-arm or Meunster cast for 4 to 6 weeks. Reevaluate the patient for tenderness and instability after 4 to 6 weeks. A cortisone injection may be employed for recalcitrant tears.
- **Rehabilitation.** Start therapy after the patient is nontender over the TFCC and the DRUJ is stable. Therapy

consists of ROM and strengthening. A wrist support may be utilized to transition the patient from a cast.

Operative Management

Codes

ICD-10 code: S63.5 Sprain of wrist joint

CPT codes: 29846 Arthroscopy wrist with excision or repair of triangular fibrocartilage and/or joint débridement

25107 Arthrotomy, distal radioulnar joint including repair of triangular cartilage complex

Indications

- Conservative measures have failed.
- Gross DRUJ instability.
- An ulnar shortening osteotomy is sometimes indicated when there is significant ulnar positive variance and evidence of ulnocarpal impaction.

Informed consent and counseling

- If surgical repair of the TFCC is indicated, the patient can expect to be immobilized for approximately 6 weeks. The type of immobilization depends on the surgical procedure performed.
- The patient will require approximately 1 to 2 months of hand therapy to restore motion and strength.
- Occasionally, some permanent stiffness in the wrist persists and may be noted in flexion, extension, supination, and pronation. Some stiffness of the wrist may be necessary in order to achieve stability of the DRUJ.

Anesthesia

- Regional anesthetic such as a brachial plexus block, with sedation or general anesthesia

Patient positioning

- Wrist arthroscopy: Supine with the arm positioned in a traction tower
- Nonsterile tourniquet on the brachium

Surgical Procedures

Arthroscopic Débridement and Repair

The affected arm is positioned in a traction tower with 15 lb of traction across the wrist. The camera is introduced into the 3-4 portal located between the third and fourth dorsal extensor compartments. A second portal is established at the 4-5 portal located between the fourth and fifth dorsal extensor compartments and probe is placed into the joint. Under direct visualization, the TFCC is inspected and probed to evaluate for injury, and characterize the size and location of the tear. A TFCC central tear is débrided with a shaver back to stable borders. A peripheral tear is débrided and then repaired with suture. There are many different techniques that may be employed to repair the TFCC. In general, the camera is placed in 6R portal (just radial to the ECU tendon) and an incision is made in line with the 6U portal (just ulnar to the ECU tendon). The dorsal ulnar sensory nerve is identified and protected. Sutures are passed through a cannula in the 1-2 or 3-4 portal and sharply into the TFCC and out through the capsule into the 6U incision. A second pass through the TFCC secures the suture in a mattress fashion and the suture ends are then tied down over the capsule. Care is taken to avoid entrapment of the **ulnar dorsal sensory nerve** under the suture. The wound is closed with suture. For TFCC repairs, the patient should be placed in a long-arm splint with the forearm supinated 45 degrees. For débridement only, a short-arm splint may be applied.

Estimated Postoperative Course

TFCC débridement

Postoperative 2 weeks:

- Perform a wound check, and remove the sutures.
- Apply a removable wrist splint, and start therapy for gentle wrist motion.

Postoperative 4 to 6 weeks:

- Wean the patient from the splint, and have the patient return to gradual activities as tolerated.

TFCC repair

Postoperative 2 weeks:

- Sutures are removed. A long-arm cast or Muenster cast with the wrist in supination is applied for 4 weeks.
- Some surgeons prefer a removable long-arm thermoplastic splint so that the patient can start to work on gradual forearm pronation.

Postoperative 6 weeks:

- Some surgeons apply a short-arm cast at this point, or they initiate splinting and motion.

Postoperative 8 to 9 weeks:

- Apply a removable splint for 4 weeks with therapy for motion and strengthening.

SUGGESTED READINGS

Adams BD: Distal radioulnar joint instability. In Wolfe SW, Hotchkiss RN, Pedersen WC, Kozin SH, editors: *Green's operative hand surgery*, ed 6, Philadelphia, 2011, Elsevier.

Ahn A, Chang D, Plate A: Triangular fibrocartilage complex tears: a review, *Bull Hosp Jt Dis* 64(3-4):114–118, 2006.

Henry MH: Management of acute triangular fibrocartilage complex injury of the wrist, *J Am Acad Orthop Surg* 16:320–329, 2008.

Rynders SD, Chhabra AB: Wrist arthroscopy. In Miller MD, Chhabra AB, editors: *Safran MR: Primer of arthroscopy*, Philadelphia, 2010, Saunders, pp 143–172.

REFERENCES

1. Lee YH, Choi YR, Kim S, Song HT, Suh JS: Intrinsic ligament and triangular fibrocartilage complex (TFCC) tears of the wrist: comparison of isovolumetric 3D-THRIVE sequence MR arthrography and conventional MRI image at 3T, *Magn Reson Imaging* 31(2):221–226, 2013.
2. Palmer AK: Triangular fibrocartilage complex lesions: a classification, *J Hand Surg Am* 14:594–606, 1989.

OSTEOARTHRITIS OF THE WRIST AND HAND

OA of the hand is a commonly encountered cause of hand pain in patients over 60 years old. The most commonly affected joints in the hand are the first CMC joint at the base of the thumb (also called basilar joint), PIP joints, and DIP joints. Less often affected are the metacarpalphalangeal (MCP) joints which are more frequently encountered in rheumatologic disease. OA of the hand can cause painful, swollen joints that may interfere with a patient's lifestyle and activities. Treatment options are vast and conservative management should be maximized prior to surgical intervention.

History

- The patient may report pain, edema, stiffness, or deformity of the affected joint.
- Pain may be worse in the morning and after repetitive activities.

- Particular to the first CMC joint, patient reports pain at the base of the thumb that is worse with pinch grasp, opening jars or door knobs, and loss of key pinch and grip strength.
- Inquire about previous injuries that could identify posttraumatic arthritis

Physical Examination

- Edema over the affected joint, limited ROM, sometimes deformity or angulation
- Tenderness to palpation over the involved joint
- Nodules over the DIP joints (Heberden nodes) or PIP joints (Bouchard nodes)
- Ganglion cysts (also called mucous cysts) over the DIP joints
- **Specific to first CMC joint OA:**
  - **First CMC grind test:** An axial load placed on the thumb in combination with circumduction elicits pain and sometimes crepitus
  - **Shoulder sign:** Prominence of the first CMC joint creating an appearance of a "shoulder" at the base of the thumb
  - Possible hyperextension or laxity of the MCP joint
  - Weakened grip or key pinch strength

Imaging: Fig. 4.36

- Order affected wrist, hand, or finger radiographs: PA, lateral, and oblique views.
- Radiographic findings of OA include joint space narrowing, subchondral sclerosis or subchondral cysts, and periarticular osteophytes.
- Symptoms of arthritis can precede radiographic findings. This is generally due to cartilage wear and synovitis that is not visible on plain x-rays.

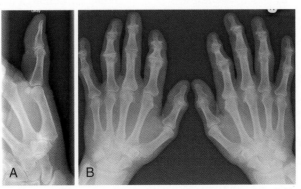

Fig. 4.36 **A** First carpometacarpal joint osteoarthritis. **B** Osteoarthritis of the hand. Note the joint space narrowing and periarticular sclerosis.

Classification
First Carpometacarpal Joint Arthritis
- Eaton stages of first CMC joint OA[1]:
  Stage 1: normal joint with exception of possible widening from synovitis
  Stage 2: joint space narrowing with debris and osteophytes smaller than 2 mm
  Stage 3: joint space narrowing with debris and osteophytes larger than 2 mm
  Stage 4: scaphotrapezial joint space involvement in addition to narrowing of the CMC joint

Differential Diagnosis
- Joint sprain or fracture
- Inflammatory arthritis such as rheumatoid arthritis
- Gout

Initial Management
- **Patient Education.** Educate patient about OA, its natural history, and options for conservative care. OA is very common and although there is no cure, effective treatment options exist. These include both non-operative and operative interventions. It is important to consider use of over-the-counter modalities and activity modification as a factor that can prolong time to surgical intervention.
- NSAIDs (used appropriately in bursts or with monitored chronic use) are helpful for pain and swelling.
- Intermittent splinting of affected joint (particularly helpful for first CMC joint arthritis). Some patients find relief with less restrictive neoprene supports or compression gloves. There are many styles of splints and supports available and none are proven better than another.
- Activity modification such as larger handles, wider grips, and assistive devices such as jar-openers can significantly help patients maintain independent and active lifestyles.
- Over-the-counter creams, balms, supplements, and oils are not well studied but may be beneficial in some patients.
- Hand therapy can assist with ancillary strengthening for joint support, stretching, and use of modalities such as moist heat or paraffin wax baths.
- Intraarticular cortisone injections may be used intermittently for arthritic joints that have failed the above measure. Cortisone injections can provide significant relief, though it is usually temporary. Prolonged and repetitive use of corticosteroid injections is not recommended (see p. 178).
- Prescription opioid medications are NOT recommended in the management of chronic OA.

Operative Management
Codes
ICD-10 codes: M19.04 Primary osteoarthritis, hand
M18.1 Unilateral primary osteoarthritis first carpometacarpal joint
CPT codes: 25447: Arthroplasty, interposition, intercarpal, or carpometacarpal joints
26860: Arthrodesis, interphalangeal joint, with or without internal fixation
26531: Arthroplasty, metacarpophalangeal joint, with prosthetic implant, each joint
26536: Arthroplasty, interphalangeal joint, with prosthetic implant each joint
Indications
- Painful or dysfunctional joint that does not respond to a trial of conservative measures
Informed consent and counseling
- Surgical management of arthritic joints generally involves removing the arthritic bone, interposing material into a joint, replacing the joint (arthroplasty), or fusing the joint (arthrodesis) to reduce pain.
- Arthrodesis is a pain-relieving surgical procedure that fuses two bones together in a position of function. This will render the affected joint permanently immobile in order to achieve permanent pain relief. There is a risk of nonunion reported in smokers; smoking is considered a relative contraindication.
- Arthroplasty is most commonly used for treatment of the PIP joint. Implants vary; the most commonly encountered implants are silicone, metal-on-polyethylene, or pyrocarbon.
- First CMC joint arthroplasty is a very common surgical procedure to treat first CMC joint OA. There are numerus described techniques but recovery time is generally 8 to 12 weeks. There is a risk for irritation to the **SSRN** that may cause temporary numbness and tingling along the thumb during the postoperative period.
- There is a risk of nail deformity with DIP joint surgical interventions.
Anesthesia
- Depends on location: DIP joint fusions can be performed under a local anesthetic or Bier block.

Surgery on multiple digits or the first CMC joint requires a regional anesthetic such as a bier block, brachial plexus block, or general anesthesia

Patient positioning

- Supine with the arm extended on a hand table
- Nonsterile tourniquet on the brachium

Surgical Procedures

First Carpometacarpal Joint Arthroplasty

The first CMC joint is identified and an incision is made overlying the joint. Care is taken to identify and protect the branches of the **superficial radial nerve** and the **dorsal branch of the radial artery.** The trapezium is identified. Generally, the trapezium is osteotomized and removed, taking care not to disrupt the **FCR** tendon which lies deep within the joint. Then an interposition arthroplasty or a suspensionplasty may be performed. During an interposition arthroplasty, part or all of the FCR is harvested and interposed into the CMC joint. During a suspensionplasty, a slip of the abductor pollicis longus (APL) tendon is suspended with suture into the joint. Adequate positioning of the thumb is confirmed with fluoroscopy and the wound is irrigated and closed. A thumb spica splint with the thumb in a position of abduction and extension is applied.

Interphalangeal Joint Arthrodesis

The PIP and DIP joints may be fused using a surgeon's preferred technique. Common fusion techniques include a tension band construct, Kirschner (K)-wires, or a compression screw. An incision is made overlying the affected joint and the joint is arthrotomized. The remaining cartilage is rongeurred from the bone ends to promote fusion of cortical bone. Intraoperative fluoroscopy confirms placement of hardware and adequate joint positioning.

Estimated Postoperative Recovery Course

First Carpometacarpal Joint Arthroplasty

Postoperative day 7 to 10:

- Patient returns to clinic for wound check and suture removal.
- X-rays (PA, lateral, oblique view of the thumb) are frequently ordered to confirm arthroplasty positioning.
- The patient is placed into a thumb spica cast with the interphalangeal (IP) joint free.

Postoperative 1 month:

- Patient returns and cast is removed.

- Apply a forearm or hand-based thumb spica removable splint (off-the-shelf or made by a therapist) and start therapy for ROM, stretching, and gradual strengthening.

Postoperative 2 months:

- Patient returns for motion check.
- Continue therapy if needed.

Postoperative 3 months:

- Patient returns for motion check.
- Most patients can be discharged with a therapy home exercise program to continue strengthening.

Interphalangeal Joint Arthroplasty

Postoperative day 7 to 10:

- Patient returns for wound check and suture removal.
- X-rays of the finger (PA, lateral, oblique) are usually obtained.
- A fabricated or custom finger splint is made that the patient should wear at all times; removal for gentle cleansing and skin hygiene is usually permitted. ROM of unaffected joints above and below the fusion site is permitted and guided hand therapy may be helpful for some patients.

Postoperative 1 month:

- Recheck x-rays and evaluate for fusion.
- Ensure patient is moving adjacent joints.

Postoperative 2 month:

- Recheck x-rays. Fusion site should be complete.
- If fused, discontinue splint.

Board Review

Heberden's nodes are nodules over the DIP joints associated with DIP joint OA.

Bouchard's nodes are nodules over the PIP joints associated with PIP joint OA.

Basilar joint arthritis causes pain at the base of the thumb worse with key pinch and grip.

SUGGESTED READINGS

Amadio PC, Shin AY. Arthrodesis and Arthroplasty of small joints of the hand. In: Greens operative hand surgery, ed 6, Philadelphia, Elsevier.

Berger AJ, Meals R: Management of osteoarthrosis of the thumb joints, *J Hand Surg Am* 40(4):843–850, 2015.

Higgenbotham C, Boyd A, Busch M, Heaton D, Trumble T: Optimal management of thumb basal joint arthritis: challenges and solutions, *Orthop Res Rev* 9:93–99, 2017.

REFERENCE

1. Eaton RG, Littler JW: Ligament reconstruction for the painful thumb carpometacarpal joint, *J Bone Surg Am* 55:1655–1666, 1973.

CARPAL TUNNEL SYNDROME

Carpal tunnel syndrome (CTS) is probably the most widely known ailment affecting the hand and is the most common compression neuropathy of the upper extremity. CTS is caused by compression of the median nerve by the transverse carpal ligament on the volar aspect of the wrist. The condition presents as numbness, tingling, and pain in the thumb, index, middle, and radial half of the ring fingers. CTS may occur due to organic compressive factors or may be related to poor ergonomics, overuse, or occupational factors. CTS is more common in women and diabetic patients, and is frequently encountered in pregnancy. CTS of pregnancy is usually related to fluid retention and resolves after delivery.

History

- Patient reports numbness, tingling, and achy pain in the thumb, index finger, middle finger, and the radial half of the ring finger. Occasionally, patients report numbness or tingling in all of the fingers and careful history taking is necessary to determine which nerve distributions are involved.
- Symptoms tend to be worse at night or when driving.
- The patient reports feeling the need to shake out the hands to get relief, also known as the "flick sign."
- The patient may note hand clumsiness and/or subjectively weakened grip strength.
- Pain may radiate to the forearm.

Physical Examination

- Inspect for thenar atrophy of the abductor pollicis brevis (suggestive of severe involvement).
- **Positive Tinel sign:** Percussion over the median nerve at the wrist flexor crease reproduces paresthesias in the fingers.
- **Positive pressure test:** Direct compression over the median nerve reproduces paresthesias in the fingers.
- **Positive Phalen test:** Wrist flexion for 1 to 2 minutes reproduces paresthesias in the fingers (note: keep the elbow extended during this test to prevent compression at the elbow).

- Two-point discrimination may be diminished in the median nerve distribution (5 mm considered normal).
- Weakness with resisted thumb abduction may be noted.

Diagnostic Testing

- Order electrodiagnostic testing: Electromyography (EMG) and nerve conduction studies (NCS). EMG evaluates either spontaneous or volitional electrical activity in the muscle; fibrillation potentials are early signs of muscle denervation. NCS evaluates motor and sensory portions of the nerve.
- Ask the electromyographer to evaluate for the differential diagnosis of carpal tunnel syndrome: "Evaluate for carpal tunnel syndrome, cubital tunnel syndrome, cervical radiculopathy, and peripheral neuropathy." Specify side and site and request for paraspinal muscle testing: "Right upper extremity EMG/NCS with paraspinal muscle testing."
- EMG/NCS may not be necessary if history and physical examination findings indicate classic findings for carpal tunnel syndrome.

Classification

- CTS is classically described on EMG/NCS as mild, moderate, or severe.

Differential Diagnosis

- Cubital tunnel syndrome
- Cervical radiculopathy
- Peripheral neuropathy associated with diabetes, renal failure, or chronic substance abuse
- Thoracic outlet syndrome

Initial Management

- Patients presenting for the first time with symptoms should be given a trial with a night-time wrist splint and NSAIDs, if appropriate.
- If symptoms persist, further evaluation and management is necessary to avoid chronic muscle denervation and permanent muscle weakness.

Nonoperative Management

Indications

- Nonoperative management is appropriate for all patients with new onset symptoms or symptoms lasting less than a few weeks to months. It is contraindicated in patients with wasting of the thenar muscles.

- Nonoperative management includes:
  - Splinting in a removable wrist splint, usually worn at night
  - NSAIDs, if appropriate
  - Cortisone injection into the carpal canal (see p. 176). Cortisone injection is thought to be most effective in patients with mild or early moderate disease and in those too ill for surgery.[1] Occasionally, cortisone injection can be used as a diagnostic tool: if a patient experiences temporary relief of symptoms after a cortisone injection, they are likely to have similar results with carpal tunnel release surgery.

Operative Management

ICD-10 code: G56.0 Carpal tunnel syndrome
CPT codes: 64721 Open carpal tunnel release
29848 Endoscopic carpal tunnel release

Indications

- CTS that has failed conservative management with splinting, NSAIDs, and possible cortisone injections
- Advanced CTS with evidence of thenar atrophy and/or denervation on nerve testing

Informed consent and counseling

- Even with appropriate treatment and good surgical release, there may be residual paresthesias, depending on the severity of disease or concurrent diagnoses such as peripheral neuropathy or cervical radiculopathy.

- Postoperative recovery time is 3 to 6 weeks depending on patient occupation or activity level, though it may take weeks to months for paresthesias to improve.
- Periincisional tenderness may occur in some patients for up to 3 months postoperatively and is commonly known as "pillar pain." Therapy can be helpful for strengthening and scar massage.

Anesthesia

- Local, or regional anesthetic with sedation
- General anesthesia may be preferable for endoscopic techniques to limit patient motion

Patient positioning

- Supine with the arm extended on a hand table
- Nonsterile tourniquet on the brachium

Surgical Procedures

Open Carpal Tunnel Release: Fig. 4.37

The location of the surgical incision is determined by drawing Kaplan's cardinal line on the palm from the hook of the hamate to the first web space. An incision is made along the radial border of the ring finger to the ulnar side of the palmaris longus tendon insertion in order to avoid injury to the palmar cutaneous branch of the median nerve. Sharp dissection is carried down through the subcutaneous tissues and the longitudinal fibers of the superficial palmar fascia to expose the transverse fibers of the transverse carpal ligament (TCL). Care is taken to protect the **recurrent motor branch of the**

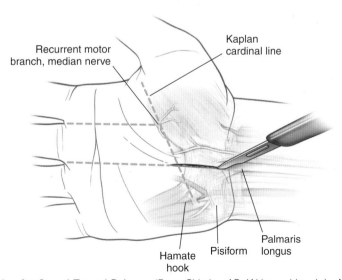

Fig. 4.37 Incision for Carpal Tunnel Release. (From Chhabra AB: Wrist and hand. In: Miller MD, Chhabra AB, Hurwitz S, et al, editors, *Orthopaedic surgical approaches*, Philadelphia, 2008, Saunders, p 177.)

media nerve which can have a variable course. Distally, the **superficial palmar arch** is protected. Once the TCL is identified, care is taken to avoid injury to the underlying median nerve and the TCL is sharply incised along the entire length proximally and distally. The wound is irrigated and closed with suture. A soft dressing or small volar splint is applied.

Endoscopic Carpal Tunnel Release

Endoscopic carpal tunnel release may provide earlier return to work and a less sensitive scar. Utilization of this technique is dependent on surgeon preference and training. During this procedure a small, volar transverse incision is made near the wrist flexor crease. The carpal canal is dilated with graduated instruments until the endoscope can be easily inserted. The median nerve is identified and protected deep to the endoscope. The endoscope blade is deployed and the TCL is incised from deep to superficial with care taken to perform a complete release and to protect the **median nerve, motor branch of the median nerve, and the superficial palmar arch.** The endoscope is withdrawn and the wound is closed with suture. A soft dressing or small volar splint is applied.

Estimated Postoperative Course

- Postoperative days 3 to 6:

Some surgeons initiate hand therapy at this point.
- Postoperative days 10 to 14:

Sutures are removed, and a wound check is performed.
- Postoperative 4 weeks:

Motion and wound checks are performed; release the patient to regular activities if they are minimally symptomatic.

Board Review

Carpal tunnel syndrome will cause numbness and tingling in the median nerve distribution of the hand, including the thumb, index, middle finger, and half of the ring finger. Physical examination findings will reveal a positive Tinel's sign and Phalen's test.

SUGGESTED READINGS

Chhabra AB: Wrist and hand. In Miller M, Chhabra B, Hurwitz S, et al.: *Orthopaedic surgical approaches*, Philadelphia, 2008, Saunders, pp 145–210.

Keith MW, Masear V, Chung K, et al.: Diagnosis of carpal tunnel syndrome, *J Am Acad Orthop Surg* 17(6):389–396, 2009.

Keith MW, Masear V, Chung K, et al.: Treatment of carpal tunnel syndrome, *J Am Acad Orthop Surg* 17(6):397–405, 2009.

Molinari III WJ, Elfar JC: The double crush syndrome, *J Hand Surg Am* 38:799–801, 2013.

REFERENCE

1. Evers S, Bryan AJ, Sanders, et al.: Corticosteroid injections for carpal tunnel syndrome: long-term follow-up in a population-based cohort, *Plast Recon Surg* 140(2):338–347, 2017.

DE QUERVAIN'S TENOSYNOVITIS

De Quervain's tenosynovitis (also known as radial styloid tenosynovitis) is a painful tendonitis of the APL and the extensor pollicis brevis (EPB) tendons which make up the first extensor compartment of the wrist. This inflammatory condition is associated with repetitive tasks involving the thumb and wrist and normal anatomic variants (such as an extra slip of tendon within the tunnel) that can predispose a patient to this condition. This condition is more common in females and racquet sports, weight-lifting, rowing, and golfing.[1] New parents are prone to developing this condition due to prolonged abnormal positioning of the wrist and thumb that occurs while holding a baby for nursing and sleeping. De Quervain's tenosynovitis is considered a "stenosing tenosynovitis." The first extensor compartment is a created by a thick sheath of tissue that surrounds the APL and EPB tendons and approximates them to the bony radial styloid. When abnormal repetitive activity or malpositioning creates increased friction within the tunnel, the tenosynovium becomes inflamed and narrows the space in which the tendons glide in the compartment, causing pain.

History

- The patient may report a history of overuse or repetitive activity, or a new baby at home.
- The patient reports pain over the radial wrist and thumb that is worse with thumb abduction and/or extension.
- Pain may initially occur only with a certain activity or a particular position but can progress to constant pain.

Physical Examination

- Inspection of the wrist may reveal edema over the radial styloid and first extensor compartment.
- Precise palpation of the first extensor compartment produces tenderness at the level of the radial styloid and may feel "boggy" from the inflammation.
- Perform a **Finkelstein's test** (Fig. 4.38): The thumb is clasped into the palm, and the wrist is passively ulnarly deviated. When De Quervain's tenosynovitis is present, the patient will experience severe pain with this maneuver.
- Pain may also be reproduced with active circular thumb motion or active radial deviation.
- Occasionally, this disorder is associated with a palpable ganglion cyst over the first dorsal compartment.

Imaging

- Not necessary for diagnosis.
- MRI can be helpful to differentiate this disorder if physical examination is inconclusive.

Differential Diagnosis

- Intersection syndrome. This is a similar condition of inflammation that occurs more proximally and dorsally on the wrist than De Quervain's tenosynovitis. Examination of Intersection syndrome will reveal tenderness and occasionally crepitus at the point where the first extensor compartment tendons cross over the second extensor compartment tendons (extensor carpi radialis longus and the extensor carpi radialis brevis tendons). It is important to differentiate De Quervain's tenosynovitis from intersection syndrome.
- First CMC joint arthritis
- Wrist arthritis
- Scaphoid fracture

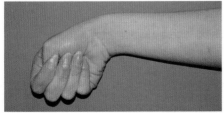

Fig. 4.38 Finkelstein Test. (From Schnur D: de Quervain's tenosynovitis. In: Miller MD, Hart JA, MacKnight JM, editors, *Essential orthopaedics,* Philadelphia, 2010, Saunders, p 326.)

- SSRN neuroma
- Radial styloid fracture

Initial Management

- Apply an off-the-shelf rigid thumb spica wrist splint and instruct patient to wear it at all times.
- Recommend activity modification and rest, ice over the radial styloid, and NSAIDs if appropriate.
- Refer to a hand specialist if pain has been present for several months or persists for several weeks after initial management measures.

Nonoperative Management

Indications

- Nonoperative management is almost always indicated for this condition, at least initially.
- Management consists of judicious use of a rigid thumb spica splint, activity modification, NSAIDs, and ice.
- Cortisone injection into the first extensor compartment (see p. 179) is indicated if the patient's symptoms have been present for several weeks or have not responded to several weeks of initial management. Counsel the patient on the possibility for skin depigmentation or subcutaneous fat atrophy after cortisone injection. Splinting after injection is recommended until symptoms abate.
- A referral to hand therapy may be helpful for local antiinflammatory modalities, stretching and tendon gliding, and activity modification recommendations.

Operative Management

ICD-10 code: M65.4 Radial styloid tenosynovitis (De Quervain's tenosynovitis)

CPT code: 25000 Incision extensor tendon sheath

Indications

- Limited or no response to conservative measures or recurrent symptoms

Informed consent and counseling

- The SSRN lies in close proximity to the first extensor compartment at the level of the wrist. Irritation can occur postoperatively resulting in temporary paresthesias over the dorsal aspect of the thumb and hand.

Anesthesia

- Local anesthetic, or regional anesthetic such as a Bier block with or without sedation

Patient positioning

- Supine with the arm extended on a hand table
- Nonsterile tourniquet on the brachium

Surgical Procedure
First Dorsal Compartment Release

The first extensor compartment is approached radially with a short longitudinal, transverse, or oblique incision. The skin is sharply incised followed by blunt dissection through the subcutaneous tissues to identify and avoid injury to the **SSRN**. The extensor retinaculum overlying the first extensor compartment is identified and sharply incised. The EPB and APL tendons are identified and any septae lying within the compartment are released so that the tendons freely glide. Any excess tenosynovitis is débrided. The wound is irrigated and closed using cutaneous sutures. A light dressing or thumb spica splint is applied.

Estimated Postoperative Course

Postoperative days 10 to 14:

- Sutures are removed, and a wound check is performed.
- A splint and therapy may be initiated in some patients; other patients can gradually return to activities as tolerated

Postoperative 4 weeks:

- All splints should be discontinued at this point.
- Motion check performed; continue therapy if stiffness persists.

Postoperative 6 to 8 weeks:

- Release the patient to all regular activities.

Board Review

- De Quervain's tenosynovitis (radial styloid tenosynovitis) will present with pain or tenderness over the radial styloid and pain reproduced with passive wrist ulnar deviation (Finkelstein's test).
- Finkelstein's test is used to diagnose De Quervain's tenosynovitis (radial styloid tenosynovitis) and a positive test is described as pain with passive wrist ulnar deviation.

SUGGESTED READINGS

Lipscomb PR: Stenosing tenosynovitis at the radial styloid process: De Quervain's tenosynovitis, *Ann Surg* 134(1):110–115, 1951.

Sarris I, Darlis NA, Musgrave D, et al.: Tenosynovitis: trigger finger, De Quervain's syndrome, flexor carpi radialis, and extensor carpi ulnaris. In Trumble TE, Budoff JE, Cornwall R, editors: *Hand, elbow, and shoulder: core knowledge in orthopaedics*, Philadelphia, 2006, Mosby, pp 212–221.

REFERENCE

1. Weiss AP, Akelman E, Tabatabi M: Treatment of De Quervain's disease, *J Hand Surg Am* 19(4):595–598, 1994.

NAIL BED INJURY

Injuries to the fingertip and nailbed are one of the most common reasons for patients to visit an emergency room or urgent care facility. These injuries usually result from a crush-type injury when the finger is pinched between two hard surfaces. Frequently, there are additional soft tissue, bone, or tendon injuries associated with nailbed injuries. The nail bed is made of the following structures: germinal matrix, sterile matrix, and dorsal nail bed. The germinal matrix is proximal to the lunula and contains specialized cells that generate the nail plate. The sterile matrix is located distal to the germinal matrix and functions to adhere the nail plate to the nail bed.[1] It is important to address nailbed injuries and even seemingly benign subungual hematomas in order to restore normal contour to the nailbed structures and prevent troubling nail plate abnormalities. Injuries to the nailbed can result in abnormal nail plate growth, partial growth, irritating ridges, grooves, or even a hook nail deformity. The nailbed should always be addressed in finger-tip amputation injuries and can be completely excised or ablated to prevent permanent nailbed abnormalities on a shortened digit.

History

- Patient reports a traumatic, crush-type injury event to the finger
- Patient reports a painful finger and possible open injury or deformity of the finger tip

Physical Examination

- Evaluate for deformity, nail plate avulsion, edema, subungual hematoma, open lacerations, or exposed bone.
- Assess vascularity and sensation, if possible.
- If a subungual hematoma is present, evaluate what percentage of the nail plate is involved.

Imaging

- Order finger radiographs: PA, lateral, and oblique to evaluate for an associated distal phalanx fracture.

Initial Management

- Assess wound and injury zone. Determine extent of nailbed injury and exactly which structures are involved.
- If an open wound is identified, a digital block may be performed for patient comfort while performing wound cleansing and care.
- Cleanse an open wound with a betadine solution or other antibacterial cleanser of choice. Remove debris, if present.
- **When to Refer:** Refer to a hand specialist if there is a displaced fracture, open fracture, tendon injury, or if there is significant soft-tissue injury or amputation.
- If an urgent referral to a hand specialist is deemed necessary, cleanse and stabilize the soft tissues with suture, if possible, and apply a bulky dressing and splint.
- Update patient's tetanus status, if necessary, and start patient on prophylactic oral antibiotics in the setting of a potentially contaminated open injury.
- **Subungual Hematoma.** If the hematoma involves less than 50% of the nail plate, trephine the nail plate with a sterile needle to allow the hematoma to drain.
- **Nailbed Laceration.** If the nail plate is lacerated or has a hematoma larger than 50%, proceed with nail bed repair immediately (see later). Nailbed repair can be done in a well-equipped emergency department or outpatient office.
- **Patient Education.** Inadequate or delayed treatment can lead to functional and/or cosmetic nail deformities. Patients should be educated that the nail plate grows at a rate of 0.1 mm/day with quicker growth in summer than in winter. After injury, nail growth does not normalize until approximately 100 days.

Operative Management

ICD-10 code: S61.3 Open wound without foreign body with injury to nail, unspecified finger
CPT codes: 11730 Removal of nail plate
11760 Repair of nail bed

Indications

- If nail is lacerated or has hematoma larger than 50%

Informed consent and counseling

- Even with appropriate treatment and good surgical repair, there is still a possibility of nail plate deformity.

Anesthesia

- Digital block

Patient positioning

- Seated, with the finger placed on a stable surface

Surgical Procedure: Fig. 4.39

Nailbed Repair

After performing a digital block, apply a finger tourniquet to prevent bleeding and improve visualization (if a tourniquet is not available, use a sterile Penrose drain wrapped around the base of finger and held tight with a hemostat). Scrub or cleanse the digit to remove debris. Irrigate any exposed bone or open fractures thoroughly. Using a hemostat, remove the remaining nail plate by elevating it from the nailbed. Take care not to avulse or injure additional areas of the nail bed during removal. If necessary, repair the skin surrounding the nail bed with 5-0 nylon sutures first. Next, repair the laceration in the nailbed itself with 6-0 chromic suture, under loupe magnification, if available. After the nailbed has been repaired, the proximal nail fold (or cuticle) should be stented open to encourage future nail plate growth. This can be accomplished by using the original minimally injured nail plate held in place with nylon suture in the corners, or a piece of nonadherent gauze (such as petroleum-impregnated gauze). The original nail plate or nonadherent gauze will eventually fall off as healing occurs. Dress the finger with a bulky dressing. A small digital splint across the DIP joint may be applied for extra support or if an associated distal phalanx fracture is present.

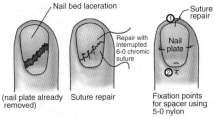

Fig. 4.39 Nail Bed Repair Technique. (From Fledman M, Isaacs JE: Nail bed injuries. In: Miller MD, Hart JA, MacKnight JM, editors, *Essential orthopaedics*, Philadelphia, 2010, Saunders, p 370.)

Estimated Postoperative Recovery Course

Postoperative days 3 to 5:

- The dressing is changed. Frequently, the dressing will adhere to the injury site due to postoperative drainage or bleeding. If this occurs, soak the finger in a water and hydrogen peroxide solution and utilize forceps to help remove the dressing. DO NOT REMOVE the material that has been placed over the nailbed repair.

Postoperative days 10 to 14:

- Any nonabsorbable sutures are removed. The nail plate or other material will adhere to matrix for 1 to 3 months until it is pushed off by the new nail.
- If a distal phalanx fracture is present, splint for a total of 3 weeks.

Postoperative week 3:

- Check wound and ROM.
- In the setting of a distal phalanx fracture, repeat radiographs to evaluate for healing, discontinue splint, and start gentle ROM if healed.

SUGGESTED READINGS

Feldman M, Isaacs JE: Nail bed injuries. In Miller MD, Hart JA, MacKnight JM, editors: *Essential orthopaedics*, Philadelphia, 2010, Saunders, pp 369–371.

Richards A, Crick A, Cole R: A novel method of securing the nail following nail bed repair, *Plast Reconstr Surg* 103(7):1983–1985, 1999.

REFERENCE

1. Zook EG, Van Beek AL, Russell RC, Beatty ME: Anatomy and physiology of the perionychium: a review of the literature and anatomic study, *J Hand Surg Am* 5(6):528–536, 1980.

BENNETT FRACTURE

A Bennett's fracture is a named fracture-dislocation that occurs at the base of the thumb metacarpal. By definition, it is an intraarticular, oblique fracture-dislocation of the ulnar-volar thumb metacarpal base, and it is inherently unstable. The abductor pollicis brevis tendon inserts on the radial side of the thumb metacarpal base and causes the metacarpal to displace proximally and radially from the stationary ulnar fragment. The ulnar fragment remains reduced due to the attachment of the anterior oblique ligament (formerly called the beak ligament).[1] This fracture pattern nearly always requires surgical intervention to reduce the fracture and restore the CMC joint surface congruity. Failure to address and reduce this fracture adequately can result in painful arthritis and thumb dysfunction.

History

- Axial loading and abduction force to the thumb (usually from a fall or sporting event)
- Patient reports thumb pain, swelling, and reduced and painful motion

Physical Examination

- Edema and/or ecchymosis in the thenar region
- Thumb possibly appearing deformed or malrotated
- Tenderness over the base of the thumb at the first CMC joint

Imaging: Fig. 4.40

- Order thumb radiographs: PA, lateral, and oblique views.

Differential Diagnosis

- Rolando fracture (three-part intraarticular fracture at the base of the thumb metacarpal; in addition to the ulnar-volar fragments seen in a Bennett fracture, also a large dorsal fragment resulting in a Y- or T-shaped fracture)
- Thumb CMC joint dislocation

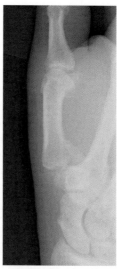

Fig. 4.40 Radiograph of a Bennett Fracture. (From Rynders SD, Chhabra AB: Thumb fractures. In: Miller MD, Hart JA, MacKnight JM, editors, *Essential orthopaedics*, Philadelphia, 2010, Saunders, p 404.)

- CMC joint OA
- Thumb MCP joint sprain
- Scaphoid fracture

Initial Management

- Most Bennett fractures are resistant to closed reduction and nonoperative treatment and often require open reduction and fixation. Additionally, surgical treatment is more likely to produce reliable results than casting. A mismanaged Bennett fracture will result in traumatic arthritis and cause impairment of thumb function. Even with surgical intervention, the injured joint is more likely to develop arthritis.
- Apply a short-arm thumb spica splint until edema subsides.
- Refer to an orthopaedic surgeon to be seen within 3 to 5 days from injury.

Nonoperative Management

- Conservative management is reserved for fractures with less than 1 mm displacement. The patient requires frequent follow up with radiographs to ensure that reduction is maintained.
- Immobilize in a thumb spica splint for 1 to 2 weeks to reduce edema. Then apply a thumb spica cast for 4 to 6 weeks. Check weekly serial x-rays to monitor for displacement.
- **Rehabilitation.** After 6 weeks of splint and cast immobilization and with evidence of healing on a radiograph, the patient can start thumb motion.
- An off-the-shelf wrist brace may be used to transition from the cast.
- The patient can return to a preinjury activity level at 6 to 8 weeks.

Operative Management

ICD-10 code: S62.21 Bennett's fracture, closed fracture base of thumb metacarpal

CPT codes: 26665 Open reduction, internal fixation of a Bennett's fracture

26650 Closed reduction percutaneous pinning of a Bennett's fracture

Indications

- Bennett fracture with at least 1 mm of articular displacement

Informed consent and counseling

- The affected joint is more likely to develop OA.

- The patient can expect to be immobilized for roughly 4 to 6 weeks postoperatively.
- The patient will require a short course of outpatient hand therapy to restore motion and strength.
- If wires or pins are utilized, these will stay in for 4 to 6 weeks prior to removal.
  ### *Anesthesia*
- Regional anesthetic such as a brachial plexus block, with sedation or general anesthesia
  ### *Patient positioning*
- Supine with the arm extended on a hand table
- Nonsterile tourniquet on the brachium

Surgical Procedure

Closed Reduction, Percutaneous Pinning: Fig. 4.41
Closed reduction and percutaneous pinning (CRPP) is less invasive than open techniques and therefore may be used preferentially for treatment of Bennett fractures. Using fluoroscopy, longitudinal thumb traction with an abduction and pronation force over the first metacarpal base is used to reduce and align the fracture. Once reduced, K-wires are placed percutaneously through the metacarpal shaft and into the trapezium and/or second metacarpal thereby securing the metacarpal base to the stationary volar-ulnar fragment. It is not always necessary to capture the Bennett fragment because reduction of the joint should reapproximate the fracture fragment. A thumb spica splint is applied.

Occasionally, the thumb metacarpal base is difficult to reduce and align using a closed procedure. This

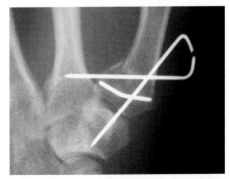

Fig. 4.41 Bennett Fracture Treated with Closed Reduction, Percutaneous Pinning. (From Markiewitz AD: Fractures and dislocations involving the metacarpal bone. In: Trumble T, Budoff J, Cornwall R, editors, *Hand, elbow, and shoulder: core knowledge in orthopaedics*, Philadelphia, 2006, Mosby, p 42.)

operation can be converted to an open reduction and internal fixation so that the metacarpal base joint surface can be reduced under direct visualization.

Estimated Postoperative Recovery Course

Postoperative days 10 to 14:
- A wound check is performed. If the procedure required an open reduction, sutures are removed.
- Obtain radiographs: thumb PA, lateral, and oblique views. Evaluate fracture reduction and hardware placement.
- Immobilization: The patient is placed into a thumb spica cast, padded to protect pin sites.

Postoperative 4 to 6 weeks:
- Obtain radiographs: thumb PA, lateral, and oblique views. Evaluate for evidence of healing.
- The decision to remove the K-wires usually occurs 4 to 6 weeks postoperatively based on radiographic evidence of healing. External K-wires can easily be removed in the office. Subcutaneous wires can be removed under fluoroscopy with a local anesthetic on board.
- *Therapy*: Once the K-wires are moved and there is evidence of osseous healing, the patient can start therapy for gentle wrist and thumb ROM and gradual strengthening.

Postoperative 3 months:
- Obtain radiographs: thumb PA, lateral, and oblique views. Evaluate for fracture healing.
- Check progress and motion and if satisfactory, the patient can resume all regular activities.

SUGGESTED READINGS

Carlsen BT, Moran SL: Thumb trauma: Bennett fractures, Rolando fractures, and ulnar collateral ligament injuries, *J Hand Surg Am* 34A:945–952, 2009.

Day CS, Stern PJ: Fractures of the metacarpals and phalanges. In Green DP, Hotchkiss RN, Pederson WC, et al.: *Green's operative hand surgery*, ed 6, Philadelphia, 2011, Churchill Livingstone, pp 239–290.

REFERENCE

1. Day CS, Stern PJ: Fractures of the metacarpals and phalanges. In Green DP, Hotchkiss RN, Pederson WC, et al.: *Green's operative hand surgery*, ed 6, Philadelphia, 2011, Churchill Livingstone, pp 239–290.

METACARPAL FRACTURES

Fractures of the hand metacarpal bones are commonly encountered injuries and account for 18% of all upper extremity injuries in the general population.[1] The most well-known metacarpal fracture is the Boxer's fracture, or fracture of the fifth metacarpal neck due to impact on a closed fist (punching motion). It is important to be able to identify, describe, and adequately examine metacarpal fractures in order to prescribe appropriate treatment. It is paramount to evaluate patients with metacarpal fractures for distal rotational or angular finger deformities that may only be apparent when the patient makes a fist or performs full finger extension. If malrotation is not identified and corrected, permanent hand dysfunction may result.

History

- Trauma due to a fall, striking an object with a closed fist, or a sudden rotational force.
- Patient reports pain, swelling, and reduced motion of the hand.

Physical Examination

- Inspect for any open injuries or a "fight bite" when the patient was involved in an altercation (see p. 171).
- Edema and/or ecchymosis is present about the hand and frequently palmar ecchymosis is noted.
- Tenderness to palpation is noted over the affected metacarpal.
- Examine the affected metacarpal's finger in flexion and extension to evaluate for angulation or rotation. It may be helpful to compare digital cascade with that of the uninjured hand.
- A local field block may help to obtain an accurate examination.
- Evaluate for tendon injury if a wound is present.
- Perform a neurovascular examination.

Imaging: Figs. 4.42 and 4.43

- Order hand radiographs: PA, lateral, and oblique views. Evaluate the fracture for rotation by inspecting and comparing the adjacent metacarpal heads.
- Evaluate metacarpal base fractures for concomitant CMC fracture-dislocation. Fourth and fifth metacarpal base fractures are more commonly associated with a fracture-dislocation pattern.

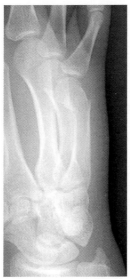

Fig. 4.42 Fifth Metacarpal Neck Fracture or Boxer Fracture.

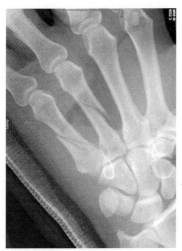

Fig. 4.43 Fourth and Fifth Metacarpal Shaft Fractures. This is considered an unstable fracture pattern.

Classification

- It is important to accurately describe a metacarpal fracture on radiographs: First, a fracture should be identified as "displaced" or "nondisplaced" and "intraarticular" or "extraarticular." Next, the involved bone should be named. The metacarpals are numbered first through fifth, starting with the thumb. The fracture pattern should be examined and described as transverse, oblique, spiral, or comminuted and the location on the bone should be identified as occurring

at the base, shaft, neck, or head of the bone. In Fig. 4.43, the fracture would be described as "minimally displaced extraarticular fourth and fifth spiral metacarpal shaft fractures."

Differential Diagnosis

- Phalanx fracture
- Carpal or radiocarpal fracture
- Hand contusion
- Compartment syndrome of the hand
- Hand space infection

Initial Management

- Reduce significantly displaced fractures under a hematoma block. Maintain fracture reduction with a molded splint. The hand should be positioned with the MCP joints in flexion, also known as the "intrinsic plus" position.
- Refer the patient to an orthopaedic surgeon to be seen within 3 to 5 days.
- All open injuries require bedside irrigation before splint application, as well as oral antibiotics.
- All "fight bite" injuries, with or without tendon injury, require operative exploration and irrigation to prevent joint infection by human oral flora.

Nonoperative Management

- Singular, closed, nondisplaced, or minimally displaced metacarpal fractures without rotation or angulation can usually be treated with splinting and casting. Instruct the patient to elevate the hand to prevent and reduce edema.
- If a fracture was initially closed-reduced, plan to obtain weekly serial x-rays to ensure proper fracture alignment.
- Immobilize the fracture in a splint for 1 to 2 weeks to allow edema to subside. Then, apply a cast based on the location of the fracture. Metacarpal base fractures can typically be treated in a short-arm cast. Fractures of a metacarpal shaft or neck should be treated in a cast that immobilizes the MCP joint, but allows PIP joint motion.
- Obtain x-rays at 4 weeks postinjury to evaluate for healing in the form of fracture consolidation and callus formation. Patients who smoke may require additional immobilization due to delayed healing.
- Once the fracture is nontender to palpation on physical examination AND there is radiographic evidence

of healing, the patient can transition to a removeable splint and start active finger and wrist motion.

- Total healing time is typically 6 to 8 weeks to return to full function.

Operative Management

ICD-10 codes: S62.2 Fracture of first metacarpal bone
S62.3 Fracture of other metacarpal bone
CPT codes: 26608: Percutaneous skeletal fixation of metacarpal fracture, each bone
26615: Open treatment of metacarpal fracture, single, includes internal fixation, when performed, each bone

Indications: Table 4.9

- Metacarpal fractures with an associated fight bite or suspected or known extensor tendon injury
- Multiple metacarpal fractures
- Fractures meeting operative criteria as defined in Table 4.9
- CMC fracture-dislocations

Informed consent and counseling

- The patient can expect to be immobilized for approximately 4 weeks, but the type of immobilization depends on the surgeon's preference and the fracture fixation.
- The patient will require outpatient hand therapy to restore motion and strength.

Anesthesia

- Regional anesthetic such as a brachial plexus block, with sedation or general anesthesia

Patient positioning

- Supine with the arm extended on a hand table
- Nonsterile tourniquet on the brachium

Surgical Procedures

Open Reduction, Internal Fixation: Fig. 4.44

Generally, a longitudinal incision is made directly overlying the affected metacarpal. The extensor tendons are retracted laterally for visualization and the periosteum is incised and elevated from the fracture site. The fracture is débrided of hematoma and reduced under fluoroscopy. Surgical fixation can be accomplished with lag screws, a plate and screws, intermedullary screws, or K-wires. Once reduced, the periosteum and skin are closed and a splint is applied (volar splint or ulnar gutter splint).

Closed or Open Reduction, Percutaneous Pinning

Alternative to open reduction, some metacarpal fractures and fracture-dislocations may be amenable to closed reduction and pinning. The metacarpal fracture is reduced under fluoroscopy and held in place by K-wires positioned intermedullary or in a transverse fashion proximal and distal to the fracture site.

Estimated Postoperative Course

Postoperative days 10 to 14:

- A wound check is performed, and sutures are removed as necessary.

TABLE 4.9	**Indications for Surgery in Metacarpal Fractures**	
Metacarpal Fracture Location	**Surgical Indication**	**Comments**
Head	1-mm step-off Fracture involving >20% articular surface	Collateral ligament injuries common in thumb, index finger, and small finger; also assess for "fight bite"
Neck	Index and long fingers: >15 degrees of angulation Ring and small fingers: >45 degrees of angulation (some surgeons allow up to 70 degrees angulation of small finger) Rotation unacceptable and treated with surgery	Acceptable degree of angulation contested in literature
Shaft	Index and long fingers: >15 degrees of angulation Ring and small fingers: >40 degrees of angulation All fingers: shortening: >5 mm	Every 10-degree shaft rotation = 2 cm of fingertip overlap with flexion
Base	Usually indicated in thumb and small finger	See section on Bennett fracture and baby Bennett fracture for thumb and small finger metacarpal base fractures

- Obtain radiographs: hand PA, lateral, and oblique views. Evaluate fracture reduction and hardware placement.
- Immobilization: A custom splint or short-arm or outrigger cast is used for approximately 4 weeks, depending on fracture fixation and surgeon preference.
- *Therapy referral:* Early controlled motion with therapy may be indicated, depending on fracture location and surgical fixation.

Postoperative 4 weeks:

- A wound check is performed, and sutures are removed as necessary.
- Obtain radiographs: hand PA, lateral, and oblique views. Evaluate for evidence of healing.
- K-wires may be considered for removal between 4 and 6 weeks postoperatively.
- Initiate therapy for ROM if the fracture shows evidence of healing, the fracture site is nontender to palpation, and once retained wires have been removed. A custom splint may be fashioned for protection.

Postoperative 6 to 8 weeks:

- The patient returns for a motion check.
- Radiographs are obtained: hand PA, lateral, and oblique views.

Board Review

A Boxer's fracture is usually referring to a fracture of the fifth metacarpal neck.

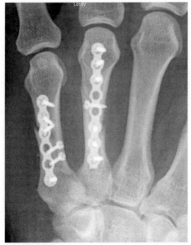

Fig. 4.44 Open Reduction and Internal Fixation of Fourth and Fifth Metacarpal Shaft Fractures.

SUGGESTED READINGS

Day CS, Stern PJ: Fractures of the metacarpals and phalanges. In Green DP, Hotchkiss RN, Pederson WC, et al.: *Green's operative hand surgery*, ed 6, Philadelphia, 2011, Churchill Livingstone, pp 239–290.

Henry MH: Fractures of the proximal phalanx and metacarpals in the hand: preferred methods of stabilization, *J Am Acad Orthop Surg* 16(10):586–595, 2008.

Kollitz KM, Hammert WC, Vedder NB, Huang JI: Metacarpal fractures: treatment and complications, *Hand* 9:16–23, 2014.

REFERENCE

1. Chung KC, Spilson SV: The frequency and epidemiology of hand and forearm fractures in the United States, *J Hand Surg Am* 39(3):474–479, 2014.

PHALANX FRACTURES AND PIP JOINT INJURIES

A "jammed" finger is a frequently used and inappropriate catch-all term that is applied to many finger injuries. The term fails to accurately describe an injured anatomic structure and suggests a poor understanding of the anatomy. Instead, the practitioner should be able to accurately examine, identify, and describe the injured anatomic structure at the PIP joint. This includes fracture, dislocation, ulnar or radial collateral ligament injury, volar plate injury, and central slip extensor tendon injury (see extensor tendon section).

Fractures of the finger phalanges are common and can occur from a simple fall, impact, twist, or "jam" (Fig. 4.45). Although the injured digit may initially appear unimpressive, a nuanced physical examination is necessary in order to evaluate for rotational abnormalities and tendon and ligament injuries. Successful functional outcome is dependent on a fracture healing in anatomic alignment. If a fracture heals in an angulated or rotated manner, a patient can experience significant loss of function and grip strength.

Intraarticular phalanx fractures and periarticular fracture-dislocations (commonly called pilon fractures) are particularly difficult to treat and often require surgical management in order to restore a congruent joint surface. Careful x-ray evaluation, particularly on lateral view x-rays, is important to evaluate for joint subluxation or dislocation.

PIP joint dislocations can occur with or without an associated fracture. Dorsal dislocations are more common and should be reduced under a local anesthetic. Injuries to the collateral ligaments, volar plate, or central slip can occur with dislocations and should not be overlooked.

History

- Trauma to the finger, often during sports, is reported.
- The patient may report a "jammed" finger, a fall with direct impact on the digit, or a twisting injury.

Physical Examination

- Inspect for abrasions or open wounds.
- Edema and ecchymosis of the affected digit may be present. ROM will be reduced or limited by pain.
- The PIP joint may appear flexed and enlarged if the joint is dislocated.
- Evaluate for obvious finger deformity, angulation, or rotation.
- Evaluate the rotation and angulation of the digit in both flexion and extension. Note any cross-over of the affected digit in flexion. Compare to the uninjured hand.
- Palpate for tenderness along the phalanges, the ulnar aspect of the PIP joint, radial aspect of the PIP joint, dorsal and volar PIP joint. Document area of tenderness.
- Perform a neurovascular examination. Check each digital nerve and capillary refill. This is especially important in the setting of a dislocation or associated laceration.

Imaging

- Order radiographs of the affected finger: PA, lateral, and oblique views. Observe the alignment of the phalanx condyles as a subtle way of detecting rotational abnormalities.

Classification: Table 4.10

Differential Diagnosis

- Phalanx fracture
- PIP joint dislocation
- PIP joint collateral ligament sprain
- Volar plate avulsion fracture
- Central slip injury
- Mallet finger
- Jersey finger
- Contusion

Management of Phalanx Fractures

- Identify level of injury and determine if there is rotation or angular deformity. Check the digit in flexion and extension.
- Evaluate PA, lateral, and oblique x-rays. See Table 4.10 for operative indications.

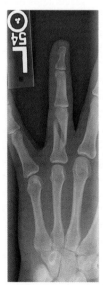

Fig. 4.45 Radiograph of a Displaced, Rotated, Extraarticular Long Oblique Fracture of the Middle Phalanx.

TABLE 4.10	**Surgical Indications for Phalanx Fractures**	
Phalanx	**Indications For Surgery**	**Comments**
Proximal	Articular step-off >2-mm shortening rotation	Oblique, comminuted, spiral fractures are unstable
Middle	Articular step-off >2-mm shortening Irreducible dislocation Injury to central slip (in volar dislocations)	Oblique, comminuted, spiral fractures are unstable
Distal	Irreducible fractures Unstable transverse fracture	See also mallet finger/jersey finger

Nonoperative Management
Indications
Nondisplaced fractures can be managed nonoperatively.
- Splint or cast one joint above and below the injury:
  - *Distal phalanx fractures* can be placed into an aluminum splint covering the distal and middle phalanx with the PIP joint free.
  - *Middle and proximal phalanx fractures* should be placed into a hand-based or forearm-based radial gutter, ulnar gutter, or resting volar splint with the MCP joints flexed into the intrinsic plus position.
- Instruct patient to keep splint on, use ice, and elevate the affected hand. Refer to a hand specialist for evaluation within 3 to 5 days.
- Follow-up care may involve weekly x-ray evaluation to ensure the fracture does not lose reduction.
- After 3 weeks of splint or cast immobilization, repeat x-rays to evaluate for healing.
  - *Distal phalanx fractures*: Discontinue splinting, start ROM.
  - *Proximal phalanx fracture*: Start protected ROM with intermittent splinting or "buddy-taping."
- A patient can be referred to a hand therapist to assist with ROM and prevent stiffness.
- A fracture should be healed and the patient should be released to most regular activities by 6 weeks postinjury.
- **Patient Education.** Some finger stiffness is anticipated and hand therapy can assist with improving motion, grip strength, and dexterity.

Operative Management
ICD-10 codes: S62.6 Phalanx fracture

CPT codes: 26727: Percutaneous skeletal fixation of unstable phalangeal shaft fracture, proximal or middle phalanx, finger or thumb, with manipulation, each

26735: Open treatment of phalangeal shaft fracture, proximal or middle phalanx, finger or thumb, includes internal fixation, when performed, each

26756: Percutaneous skeletal fixation of distal phalangeal fracture, finger or thumb, each

26765: Open treatment of distal phalangeal fracture, finger or thumb, includes internal fixation, when performed, each

Surgical Procedure: Fig. 4.46
Surgery can be performed under a local or regional anesthetic. The operative goal is to reduce and stabilize the fracture with as minimally invasive a procedure as possible. Closed reduction and percutaneous pinning, when indicated, is preferable to open reduction and internal fixation because of the risk of tendon adhesions and finger stiffness with open procedures. Many different surgical techniques have been described, and procedure selection is based on the location and character of the fracture. Regardless of the procedure, the patient can expect to participate in a postoperative rehabilitation program to restore ROM.

Estimated Postoperative Recovery Course
Postoperative 7 to 10 days:
- Patient returns for wound check, suture removal (if indicated) and postoperative x-rays.
- Apply a splint, cast, or custom therapy splint that the patient should wear at all times.
- Encourage active ROM of unaffected joints.

Postoperative 3 to 4 weeks:
- Obtain x-rays to evaluate for fracture healing.
- K-wires are usually left in place for 3 to 4 weeks and can be removed in the clinic or if subcutaneous, under a local anesthetic.
- Initiate protected ROM with a hand therapist. Therapy can progress and splints can be discontinued by 6 weeks postoperative. All patients will require extensive hand therapy to restore ROM.

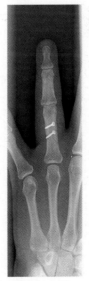

Fig. 4.46 Open Reduction and Internal Fixation with Lag Screws of the Same Fracture as in *Fig. 4.46*.

Management of PIP Joint Dislocation[1]:
Fig. 4.47
- If the PIP joint is dislocated, attempt reduction under a digital block:
  - Apply a constant dorsal pressure over the prominent dislocated middle phalanx. Simultaneously apply longitudinal traction on the affected digit with the other hand and flex the PIP joint until it reduces.
  - Once reduced, obtain postreduction x-rays to ensure alignment and evaluate for fractures.
  - An irreducible PIP joint may indicate interposition of adjacent tissue such as the volar plate. Should this occur, contact a hand surgeon for immediate treatment as open reduction may be required.
- Check PIP joint stability postreduction:
  - While the digit is anesthetized, ask the patient to actively flex and extend the digit and evaluate for instability and redislocation. Then, passively stress the ulnar and radial collateral ligaments of the PIP joint in 30 degrees of flexion and again in extension. If there is a stable endpoint and no redislocation event, the finger can be "buddy-taped" to an adjacent finger and the patient can start protected ROM. Refer to a hand surgeon for evaluation in 7 to 10 days.

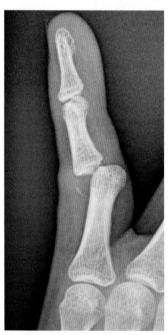

Fig. 4.47 X-ray, lateral view, of a dorsal proximal interphalangeal joint dislocation. (Original Image.)

- If instability or significant ligamentous laxity is present, splint the finger with a dorsal-blocking splint in a position of flexion in which the PIP joint remains reduced. Instruct patient to leave splint in place at all times and refer to a hand surgeon in 3 to 5 days.
- Most PIP joint dislocations can be managed without surgery. Early protected ROM is ideal for stable injuries, whereas a short period of splinting followed by protected ROM is usually sufficient to treat more severe cases.
- **Patient Education.** The PIP joint is prone to stiffness and flexion contracture. Hand therapy may be indicated to prevent loss of motion. The PIP joint may appear enlarged or edematous for a prolonged period of time after injury due to inflammation, thickening, and scarring of the periarticular tissues.

Management of PIP Joint Collateral Ligament Sprain
- Sprain of the radial or ulnar collateral ligaments of the PIP joint occurs from an impact or "jamming" mechanism.
- The patient will present with a painful, edematous PIP joint with limited ROM due to pain or swelling.
- X-rays will appear normal or demonstrate a small avulsion fracture on the lateral aspect of the PIP joint.
- First, identify the injured structure. Evaluate for tenderness to palpation over the radial and ulnar aspect of the PIP joint.
- Next, test the stability of each collateral ligament with the finger in extension and in 30 degrees of flexion. A sprain may be mild, moderate, or severe:
  - Mild: pain with no laxity
  - Moderate: pain and laxity but a firm endpoint on testing
  - Severe: pain and laxity with no firm endpoint
- Most injuries, even those with pain and laxity, respond well to "buddy-taping" and early protected motion. Grossly unstable injuries may require surgical intervention including repair of the ligament and possible temporary pinning of the joint.

Management of PIP Joint Volar Plate Injury
- The volar plate is a thick fibrocartilaginous structure on the volar aspect of the PIP joint that acts as a checkrein to prevent hyperextension of the PIP joint.

- The volar plate can be injured when a finger is "jammed" or hyperextended and can present as a strictly soft tissue injury, or involve a small bony avulsion fracture from the volar base of the middle phalanx.
- Check x-rays: PA, lateral, oblique views. Evaluate for an avulsion fracture of the base of the middle phalanx. If a fracture is present, determine the percentage of joint surface involved and if there is a subluxation of the middle phalanx (Fig. 4.48).
- Most volar plate avulsion fracture injuries can be managed initially in a dorsal blocking splint for 1 to 2 weeks followed by protected ROM with "buddy-taping."

SUGGESTED READINGS

Meals C, Meals R: Hand Fractures: A review of current treatment strategies, *J Hand Surg Am* 38:1021–1031, 2013.
Merrell G, Slade JF: Dislocations and ligament injuries in the digits. In Wolfe SW, Hotchkiss RN, Pedersen WC, Kozin SH, editors: *Green's operative hand surgery*, ed 6, Philadelphia, 2011, Elsevier.

Shah CM, Sommerkamp TG: Fracture dislocation of the finger joints, *J Hand Surg Am* 39:792–802, 2014.
Slade JF, Magit DP: Phalangeal fractures and dislocations. In Trumble TE, Budoff JE, Cornwall R, editors: *Hand, elbow, and shoulder: core knowledge in orthopaedics*, Philadelphia, 2006, Mosby, pp 22–37.

REFERENCE

1. Merrell G, Slade JF: Dislocations and ligament injuries in the digits. In Wolfe SW, Hotchkiss RN, Pedersen WC, Kozin SH, editors: *Green's operative hand surgery*, ed 6, Philadelphia, 2011, Elsevier.

THUMB ULNAR COLLATERAL LIGAMENT SPRAIN

The ulnar collateral ligament (UCL) at the thumb MCP joint (hereon referred to as the thumb UCL) is an important anatomic structure for key grasp and pinch grasp. An

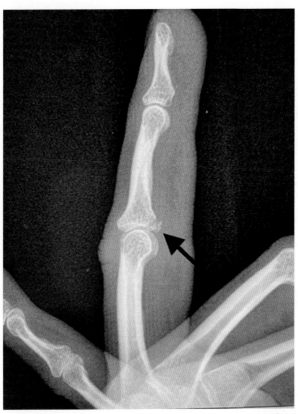

Fig. 4.48 X-ray, lateral view, of a volar plate avulsion fracture *(arrow)*. (Original Image.)

injury to the ligament will result in significant hand dysfunction. A sprained UCL is also known as a Skier's thumb (acute injury) or Gamekeeper's thumb (chronic injury). Skier's thumb is caused by a sudden hyper-abduction force on the thumb MCP joint, such as a fall. Gamekeeper's thumb is due to chronic low force trauma across the thumb UCL resulting in gradual development of instability.

The thumb UCL is made up of the proper and accessory collateral ligaments. Physical examination is key to determining whether a UCL tear is partial or complete and will determine whether an injury should be managed surgically. X-rays are also imperative to evaluate for an associated avulsion fracture from the proximal phalanx. Advanced imaging such as ultrasound or MRI may be used when the diagnosis is uncertain.

History

- Patient may report a fall or abrupt abduction force across the thumb UCL. Patient may state "my thumb bent backwards."
- Often associated with activities such as skiing and contact or ball-handling sports.
- In cases of gamekeeper's thumb, the patient may report gradual loss of key pinch strength and pain with key pinch.

Physical Examination

- Edema and ecchymosis at the thumb MCP joint
- Tenderness at the ulnar aspect of the thumb MCP joint
- An area of thickened tissue over the UCL may represent a Stener's lesion (see classification)

Ulnar Collateral Ligament Stress Test: Fig. 4.49

Apply valgus stress across the thumb MCP joint in extension *and* in 30 degrees of flexion. Laxity of more than 30 degrees in either plane when compared with the contralateral thumb with or without pain is diagnostic

> **! CLINICAL ALERT**
>
> Always obtain radiographs before the stress test to evaluate for the presence of an avulsion fracture. If a fracture is present, the injury is considered a complete ligament tear even though the defect is at the bony insertion and not within the substance of the ligament. If stressed before radiography, the bony fragment could displace, and a nonoperative injury could become operative.

of a complete UCL rupture.[1] If there is a definitive end point with pain, the injury is likely partial.

Imaging: Fig. 4.50

- Order thumb radiographs prior to stress testing: PA, lateral, and oblique views.
- The image may appear normal or may have an associated avulsion fracture.
- If no fracture is present, stress views can be helpful. Often this is done under a local anesthetic. Obtain a radiograph while applying valgus stress to the thumb

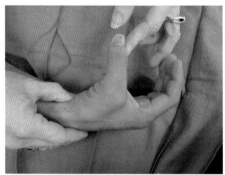

Fig. 4.49 Ulnar Collateral Ligament Stress Test. (From Ignore J, Blum G: Ulnar collateral ligament injuries of the thumb [gamekeeper's thumb, skier's thumb. In: Miller MD, Hart JA, MacKnight JM, editors, *Essential orthopaedics*, Philadelphia, 2010, Saunders, p 346.)

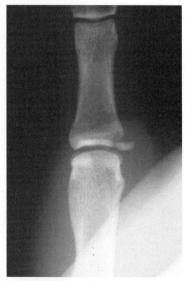

Fig. 4.50 Avulsion Fracture Associated with an Ulnar Collateral Ligament Sprain.

MCP and compare it with the uninjured thumb. A positive stress view will reveal greater laxity of the injured digit compared to the uninjured side.

- MRI may be helpful if radiographs are negative for an avulsion fracture and the physical examination is equivocal for a complete or partial tear. MRI has been found to be 100% specific and sensitive for identifying thumb UCL tears.[2] Some institutions may use ultrasound as a diagnostic tool, but its sensitivity and specificity are user dependent.

Classification

- Complete tear
- Partial tear
- With or without avulsion fracture
- Stener lesion: A palpable mass just proximal to the MCP joint may represent a Stener lesion. This occurs when the torn aspect of the UCL displaces outside the adductor aponeurosis. A Stener lesion does not occur with partial tears and can only be diagnosed definitively by MRI or intraoperatively. When this lesion occurs, it always requires operative intervention.

Differential Diagnosis

- Radial collateral ligament injury
- Proximal phalanx fracture without ligament injury
- MCP joint capsular sprain
- Trigger finger

Initial Management

- Assess with x-rays to evaluate for avulsion fracture prior to stress testing.
- Perform a physical examination as described earlier.
- A digital block can be performed for patient comfort prior to stress testing the UCL.
- Apply a thumb spica splint and refer to a hand specialist within 7 to 10 days from injury.
- Encourage ice, elevation, and rest of the extremity.

Nonoperative Management
Indications
- Partial ligament tears and stable nondisplaced avulsion fractures that do not involve more than 10% of the articular surface.
- Immobilize in a thumb spica splint for 1 to 2 weeks postinjury to allow edema to subside.
- Transition patient from a splint to a thumb spica cast until 4 to 6 weeks from the injury date.

- Four to six weeks after injury, replace the cast with a removable hand-based thumb spica splint and allow the patient to remove the splint to start gentle thumb motion.
- A guided hand therapy program may be indicated to improve ROM and strength.

Operative Management
ICD-10 code: S53.30 Traumatic rupture of UCL
S63.642 Left thumb MCP joint sprain
S63.641 Right thumb MCP joint sprain
CPT codes: 26540: Repair of collateral ligament, metacarpophalangeal or interphalangeal joint
26541: Reconstruction, collateral ligament, metacarpophalangeal joint, single; with tendon or fascial graft (includes obtaining graft)
26542: Reconstruction, collateral ligament, metacarpophalangeal joint, single; with local tissue e.g., adductor advancement)
Indications
- Acute, complete tear of the thumb MCP joint UCL
- Partial tear that does not respond to nonoperative management
- A displaced avulsion fracture at the ulnar base of proximal phalanx that involves more than 10% of the articular surface
- Chronic tears, which may require reconstruction with a tendon graft
Informed consent and counseling
- The patient can expect to be immobilized for roughly 3 to 4 weeks postoperatively.
- The patient will require outpatient hand therapy to restore motion and strength.
Anesthesia
- Regional anesthetic such as a brachial plexus block, with sedation or general anesthesia
Patient positioning
- Supine with the arm extended on a hand table
- Nonsterile tourniquet on the brachium

Surgical Procedure
Thumb Ulnar Collateral Ligament Repair
An incision is made on the midlateral ulnar thumb, curved over the MCP joint, and extended proximally, just ulnar to the extensor pollicis longus tendon. Careful dissection is used through the subcutaneous fat to identify and protect any branches of the **dorsal sensory nerve.** The MCP joint is identified through the layers of fascia and extensor hood.

If present, a Stener lesion may be visible at this point. The joint capsule and injured ligament are identified, divided, and characterized. An intrasubstance tear of the UCL may be directly repaired; an avulsion of the ligament from its insertion on the proximal phalanx is frequently repaired using a suture anchor or internal bracing system; an avulsion fracture fragment is frequently stabilized with a screw or wire. Once the repair is complete the tissues are irrigated and closed in layers. Skin suture using a 4-0 or 5-0 suture are performed and a thumb spica splint is applied.

Thumb Ulnar Collateral Ligament Reconstruction

Several different surgical techniques have been described. Frequently, a tendon graft from the patient's palmaris longus tendon or a slip of the FCR tendon is used to reconstruct the UCL.

Estimated Postoperative Recovery Course

Postoperative days 10 to 14:
- Sutures are removed, and a wound check is performed.
- Obtain x-rays if a bony repair was performed or if K-wires are present.
- A thumb spica cast is applied for about 4 weeks.

Postoperative 4 weeks:
- The cast is removed, and a supportive, hand-based thumb spica splint is applied.
- Start therapy for thumb motion and initiate strengthening over the next several weeks.
- If a K-wire is present, it is generally removed around 4 weeks postoperative.

Postoperative 3 months:
- Return to activities is unrestricted.

SUGGESTED READINGS

Heymen P: Injuries to the ulnar collateral ligament of the thumb metacarpophalangeal joint, *J Am Acad Orthop Surg* 5:224–229, 1997.

Merrell G, Slade JF: Dislocations and ligament injuries in the digits. In Wolfe SW, Hotchkiss RN, Pedersen WC, Kozin SH, editors: *Green's operative hand surgery*, ed 6, Philadelphia, 2011, Elsevier.

REFERENCES

1. Heymen P: Injuries to the ulnar collateral ligament of the thumb metacarpophalangeal joint, *J Am Acad Orthop Surg* 5:224–229, 1997.

2. Hergan K, Mittler C, Oser W: Ulnar collateral ligament: differentiation of displaced and nondisplaced tears with US and MR imaging, *Radiology* 194(1):65–71, 1995.

EXTENSOR TENDON INJURIES

It is important to understand the anatomy of the extensor tendon hood in the finger in order to properly identify, diagnose, and treat injuries of the finger (Fig. 4.51). Extensor tendon injuries can result from an open laceration or a closed traumatic event. Specifically, this section will focus on injury of the extensor tendon central slip and terminal extensor tendon (also known as mallet finger). These injuries are important to identify because a missed diagnosis or delayed treatment can result in a Boutonnière deformity and swan neck deformity, respectively. Other zones of extensor tendon injury and recommended treatment will be mentioned briefly.

Central Slip Injury

The central slip of the extensor communis tendon inserts on the dorsal base of the middle phalanx. The central slip may be injured due to an open laceration over the dorsal PIP joint or from a sudden traumatic event such as a volar PIP joint dislocation (the middle phalanx is displaced volar to the proximal phalanx; volar PIP dislocations are not as common as dorsal PIP joint dislocations). If the injury is not identified the patient may be develop a Boutonnière deformity of the digit.

History

- Injury or laceration near the dorsal PIP joint
- Associated with volar PIP joint dislocations
- Patient may report an inability to fully extend the finger

Physical Examination

- Observe for lacerations or deformity of the digit.
- Observe if there is an extension lag in the affected digit.
- Assess the neurovascular status of both digital nerves.
- Examine the patient's ability to extend each finger individually while the adjacent fingers remain flexed at the MCP joint. This maneuver eliminates pull from a juncturae tendinum that can confuse the examination:
  - Juncturae tendinum are variable interconnections between the extensor tendons at the level of the hand metacarpals. If an extensor tendon

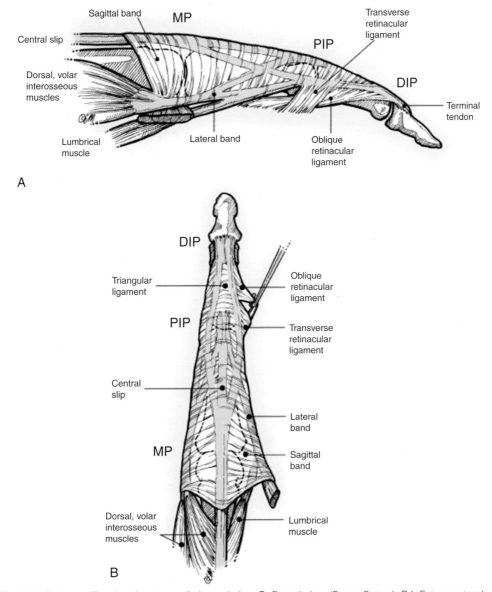

Fig. 4.51 Extensor Tendon Anatomy. A. Lateral view **B.** Dorsal view (From: Strauch RJ: Extensor tendon injury. In: Wolfe, Hotchkiss, Pedersen, Kozin, editors, *Greens operative hand surgery*, ed 6, Philadelphia, 2011, Elsevier, Figure 6.5A&B, p. 162)

laceration is proximal to the juncturae, the adjacent intact extensor tendon can extend the finger, and an extensor tendon laceration can be missed.

- Apply strength against resistance of the affected digit in extension; a weak or painful test may indicate a partial or full central slip injury.
- Perform an **Elson test** (Fig. 4.52):

- Rest the patient's hand on a table with the affected finger flexed at the PIP joint over the edge of the table.
- Hold the PIP joint fixed at 90 degrees while the patient attempts to extend at the PIP joint.
- If the DIP joint is supple during active extension, the central slip is intact.

Elson's Test

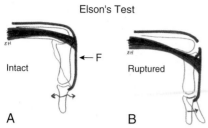

Intact   Ruptured

A   B

Fig. 4.52 A and B, The Elson test for acute rupture of the central slip. *F*, Static force. (From Lattanza LL, Hattwick EA: Extensor tendon repair and reconstruction. In: Trumble T, Budoff J, Cornwall R, editors, *Hand, elbow, and shoulder: core knowledge in orthopaedics*, Philadelphia, 2006, Mosby, p 206.)

- If the DIP joint is rigid during active extension, the central slip is likely completely ruptured. This occurs because the patient will inadvertently try to extend the finger by using the intact lateral bands and terminal extensor tendon that inserts onto the distal phalanx, thereby making the DIP joint rigid (see Fig. 4.5 for anatomy).

Imaging

- Order finger radiographs: PA, lateral, and oblique views to evaluate for concomitant fracture or joint subluxation/dislocation.
- MRI or ultrasound can help evaluate for tendon ruptures or lacerations if the diagnosis cannot be made based on physical examination alone.

Classification

- There are 8 zone of extensor tendon injury plus the thumb (Fig. 4.53).

Differential Diagnosis

- Partial extensor tendon injury
- PIP joint sprain
- PIP joint dislocation
- Volar plate injury/avulsion
- Joint contracture

Initial Management

- If a laceration is present, perform a digital block and thoroughly cleanse the wound. Observe the extensor tendon during laceration repair and note if the injury is full or partial (e.g., 50% laceration, 25% laceration). Close the wound with suture and refer to a

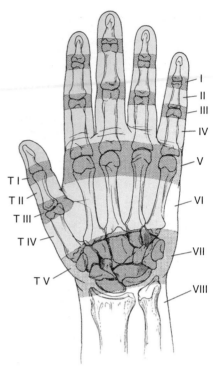

Fig. 4.53 Zones of the Extensor Tendon System. *T*, Thumb. (From Lattanza LL, Hattwick EA: Extensor tendon repair and reconstruction. In: Trumble T, Budoff J, Cornwall R, editors, *Hand, elbow, and shoulder: core knowledge in orthopaedics*, Philadelphia, 2006, Mosby, p 203.)

hand specialist. Tetanus status update and prophylactic antibiotics may be indicated.
- If a dislocation is present, perform closed reduction under a digital block and splint in extension. Refer to a hand specialist for evaluation.
- If the injury is reduced and closed, splint the finger in extension and refer to a hand specialist for further evaluation.
- **Patient Education.** If an injury to the central slip is not properly treated the patient will develop a flexion contracture of the PIP joint called a Boutonnière deformity.

! CLINICAL ALERT

The patient with a central slip injury MUST wear their splint 24/7 in order to facilitate tendon healing. If the PIP joint is allowed to bend at any point, the time to complete healing restarts.

Nonoperative Management

Indications

- Open or closed partial central slip injuries
- Acute closed central slip injuries

Apply a PIP joint extension splint (the DIP and MCP joints should remain mobile) and instruct the patient to wear the splint continuously for a minimum of 6 weeks. The splint cannot be removed and the PIP joint cannot be allowed to flex during this time.

After 6 weeks of continuous mobilization, start intermittent and night splinting for an additional 4 to 6 weeks and monitor for development of an extensor lag or Boutonnière deformity at the PIP joint. Counsel the patient that if a lag develops, additional splinting or surgery may be indicated.

Operative Management

ICD-10 Code: S66.9 Laceration of unspecified muscle, fascia, and tendon at wrist and hand level

M20.0 Boutonnière deformity

CPT codes: 26426 Extensor tendon repair, central slip repair, secondary (Boutonnière deformity); using local tissue

Indications

- Central slip injury with displaced avulsion fracture
- Acute injuries with joint instability or subluxation
- Failure of nonoperative management

Informed consent and counseling

- Repair of the central slip may result in some degree of permanent finger stiffness. Compliance with postoperative instructions and therapy is paramount to a good result.

Anesthesia

- Local anesthetic such as a digital block or regional anesthetic such as a Bier block with or without sedation

Patient positioning

- Supine with arm extended on a hand table

Surgical Procedure

A straight dorsal approach to the PIP joint is typically used. The extensor hood and the zone of injury within the central slip is identified and freed of adhesions. If a fracture is present, K-wires are used to reduce the fracture under fluoroscopic guidance. The central slip can be repaired primarily with suture or a suture anchor. Frequently, a temporary K-wire is placed across the PIP joint to hold it in extension.

The wound is irrigated and closed and the finger is splinted in full extension.

Estimated Postoperative Recovery Course

Postoperative 1 to 2 weeks:

- Wound check and resplint. Some prefer to transition the patient to a custom PIP joint extension splint fabricated by a hand therapist. Ensure the patient is moving adjacent joints and fingers to prevent stiffness. If wire present, perform x-rays and teach pin-site care.

Postoperative 6 weeks:

- Transarticular wires are removed, if present. The patient will start a graduated therapy program with intermittent and night time splinting for the next 2 to 4 weeks. Dynamic splinting and therapy techniques may also be employed in order to regain finger flexion.

Postoperative 12 weeks:

- Assess and document PIP joint motion. Continue therapy if needed.

MALLET FINGER

A mallet finger is a commonly encountered injury that results from a sudden axial force at the fingertip such as "jamming" the finger into an object. The injury mechanism results in a disruption of the terminal extensor tendon from its insertion on the distal phalanx and subsequently the patient develops an extensor lag, or an inability to extend the finger actively at the DIP joint. The injury may be isolated to the extensor tendon (soft tissue) or result in a bony avulsion from the dorsal distal phalanx (bony).

History

- The mechanism of injury is forced flexion of an extended finger at the DIP joint.
- The injury may be associated with an open laceration dorsally.

Physical Examination: Fig. 4.54

- The finger may be edematous, ecchymotic, and painful at the DIP joint.
- Loss of active extension is noted at the DIP joint, but passive extension is intact.
- The finger is often held in a flexed position at the DIP joint.
- Nail hematoma is possible.

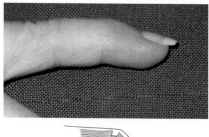

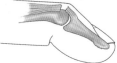

Fig. 4.54 Mallet Finger Position Resulting from Rupture of the Terminal Extensor Tendon. (From Henry SL, Ingari J: Mallet finger. In: Miller MD, Hart JA, MacKnight JM, editors, *Essential orthopaedics*, Philadelphia, 2010, Saunders, p 362.)

Imaging
- Order finger radiographs: PA, **unsupported** lateral, and oblique views. Evaluate for an avulsion fracture. Evaluate for subluxation of the distal phalanx.

Classification: Figs. 4.55 and 4.56
- Soft tissue or bony
- Type 1: closed mallet finger
- Type 2: open mallet finger (laceration at the dorsum of the DIP joint)
- Type 3: open with loss of skin and tendon
- Type 4: involving large mallet fragments

Differential Diagnosis
- Arthritis of the DIP joint
- Other fracture or dislocation of the DIP joint

Initial Management
- This common injury can usually be treated without surgery but patient education and compliance is key to a successful and timely outcome.
- Splint the DIP joint in extension (allow PIP joint motion) and refer to a hand surgeon to be seen within 7 to 10 days (Fig. 4.57).
- Open injuries should be anesthetized, cleansed and sutured, and splinted with the DIP joint in extension. Refer to a hand surgeon for evaluation within 3 days.
- **Patient Education.** It is important to clearly inform the patient NOT to remove the splint and that

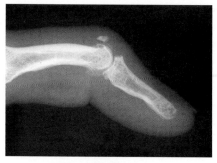

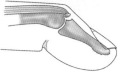

Fig. 4.55 Bony mallet finger involving a small avulsion fracture. This injury will usually heal with splinting. (From Henry SL, Ingari J: Mallet finger. In: Miller MD, Hart JA, MacKnight JM, editors, *Essential orthopaedics*, Philadelphia, 2010, Saunders, p 362.)

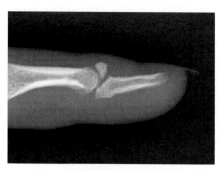

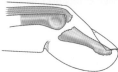

Fig. 4.56 Bony mallet finger with a large fracture fragment that encompasses 50% of the articular surface with subluxation of the distal phalanx. This requires operative intervention. (From Henry SL, Ingari J: Mallet finger. In: Miller MD, Hart JA, MacKnight JM, editors, *Essential orthopaedics*, Philadelphia, 2010, Saunders, p 363.)

treatment requires that it be worn CONTINUOUSLY for 6 to 8 weeks.
- Even with appropriate treatment, a small extensor lag may persist, and a less than 15-degree extensor lag after treatment is acceptable.

> **! CLINICAL ALERT**
>
> If left untreated, a mallet finger will result in a permanent swan neck deformity.

Nonoperative Management

Indications

- Conservative management is reserved for closed soft tissue mallet fingers or bony mallets with an articular fragment smaller than 40% of the joint surface and no joint subluxation.
- Immobilize type 1 injuries for 6 to 8 weeks in a DIP joint hyperextension splint, and allow PIP motion (see Fig. 4.57).
  - The finger must remain in the splint at all times. If the splint is removed at any point, the clock is restarted for splinting.
  - Education regarding skin care and the importance of keeping the finger extended at all times is essential.
- Mallet injuries up to 3 months old may be treated in a splint.
- If an extensor lag is still present after 6 weeks of splinting, an additional 2-week period of nighttime splinting in extension is indicated.
- **Rehabilitation.** After 6 to 8 weeks of splinting, the patient can start gradual ROM and use the splint intermittently.

Operative Management

ICD-10 code: M20.01 Mallet finger

CPT codes: 26432 Closed treatment of distal extensor tendon with or without percutaneous pinning

26433 Tendon repair, distal insertion (mallet finger), open, primary, or secondary repair; without graft

Indications

- Surgery is indicated if there is subluxation of the distal phalanx or if there is a bony articular fragment greater than 40% of joint surface (both seen on lateral radiograph).
- Type 2 injuries:

Acute primary repair is performed with nonabsorbable suture sewn in a figure-of-eight fashion. This repair can often be done by incorporating the skin and tendon into the repair. A DIP joint extension splint is still required for 6 to 8 weeks.

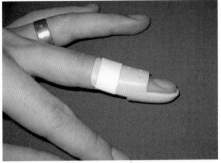

Fig. 4.57 Stack splint used to hold the distal interphalangeal joint in extension while allowing proximal interphalangeal joint motion. (From Henry SL, Ingari J: Mallet finger. In: Miller MD, Hart JA, MacKnight JM, editors, *Essential orthopaedics*, Philadelphia, 2010, Saunders, p 364.)

- Type 3 injuries:

These injuries require soft tissue coverage in the operating room.

- Type 4 injuries:

These injuries require open reduction, internal fixation with screw or wire.

Informed consent and counseling

- The K-wire may stay in place for 4 to 6 weeks and if visible should be kept clean with routine pin site care in order to reduce the risk for infection.
- Stiffness of the DIP joint can develop after surgery, and the patient will require hand therapy to improve terminal finger flexion.

Anesthesia

- Digital block with sedation

Patient positioning

- Supine with the arm extended on a hand table
- Nonsterile tourniquet on the brachium

Surgical Procedure

Closed Reduction, Percutaneous Pinning of the Distal Interphalangeal Joint

- The DIP joint is hyperflexed, and a wire is inserted into the head of the middle phalanx.
- The distal phalanx is then extended until the fracture fragment abuts the wire. The wire acts as an extension block and facilitates reduction.
- Following reduction, a second wire is driven through the end of the finger and across the DIP joint for internal fixation. The patient is placed in a hyperextension finger splint.

Estimated Postoperative Course

- The affected digit is splinted in extension and the PIP joint is allowed to move.
- X-rays are obtained postoperatively to evaluate and document that the joint remains reduced and any fracture fragments, if present, demonstrate healing over time.
- The K-wire is removed under a digital block after 6 to 8 weeks.
- In some cases, nighttime splinting is recommended for an additional 4 weeks after the wire is removed.

! **CLINICAL ALERT**

"Fight bites" are lacerations that occur over the dorsal MCP joint and result in an open, contaminated wound and a partial or complete extensor tendon laceration. Typical isolated organisms are *Eikenella, Streptococcus, or Staphylococcus* species. If the patient is presenting early, thorough irrigation and débridement and initiation of broad-spectrum antibiotics are key to preventing infection. A thorough evaluation that includes x-rays to evaluate for retained tooth fragments and fracture is required. The wound should be left open to allow for drainage and to prevent the development of abscess and the MCP joints should be splinting in extension. The patient should be referred to a hand surgery within 3 days for evaluation and treatment.

Board Review

1. An injury to the extensor tendon central slip at the PIP joint can result in a Boutonnière deformity.
2. A Boutonnière deformity is defined as flexion of the PIP Joint with paradoxical hyperextension of the DIP joint.
3. An injury to the terminal extensor tendon at the DIP joint is called a mallet finger and results in an extensor lag (or flexed posture) of the DIP joint.
4. A swan neck deformity can result from an untreated mallet finger.
5. A swan neck deformity is defined as hyperextension of the PIP joint with paradoxical flexion of the DIP joint.

SUGGESTED READINGS

Hanz KR, Saint-Cyr M, Semmler M, et al.: Extensor tendon injuries: acute management and secondary reconstruction, *Plast Reconstr Surg* 121:109e–120e, 2008.

Henry SL, Ingari J: Mallet finger. In Miller MD, Hart JA, MacKnight JM, editors: *Essential orthopaedics*, Philadelphia, 2010, Saunders, pp 361–366.

Lattanza LL, Hattwick EA: Extensor tendon repair and reconstruction. In Trumble TE, Budoff JE, Cornwall R, editors: *Hand, elbow, and shoulder: core knowledge in orthopaedics*, Philadelphia, 2006, Mosby, pp 201–211.

Matzon JL, Bozentka DJ: Extensor tendon injuries, *J Hand Surg Am* 35:854–861, 2010.

Newport ML: Extensor tendon injuries in the hand, *J Am Acad Orthop Surg* 5(2):59–66, 1997.

Rockwell WB, Butler PN, Byrne BA: Extensor tendon: anatomy, injury and reconstruction, *Plast Reconstr Surg* 106:1592–1603, 2000.

FLEXOR TENDON INJURIES

History

- Laceration to the volar surface of the wrist, hand, or finger is present.
- The patient may report an inability to flex a digit or digits.
- The patient may report decreased sensation if there is concomitant nerve injury.
- Ruptures may occur in the setting of chronic attrition (seen in inflammatory conditions such as rheumatoid arthritis).

Physical Examination

- Inspect the wound (do not probe).
- Assess capillary refill in the digits.
- Assess sensation to light touch on *both* ulnar and radial sides of the digits *before* digital block anesthetic is administered.
- Evaluate the flexor tendons (Figs. 4.58 and 4.59). There are two tendons to each finger, and each must be tested individually. (See the note later in this section about the thumb tendon.)

Flexor Digitorum Profundus Tendon: Fig. 4.59
- The flexor digitorum profundus (FDP) tendon controls motion of the DIP joint.
- Place the patient's hand on the examining table with the palm up. Apply pressure over the middle phalanx, and ask the patient to flex the DIP joint. If the FDP is injured, the patient will not be able to flex the DIP joint. (If the FDS is still intact, the patient will be able to flex at the PIP joint.)

Flexor Digitorum Superficialis Tendon: Fig. 4.59

- The flexor digitorum superficialis (FDS) tendon controls motion of the PIP joint.
- Isolated FDS injuries may be more difficult to identify because the FDP will flex the entire digit. Again, place the patient's hand on the examining table with the palm up. Ask the patient to flex the digit. The patient will often have pain, weakness, or incomplete flexion if the FDS is injured.

Flexor Pollicis Longus Tendon

- **Note:** There is only one flexor tendon to the thumb: the flexor pollicis longus (FPL).
- Test the FPL by applying pressure over the proximal phalanx and asking the patient to flex the thumb at the IP joint. An inability to flex the distal phalanx indicates an FPL injury.

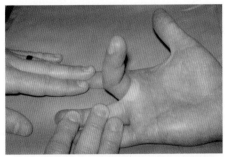

Fig. 4.58 Testing for Flexor Digitorum Superficialis Tendon Injury. (From Chadderdon RD, Isaacs, JE: Flexor tendon injuries. In: Miller MD, Hart JA, MacKnight JM, editors, *Essential orthopaedics*, Philadelphia, 2010, Saunders, p 354.)

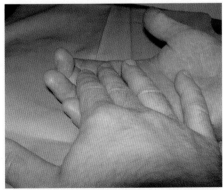

Fig. 4.59 Testing for Flexor Digitorum Profundus Tendon Injury. (From Chadderdon RD, Isaacs, JE: Flexor tendon injuries. In: Miller MD, Hart JA, MacKnight JM, editors, *Essential orthopaedics*, Philadelphia, 2010, Saunders, p 354.)

- Pain with flexion against resistance may indicate a partial tendon injury.

Imaging

- Order wrist, hand, and finger radiographs: PA, lateral, and oblique views to evaluate for concomitant fracture.

Classification: Fig. 4.60

Initial Management

- Wounds should be anesthetized and cleansted and sutured AFTER a complete neurovascular exam. Prophylactic antibiotics may be prescribed.
- A dorsal-blocking splint is applied to prevent proximal tendon migration.
- Refer the patient to a hand surgeon to be seen within 3 to 5 days of injury. Complete tendon injuries require immediate repair within 7 to 10 days.
- **Patient Education.** This injury does not heal without surgery. Successful outcomes depend on the patient's compliance with postoperative therapy.

Operative Management

Principles of flexor tendon repairs:

- Easy placement of sutures
- Secure suture knots
- Smooth juncture at tendon ends
- Minimal gapping at the repair site
- Minimal interference with tendon vascularity
- Sufficient strength throughout healing to allow early motion

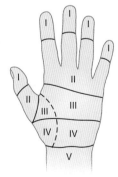

Fig. 4.60 Zones of the Flexor Tendons. (From Boyer MI: Flexor tendon injuries. In: Green DP, Hotchkiss RN, Pederson WC, et al., editors, *Green's operative hand surgery*, Ed 5, Philadelphia, 2005, Churchill Livingstone. Copyright Elizabeth Martin, p 221.)

ICD-10 codes: M66.92 Laceration of muscle, fascia, tendon at wrist and hand level

CPT codes: 25260 Repair, flexor tendon primary

25263 Repair, tendon, secondary

26350 Repair, flexor tendon not in "no man's land"

26356 Repair, flexor tendon in no man's land

26370 Profundus tendon repair, with intact sublimis, primary

Zone I Injuries

- Jersey finger (see the next section, on jersey finger)

Zone II Injuries

- This zone is referred to as "no man's land" because stiffness after injury is very common, and surgery in this area is difficult because of the relationship of the two flexor tendons within the flexor tendon sheath:
  - Camper chiasm occurs at this level (the FDS splints to allow the FDP to continue distally), as does the A2 pulley, which must be repaired to prevent bowstringing of the tendons. Tendon adhesions occur very easily in this area.
- Many techniques have been described, and the type of repair is based on the surgeon's preference.

Zone III Injuries

- Surgical exposure of tendons in this area is easier than in zone II because of the lack of the tendon sheath at this level. Surgical repairs at this level are usually less prone to the stiffness seen in zone II injuries.

Zone IV Injuries

- The tendon is repaired in similar fashion to zone III injuries.
- Repair of the median nerve may also be necessary at this level.

Zone V Injuries

- These injuries can be difficult to repair because muscle tissue will not hold suture.
- Often, mattress sutures are used.

Thumb Flexor Pollicis Longus Tendon Injuries

- Preserve the oblique pulley and the A2 pulley.
- If the FPL tendon has retracted proximally, an incision at the level of the wrist is recommended rather than an incision in the thenar region.
- Repair is similar to that of other flexor tendons, based on the level of injury.

Estimated Postoperative Course

A successful outcome of flexor tendon repair is directly related to strict compliance with a hand therapy program. Many postoperative rehabilitation protocols exist, and the one chosen is based on the type of surgical repair and the experience and preference of the surgeon. Protocols that favor early passive flexion exercise within 3 to 5 days of surgery may have improved functional outcomes.

SUGGESTED READINGS

Boyer M, Taras JS, Kaufman RA: Flexor tendon injury. In Green DP, Hotchkiss RN, Pederson WC, et al.: *Green's operative hand surgery*, ed 5, Philadelphia, 2005, Churchill Livingstone, pp 219–276.

Chadderdon RC, Isaacs JE: Flexor tendon injuries. In Miller MD, Hart JA, MacKnight JM, editors: *Essential orthopaedics*, Philadelphia, 2010, Saunders, pp 352–356.

Lilly SI, Messer TM: Complications after treatment of flexor tendon injuries, *J Am Acad Orthop Surg* 14(7):387–396, 2006.

Rekant M: Flexor tendon injuries. In Trumble TE, Budoff JE, Cornwall R, editors: *Hand, elbow, and shoulder: core knowledge in orthopaedics*, Philadelphia, 2006, Mosby, pp 189–200.

Strickland JW: Development of flexor tendon surgery: twenty-five years of progress, *J Hand Surg Am* 25(2):214–235, 2000.

JERSEY FINGER

A Jersey Finger is a rupture of the FDP tendon from its insertion on the distal phalanx and results in an inability to flex the finger at the DIP joint.

History

- Forced hyperextension of the distal phalanx from a flexed position (Fig. 4.61).
- Jersey finger often results from an athletic injury.
- The patient may report hearing a "pop" in the finger.
- The ring finger is the most commonly injured.

Physical Examination

- Tenderness to palpation at the volar base of the DIP joint
- Edema and/or ecchymosis surrounding the volar DIP joint
- Inability to flex at the DIP joint actively, with intact passive flexion

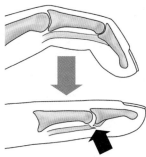

Fig. 4.61 Jersey Finger: Flexor Digitorum Profundus Rupture. Tendon rupture occurs when a flexed digit in forcibly extended. (From Ingari J: Jersey finger [flexor digitorum profundus avulsion]. In: Miller MD, Hart JA, MacKnight JM, editors, *Essential orthopaedics*, Philadelphia, 2010, Saunders, p 368.)

- Possible tenderness to palpation at the location of a retracted tendon stump

Imaging

- Order finger radiographs: PA, lateral, and oblique views.
- Avulsion fracture can accompany tendon injury.

Additional Imaging

- Ultrasonography or MRI can help to identify rupture of the flexor tendon or localize the proximal stump for surgical planning.

Classification

- Type 1: The FDP stump has retracted into the palm.
- Type II: The FDP stump has retracted to the level of the PIP joint.
- Type III: The FDP avulsion is attached to a large fracture fragment.

Differential Diagnosis

- Fracture not associated with an FDP avulsion
- Nerve injury or palsy (e.g., anterior interosseous nerve palsy)
- Flexor tendon rupture outside zone 1

Initial Management

- A dorsal blocking splint that includes all the digits should be applied to try to prevent further proximal migration of the tendon stump.
- The patient should be referred to a hand surgeon with 3 to 5 days of injury for a timely repair within 7 to 10 days of injury.

- **Patient Education.** A jersey finger injury always requires surgical intervention.

Operative Management

ICD-9 Code: M66.34 spontaneous rupture of flexor tendon, hand
CPT code: 26350 Repair of flexor tendon

Type 1 injury
- The blood supply is compromised, and the tendon should be repaired within 7 days.

Type II and III injuries
- These injuries can be repaired even after a delay in treatment of several weeks.

Informed consent and counseling
- The patient can expect to be immobilized in some fashion for 4 to 6 weeks.
- The patient will require approximately 3 to 4 months of outpatient hand therapy to restore motion and strength. This therapy is essential for a good outcome.
- Even with good surgical repair and compliance with a therapy program, stiffness may persist.

Anesthesia
- Regional anesthetic such as a brachial plexus block, with sedation or general anesthesia

Patient positioning
- Supine with the arm extended on a hand table
- Nonsterile tourniquet on the brachium

Surgical Procedure

Flexor Digitorum Profundus Repair with Button Technique or Suture Anchor

A Bruner-type incision is made on the volar aspect of the finger in order to prevent scar contracture. The avulsion site on the volar distal phalanx is identified and débrided. Then, the proximal end of the tendon is retrieved. Core sutures are placed in the tendon stump for subsequent passage into the tendon sheath. The A2 and A4 pulleys are protected and preserved. Keith needles are driven from proximal to distal and volar to dorsal through the distal phalanx, exiting dorsally in the nail plate and temporarily left in place. The sutures are threaded through the needles and pulled out dorsally. A surgical button is applied, the finger is flexed, and the sutures are tied tightly over the button. Alternatively, suture anchors into the distal phalanx may be used. The patient is placed in dorsal blocking splint with wrist in slight flexion.

Estimated Postoperative Course

Postoperative days 10 to 14:
- Sutures are removed from the volar finger incision; the button or suture over the nail remains in place for 4 to 6 weeks.
- Immobilization: The patient is given a dorsal blocking splint.
- *Therapy referral:* Start a flexor tendon protocol (many exist, it will be the surgeon's choice).

Postoperative 4 to 6 weeks:
- The button or suture is removed, and the therapy protocol progresses.

Postoperative 12 and 16 weeks:
- The patient returns for a motion check.
- Progress with therapy is made according to the protocol.

SUGGESTED READINGS

Ingari J: Jersey finger (flexor digitorum profundus avulsion). In Miller MD, Hart JA, MacKnight JM, editors: *Essential orthopaedics*, Philadelphia, 2010, Saunders, pp 367–368.

Rekant M: Flexor tendon injuries. In Trumble TE, Budoff JE, Cornwall R, editors: *Hand, elbow, and shoulder: core knowledge in orthopaedics*, Philadelphia, 2006, Mosby, pp 189–200.

Tuttle HG, Oley SP, Stern PJ: Tendon avulsion injuries of the distal phalanx, *Clin Orthop Relat Res* 445:157–168, 2006.

Murphy BA, Mass DP: Zone 1 flexor tendon injuries, *Hand Clin* 21:167–171, 2005.

FINGER INFECTIONS: PARONYCHIA AND FELON

A paronychia is common type of finger infection that results in infection and abscess along the nailfold (Fig. 4.62). It is usually associated with hang nails, biting of the nails, or contamination from manicures.

A felon is an infection of the finger pulp, the septated spongy tissue on the volar aspect of the digit (Fig. 4.63). A felon can result from a laceration or puncture.

Both are associated with *Staphylococcus aureus* or *Streptococcus* species, though cultures should be taken to help guide antibiotic treatment. Felon and paronychia can occur simultaneously, and both require surgical incision and drainage.

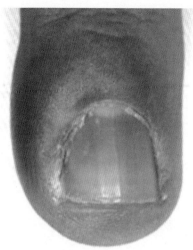

Fig. 4.62 Paronychia. (From Waugh RP, Zlotolow: Hand infections. In: Miller MD, Hart JA, MacKnight JM, editors, *Essential orthopaedics*, Philadelphia, 2010, Saunders, Figure 94.3A, p 383)

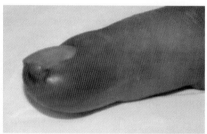

Fig. 4.63 Felon. (From Waugh RP, Zlotolow: Hand infections. In: Miller MD, Hart JA, MacKnight JM, editors, *Essential orthopaedics*, Philadelphia, 2010, Saunders, Figure 94.3B, p 383)

History
- The patient may or may not recall a traumatic event prior to the onset of symptoms.
- The patient reports pain and tenderness localized to the nailfold (paronychia) or the finger pulp (felon).

Physical Examination
- There may be erythema, enlargement, and edema of the affected area
- A visible abscess may be present, especially with a paronychia
- Finger ROM is generally preserved but mild limitation due to pain may be present
- There is NO tenderness related to the DIP joint or flexor tendon sheath

Imaging

- Usually not necessary unless the infection has been prolonged or fulminant and there is concern for bone or joint involvement.

Differential Diagnosis

- Cellulitis
- Infectious flexor tenosynovitis
- Gouty arthritis
- Septic arthritis
- Foreign body reaction

Initial Management

- Paronychia that is caught early in the stages of cellulitis and lacks abscess could potentially be managed with warm water and Epson salt soaks and oral antibiotics. Close follow up to ensure response to treatment is recommended.
- Incision and drainage is the recommended treatment for paronychia and felons.
- **Patient Education.** Wounds are typically packed open and follow-up wound care may be necessary. Provide counsel on avoiding biting of the nails or contaminated manicures.

Operative Management

ICD-10 Code. L02.51 Cutaneous abscess of finger
CPT Code. 20600 Incision and drainage of finger abscess

Indications

- Active or evolving paronychia or felon.

Informed consent and counseling

- The patients wound will be packed open to allow for continued drainage and postoperative wound care will be necessary. Oral antibiotics should be taken to treat the infection.

Anesthesia

- This procedure can be performed in a clinic or small-procedure setting under a local digital block

Surgical Procedure
Incision and Drainage

Finger Abscess. Once the finger is anesthetized under a digital block, a finger tourniquet is placed to prevent bleeding and improve visualization.

Paronychia. A #15 blade is used to incise the affected area in a longitudinal fashion along the nailfold. Cultures can be obtained. Hemostats are used to spread tissue to ensure complete drainage and the wound is copiously irrigated with normal saline. Sterile gauze packing may be placed into the wound. A dressing is applied and the tourniquet is released.

Felon. A #15 blade is used to create a 1-cm incision on the radial or ulnar aspect of the affected digit. Consideration should be taken if the finger is a "border digit" as sensitivity can occur. For felons affecting the index finger, the incision should be placed on the ulnar aspect of the pulp. For infections affecting the small finger, the incision should be placed on the radial aspect of the digit. It is paramount to use a hemostat to penetrate the deeper tissue of the finger pulp in order to open the individual septae of the pulp. Cultures may be obtained and the wound is copiously irrigated and packed open. A dressing is applied and the tourniquet is released.

Estimated Postoperative Recovery Course

Postoperative day 1 to 2:
- Perform a wound check to ensure infection is improving.
- Remove packing and perform local wound care. Repeat packing may be necessary, depending on severity of infection.
- Check cultures and adjust antibiotics as needed.

Postoperative day 7 to 10:
- Infection should be resolved and the patient should begin to return to regular activities.

Board Review

A paronychia is an infection of the nailfold.
   A felon is an infection of the finger pulp.

SUGGESTED READINGS

Jebson P: Infections of the fingertip: paronychias and felons, *Hand Clin* 5:547–555, 1998.
Osterman M, Draeger R, Stern P: Acute hand infections, *J Hand Surg Am* 39(8):1628–1635, 2014.

ORTHOPAEDIC PROCEDURES

Carpal Tunnel Injection
Code

CPT code: 20526

Indications
- Median nerve compression (i.e., CTS) that has not responded to conservative treatment

Contraindications
- Allergy to an intended medication
- Local skin rash or active skin lesion over the injection site

Equipment Needed
- Alcohol swabs and povidone-iodine swab sticks or other antiseptic of choice
- 5-mL syringe
- 25-gauge needle, 1 to 1.5 inches
- Injectate: 3 mL 1% lidocaine without epinephrine and 1 mL corticosteroid
- Adhesive bandage
- Optional: ethyl chloride spray

Procedure
1. Identify anatomic landmarks.
   - Have the patient pinch all fingertips together while the wrist is in a neutral position to identify the palmaris longus (PL) tendon.
   - Identify the proximal wrist crease.
   - In patients without a PL tendon, use the ulnar midline of the wrist.
2. Clean and prepare skin at the site of injection.
3. Spray with ethyl chloride.
4. Wipe once more with an alcohol pad.
5. Insert the needle just ulnar to the PL tendon at the level of the proximal wrist crease at a 30- to 45-degree angle, directed toward the ring finger (Fig. 4.64).
6. If the needle meets obstruction or the patient experiences nerve pain, withdraw the needle and redirect in a slightly more ulnar location.
7. Inject slowly with constant pressure.
8. Remove the needle, and hold pressure with gauze.
9. Place a bandage over the injection site.

Aftercare Instructions
1. If the patient has diabetes mellitus, caution that glucose levels may increase for up to 5 to 7 days.
2. The patient should avoid strenuous activity with the hand for 24 to 48 hours after injection.
3. Pain or discomfort at the injection site may occur, but it typically subsides within 24 to 48 hours. This pain may be treated with ice and/or NSAIDs.

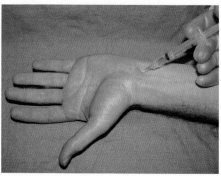

Fig. 4.64 Carpal Tunnel Wrist Injection. The needle is inserted just ulnar to Palmaris longus at the wrist crease. (From Schnur D: Carpal tunnel injection. In: Miller MD, Hart JA, MacKnight JM, editors, *Essential orthopaedics*, Philadelphia, 2010, Saunders, p 441.)

Trigger Finger Injection
Code
CPT code: 20526

Indications
- Symptomatic trigger finger
- Noninfectious flexor tenosynovitis (found in rheumatoid arthritis)

Contraindications
- Allergy to intended medication
- Local skin rash or active skin lesion over the injection site

Equipment Needed
- Alcohol swabs and povidone-iodine swab sticks or other antiseptic of choice
- 3-mL syringe
- 25- or 27-gauge needle, 1 to 1.5 inches
- Injectate: 1 mL 1% lidocaine without epinephrine and 1 mL of corticosteroid
- Adhesive bandage
- Optional: ethyl chloride spray

Procedure: Figs. 4.65 and 4.66
1. Identify anatomic landmarks, and inject at the level of the A1 pulley.
2. Clean and prepare the skin at the site of injection.
3. Spray with ethyl chloride.
4. Wipe once more with an alcohol pad.
5. Insert the needle at the level of the A1 pulley with the needle pointing toward the affected finger.

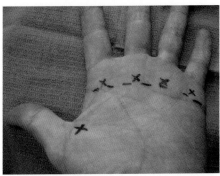

Fig. 4.65 X Marks the Sites of Injection for Trigger Digits. (From Ingari J: Trigger finger injection. In: Miller MD, Hart JA, MacKnight JM, editors, *Essential orthopaedics,* Philadelphia, 2010, Saunders, p 446.)

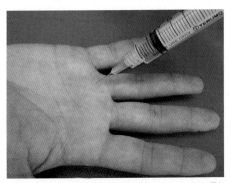

Fig. 4.66 Trigger Finger Injection. (From Ingari J: Trigger finger injection. In: Miller MD, Hart JA, MacKnight JM, editors, *Essential orthopaedics*, Philadelphia, 2010, Saunders, p 446.)

6. If the needle meets obstruction or the patient experiences nerve pain, withdraw the needle slightly and inject again.
7. Inject slowly with constant pressure.
8. Remove the needle, and hold pressure with gauze.
9. Place a bandage on the injection site.

Aftercare Instructions
1. If the patient has diabetes mellitus, caution that glucose levels may increase for up to 5 to 7 days.
2. The patient should avoid strenuous activity with the hand for 24 to 48 hours after injection.
3. Pain or discomfort at the injection site may occur, but it typically subsides within 24 to 48 hours. This pain may be treated with ice and/or NSAIDs.

First Carpometacarpal Joint Injection
Code
CPT code: 20526

Indications
• First CMC joint OA not responsive to conservative measures

Contraindications
• Allergy to intended medication
• Local skin rash or active skin lesion over the injection site

Equipment Needed
• Fluoroscopy to help guide the injection site, if available
• Alcohol swabs and povidone-iodine swab sticks or antiseptic of choice
• 3-mL syringe
• 25- or 27-gauge needle, 1 to 1.5 inches
• Injectate: 1 mL 1% lidocaine without epinephrine and 1 mL corticosteroid
• Adhesive bandage
• Optional: ethyl chloride spray

Procedure: Figs. 4.67 and 4.68
1. Identify anatomic landmarks.
   • Place the patient's hand dorsal side down.
   • Palpate the joint space between the trapezium and the first metacarpal.
1. Clean and prepare the skin at the site of injection.
2. Spray with ethyl chloride.
3. Wipe once more with an alcohol pad.
4. Insert the needle at the first CMC joint; use fluoroscopy if available. Traction may be applied to the thumb to open the joint space further.
5. If the needle meets obstruction, withdraw the needle slightly and inject again.
6. Inject slowly with constant pressure.
7. Hold pressure with gauze.
8. Place a bandage on the injection site.

Aftercare Instructions
1. If the patient has diabetes mellitus, caution that glucose levels may increase for up to 5 to 7 days.
2. The patient should avoid strenuous activity with the hand for 24 to 48 hours after injection.
3. Pain or discomfort at the injection site may occur, but it typically subsides within 24 to 48 hours. This pain may be treated with ice and/or NSAIDs.

Wrist Injection and Aspiration
Code
CPT code: 20605

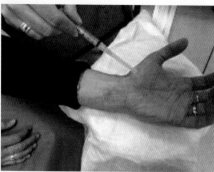

Fig. 4.67 Volar Approach to First Carpometacarpal (CMC) Injections.

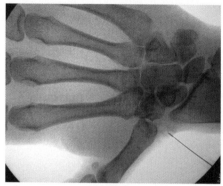

Fig. 4.68 Fluoroscopic Confirmation of Needle Placement for a First Carpometacarpal (CMC) Injection.

Indications
- Injection
  - Radiocarpal wrist arthritis
  - SLAC
  - Scaphoid nonunion advanced collapse
  - Kienbock disease
  - Hematoma block for fracture reduction
- Aspiration to aid in diagnosis of:
  - Septic arthritis
  - Crystalline arthropathy (i.e., gout or pseudogout)

Contraindications
- Allergies to cortisone or its derivative
- Local skin rash or active skin lesion over the injection site
- Suspected wrist infection

Equipment Needed
- Alcohol swabs and povidone-iodine swab sticks or antiseptic of choice

- Bandage strip and gauze pad
- Optional: ethyl chloride spray
  Injection
- 5-mL syringe
- 25- or 27-gauge needle, 1 to 1.5 inches
- Injectate: 3 mL 1% lidocaine without epinephrine and 1 mL of corticosteroid
  Aspiration
- 10-mL empty syringe
- 18- to 21-gauge needle

Procedure: Figs. 4.69 and 4.70
1. Identify anatomic landmarks for the radiocarpal joint.
2. Palpate Lister tubercle; about 1 to 2 cm distal to this is the SL interval.
3. Clean and prepare the skin at the site of injection.
4. Spray with ethyl chloride.
5. Wipe once more with an alcohol pad.
6. Insert the needle into the radiocarpal joint at the previously described interval. Traction may be applied to wrist to open the joint space further.
7. If the needle meets obstruction, withdraw the needle slightly and redirect it.
8. Inject slowly with constant pressure.
9. Hold pressure with gauze.
10. Place a bandage on the injection site.
11. Aspiration is performed in a similar manner.

Aftercare Instructions
1. If the patient has diabetes mellitus, caution that glucose levels may increase for up to 5 to 7 days.
2. The patient should avoid strenuous activity with the wrist for 24 to 48 hours after injection.
3. Pain or discomfort at the injection site may occur, but it typically subsides within 24 to 48 hours. This pain may be treated with ice and/or NSAIDs.

De Quervain's Tenosynovitis Injection
Code
CPT code: 20550

Indications
- Pain from de Quervain's tenosynovitis that has not responded to conservative measures

Contraindications
- Allergy to intended medication

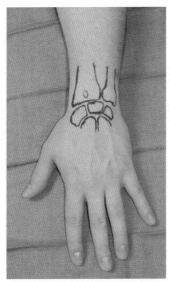

Fig. 4.69 Landmarks for Radiocarpal Injection. (From Zlotolow DA: Radiocarpal joint injection. In: Miller MD, Hart JA, MacKnight JM, editors, *Essential orthopaedics*, Philadelphia, 2010, Saunders, p 438.)

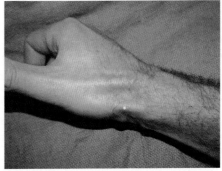

Fig. 4.71 With the thumb abducted and extended, note the tendons of the first dorsal compartment make up the radial border of the snuffbox. (From Zlotolow DA: Radiocarpal joint injection. In: Miller MD, Hart JA, MacKnight JM, editors, *Essential orthopaedics*, Philadelphia, 2010, Saunders, p 436.)

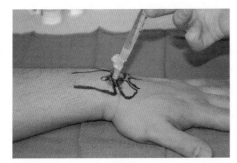

Fig. 4.70 Injection of the Radiocarpal Joint. (From Zlotolow DA: Radiocarpal joint injection. In: Miller MD, Hart JA, MacKnight JM, editors, *Essential orthopaedics*, Philadelphia, 2010, Saunders, p 438.)

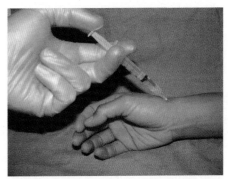

Fig. 4.72 The First Dorsal Compartment Injected at the Level of the Radial Styloid. (From Zlotolow DA: Radiocarpal joint injection. In: Miller MD, Hart JA, MacKnight JM, editors, *Essential orthopaedics*, Philadelphia, 2010, Saunders, p 436.)

- Local skin rash or active skin lesion over the injection site

Equipment Needed
- Alcohol swabs and povidone-iodine swab sticks or other antiseptic of choice
- 5-mL syringe
- 25- or 27-gauge needle, 1 to 1.5 inches
- Injectate: 2 mL 1% lidocaine without epinephrine and 1 mL of corticosteroid
- Adhesive bandage
- Optional: ethyl chloride spray

Procedure: Figs. 4.71 and 4.72
1. Identify anatomic landmarks.
2. With the patient's thumb abducted and extended, palpate the APL and EPB.
3. Clean and prepare the skin at the site of injection.
4. Spray with ethyl chloride.
5. Wipe once more with an alcohol pad.
6. Place the needle in the first extensor compartment, direct it proximally toward the radial styloid, and slide it parallel to the abductor and extensor tendons; observe filling in the sheath.
7. Inject slowly with constant pressure.
8. Hold pressure with gauze.
9. Place a bandage at the injection site.

Aftercare Instructions

1. If the patient has diabetes mellitus, caution that glucose levels may increase for up to 5 to 7 days. Subcutaneous fat atrophy and skin hypopigmentation may occur at the injection site. These changes are usually reversible but may take up to 1 year to resolve.
2. The patient should avoid strenuous activity with the wrist for 24 to 48 hours after injection and should wear a wrist splint continuously except for bathing.
3. Pain or discomfort at the injection site may occur, but it typically subsides within 24 to 48 hours. This pain may be treated with ice and/or NSAIDs.

Dorsal Ganglion Cyst Aspiration (Volar Not Recommended Secondary to Close Proximity of Neurovascular Structures)

Code
CPT code: 20612

Indications
- Painful dorsal wrist or hand cyst
- Cosmetically displeasing cyst

Contraindications
- Allergy to intended medication
- Local skin rash or active skin lesion over the injection site

Equipment Needed
- Alcohol swabs and povidone-iodine swab sticks or antiseptic of choice
- 10- to 20-mL empty syringe
- 18-gauge needle for aspiration
- Local anesthetic: 2–5 mL 1% lidocaine without epinephrine
- 3-mL syringe with 25- or 27-gauge needle, 1 to 1.5 inches for lidocaine administration
- Adhesive bandage
- Compressive wrap
- Optional: ethyl chloride spray

Procedure: Fig. 4.73
1. Identify anatomic landmarks.
2. Palpate the cyst boundaries.

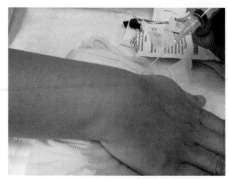

Fig. 4.73 Aspiration of a Dorsal Ganglion Cyst.

3. Clean and prepare the skin at the site of aspiration.
4. Spray with ethyl chloride.
5. Wipe once more with an alcohol pad.
6. Anesthetize the area just proximal to the cyst with 2–5 mL 1% lidocaine without epinephrine.
7. Using an 18-gauge needle and a 10- to 20-mL syringe, aspirate the ganglion cyst. The practitioner may need to encourage aspiration of fluid with digital pressure over the cyst. After the needle is removed, deep palpation may be used for continued release of the cyst.
8. Hold pressure with gauze.
9. Place an adhesive bandage at the injection site, and apply a compressive dressing.

Aftercare Instructions
1. Remove the pressure dressing after 12 to 24 hours.
2. Patients should be aware of the risk of possible cyst recurrence after aspiration.
3. Patients should avoid strenuous activity with the wrist for 24 to 48 hours after aspiration.
4. Pain or discomfort at the injection site may occur, but it typically subsides within 24 to 48 hours. This pain may be treated with ice and/or NSAIDs.

ACKNOWLEDGMENTS

The authors would like to acknowledge the contribution of the previous edition author, Amy Radian.

5

Pelvis

Chad Wilson

ANATOMY: FIG. 5.1

See Chapter 6 (Hip and Femur) for additional images.

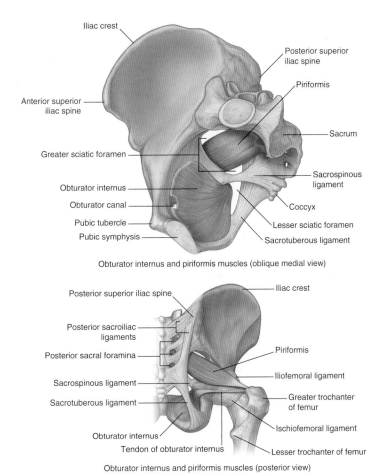

Obturator internus and piriformis muscles (oblique medial view)

Obturator internus and piriformis muscles (posterior view)

Fig. 5.1 Pelvic Ligaments. (Elsevier illustration from www.elsevierimages.com. Copyright, Elsevier Inc. All rights reserved.)

PHYSICAL EXAMINATION

Inspect for deformity, lower extremely malrotation, leg length discrepancy, increased/decreased lordosis, pelvic obliquity

Palpate anterior and posterior landmarks

- Iliac crest
- Iliac tubercle
- Pubic tubercle
- Anterior superior iliac spine (ASIS)
- Posterior superior iliac spine (PSIS)
- Sacroiliac (SI) joint
- Coccyx
- Ischial tuberosity
- Greater trochanter
- Iliopsoas tendon
- Piriformis
- Inguinal ligament
- Symphysis
- Pubic rami
- Abdomen for hernia or masses

Neurovascular Examination: Table 5.1
Special Tests

- **FABER test,** Flexion ABduction External Rotation: Tests for SI joint or hip pathology. With the patient lying supine, the femur is flexed, abducted, and externally rotated by placing the foot of the involved side on the opposite knee. If inguinal pain is elicited, this suggests hip pathology. The examiner then places one hand on the flexed and abducted knee and the other hand on the patient's ASIS. Pressure is applied; increased pain during this maneuver suggests SI joint pathology.
- **Trendelenburg sign:** Tests for hip abductor muscle (gluteus medius and minimus) dysfunction or weakness. The patient assumes a one-legged stance on the affected leg (lifts unaffected leg). A positive sign is when the pelvis drops on the contralateral side (the side with the leg lifted).
- **Fair test,** Flexion Adduction Internal Rotation: Tests for piriformis syndrome. The patient is placed in the lateral recumbent position with the affected side up. The femur is passively flexed, adducted, and internally rotated. A positive test occurs when pain is reproduced in the gluteus.

Differential Diagnosis: Table 5.2

SACROILIAC DYSFUNCTION

SI joint dysfunction is common amongst patients who experience axial low back pain. Diagnosis can be difficult as imaging alone is not sufficient. Local anesthetic blocks are beneficial in confirming the diagnosis. Long term treatment remains challenging.

History

- Pregnancy
- Leg length discrepancy
- Scoliosis

TABLE 5.1	Neurovascular Examination
Nerve/Vessel	**Location**
Femoral artery	Inferior to inguinal ligament; halfway between the anterior superior iliac spine and the pubic tubercle
Cluneal nerve	Iliac crest between the posterior superior iliac spine and the iliac tubercle
Sciatic nerve	Midway between the greater trochanter and the ischial tuberosity

TABLE 5.2	Differential Diagnosis
Anterior pelvic pain	Pubic rami fracture, acetabular fracture, femur fracture, pubic symphysis disruption, iliopsoas tendonitis/bursitis, hip arthritis, femoral acetabular impingement (FAI), lumbar radiculopathy, nonorthopaedic causes (e.g., intraabdominal, gynecologic, genitourinary)
Lateral pelvic pain	Greater trochanter bursitis, FAI
Posterior pelvic pain	Sacral fractures, sacroiliac joint arthritis/dislocation/fracture, piriformis syndrome, lumbar radiculopathy

- Trauma
- Inflammatory arthritis
- Bacterial infection
- Malignancy
- Complaints of pain in the lower back exacerbated by prolonged sitting, twisting, or hyperextending the back
- Difficulty getting in or out of a car, putting on shoes, or turning over in bed
- Pain is typically unilateral
- Pain may radiate to the buttocks

Physical Examination

- Patient is tender to palpation at the SI joint unilaterally, or bilaterally.
- Perform a Gillet or Stork test. This tests for SI joint dysfunction and is performed bilaterally for comparison. The patient stands with his or her back to the examiner. The examiner places one thumb inferior/medial to the PSIS and one thumb on the base of the sacrum at S2. The patient flexes the hip to 90 degrees. An abnormal or positive test occurs when the examiner's thumb near the PSIS of the flexed hip either remains in place or moves cranially. If the thumb moves caudally, this indicates a normal or negative test.

Imaging: Fig. 5.2

- Pelvis radiograph: Anteroposterior (AP) and lateral to evaluate for sclerosis at the SI joint.
- Bone scans may indicate areas of stress, magnetic resonance imaging (MRI) may reveal synovitis or tumors.

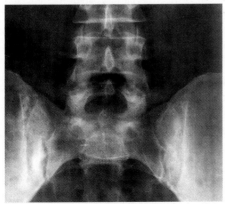

Fig. 5.2 Sclerosis and Pseudowidening at the Sacroiliac Joint. (From Goldman L, Schafer AI: *Goldman's Cecile Medicine,* ed 24, Philadelphia, 2012, Saunders.)

Additional Imaging

- The gold standard is a lidocaine/steroid injection under fluoroscopy to the SI joint, which may be both diagnostic and therapeutic.

Differential Diagnosis

- Intraarticular hip pain
- Lumbar spine disease

Initial Management

- Rest, ice, and mobilization with heat in the acute phase (1–3 days)
- Pelvic belt can also be used in the acute phase but rapid weaning is recommended to reduce weakness and muscular dependence

Nonoperative Management

- Physical therapy to improve pain, strength, flexibility, proprioception
- Intraarticular injections with local anesthetic and corticosteroids have the strongest evidence supporting their use; fluoroscopy is recommended to ensure accuracy
- Prolotherapy can be used to create scarring to minimize motion at the joint if notable laxity at the SI joint

Operative Management

ICD-10 Code: M53.3

Indications

- Failure of all conservative modalities, continued severe pain, and associated functional limitation
- To solidify diagnosis and appropriateness of surgical intervention, patient should experience greater than 75% pain relief from fluoroscopic lidocaine/steroid injection

Informed consent and counseling

- Currently, most private insurances do not cover the cost of surgery
- Many patients will continue to experience some pain after surgery and may ultimately require repeat surgery

Anesthesia

- General anesthesia
- Prone position

Surgical Procedure

- SI arthrodesis is the only described surgical option for SI dysfunction.
- Can be done open or using a percutaneous approach.

- Percutaneous surgical approaches are becoming first-line surgical treatment for SI arthrodesis. Potential advantages include a short hospital stay, decreased limitation of postoperative weight bearing, decreased morbidity, and a small incision.
- There are two open approaches that are commonly utilized: anterior and posterior.
- The anterior approach provides direct access to the ventral and superior portions of the SI joint without notable ligamentous disruption, though this approach can be complicated by greater danger to important neurovascular structures.
- The posterior approach may be a safer approach, but a bony overhang from the posterior iliac crest limits access to the joint, and the incision is located in a dependent position which can lead to wound complications.

Estimated Postoperative Recovery Course

Immediate postoperative:

- Weight bearing as tolerated, no brace required (may depend on approach).

Postoperative week 3:

- First postoperative visit: clinical assessment of wound healing and x-ray to assess implant position and stability.

Postoperative month 3:

- Final routine postoperative visit: repeat x-ray to assess fusion and healing.

Board Review

Image-guided injections are the gold standard in identifying SI joint dysfunction.

SUGGESTED READINGS

Schmidt GL, Bhandutia AK, Altman DT: Management of sacroiliac joint pain, *J Am Acad Orthop Surg* 26(17):610–616, 2018.

Telli H, Telli S, Topal M: The validity and reliability of provocation tests in the diagnosis of sacroiliac joint dysfunction, *Pain Physician* 21(4):E367–E376, 2018. PMID: 30045603.

Polly Jr DW: The sacroiliac joint, *Neurosurg Clin N Am* 28(3):301–312, 2017.

OSTEITIS PUBIS

Osteitis pubis is the inflammation of the pubic symphysis. The etiology is unclear, although it was first described in patients who had undergone suprapubic surgery and later linked to athletes. Inflammation is caused by microtrauma to the adductors or lower rectus muscles, which increases shear forces across the pubic symphysis.

History

- May follow urologic surgery.
- May be associated with athletes involved in soccer, track (sprinters), ice hockey, and football.
- Patient will complain of pain in the groin, hip, perineum, or testicles. The pain may also manifest as lower abdominal pain that radiates to the pubis.
- Pain is worse with running, kicking, or pushing off.

Physical Examination

- A waddling gait is noticeable.
- Tenderness to palpation presents over the pubic symphysis.
- A "single leg hop" may reproduce pain.
- Compression of greater trochanters bilaterally causes pain at the pubic symphysis.
- Weakness at hip adductors or flexors is evident.
- Evaluate for SI joint dysfunction, which can contribute to instability of the pubic symphysis.

Imaging

- AP radiographs of the pelvis may show sclerotic bone, osteolysis, widening, or instability, but positive findings are not seen until more than 4 weeks after the onset of symptoms:
  - Widening of cleft = 10 mm
  - Instability = greater than 2 mm cephalad translation with the patient standing alternately on one leg
- MRI is useful in the acute setting and may demonstrate subchondral bone edema.

Differential Diagnosis

- Intraarticular hip pain
- Genitourinary disorders
- Lumbar radiculopathy
- Sports/inguinal hernia

Initial Management

- REST: Athletes should refrain from sports for at least 1 week.
- Start nonsteroidal antiinflammatory drugs (NSAIDs) to reduce inflammation, massage, and ultrasound.

Nonoperative Management

- Rehabilitation program/physical therapy: aims to correct muscular imbalance around the pubic symphysis. It usually consists of a progressive exercise program, involving stretching and pelvic musculature strengthening to improve pain and prevent recurrence.
- If there is no improvement of pain, corticosteroid injections to the pubic symphysis may be considered. After injection, the athlete must continue to rest and refrain from activity for another week.

Operative Management

- Surgery is rarely indicated but options include curettage of symphyseal fibrocartilage, symphyseal fusion, wedge resection of the symphysis with or without fusion.
- Osteitis pubis is typically self-limiting.

Estimated Recovery Course

- Follow up in clinic in 1 month; if pain free, recommend starting formal rehabilitation program.
- The average time to start squad training is 2 months, while an average of 3 months is required to return to competition.
- Most of the athletes return to preinjury levels within 3 months (from 4 to 14 weeks). Moreover, a successful long-term follow up was reported between 6 and 48 months for all patients.

Board Review

Osteitis is a rare source of groin pain, but most commonly occurs in athletes, specifically, soccer players and runners.

SUGGESTED READINGS

Choi H, McCartney M, Best TM: Treatment of osteitis pubis and osteomyelitis of the pubic symphysis in athletes: a systematic review, *Br J Sports Med* 45(1):57–64, 2011.

Dirkx M, Vitale C: Osteitis pubis. 2020 Mar 5. In *StatPearls [Internet]*, Treasure Island (FL), 2020, StatPearls Publishing.

Via AG, Frizziero A, Finotti P, Oliva F, Randelli F, Maffulli N: Management of osteitis pubis in athletes: rehabilitation and return to training - a review of the most recent literature, *Open Access J Sports Med* 10:1–10, 2018.

APOPHYSITIS AND HIP POINTERS

Apophysitis: an overloading injury at a tendon insertion site; may be acute or chronic and may be associated with avulsion fracture; most commonly affects adolescents

Hip pointers: an injury to the iliac crest or greater trochanter, often due to a direct fall or blow which often resolves entirely with rest

History

- *Apophysitis:* Mechanism of injury (MOI) is a sudden contraction of the muscle followed by acute pain, swelling, and weakness at the insertion point. Symptoms are usually acute but may develop gradually. It is rarely due to a direct blow.
- *Hip pointers:* Direct blow, fall to the hip area. Patient will complain of pain, swelling, or bruising at the site of injury. Symptoms are acute, although they may take 24 to 48 hours to develop after initial injury.

Physical Examination

- Tenderness to palpation, edema, and/or ecchymosis noted along insertion site of hip tendons or bony landmarks
- Antalgic gait
- Pain may limit range of motion
- In apophysitis, pain is reproduced with initiation of the MOI

Imaging

- Plain radiograph of the AP/lateral pelvis may show an avulsion fracture or myositis ossificans, but may also be unremarkable.
- Bone scan/MRI may both be useful in revealing stress/avulsion fracture.

Differential Diagnosis

- Intraarticular hip injury (fracture, avascular necrosis)
- Chronic exertional compartment syndrome

Initial Management

- Recommend ice, rest, NSAIDs, and the use of crutches to facilitate walking if needed.
- Avoidance of aggravating activity. Athletes need to refrain from play until they are pain free to avoid further injury.
- See the patient in follow-up clinic at 2-week intervals until they are pain free with ambulation and range of motion.
- If a hematoma develops, an aspiration can be performed to prevent neurovascular compromise and reduce the risk for developing myositis ossificans. Evacuation of the hematoma could also be performed

surgically if necessary. If pain persists for more than 2 weeks or an avulsion fracture is suspected, refer the patient to an orthopaedic surgeon.

Nonoperative Management
- Local anesthetic injections with/without cortico-steroids may provide short-term pain relief

Operative Management
In the absence of fracture or development of expanding hematoma, surgery is not required.

SUGGESTED READINGS

Paluska SA: An overview of hip injuries in running, *Sports Med* 35(11):991–1014, 2005.

Hall M, Anderson J: Hip pointers, *Clin Sports Med* 32(2):325–330, 2013.

Varacallo M, Bordoni B: Hip pointer injuries. In *StatPearls [Internet]*, Treasure Island (FL), 2020, StatPearls Publishing; 2020.

> **! CLINICAL ALERT**
>
> Rule out expanding hematoma which can lead to myositis ossificans if left untreated.

PIRIFORMIS SYNDROME

Piriformis syndrome is typically characterized as peripheral neuritis of the sciatic nerve caused by inflammation or an abnormal condition of the piri-formis muscle or surrounding musculature at the level of the ischial tuberosity. It is sometimes called deep gluteal syndrome.

History
- Increase in seated or forward-moving activities such as running or cycling
- Trauma to the hip or buttock area
- Patient reports pain in gluteal region
- Symptoms can include numbness and tingling but may improve with external rotation of hip

Physical Examination
- No obvious signs on inspection.

- Palpable tenderness along piriformis and sciatic notch.
- Positive FAIR test: The patient is placed in the lateral recumbent position with the affected side up. The femur is passively flexed, adducted, and internally rotated. A positive test is when pain is reproduced in the gluteus.
- May have positive straight leg raise: The affected leg is held straight and the examiner passively lifts the leg, flexing at the hip. The ankle may be dorsiflexed as well. A positive test elicits pain in the posterolateral affected leg.
- Pertinent negatives include no palpable tenderness, painless range of motion of hip, normal dermatomal sensation.

Imaging
- Limited applicability in diagnosis, but MRI is thought to be the preferred imaging tool used primarily to exclude radiculopathy or spinal stenosis as a cause of sciatica or buttock pain.
- Ultrasound can also be used to identify the location of myofascial trigger points.

Differential Diagnosis
- Lumbar radiculopathy
- Primary sacral dysfunction
- Hip joint pathology

Initial Management
- Nonsurgical multidisciplinary care is the mainstay of treatment
- Condition is often self-limited
- Use of over-the-counter NSAIDs, muscle relaxants, and neuropathic medications such as gabapentin can be helpful in providing symptomatic relief
- Physical therapy for strengthening, isometric stretching, and pain-relieving modalities

Nonoperative Management
- Injections (local anesthetic with or without cortico-steroids) into the body of the piriformis muscle or nerve sheathe can be both diagnostic and therapeutic. Advanced imaging with fluoroscopy or ultrasound can improve accuracy.

Operative Management
Surgery is rarely required, but surgical release/tenotomy of the piriformis muscle can be considered in refractory cases.

SUGGESTED READINGS

Hopayian K, Danielyan A: Four symptoms define the piriformis syndrome: an updated systematic review of its clinical features, *Eur J Orthop Surg Traumatol* 28(2):155–164, 2018.

Jankovic D, Peng P, van Zundert A: Brief review: piriformis syndrome: etiology, diagnosis, and management, *Can J Anaesth* 60(10):1003–1012, 2013.

Probst D, Stout A, Hunt D: Piriformis syndrome: a narrative review of the anatomy, diagnosis, and treatment, *PM R* 11(Suppl 1):S54-S63, 2019.

> **! CLINICAL ALERT**
>
> Emergent causes of sciatica should be ruled out. Loss of bowel or bladder control or weakness of the lower extremity may be signs of cauda equina syndrome or significant nerve damage and should be evaluated urgently.

PELVIC FRACTURE

Pelvic fractures can be relatively benign and be the result of low energy trauma in the elderly. They can also be life threatening and the result of high energy forces. Determining the stability of the pelvis is the most important diagnostic factor.

History

- High velocity trauma can result in unstable pelvic ring fractures
- Low impact injuries (ground level falls) can cause avulsion fractures or pelvic wing fractures in adolescents or stable pelvic ring fractures or insufficiency fractures of the sacrum in the elderly
- Patient reports inability to ambulate without significant pain
- Specific symptoms depend on the location of the fracture

Physical Examination

- Inability to ambulate due to pain
- Inspect patient, palpate perineum, rectum for potential open fractures
- Use compression, distraction to determine stability of the pelvis. If the iliac crests can be pressed together or pulled apart, the pelvis is unstable
- Palpate sacrum, iliac wings, and pubic symphysis

- Complete physical examination: high velocity pelvic injuries are often associated with other injuries, so a complete skeletal survey is imperative.

Imaging: Fig. 5.3

- Obtain pelvic radiographs (AP, inlet, outlet) for screening (90% of pelvic injuries will be revealed on AP view).
- Radiographs are usually repeated after patient mobilizes to assess stability.
- Obtain computed tomography (CT) scan to further determine the extent of the fracture and stability of the pelvis.

Initial Management

- Initial trauma survey to assess extent of injuries.
- Determine stability of the fracture with radiographs and CT scan.
- If unstable fracture pattern (see Operative Indications), patient should be hospitalized to determine further management.
- Determine hemodynamic stability and rule out active bleeding. This may require vascular and general surgery consults.
- Pelvic binders are used in the ED when there is suspicion for unstable pelvic fractures and/or associated major hemorrhage.

Nonoperative Management

- Nonoperative management is reserved for stable fracture patterns or when a patient is too ill for surgery
- Most stable pelvic fractures will heal without surgery
- Hospitalization may be required for pain management, otherwise oral analgesics can be used at home

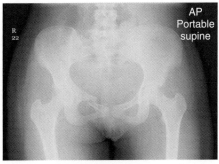

Fig. 5.3 Pelvic Fracture.

- The patient may weight bear as tolerated with assistive device and strict fall precautions
- The patient may need assistance with activities of daily living

Operative Management

ICD-10 Code: S32.9XXA Closed pelvic fracture
S32.9XXB Open pelvic fracture
CPT Codes: 20690 Application of external fixator
27218 Open reduction, internal fixation (ORIF) pelvis, posterior bone fractures, and/or dislocation which disrupt the pelvic ring

Indications

- Fractures resulting in a pubic diastasis of more than 2.5 cm
- Fracture of the pubic rami resulting in more than 2 cm of displacement
- Rotationally unstable fractures causing more than a 1.5 cm leg length discrepancy
- SI joint displacement more than 5 mm in any plane
- Posterior pelvic ring fracture gap more than 1 cm
- Lateral border sacrum fracture, ischial spine fracture, all open fractures, rotational deformities

Anesthesia

- General anesthesia
- Supine or prone depending on body habitus and fracture pattern

Surgical Procedure

- Surgical technique and approach vary greatly depending on the patient and nature of the fracture.
- ORIF is commonly used for open fractures requiring aggressive débridement. The benefits include better fracture reduction, superior biomechanical stability, and earlier patient ambulation.
- External fixation using pins is a technique used for provisional fixation to stabilize bleeding bone surfaces, venous plexus to encourage clot formation, especially useful when the risk for infection is exceedingly high, though fixation not sufficient to stabilize combined rotationally and vertically unstable injuries to allow the patient to get out of bed.

- Percutaneous pinning is a minimally invasive option in cases of traumatized posterior skin that are prone to breakdown with open reduction.

Estimated Postoperative Recovery Course

Postoperative day 10 to 14:
- First postoperative visit—wound assessment, toe touch weight bearing, in home physical therapy.

Postoperative week 6:
- Pelvis x-ray to assess fracture healing and implant position, transition to weight bearing as tolerated, out-patient physical therapy.

Postoperative month 3:
- Pelvis x-ray to assess for fracture healing.

Board Review

The Young-Burgess classification system is the most commonly used pelvic fracture classification system.

SUGGESTED READINGS

Davis DD, Foris LA, Kane SM, Waseem M: Pelvic fracture. In *StatPearls [Internet]*, Treasure Island (FL), 2020 Nov 20, StatPearls Publishing; 2020.

Perry K, Chauvin BJ: Pelvic ring injuries. In *StatPearls [Internet]*, Treasure Island (FL), 2020 Aug 15, StatPearls Publishing; 2020.

ACKNOWLEDGMENTS

The authors would like to acknowledge the contribution of the previous edition authors, Deana Bahrman and Katherine Sharpe.

> **! CLINICAL ALERT**
>
> Because of the extensive soft tissue disruption associated with pelvic ring injuries, associated vascular, neurologic, and visceral injuries are common and should be ruled out.

6

Hip and Femur

Nicholas Calabrese

ANATOMY

Bones: Figs. 6.1 and 6.2

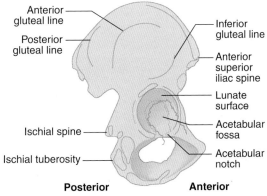

Anterior gluteal line

Posterior gluteal line

Inferior gluteal line

Anterior superior iliac spine

Lunate surface

Acetabular fossa

Ischial spine

Acetabular notch

Ischial tuberosity

Posterior   **Anterior**

Fig. 6.1 External Surface of the Hip Bones. (From Bogart BI, Ort VH: *Elsevier's integrated anatomy and embryology*, Philadelphia, 2007, Mosby.)

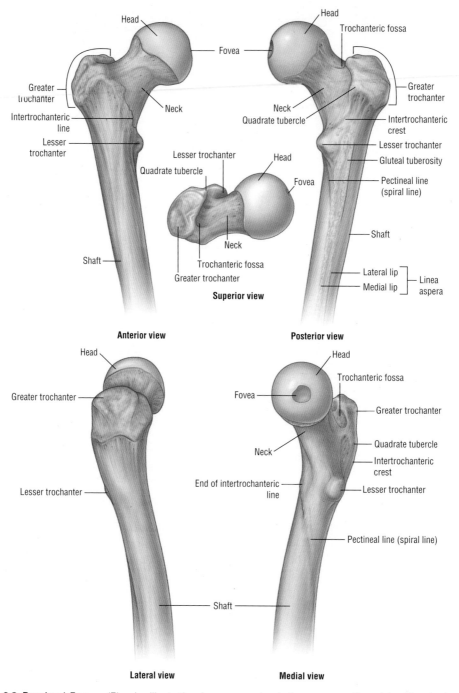

Fig. 6.2 Proximal Femur. (Elsevier illustration from www.elsevierimages.com. Copyright, Elsevier Inc. All rights reserved.)

Ligaments: Fig. 6.3

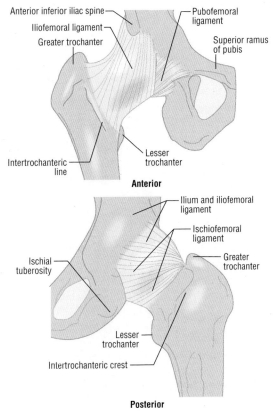

Fig. 6.3 Ligaments of the Hip. (From Bogart BI, Ort VH: *Elsevier's integrated anatomy and embryology*, Philadelphia, 2007, Mosby.)

Muscles and Tendons: Figs. 6.4 and 6.5

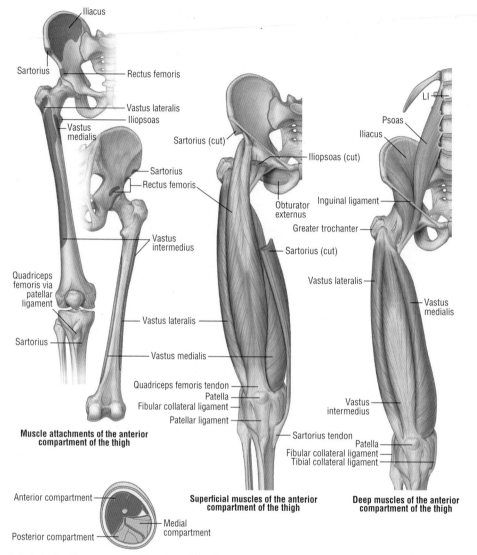

Iliacus

Sartorius

Rectus femoris

Vastus lateralis
Iliopsoas

Vastus medialis

Sartorius (cut)

Sartorius

Iliopsoas (cut)

Rectus femoris

Obturator externus

Sartorius (cut)

Vastus intermedius

Quadriceps femoris via patellar ligament

Vastus lateralis

Sartorius

Vastus medialis

Quadriceps femoris tendon
Patella
Fibular collateral ligament
Patellar ligament

Muscle attachments of the anterior compartment of the thigh

LI

Psoas
Iliacus

Inguinal ligament

Greater trochanter

Vastus lateralis

Vastus medialis

Vastus intermedius

Sartorius tendon
Patella
Fibular collateral ligament
Tibial collateral ligament

Superficial muscles of the anterior compartment of the thigh

Deep muscles of the anterior compartment of the thigh

Anterior compartment

Posterior compartment

Medial compartment

Fig. 6.4 Anterior Compartment Muscles of the Thigh. (Elsevier illustration from www.elsevierimages.com. Copyright, Elsevier Inc. All rights reserved.)

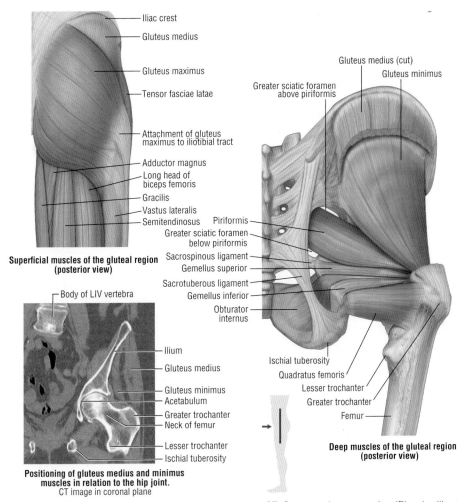

Iliac crest
Gluteus medius
Gluteus maximus
Tensor fasciae latae
Attachment of gluteus maximus to iliotibial tract
Adductor magnus
Long head of biceps femoris
Gracilis
Vastus lateralis
Semitendinosus

Superficial muscles of the gluteal region (posterior view)

Gluteus medius (cut)
Gluteus minimus
Greater sciatic foramen above piriformis
Piriformis
Greater sciatic foramen below piriformis
Sacrospinous ligament
Gemellus superior
Sacrotuberous ligament
Gemellus inferior
Obturator internus
Ischial tuberosity
Quadratus femoris
Lesser trochanter
Greater trochanter
Femur

Deep muscles of the gluteal region (posterior view)

Body of LIV vertebra
Ilium
Gluteus medius
Gluteus minimus
Acetabulum
Greater trochanter
Neck of femur
Lesser trochanter
Ischial tuberosity

Positioning of gluteus medius and minimus muscles in relation to the hip joint.
CT image in coronal plane

Fig. 6.5 Gluteal Region: Superficial and Deep Muscles. *CT,* Computed tomography. (Elsevier illustration from www.elsevierimages.com. Copyright, Elsevier Inc. All rights reserved.)

Nerves and Arteries: Fig. 6.6 and Table 6.1

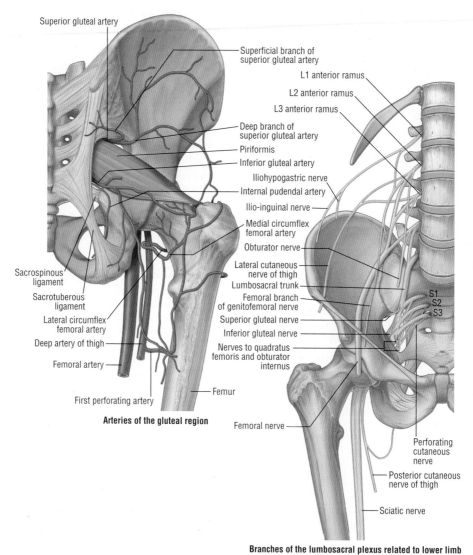

Superior gluteal artery

Superficial branch of
superior gluteal artery

L1 anterior ramus

L2 anterior ramus

L3 anterior ramus

Deep branch of
superior gluteal artery

Piriformis

Inferior gluteal artery

Iliohypogastric nerve

Internal pudendal artery

Ilio-inguinal nerve

Medial circumflex
femoral artery

Obturator nerve

Lateral cutaneous
nerve of thigh

Lumbosacral trunk

Femoral branch
of genitofemoral nerve

Superior gluteal nerve

Inferior gluteal nerve

Nerves to quadratus
femoris and obturator
internus

Sacrospinous
ligament

Sacrotuberous
ligament

Lateral circumflex
femoral artery

Deep artery of thigh

Femoral artery

First perforating artery

Femur

Arteries of the gluteal region

Femoral nerve

S1
S2
S3

Perforating
cutaneous
nerve

Posterior cutaneous
nerve of thigh

Sciatic nerve

Branches of the lumbosacral plexus related to lower limb

Fig. 6.6 Gluteal Region: Arteries and Nerves. (Elsevier illustration from www.elsevierimages.com. Copyright, Elsevier Inc. All rights reserved.)

TABLE 6.1   Nerves of the Hip and Thigh

Nerve	Branch	Motor	Test	Sensory
Lumbar plexus (anterior division) L1-2	Genitofemoral	None		Proximal anteromedial thigh
Lumbar plexus (anterior division) L2-4	Obturator	Gracilis (anterior division) Adductor longus (anterior division) Adductor brevis (anterior and posterior divisions) Adductor magnus (posterior division) Obturator externus	Hip adduction, flexion, internal and external leg rotation	Inferomedial thigh; via cutaneous branch of obturator nerve
Lumbar plexus (posterior division) L2-3	Lateral femoral cutaneous	None		Lateral thigh
Lumbar plexus (posterior division) L2-4	Femoral	Psoas Sartorius Articularis genu Pectineus Quadriceps (rectus femoris, vastus lateralis, vastus intermedius, vastus medialis)	Hip flexion, leg external rotation, leg extension, leg adduction	Anteromedial thigh; via anterior and intermediate cutaneous nerves
Sacral plexus (anterior division) L4-S3	Tibial (descends as sciatic in posterior thigh)	Posterior thigh (biceps femoris [long head], semitendinosus, semimembranosus)	Hip extension, leg flexion	None
Sacral plexus (posterior division) L4-S1	Common peroneal (descends as sciatic in posterior thigh	Biceps femoris (short head)	Hip extension, leg flexion	None (in thigh)
Sacral plexus (posterior division) S1-3	Posterior femoral cutaneous	None		Posterior thigh

Surface Anatomy: Fig. 6.7

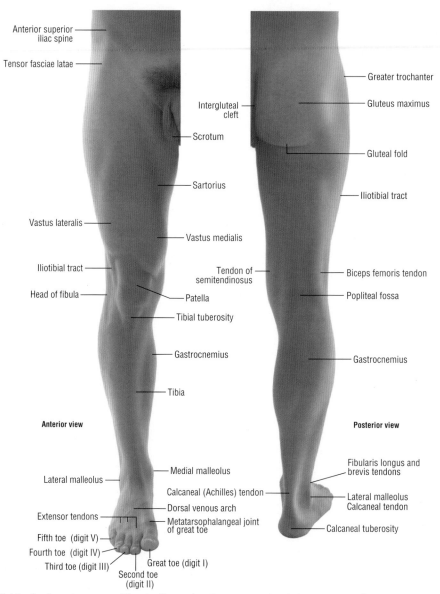

Anterior superior iliac spine

Tensor fasciae latae

Intergluteal cleft

Scrotum

Sartorius

Vastus lateralis

Vastus medialis

Iliotibial tract

Head of fibula

Patella

Tibial tuberosity

Tendon of semitendinosus

Gastrocnemius

Tibia

Greater trochanter

Gluteus maximus

Gluteal fold

Iliotibial tract

Biceps femoris tendon

Popliteal fossa

Gastrocnemius

Anterior view

Posterior view

Lateral malleolus

Medial malleolus

Calcaneal (Achilles) tendon

Dorsal venous arch

Extensor tendons

Metatarsophalangeal joint of great toe

Fifth toe (digit V)

Fourth toe (digit IV)

Third toe (digit III)

Great toe (digit I)

Second toe (digit II)

Fibularis longus and brevis tendons

Lateral malleolus
Calcaneal tendon

Calcaneal tuberosity

Fig. 6.7 Hip Surface Anatomy. (Elsevier illustration from www.elsevierimages.com. Copyright, Elsevier Inc. All rights reserved.)

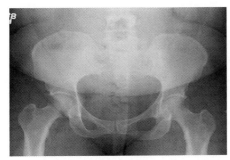

Fig. 6.8 Normal Radiograph of the Hip.

Normal Radiographic Findings: Fig. 6.8

PHYSICAL EXAMINATION

Inspect the patient's gait and look for deformity.
Palpate: Fig. 6.2

- Greater trochanter
- Iliotibial band
- Anterior superior iliac spine
- Iliopsoas tendon
- Sacroiliac joint

Normal Range of Motion (ROM): Table 6.2

Neurovascular Examination: Table 6.3

Special Tests

- **FABER test,** Flexion, ABduction, External Rotation: This maneuver tests for hip osteoarthritis (OA) and sacroiliac (SI) joint dysfunction or arthritis. The patient lies supine while the examiner flexes hip and knee and places the lateral malleolus across the contralateral knee. The examiner then extends the hip by pushing the flexed knee toward the table. A

TABLE 6.2 **Normal Range of Motion of the Hip**	
Extension	115 degrees
Flexion	125 degrees
External rotation	45 degrees
Internal rotation	45 degrees
Abduction	45 degrees
Adduction	45 degrees

positive test result is when this maneuver elicits severe pain or restriction.

- **Stinchfield test:** This test is to evaluate for intraarticular hip pathology or iliopsoas dysfunction. Ask the supine patient to raise their leg off the table, while keeping the knee in full extension, against resistance provided by the examiner pressing a hand against the lower shin. The test is positive if it elicits pain in the groin and/or weakness indicative of intraarticular hip or iliopsoas pathology.

Differential Diagnosis: Table 6.4

SUGGESTED READINGS

Musculoskeletal examination of the hip and groin. UpToDate.
American Academy of Orthopedic Surgeons: *OrthoInfo* (Website). Osteoarthritis of the Hip. https://orthoinfo.aaos .org/en/diseases--conditions/osteoarthritis-of-the-hip/.
Hansen JT: In *Netter's clinical anatomy*, ed 2, Philadelphia, 2010, Saunders.

DEGENERATIVE JOINT DISEASE OF THE HIP

Also known commonly as hip arthritis, degenerative joint disease of the hip is a commonly encountered cause

TABLE 6.3 **Neurovascular Examination**		
Nerves and Arteries	**Location of Test**	**Tests**
Femoral nerve		Check of dorsiflexion, plantar flexion, extensor hallucis longus, inversion, eversion of foot
Sciatic nerve		Numbness and tingling at low back radiating to foot
Femoral artery	Groin; medial to femoral nerve	Palpation
Dorsalis pedis and posterior tibial arteries	Along the dorsal first metatarsal and posterior to medial malleolus	Palpation and comparison with contralateral side

TABLE 6.4   Differential Diagnosis of Hip and Thigh Pain

Buttock pain	Ischial bursitis
	Sciatica
	Hamstring strain
	Piriformis syndrome
	Gluteal tear
	Sacroiliac dysfunction
Groin pain	Hip arthritis
	Avascular necrosis
	Femoral acetabular impingement
	Adductor strain
	Femoral neck fracture
	Sacroiliac dysfunction
	Osteitis pubis
Lateral hip pain	Trochanteric bursitis
Posterior thigh pain	Sciatica
Anterior thigh pain	Iliopsoas tendinitis/bursitis
	Hip arthritis
	Hamstring strain
	Femoral shaft fracture

of hip pain in the general population. Hip and groin pain, limited ROM, and antalgic gait are all hallmark findings of this condition. Hip replacement surgery has drastically improved the quality of life for patients suffering with this condition.

History

- Acute or chronic groin pain and/or deep buttocks pain
- Groin pain radiating down the thigh to the knee (rarely beyond the knee)
- Reported restricted hip ROM (i.e., difficulty putting socks and shoes on)

> **! CLINICAL ALERT**
>
> Always examine the hip in a patient with knee pain as hip pain commonly refers to the knee due to the similar innervation with the obturator nerve.

- Limping gait
- Sensation of leg length difference
- Common causes of degenerative joint disease (DJD) of the hip
  - Femoral acetabular impingement (FAI)
  - Congenital/developmental dysplasia of the hip (DDH) (~80% female)

- Trauma (three times more likely to develop DJD of hip)
- Slipped capital femoral epiphysis (SCFE) – common cause of FAI in males
- Legg-Calvé-Perthes disease
- Osteonecrosis (commonly from systemic steroids [IV or oral], EtOH abuse, and trauma with hip dislocation) – Association Research Circulation Osseous (ARCO) classification/staging
- Elevated bone density (Paget's disease)
- Inflammatory disorders (rheumatoid arthritis, juvenile rheumatoid arthritis, ankylosing spondylitis)
- Septic arthritis (complaint of sharp pain in the groin or anterior hip, worse with weight bearing; night pain in in patients with severe DJD)

Physical Examination

- Antalgic gait leaning over the affected side with or without use of an assistive device
- Pain with active and passive ROM especially with hip flexion and internal rotation
- Restricted hip active and passive ROM
- Check of distal pulses (dorsalis pedis and posterior tibial)

Imaging: Fig. 6.9

- Order radiographs: pelvis and OR lateral of affected hip(s). OR lateral view of the affected hip requires the patient to rotate the hip internally approximately 10 to 15 degrees to provide a true lateral view because of the natural anteversion of the femoral neck in relation to the acetabulum. Consider a frog leg view to assess for FAI or osteonecrosis (evaluating for subchondral collapse of the femoral head).
- FAI: Order magnetic resonance imaging (MRI) without contrast to assess for soft tissue and labral damage. If labral damage is present with associated cartilage damage, the patient will need total hip arthroplasty (THA); if not, consider surgical débridement of the femoral head/neck junction.
- Osteonecrosis: Order MRI without contrast to assess the extent of necrosis. If the femoral head has subchondral bone collapse or greater than 50% involvement, patient will benefit most from THA; if not, consider core decompression to restore the blood supply.
- Order a computed tomography (CT) scan for complex cases with bony erosion to assess the integrity

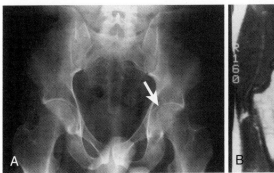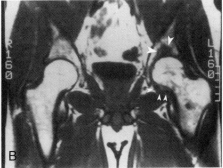

Fig. 6.9 Osteoarthritis of the left hip on radiography (**A**, *arrow*) and magnetic resonance imaging (**B**, *arrowheads*). (From Haaga JR, Lanzieri CF, Gilkeson RC, editors: *CT and MR imaging of the whole body*, ed 4, St. Louis, 2003, Mosby.)

of the anterior and posterior columns for surgical planning.

Initial Management

- **Patient Education.** DJD is a progressive condition with three main risk factors: aging, obesity, and trauma. It is irreversible; treatment is geared toward pain control with conservative methods, and surgery is a last resort. THA is contraindicated in patients with a body mass index (BMI) greater than 40.

Nonoperative Management

- Activity modification – avoiding high impact exercise and activities
- Nonsteroidal antiinflammatory drugs (NSAIDs)
- Weight loss
- Physical therapy (PT): possibly helpful for muscle weakness and gait, but discontinued if symptoms increase
- Intraarticular steroid injections (may repeat steroid at most every 3 months to prevent cartilage damage)
- Follow up in 3 months to assess effectiveness

Operative Management

Codes

ICD-10 codes:
- M16.10 Unilateral primary osteoarthritis, unspecified hip (M16.11 – Right; M16.12 – Left)
- M16.5 Unilateral posttraumatic osteoarthritis, unspecified hip (M16.51 – Right; M16.52 – Left)

CPT code:
- 27130 Total hip arthroplasty
- 27132 *Conversion* of previous hip surgery to *total hip arthroplasty*

Indications

- Night pain
- BMI lower than 40
- Failed conservative treatment
- Pain affecting activities of daily living (ADLs) and quality of life (QOL)

Informed consent and counseling

- Risks include bleeding, infection, blood clots, intraoperative femur fracture, and leg length discrepancy (LLD).
- The patient will need medical clearance by their primary care provider and appropriate medical subspecialists (i.e., Cardiology, Pulmonology, Hematology/Oncology, etc.).
- The average hospital stay lasts 1 to 2 days.
- Postoperative venous thromboembolism chemoprophylaxis/anticoagulation management varies by institution.
- Expect 6 weeks of healing, PT, and strict hip precautions to prevent dislocation (no flexion >90 degrees or adduction) if the posterolateral approach is used; if the direct anterior approach is chosen, no hip precautions are necessary.
- Expect to wait about 3 months before returning to work. General return to work guidelines are to avoid repetitive lifting greater than 50 to 100 pounds to avoid excess force through the implant.
- It may take 1 year for full recovery following total hip arthroplasty.

Anesthesia

- Regional anesthetic, such as spinal block with sedation, or general anesthesia with endotracheal intubation

Patient positioning

- Supine or lateral decubitus, with the operative side up depending on surgical approach.

Surgical Procedures

- **Direct anterior approach:** The anterior approach, also called the Smith-Petersen approach, gains exposure to the hip anteriorly without the need to detach any of the surrounding muscles. A space is created between the tensor fascia lata and the sartorius muscles. The hip joint is accessed through the anterior hip capsule.
- **Posterolateral approach:** This approach involves an incision on the side of the hip and subsequently splitting through the gluteus maximus to access the hip joint. The piriformis and gemelli tendons, which attach to the tip of the greater trochanter, are then released to allow for hip dislocation posteriorly. These tendons and the posterior capsule are later repaired with a braided nonabsorbable suture through drill holes in the greater trochanter.
- **Implant selection:** There are various systems available on the market. Routinely press-fit/cementless designs are used to allow for bony on-growth and reduction of interfaces to minimize risk for implant loosening.
- **Wound closure:** The deep fascia is routinely closed with a continuous barbed suture to ensure a watertight seal to prevent seroma or hematoma formation. Subsequently the dermis is closed with interrupted buried knot suture. Subcuticular closure varies from surgeon to surgeon. Either buried knot interrupted stitches or continuous subcuticular suture can be utilized. Additionally, topical skin adhesives may be used to seal the wound following closure of the superficial skin layer. The wound can be covered by 4 × 4 gauze or a padded bandage for the first few days following surgery to protect the incision and ensure early healing.
- **Minimizing blood loss:** Tranexamic acid (TXA), an antifibrinolytic agent, is increasingly used for joint arthroplasty to help minimize blood loss. A common regimen is 1 g intravenously before incision and 1 g intravenously during closure.

Estimated Postoperative Course

Postoperative day 14:

- Sutures are removed, and a wound check is performed.

- PT is begun for hip ROM, strengthening, balance, and gait training. The patient is weight bearing as tolerated.

Postoperative 6 weeks:

- The patient returns to the clinic for radiographs of the pelvis and the operative hip. Evaluation of ROM, as well as abductor and quadriceps strength.
- Continue to wean the patient off assistive devices (walker, cane) with progressive PT.
- The patient may drive, if he or she is not taking narcotics. Stop anticoagulation.

Postoperative 3 months, 6 months, and 1 year:

- The patient returns to the clinic for radiographs of the pelvis and hip.
- Assess for continued improvement in pain, gait, and strengthening. Assess for trochanteric bursitis or LLD. After 1 year of PT, if the patient complains of LLD, referral for a shoe lift fitting may be indicated.

SUGGESTED READINGS

Boettner F, Altneu EI, Sculco TP: Mini-posterior total hip arthroplasty. In Brown TE, Cui Q, Mihalko WM, et al.: *Arthritis and arthroplasty: the hip*, Philadelphia, 2009, Saunders, pp 204–210.

McCarthy M, Brown TE, Saleh KJ: Etiology of hip arthritis. In Brown TE, Cui Q, Mihalko WM, et al.: *Arthritis and arthroplasty: the hip*, Philadelphia, 2009, Saunders, pp 3–11.

Miller CD, Stiltner AR, Cui Q: Preoperative planning for hip surgery. In Brown TE, Cui Q, Mihalko WM, et al.: *Arthritis and arthroplasty: the hip*, Philadelphia, 2009, Saunders, pp 24–36.

Total hip arthroplasty. UpToDate (website).

MUSCLE STRAINS AND INJURIES (ADDUCTORS, HAMSTRING, QUADRICEPS)

The hamstrings (three muscles), quadriceps (four muscles), and adductors (five muscles) comprise the musculature of the thigh. Strains are tears in the muscle and are quite common in active individuals. The hamstrings and quadriceps are especially prone to injury because they cross the knee joint. These injuries are managed well with conservative treatment, and surgical intervention is exceedingly rare.

History

- Higher risk in active individuals and athletes.
- Typically, the result of eccentric contraction.
- Patient-reported acute onset, popping sound, or snapping sensation at point of injury, followed by severe pain, possible swelling, tenderness to palpation, and ecchymosis.

Physical Examination

- Antalgic gait
- Pain reproduced with active ROM of the affected muscle
- Ecchymosis evident
- Swelling, palpable mass, or gap in muscle noted
- Tenderness to palpation noted at the point of injury

Imaging

- MRI may assess for fluid collections or severity of tear, but the diagnosis is based on history and clinical presentation.

Classification

Point of Injury

- Origin of muscle
- Musculotendinous junction
- Muscle belly
- Insertion of muscle

American Medical Association Grades for Muscle Strain

- First-degree: tears of a few muscle fibers
- Second-degree: more severe tear
- Third-degree: complete disruption of the musculotendinous unit

Initial Management

- Cease play and aggravating activity
- Rest, elevate if possible, and ice the affected area

Nonoperative Management

Phases of muscle strain recovery

Acute phase (up to 5 days):

- Rest, ice, compression, elevation.

Subacute phase (3 weeks):

- Beginning active ROM exercises.

Remodeling phase (6 weeks):

- When the patient can do active ROM without pain, start increasing sport-specific activity and strengthening.

- Massage, ultrasound, and STIM (electric stimulation therapy) treatment help prevent scar tissue buildup.

Functional phase (2 weeks to 6 months):

- When the patient can run for 20 to 30 minutes and perform sport movements without disability.
- Patients with second- and third-degree strains unlikely to return to play before 5 weeks.

Rehabilitation

- Therapy is geared toward prevention by improving balance between opposing muscles (i.e., hamstrings and quadriceps), stretching techniques, and muscle conditioning.

SUGGESTED READINGS

Heftler JM: Hamstring strain. Medscape (website). https://emedicine.medscape.com/article/307765-overview.

American Academy of Orthopedic Surgeons: Muscle strains in the thigh. OrthoInfo (website). https://orthoinfo.aaos.org/en/diseases--conditions/muscle-strains-in-the-thigh/.

GREATER TROCHANTERIC BURSITIS

Inflammation of the bursa overlying the femur greater trochanter is a cause of lateral hip pain. Classically a patient will complain of lateral hip pain, worse when lying on the affected side. Intrabursal steroid injection is usually successful in managing greater trochanter bursitis.

History

- Insidious onset of lateral hip pain characterized as tenderness and burning
- Commonly an overuse injury
- Concomitant abductor tendinopathy (gluteus medius and gluteus minimus)
- Intermittent or constant lateral hip pain that can radiate down the lateral thigh
- Pain when lying on the affected side

Physical Examination

- Normal gait in early presentation.
- Trendelenburg gait secondary to abductor weakness and/or advanced tendinopathy.
- No obvious skin color changes or swelling.

- Tenderness to palpation over the lateral or posterior aspect of the greater trochanter.
- Pain with extreme hip abduction and external rotation.

Imaging

- Anteroposterior (AP) pelvis and lateral hip radiographs should be performed to rule out other disorders.

Initial Management

- **Patient Education.** This condition usually resolves with conservative measures such as activity modification, rest, ice/heat, over-the-counter (OTC) NSAIDs, and physical therapy. It may be intermittent or chronic. Pain may increase and activity may be impaired if the condition is untreated.

Nonoperative Management

- Oral NSAIDs, if appropriate
- Physical therapy to focus on stretching of the iliotibial band and strengthening of the muscles around the hip
- Greater trochanteric bursa corticosteroid injection
- Improvement expected within 6 months of conservative management, although symptoms possible
- Follow up as needed

Operative Management

- Operative intervention is rare.
- Recommend MRI without contrast to characterize the involvement of the muscles and tendons surrounding the affected hip before consulting with a surgeon regarding operative management.

SUGGESTED READINGS

Redmond JM, Chen AW, Domb BG: Greater trochanteric pain syndrome, *J Am Acad Orthop Surg* 24(4):231–240, 2016.

Barratt PA, Brookes N, Newson A: Conservative treatments for greater trochanteric pain syndrome: a systematic review, *Br J Sports Med* 51(2):97–104, 2017.

SNAPPING HIP

Snapping may be associated with the iliotibial band moving over the greater trochanter (external) or the iliopsoas tendon moving over the iliopectineal eminence. It can also be associated with a loose body, labral tear, or another disorder within the hip joint. Asymptomatic snapping does not require treatment. Painful snapping usually improves with NSAIDs and physical therapy.

History

- Commonly in female athletes
- Lateral or anterior hip pain associated with an audible "click"
- Pain and click noticed with repetitive hip flexion, extension, and abduction

Physical Examination

- Lateral snapping may be reproduced and felt with flexion and extension of the affected hip.
- Anterior snapping may improve with direct pressure over the iliopsoas tendon at the level of the femoral head.
- Pain or snapping with internal or external rotation of the affected hip may suggest an intraarticular process.

Imaging

- No standard imaging is recommended.
- Radiographs and MRI may be helpful in ruling out other disorders.

Initial Management

- Determine the severity of pain and impact on ADLs.
- Encourage activity modification to help with symptom reduction

Nonoperative Management

- Referral to physical therapy for stretching and strengthening
- NSAIDs (OTC or Rx)
- Steroid injection to the identified source of pain
- Follow up 6 weeks after initiation of treatment, to determine effectiveness
- Continue activity as tolerated with modification as appropriate
- Radiographs or MRI considered if no improvement with conservative management or suspicious for intraarticular process

Operative Management

- Surgical treatment is not usually indicated.

SUGGESTED READINGS

Badowski E: Snapping hip syndrome, *Orthop Nurs* 37(6):357–360, 2018.

American Academy of Orthopedic Surgeons: Snapping hip. OrthoInfo (website). https://orthoinfo.aaos.org/en/diseases--conditions/snapping-hip/.

HIP FRACTURES

Hip fractures are the most frequent operative fracture and can be very debilitating. Only 25% of patients with hip fractures regain their prefracture function. Hip fractures include fractures in the femoral neck, the intertrochanteric, and subtrochanteric regions. If these injuries are not treated appropriately, they have a 10% to 45% rate of osteonecrosis and a 10% to 30% rate of nonunion.

History
- Fall
- Pain in the groin, lateral hip, buttock, or low back
- Pain with weight bearing

Physical Examination
- Lower extremity malrotation and/or shortening
- Pain with ROM of the hip

Imaging: Fig. 6.10
- AP pelvis and cross-table lateral radiographs are obtained.
- If radiographic findings are negative but suspicion is high, proceed with MRI.

Classification
- The Garden classification for femoral neck fractures is based on the degrees of displacement and has a prognostic value for the incidence of osteonecrosis.
  - Type 1: valgus impaction of the femoral head
  - Type 2: nondisplaced, but complete
  - Type 3: displaced and complete, but less than 50%
  - Type 4: displaced, complete and greater than 50%
- The Boyd and Griffin classification is used for intertrochanteric fractures.
  - Type 1: fracture extending from the lesser to the greater trochanter along the intertrochanteric line

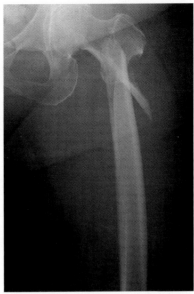

Fig. 6.10 Radiographic Appearance of Classic Hip Fracture.

- Type 2: comminuted fracture along the intertrochanteric line with multiple fractures in the cortex
- Type 3: subtrochanteric fractures with at least one fracture crossing the proximal femur just distal to or at the lesser trochanter
- Type 4: fracture in the trochanteric region and the proximal shaft in at least two planes, one usually in the sagittal plane

Initial Management
- Referral to an orthopaedic surgeon and transfer for hospital admission
- Immediate non–weight bearing

Nonoperative Management
- Reserved for non-ambulators or patients too ill to undergo surgical intervention
- Non–weight bearing
- Attentive care for position change to prevent skin breakdown
- Careful attention to pain management and nutrition
- Deep vein thrombosis (DVT) prophylaxis based on the patient's other comorbidities
- Follow up to nonoperative management variable, based on disposition
- Follow up in 2 weeks to evaluate pain management
- Follow up at 6 weeks (patient should be pain free)

Rehabilitation

- The patient should begin ROM and strengthening of other extremities

> **! CLINICAL ALERT**
>
> Among patients with hip fracture who are more than 70 years old, 20% to 30% will die in the first year after fracture.

Operative Management

Codes

ICD-10 codes: S72.019A Femoral neck fracture
S72.143A Intertrochanteric fracture
S72.23XA Subtrochanteric fracture
CPT codes: 27235 Percutaneous fixation
   27244 Open reduction, internal fixation

Indications

- Surgical fixation, fracture repair, or joint reconstruction is indicated in ambulatory patients who are medically stable for surgical intervention.
- Minimally displaced femoral neck fractures, intertrochanteric fractures, or subtrochanteric fractures can be managed with ORIF.
- Femoral neck fractures with significant displacement or increased concern for nonunion or osteonecrosis are managed with prosthetic replacement; a hemiarthroplasty may be performed if there is no evidence of acetabular arthritis in a minimally ambulatory patient; otherwise, total hip arthroplasty is indicated.

Informed consent and counseling

- Despite appropriate surgical treatment and good technique, hardware failure, nonunion, malunion, and osteonecrosis may occur.
- Discuss risk for blood loss, postoperative joint infection, periprosthetic fracture, DVT, and pulmonary embolism (PE).
- Smoking increases the risk of nonunion.
- After surgical fixation, the patient will need to be protecting weight bearing or non–weight bearing, depending on the adequacy of fixation, for a period of 6 to 12 weeks.
- The patient may require PT for strengthening and gait training.

Anesthesia

- General
- Possibility of epidural with sedation in patients unable to tolerate general.

Patient positioning

- The patient is in a supine position on a fracture table with the uninjured leg flexed and abducted at the hip in a well leg holder with a padded peroneal nerve.
- The big C-arm is draped in a sterile fashion and is utilized throughout the case to ensure appropriate fracture reduction/alignment and hardware placement.

Surgical Procedures

Open Reduction, Internal Fixation

- Hardware includes cannulated screws (femoral neck fractures), sliding compression hip screws with side plate (intertrochanteric fractures), and a regular interlocking intramedullary (IM) nail (subtrochanteric fractures).
- Lateral approach for both femoral neck and intertrochanteric fracture fixation.
- Postoperative AP and lateral radiographs are obtained in the postanesthesia care unit to confirm reduction and hardware placement.

Prosthetic Hip Replacement with Hemiarthroplasty

- Hardware includes the hemiarthroplasty component:
  - Press-fit versus cemented femoral component – determined by bone anatomy and density.
  - Unipolar vs bipolar femoral head – determined based on dislocation risk. Patients with Press-fit or cemented femoral component.
- Approaches for hip hemiarthroplasty are similar to total hip arthroplasty discussed earlier in this chapter. Patient factors such as dementia, seizure disorder, or multiple sclerosis, which increase risk for dislocation will favor direct anterior and anterolateral approaches.

Estimated Postoperative Course

Postoperative hospital course:

- Weight bearing will vary.
- The patient is out of bed with early mobilization to avoid DVT.
- Postoperative anticoagulation: The length of time and pharmacologic agent vary based on the preference of the surgeon and facility. PT is begun.

Postoperative 10 to 14 days:

- Suture removal is performed.
- The incision and lower extremity are evaluated.
- Continue PT for strengthening and gait training.

Postoperative 6 weeks:
- AP and lateral pelvis radiographs are obtained to evaluate hardware and component positions.
- Full weight bearing is allowed if initial restrictions were placed.

Postoperative 3 months:
- AP and lateral pelvis radiographs are obtained to evaluate hardware and component positions.
- A pain-free patient may resume normal activity.
- If pain persists, evaluate for nonunion or osteonecrosis with MRI of the osseous pelvis.

SUGGESTED READINGS

Beaty LH, Canale ST, editors: *Campbell's operative orthopaedics*, ed 11, Philadelphia, 2007, Mosby.

Fernandez MA, Griffin XL, Costa ML: Management of hip fracture, *Br Med Bull* 115(1):165–172, 2015.

FEMUR FRACTURE

The femur is the longest and strongest bone in the body. Fractures in younger patients usually occur due to a high-energy injury, whereas older, frail patients are also susceptible from even a low-energy fall. A complete trauma skeletal survey is necessary at the time of presentation. Femur fractures can be life-threatening and require surgical repair.

History

- High-kinetic trauma (male patients <25 years old)
- Low-impact injury (female patients >65 years old)
- Acute, severe pain, with possible deformity in the thigh or leg shortening on the affected side

Physical Examination

- Remember the basic life support priorities: circulation, airway, breathing. The patient can bleed out from a femur fracture, and 40% of patients with femur fractures will require blood transfusion.
- Obvious deformity and ecchymosis are evident.
- Patients have severe pain with movement of the affected limb or with palpation.
- Check distal pulses, and assess for hematoma or bruits indicating vascular injury.
- Check for neurologic injury.
- Check for fracture of the ipsilateral knee and for femoral neck fracture.

Imaging

- AP and lateral radiographs of the femur, hip, and knee are obtained.
- CT scan may give further information.
- Angiogram is indicated if vascular injury is suspected.

Classification: Fig. 6.11

- Transverse, oblique, spiral
- Comminuted
- Open

Initial Management

Stabilization

- Skeletal traction or an external fixator is applied to keep anatomic alignment and prevent neurovascular injury until surgery is possible (Fig. 6.12).
- Refer the patient to a vascular surgeon or a plastic surgeon in cases of vascular compromise or extensive soft tissue damage, respectively.

Nonoperative Management

Conservative treatment is rare and is typically reserved only for pediatric patients.

! CLINICAL ALERT

Be aware of the risk of *fat embolus* causing acute respiratory distress syndrome (ARDS) in trauma victims with diaphyseal femur fractures.

Operative Management

Codes

ICD-10 code: S72.3 Closed femur shaft fracture
CPT code: 27245 Intramedullary femoral nail
76000.26 Fluoroscopy time

Indications

- Once the patient is hemodynamically stable, the optimal time to surgery is less than 24 hours after fracture occurs.
- Open fractures should be considered emergencies, and surgical intervention is optimal at less than 8 hours.

Informed consent and counseling

- Even with appropriate surgical management, there is a 1% rate of nonunion after IM nailing.

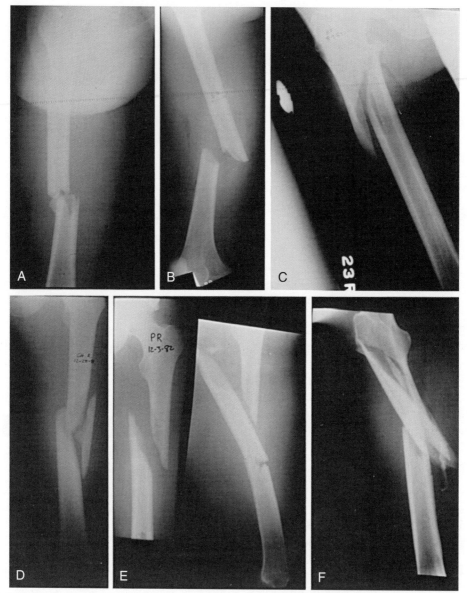

Fig. 6.11 A to F, Classification of femoral shaft fractures. (From Townsend CM Jr, Beauchamp RD, Evers BM, et al, editors: *Sabiston textbook of surgery*, ed 18, Philadelphia, 2008, Saunders.)

- Other risks include infection, DVT, and compartment syndrome.
- The patient should expect 6 weeks of healing with non–weight-bearing status.
- The rate of leg-length discrepancy after femur fracture is 7%.
  Anesthesia
- General

Patient Positioning
- Supine

Surgical Procedures

- IM nailing is the gold standard because of its 99% rate of union and 1% rate of infection.
- Plating has more complications and is generally not indicated for diaphyseal fractures.

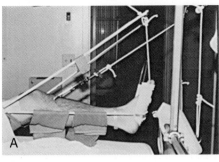

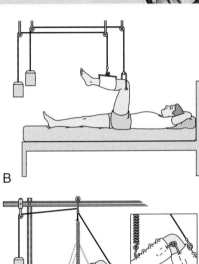

Fig. 6.12 A to C, Skeletal traction of the femur. (From Townsend CM Jr, Beauchamp RD, Evers BM, et al, editors: *Sabiston textbook of surgery*, ed 18, Philadelphia, 2008, Saunders.)

Intramedullary Nailing

- Hardware includes a titanium IM nail and interlocking screw(s).
- Intraoperative fluoroscopy is required during this procedure.
- Antegrade IM nailing is the standard, but retrograde placement is becoming more favorable, especially in obese patients. Fluoroscopic pictures should be obtained.
- Layered closure of the incision.
- Postoperative AP and lateral radiographs are obtained in the postanesthesia care unit to confirm reduction and hardware position.

Estimated Postoperative Course
- The patient will need to use crutches and remain non–weight bearing until 6 weeks postoperatively.

Postoperative days 10 to 14:
- Remove the sutures, and perform a wound check.

Postoperative 6 weeks:
- The patient returns to the clinic for AP and lateral femur radiographs.
- Callus formation, union of fracture, the absence of radiolucency around screws, and the patient's lack of pain with touch toe weight bearing indicate that the fracture is healing or has healed. The patient may progress to toe-touch weight bearing and PT for ROM and strengthening.

Postoperative 3 months:
- The patient returns to the clinic for repeat radiographs.
- If the patient has no pain with touch toe weight bearing, progress to weight bearing as tolerated. PT is given if needed.

Postoperative 6 months:
- Nonunion occurs at 6 months. If the fracture is not healing radiographically or the patient has pain with weight bearing, consider further surgical intervention.

Postoperative 1 year:
- Repeat the radiographs.

SUGGESTED READINGS

Romeo, NM et al. Femur injuries and fractures treatment and management. Medscape (website). http://emedicine.medscape.com/article/90779-treatment#aw2aab6b6b2.

Eastwood B. Diaphyseal femur fractures treatment & management. Medscape (website). http://emedicine.medscape.com/article/1246429-treatment#a1128.

FEMORAL STRESS FRACTURE

Femoral stress fractures result from the repetitive loading of the femur bone. This injury is seen in young athletes and in older persons with osteoporosis. Most stress fractures heal without surgery; however, if the fracture progresses, surgical repair will be required. Compliance with treatment is important to prevent progression of the fracture.

History

- Young athletes, typically runners
- Older patients with metabolic bone disorder
- Localized hip pain as the primary complaint
- Pain worse with activity and improved with rest
- Pain typically in the groin and possibly radiating into the thigh and knee
- Possible report of a new activity or an increase in the intensity of activity
- Night pain common

Physical Examination

- No abnormality on visual inspection
- No palpable tenderness
- Possible pain with ROM of the hip

Imaging

- Initial or late radiographs may not reveal fracture. Diagnosis often requires MRI or bone scan.

Classification

- Tension fractures: Superior aspect of the femoral neck causing a transverse fracture across the femoral neck; more common in older patients; more likely to progress and displace.
- Compression fractures: Inferior aspect of the femoral neck; more common in younger population and athletes.

Initial Management

- Non–weight bearing to the affected side
- Crutches or a walker to facilitate ambulation with this restriction

Nonoperative Management

- The patient is non–weight bearing.
- Follow up every 4 weeks for repeat radiographs to ensure no change in fracture pattern or symptoms and to evaluate callus formation.
- The fracture usually requires 3 to 6 months to heal.
- Bone scan should be performed at 3 to 6 months to confirm complete resolution, at which time patient may resume normal activity.
- A fracture that displaces or progresses should be fixed operatively.
- Osteonecrosis or nonunion may result if a stress fracture progresses or is missed.
- Once the fracture is healed, the patient may begin PT for general strengthening and gait training.

Operative Management

Codes

ICD-10 code: M84.359A Stress fracture of femoral neck

CPT code: 27235 Closed reduction, internal fixation

Indications

- Displacement of the diastasis or no evidence of healing on radiographs
- Nondisplaced fractures in patients who cannot be compliant with conservative management

Informed consent and counseling

- Fixation may be achieved with closed reduction, internal fixation, but it may require open reduction, internal fixation.
- There is still a risk of osteonecrosis despite good reduction and fixation.
- Nonunion may occur despite adequate fixation.
- Smoking increases the risk of nonunion.
- After surgical fixation, the patient will need to be protecting weight bearing or non–weight bearing, depending on the adequacy of fixation, for a period of 6 to 12 weeks.
- The patient may require physical therapy for strengthening and gait training.

Anesthesia

- General

Patient positioning

- The patient is supine on a fracture table with the uninjured leg flexed and abducted at the hip in a well leg holder with a padded peroneal nerve.
- The C-arm image intensify is positioned between the patient's legs, and the C-arm is kept on the nonsterile side of the transparent drape.

Surgical Procedure

Closed Reduction, Internal Fixation

- Hardware includes cannulated screws.
- If reduction is required, closed reduction can be attempted first and, one hopes, achieves adequate reduction. Before preparing the patient, while the patient is in the supine position on the fracture table, tie the unaffected extremity to the footplate. Tie the fractured extremity to the other footplate in an externally rotated position. While the extremity is externally rotated, abduct approximately 20 degrees, and apply enough traction to regain normal length. The extremity is then internally rotated until the patella is internally rotated 20 to 30 degrees. AP and lateral

fluoroscopic images should be obtained to ensure proper alignment.

- A standard 1-inch lateral incision is made, centered at the level of the lesser trochanter. This will allow for appropriate superomedial trajectory of the screws.
- Postoperative AP and lateral radiographs are obtained in the postanesthesia care unit to confirm reduction and hardware position.

Estimated Postoperative Course

- The patient is out of bed on postoperative day 1 with weight-bearing status determined by the surgeon.
- Ambulation with weight-protected or non–weight-bearing restrictions depend on the fixation procedure and the patient's bone quality.
- Physical therapy should start postoperative day 1 and continue as needed and appropriate.
- Follow up 10 to 14 days after discharge from the hospital to evaluate the incision and remove the sutures or staples.
- Follow up at 4 to 6 weeks for repeat AP and lateral pelvic radiographs. If the patient has no pain, gradually advance weight-bearing status to weight bearing as tolerated.
- Follow up at 3 months for repeat AP and lateral pelvic radiographs.
- If pain persists, consider an MRI or CT scan for evaluation of osteonecrosis or nonunion.

SUGGESTED READINGS

Matcuk Jr GR, Mahanty SR, Skalski MR, Patel DB, White EA, Gottsegen CJ: Stress fractures: pathophysiology, clinical presentation, imaging features, and treatment options, *Emerg Radiol* 23(4):365–375, 2016.

Wildstein MS: Femoral neck stress and insufficiency fractures, *Medscape website. Updated*, 2020. Mar 18.

Robertson GA, Wood AM: Femoral neck stress fractures in sport: a current concepts review, *Sports Med Int Open* 1(2):E58–E68, 2017.

ACKNOWLEDGMENTS

The author would like to acknowledge the contribution of the previous edition authors, Deana Bahrman and Katherine Sharpe. Thank you to Sara Rynders, PA-C and Jennifer Hart, PA-C for this opportunity to contribute this information to aid in the education of students and colleagues.

7

Knee and Lower Leg

Jennifer A. Hart

ANATOMY

Bones: Fig. 7.1

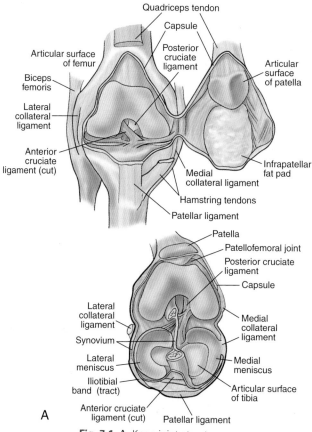

A

Fig. 7.1 A, Knee joint structures.

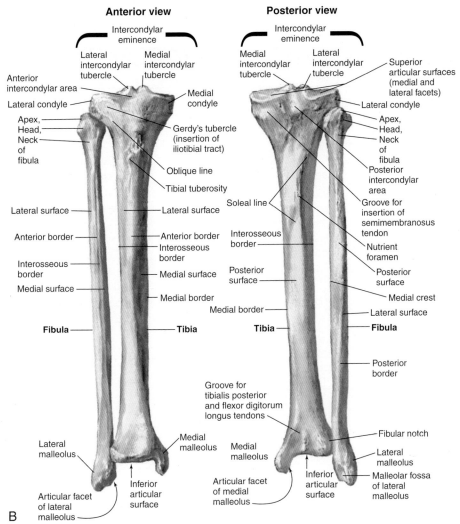

Anterior view

Intercondylar eminence

Lateral intercondylar tubercle

Medial intercondylar tubercle

Anterior intercondylar area

Lateral condyle

Medial condyle

Apex,
Head,
Neck
of
fibula

Gerdy's tubercle (insertion of iliotibial tract)

Oblique line

Tibial tuberosity

Lateral surface

Lateral surface

Anterior border

Anterior border

Interosseous border

Interosseous border

Medial surface

Medial surface

Medial border

Fibula

Tibia

Lateral malleolus

Medial malleolus

Inferior articular surface

Articular facet of lateral malleolus

Posterior view

Intercondylar eminence

Medial intercondylar tubercle

Lateral intercondylar tubercle

Superior articular surfaces (medial and lateral facets)

Lateral condyle

Apex,
Head,
Neck
of
fibula

Posterior intercondylar area

Soleal line

Groove for insertion of semimembranosus tendon

Interosseous border

Nutrient foramen

Posterior surface

Posterior surface

Medial crest

Medial border

Lateral surface

Tibia

Fibula

Posterior border

Groove for tibialis posterior and flexor digitorum longus tendons

Medial malleolus

Fibular notch

Lateral malleolus

Inferior articular surface

Malleolar fossa of lateral malleolus

Articular facet of medial malleolus

B

Fig. 7.1, cont'd B, The tibia and fibula are the bones in the leg. (From Miller MD, Hart JA, MacKnight JM, editors: *Essential orthopaedics,* Philadelphia, 2010, Saunders.)

Ligaments: Table 7.1

TABLE 7.1   Location and Function of Knee Ligaments

Ligament	Location	Function
Anterior cruciate ligament (ACL)	Originates on the tibia just anterior to the area between the tibial eminences and runs obliquely to the lateral femoral condyle	Primary restraint to anterior translation of the tibia; also rotational stability
Posterior cruciate ligament (PCL)	Originates on lateral border of the medial femoral condyle and inserts on the posterior rim of the tibia	Primary restraint to posterior translation of the tibia
Medial collateral ligament (MCL)	Originates on the medial femoral epicondyle and inserts on the medial proximal tibia	Primary restraint to valgus force
Lateral collateral ligament (LCL)	Originates on the lateral femoral epicondyle and inserts on the anterolateral fibula	Primary restraint to varus stress
Posteromedial corner (PMC): posterior oblique ligament	Located deep and posterior to the MCL	Restraint to tibial internal rotation and valgus force
Posterolateral corner (PLC): biceps, iliotibial band, popliteus, popliteofibular ligament, and joint capsule	Located posterior to the LCL	Resistance to external rotation of the knee

Muscles, Nerves, and Arteries: Fig. 7.2 and Tables 7.2 and 7.3

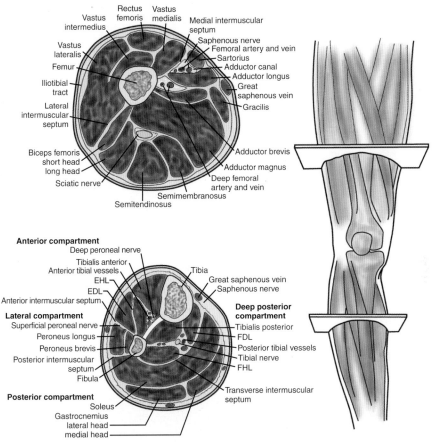

Fig. 7.2 Cross-Sectional Anatomy of the Thigh and Leg. *EDL,* Extensor digitorum longus; *EHL,* extensor hallucis longus; *FDL,* flexor digitorum longus; *FHL,* flexor hallucis longus. (From Miller MD, Hart JA, MacKnight JM, editors: *Essential orthopaedics,* Philadelphia, 2010, Saunders.)

TABLE 7.2	**Muscle Compartments of the Thigh**			
Compartment	**Muscles**	**Innervation**	**Blood Supply**	**Action**
Anterior	Vastus lateralis, vastus medialis obliquus, vastus intermedius, rectus femoris, sartorius	Femoral nerve	Superficial femoral artery	Extension of the knee
Medial	Adductors (longus, magnus, brevis) and gracilis	Obturator and sciatic nerves	Deep femoral artery	Adduction of the leg
Posterior	Semimembranosus, semitendinosus, biceps femoris	Sciatic nerve	Inferior gluteal and perforating branches of the femoral artery	Flexion of the knee and extension of the hip

TABLE 7.3	**Muscle Compartments of the Lower Leg**			
Compartment	**Muscles**	**Innervation**	**Blood Supply**	**Action**
Anterior	Tibialis anterior, extensor hallucis longus, extensor digitorum longus	Deep peroneal nerve	Anterior tibial artery	Extension and inversion of the foot and ankle, toe extension
Lateral	Peroneus brevis, peroneus longus, peroneus tertius	Superficial peroneal nerve	Peroneal artery	Eversion and plantar flexion of the foot and ankle
Superficial posterior	Gastrocnemius, soleus, plantaris	Tibial nerve	Sural arteries	Plantar flexion of the foot and flexion of the knee
Deep posterior	Flexor hallucis longus, flexor digitorum longus, tibialis posterior, popliteus	Tibial nerve	Posterior tibial artery, popliteal artery (popliteus only)	Plantar flexion and inversion of the foot and ankle, flexion of the toes

Normal Radiographic
Appearance: Figs. 7.3 and 7.4

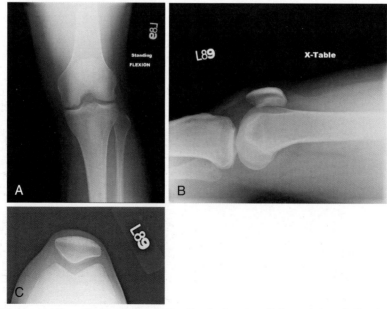

Fig. 7.3 Normal Knee Radiographs. A, Standing flexion view. **B,** Lateral view. **C,** Sunrise view.

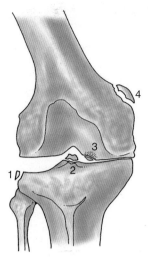

Fig. 7.4 Illustration Showing Multiple Radiographic Findings. *1,* Segond fracture (lateral capsular sign); *2,* tibial eminence fracture; *3,* osteochondritis dissecans; *4,* Pellegrini-Stieda lesion. (From Miller MD, Hart JA, MacKnight JM, editors: *Essential orthopaedics,* Philadelphia, 2010, Saunders.)

TABLE 7.4	**Lower Extremity Neurologic Examination**	
Nerve	**Motor Function**	**Sensory Distribution**
Sural	Foot plantar flexion	Lateral heel
Saphenous	None	Medial leg and ankle
Superficial peroneal	Foot eversion	Dorsum of the foot
Deep peroneal	Great toe flexion	First web space
Tibial	Toe plantar flexion	Sole of the foot

PHYSICAL EXAMINATION

Observe: gait (antalgic, assistive devices), alignment (valgus, varus), and feet (pes planus or cavus), ecchymosis, abrasion, gross deformity, effusion, quadriceps atrophy, and leg length discrepancy

Palpate: quadriceps muscle and tendon, patella (all poles, tendon, and fat pads), medial collateral ligament (MCL) and medial joint line, lateral collateral ligament (LCL) and lateral joint line, bursa (prepatellar and infrapatellar, pes anserine), and popliteal fossa

Normal range of motion (ROM): up to 10 degrees of hyperextension and 130 degrees of flexion

Neurovascular Examination: Table 7.4

Assessment of sensation and motor function of the foot; palpation of dorsalis pedis, posterior tibial, and popliteal pulses; test of patellar reflex

Special Tests
Patella

- **Patellar apprehension test:** The patient lies supine with the knee in 20 to 30 degrees of flexion and the quadriceps relaxed. Carefully glide the patella laterally. A positive test result is the presence of a reactive contraction of the quadriceps muscles by the patient in an attempt to avoid a recurrence of the dislocation or a sense of apprehension or fear that the patella will dislocate.
- **Patellar grind test:** The patient lies supine with knee fully extended. Push the patella distally in the trochlear groove. Have the patient tighten the quadriceps against patella resistance. Pain with or without crepitus is considered a positive test result.

Ligament Examination: Table 7.5 and Figs. 7.5 and 7.6

Meniscal Examination

- **McMurray test:** With patient supine, take hold of the heel with one hand and flex the leg. Place the free hand on the knee with fingers along the medial joint line and the thumb and thenar eminence on the lateral joint line. Apply valgus force, and externally rotate the lower leg, and then maintain valgus force while internally rotating. A palpable or audible click is considered a positive finding.

Differential Diagnosis: Table 7.6

- The differential diagnosis for immediate effusion, in order of frequency, is as follows: anterior cruciate ligament (ACL) tear, patella dislocation, osteochondral fracture, and peripheral meniscus tear.

ANTERIOR CRUCIATE LIGAMENT INJURY

History

- The mechanism is typically a noncontact pivoting injury.
- The patient often reports feeling or hearing a "pop" at the time of injury.
- Immediate effusion is noted.

TABLE 7.5	**Special Tests to Assess for Ligament Injury**
Ligament or Structure	**Special Test**
Anterior cruciate ligament (ACL)	**Lachman test:** With the patient in the supine position with knee at 30 degrees of flexion (placing a pillow under the knee may help the patient relax), place one hand slightly superior to the knee to stabilize the thigh, and use the other hand to apply anterior pressure to the proximal tibia. Increased anterior translation compared with the unaffected side is a positive finding.
	Anterior drawer test: With the patient lying supine with the hip flexed to 45 degrees and the knee to 90 degrees, grasp the tibia just below the joint line. Place the thumbs on either side of the patellar tendon. Use the index fingers to palpate the hamstring tendons to ensure that the tendons are relaxed. Pull forward on the tibia. Increased anterior translation compared with the unaffected side is a positive finding.
	Pivot shift test: The patient is in the supine position, the knee is extended, and the foot is internally rotated. Apply valgus stress while flexing the knee. Pivoting of the tibia is a positive finding. It is easiest to perform this test while the patient is under anesthesia.
Posterior cruciate ligament (PCL)	**Posterior drawer test:** With the patient lying supine with the hip flexed to 45 degrees and the knee to 90 degrees, grasp the tibia just below the joint line. Place the thumbs on either side of the patellar tendon. Use the index fingers to palpate the hamstring tendons to ensure that they are relaxed. Apply posterior force on the tibia. Increased posterior translation compared with the unaffected side is a positive finding.
Medial collateral ligament (MCL)	**Valgus stress test:** With the patient supine with the knee flexed to 30 degrees, apply valgus force and assess for medial opening. Repeat in full extension. Medial opening and pain are positive findings; opening in full extension indicates possible concurrent ACL injury.
Lateral collateral ligament (LCL)	**Varus stress test:** With the patient supine with the knee flexed to 30 degrees, apply varus force and assess for lateral opening. Repeat in full extension. Lateral opening and pain are positive findings.
Posterolateral corner (PLC)	**Dial test (external rotation asymmetry):** With the patient prone with the knees flexed at 30 degrees, stabilize the knees and externally rotate the feet. Repeat at 90 degrees of flexion. Asymmetry of ≥15 degrees in 30 degrees of flexion indicates isolated PLC injury; asymmetry at 90 degrees indicates combined PCL and PLC injury.
Posteromedial corner (PMC)	**Slocum test:** An anterior drawer test is performed with the patient's foot in neutral position and with the foot externally rotated. Anterior displacement should be reduced in the externally rotated position unless there is a PMC injury.

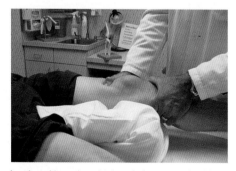

Fig. 7.5 The Lachman Examination. Note that the hand closest to the head of the patient grasps the thigh, and the opposite hand performs the examination with the thumb close to the joint line. A pillow can be placed under the knee to help the patient relax. (From Miller MD, Hart JA, MacKnight JM, editors: *Essential orthopaedics,* Philadelphia, 2010, Saunders.)

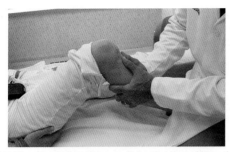

Fig. 7.6 The Posterior Drawer Examination. Note that the starting point is evaluated by palpating the medial tibial plateau in relation to the medial femoral condyle before a posteriorly directed force is applied. (From Miller MD, Hart JA, MacKnight JM, editors: *Essential orthopaedics*, Philadelphia, 2010, Saunders.)

TABLE 7.6	**Differential Diagnosis Based on Location of Knee Pain**
Location	**Differential Diagnoses**
Anterior	Patellofemoral chondromalacia, prepatellar bursitis, patellar tendinitis, patellar fracture, patellofemoral osteoarthritis
Medial	Meniscus tear, MCL injury, osteoarthritis, pes anserine bursitis
Lateral	Meniscus tear, LCL injury, osteoarthritis, iliotibial band syndrome
Posterior	Tear of posterior horn of medial or lateral meniscus, neurovascular injury (popliteal artery or nerve), PLC injury

LCL, Lateral collateral ligament; *MCL,* medial collateral ligament; *PLC,* posterolateral corner.

- The patient is typically unable to continue activity or complete a sporting event.
- Instability with pivoting and swelling after activity are seen in chronic ACL tears.

Physical Examination

- **Observe:** Note effusion, abrasion, and deformity.
- **Palpate:** Patellar ballottement is performed to assess for effusion. Joint line tenderness may be present secondary to concurrent meniscus tear.
- **ROM:** Decreased ROM may result from effusion. The lack of ability to extend the knee fully may occur with a concurrent displaced bucket handle meniscus tear.

> **! CLINICAL ALERT**
>
> Loss of full extension may indicate a "locked knee," indicating a flipped bucket handle tear of the meniscus. This is an urgent finding and should prompt magnetic resonance imaging for possible early surgical meniscal repair if appropriate.

Special Tests

- Lachman, anterior drawer, and pivot shift tests (Fig. 7.5)
- Posterior drawer test to evaluate for posterior cruciate ligament (PCL) injury (Fig. 7.6)
- McMurray test to evaluate for meniscus tear
- Dial test to evaluate for posterolateral corner (PLC) injury
- Valgus and varus stress to evaluate the collateral ligaments
- Patella apprehension and patella glide tests to evaluate for possible patella dislocation

Imaging

- Radiographs
  - Obtain standing flexion, lateral, and sunrise views.
  - Findings are often unremarkable; however, lateral tibial avulsion (Segond fracture) is highly suggestive of an ACL tear.
- Magnetic resonance imaging (MRI) of the knee without contrast (Fig. 7.7)
  - Scans show disruption of the ACL and can also identify other ligamentous, osseous, or meniscal injuries.
  - Bony contusions of the lateral femoral condyle and posterior tibia are classic in ACL tears.

Classification

- ACL tears are classified by the amount of anterior translation noted with the Lachman test:
  Grade I: less than 5 mm
  Grade II: 5 to 10 mm
  Grade III: more than 10 mm

Differential Diagnoses

- Other ligamentous knee injury (posterior cruciate or collateral ligament)
- Patella dislocation
- Meniscus tear
- Patella/quadriceps tendon rupture

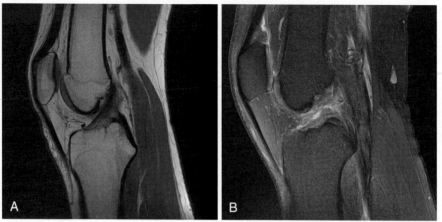

Fig. 7.7 Magnetic resonance imaging demonstrating (**A**) intact and (**B**) ruptured anterior cruciate ligament.

Initial Management

- Rest, ice, compression, and elevation are indicated.
- Aspiration may be performed to decrease effusion.
- Maintaining ROM is vital; do not place the patient in a knee immobilizer unless occult fracture is suspected.
- Crutches may be used if the patient cannot bear weight comfortably and in the absence of associated fracture.
- **Patient Eduction.** Graft selection for surgical reconstruction is made based on a variety of factors. In most cases, it is preferable to use a patient's own tissue (autograft). Allograft (cadaveric tissue) is used when autograft is not available or to supplement inadequate autograft. The most common sources of autograft are the hamstring tendons (typically gracilis and semitendinosus), quadriceps tendon, or a bone patella tendon bone (BPTB) graft (central third of the inferior patella, patella tendon, and a small portion of the tibial tuberosity).

Nonoperative Management

- Conservative management may be appropriate for patients with a low activity level and less than 5 mm of laxity compared with the unaffected side.
- Physical therapy (PT) for ROM and quadriceps strengthening is indicated.
- Without surgery, the patient may have recurrent instability and be at increased risk for meniscus tears and chondral injury or degeneration.

Operative Management

Codes

ICD-10 code: S83.519A Anterior cruciate ligament tear

CPT code: 29888 Anterior cruciate ligament reconstruction

Indications

- Most active patients with symptomatic instability who wish to continue with sports or significant physical activity require surgery to reconstruct the ACL.

Informed consent and counseling

- Possible complications include instrument breakage, aberrant tunnels, cartilage injury, hardware failure, loss of motion, residual laxity, paresthesia, effusion, deep vein thrombosis (DVT), and infection. Persistent anterior knee pain, patella tendon rupture, and patella fracture are potential complications if BPTB autograft is used.
- Anesthesia risks include paralysis, cardiac arrest, brain damage, and death.
- Postoperative PT is essential to regain motion and return to sports or physical activities.
- Return to sports is usually not expected until 6 months postoperatively.

Anesthesia

- General anesthesia with regional nerve block

Patient positioning

- Supine with a knee holder or post, with a tourniquet

Surgical Procedures

Anterior Cruciate Ligament Reconstruction

- Prepare and drape the lower extremity in a sterile fashion.
- Diagnostic arthroscopy is used to visualize the ACL and confirm injury, as well as to evaluate and treat meniscus tears, loose bodies, and chondral defects.
- Graft harvesting: Techniques vary based on graft choice. A midline incision is made for BPTB graft, and a small oscillating saw is used to cut bone plugs from the patella and tibial tubercle. A medial vertical incision approximately 5 cm below the joint line is made for harvest of a hamstring graft. The semitendinosus and gracilis are identified and harvested with a tendon stripper.
- Graft preparation: This varies based on the graft source. All grafts should be handled carefully and are prepared by a qualified assistant at an area separate from the operative field.
- Débridement and notchplasty: Excess fibrous tissue and the ACL stump are débrided with a motorized shaver and bur to allow for better visualization of the back of the notch and to provide clearance for the graft.
- Tunnel placement: The technique for tibial and femoral tunnel placement is determined by the surgeon's preference. The goal is to recreate the normal anatomic position of the ACL.
- Graft passage: Sutures that are attached to both ends of the graft are passed through the tunnels.
- Graft fixation: If BPTB graft is used, the graft is fixed with interference screws. For hamstring graft, an implant designed for soft tissue fixation is used.
- Wound closure: Multilayer closure is augmented with Steri-Strips; then a sterile dressing and an elastic compression (ACE) wrap are applied.

Estimated Postoperative Course

- Postoperative day 0 to 6 weeks:
  - The patient may remove the wound dressing the second day after surgery and replace it with self-adhesive bandages, gauze, and an elastic compression (ACE) wrap.
  - Ice, elevation, and pain medication as needed (PRN) are indicated for comfort.
  - The patient uses a cane or crutches for the first few days to two weeks for comfort.
  - Begin PT on postoperative day 1 or 2. Early-stage PT focuses on ROM, edema control, scar management, isometric quadriceps strengthening, and normalization of gait.
  - A wound check, suture removal, and assessment of ROM and stability are performed at 10 to 14 days postoperatively.
- Postoperative 6 weeks to 3 months:
  - Obtain radiographs to assess tunnels and the position of the graft fixation device.
  - Evaluate healing of the surgical site, ROM, and stability of reconstruction.
  - Advance PT.
- Postoperative 3+ months:
  - Evaluate ROM and stability of reconstruction.
  - The patient may begin straight ahead running at 3-4 months under the guidance of a physical therapist or a certified athletic trainer (ATC).
  - The patient may return to sports atleast 6 months if able to pass functional testing with the athletic trainer or the physical therapist.

Board Review

A noncontact pivoting injury to the knee with a "pop" and rapid effusion development is most commonly an ACL injury. Patella dislocation is the second most common cause of rapid knee swelling.

SUGGESTED READINGS

Kaplan Y, Witvrouw E: When is it safe to return to sport after ACL reconstruction? Reviewing the criteria. *Sports Health* 11(4):301–305, 2019.

Michelic R, Jurdana H, Jotanovic Z, et al.: Long-term results of anterior cruciate ligament reconstruction: a comparison with non-operative treatment with a follow-up of 17-20 years, *Int Orthop* 35:1093–1097, 2011.

Miller MD: Anterior cruciate ligament injury. In Miller MD, Hart JA, MacKnight JM, editors: *Essential orthopaedics*, Philadelphia, 2010, Saunders, pp 611–615.

Musahl V, Karlsson J: Anterior cruciate ligament tear, *N Engl J Med* 380(24):2341–2348, 2019.

POSTERIOR CRUCIATE LIGAMENT INJURY

History

- The mechanism of injury is typically a blow to the anterior tibia (i.e., dashboard injury) or a fall on a plantar flexed foot. Hyperextension or hyperflexion injuries also lead to PCL tear.
- Effusion is noted.
- Frank instability may or may not be present.

- Anterior and medial knee pain may be reported in chronic injury.
- Isolated PCL rupture is rare; it more commonly occurs in the multiligament knee injury.

Physical Examination

- **Observe:** Note effusion, ecchymosis, abrasion, and obvious deformity.
- **Palpate:** Patellar ballottement is performed to assess for effusion. Joint line tenderness may be present because of concurrent meniscus tear.
- **ROM:** Decreased ROM may result from effusion.

Special Tests: Figs. 7.8 and 7.9

- **Posterior drawer test:** See the classification section.
- **Posterior sag test:** With the knee and hip at 90 degrees of flexion, look for posterior sag of the tibia.
- **Dial test:** This is used to assess the PLC.
- Complete a thorough knee examination to rule out other ligamentous, meniscal, or patellar disorders.

Imaging

- Radiographs: Standing flexion, lateral, and sunrise views are often unremarkable, but they may show a PCL avulsion fragment. Stress views are obtained by applying posterior force to the proximal tibia either manually or with a Telos device.
- MRI: Imaging helps to identify the degree of injury (partial versus complete tear) and associated ligament, meniscus, and chondral injuries.

Classification

- Classification is based in the degree of posterior subluxation of the tibia in relation to the femoral condyles:

  Grade I: partial tear; posterior drawer demonstrating posterior tibial displacement that is anterior to the anterior aspect of the femoral condyles

  Grade II: posterior drawer demonstrating posterior tibial displacement that is flush with the anterior aspect of the femoral condyles

  Grade III: complete tear; posterior drawer demonstrating posterior tibial displacement posterior to the anterior aspect of the femoral condyles

Differential Diagnoses

- Other ligamentous knee injury (anterior cruciate or collateral ligament)
- Meniscus tear

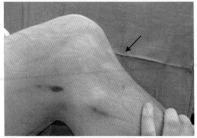

Fig. 7.8 Positive Posterior Sag Test. Note the position of the tibia *(arrow)*. (From Miller MD, Hart JA, MacKnight JM, editors: *Essential orthopaedics*, Philadelphia, 2010, Saunders.)

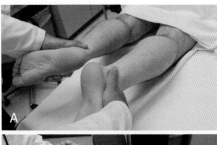

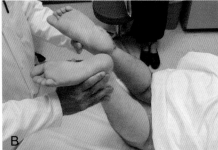

Fig. 7.9 External Rotation Asymmetry. With the knees stabilized, both feet are passively externally rotated and the thigh-foot angle is measured. Asymmetry of 15 degrees or more implies injury to the posterolateral corner structures. The test is performed in both 30 degrees **(A)** and 90 degrees **(B)** of knee flexion. Asymmetry in both 30 and 90 degrees implies injury to both the posterolateral corner and the posterior cruciate ligament. (From Miller MD, Hart JA, MacKnight JM, editors: *Essential orthopaedics*, Philadelphia, 2010, Saunders.)

Initial Management

- Elevation, ice, and nonsteroidal antiinflammatory drugs (NSAIDs) to decrease pain and effusion
- **Patient Education.** Unlike the ACL, the PCL has some healing potential. Not all PCL injuries require surgical reconstruction. Nonoperative management consists of intensive PT. Some research indicates an increased risk of developing degenerative changes in the PCL-deficient knee, especially in the patellofemoral compartment.

Nonoperative Management

- Grade I and II injuries with no or small bone fragment can be managed with PT. The focus of PT is on quadriceps strengthening and ROM.
- Patients may return to sports when quadriceps strength is near normal, approximately 4-6 weeks after injury.

Operative Management

Codes

ICD-10 code: S83.529A Posterior cruciate ligament tear
CPT code: 29889 Posterior cruciate ligament reconstruction

Indications

- Grade I or II injury with large bone fragment
- Grade III injury
- Chronic grade II or grade III injuries that do not respond to extensive (>6 months) PT.
- Multiligament injury

Informed consent and counseling

- Possible complications include residual laxity, instrument breakage, aberrant tunnels, avascular necrosis of the medial femoral condyle, cartilage injury, heterotopic ossification, hardware failure, loss of motion, neurovascular injury, paresthesia, effusion, DVT, and infection. Anesthesia risks include paralysis, cardiac arrest, brain damage, and death.
- Postoperative PT is essential to regain full ROM, strengthen quadriceps, and return to sport or physical activities.
- Full recovery may take up to 1 year.

Anesthesia

- General with regional nerve block

Patient positioning

- Supine with a knee holder or post or lateral decubitus, with a tourniquet

Surgical Procedure: Fig. 7.10

- Autograft (patellar tendon, quadriceps tendon, or hamstring tendons) or allograft (patellar tendon, quadriceps tendon, Achilles tendon, and hamstring tendons) may be used.

Transtibial Single-Bundle Technique

- The extremity is prepared and draped in standard sterile fashion. The tibial tunnel is drilled at the anterolateral cortex of the proximal tibia. The knee

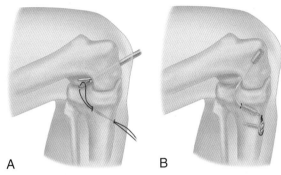

Fig. 7.10 Posterior Cruciate Ligament Reconstruction. **A,** The graft is passed from tibia to femur. **B,** Fixation is established with interference screws, and back-up fixation may be used if desired. (From Miller MD, Hart JA, editors: *SMART: sports medicine assessment and review textbook,* Philadelphia, 2011, Saunders.)

is flexed to 110 degrees while the proximal tibia is pushed in posteriorly. A plastic sheath is placed in contact with the lateral femoral condyle, and then a femoral tunnel is created 2 to 3 mm proximal to the articular junction at the 1 o'clock position in the right knee or the 11 o'clock position in the left. A fixation device (chosen based on surgeon preference) is attached to the graft with a whipstitch. The graft is passed through both tunnels and secured with interference screws. The incisions are irrigated, then closed, and a sterile dressing is applied.

Arthroscopic Tibial Inlay Technique (Single- or Double-Bundle)

- The extremity is prepared and draped in standard sterile fashion. Anterolateral and anteromedial portals are established. Diagnostic arthroscopy is performed; meniscal and cartilage disorders are addressed. Next, a posteromedial portal is established for instrument passage. The PCL stump is débrided, while preserving the anterior edge of the PCL footprint to serve as a reference point for the inlay. The tibial tunnel is prepared with the knee in flexion. An arthroscopic PCL guide is used to position a pin in the proximal aspect of the PCL footprint. A flip cutter is used to create the tibial socket in an inside-out fashion. A C-arm and the arthroscope are used for guidance. The femoral tunnels are created using a PCL guide centered over the medial femoral condyle at the border of the vastus medialis. For single-bundle reconstruction, the femoral tunnel is drilled at the 11 o'clock position; for double-bundle reconstruction, tunnels are drilled at 9 o'clock and 11 o'clock positions. Grafts are passed with the knee flexed at 90 degrees. The grafts are fixed (various fixation devices are available). The incisions are irrigated, then closed, and a sterile dressing is applied.

Estimated Postoperative Course
* Postoperative day 0 to 6 weeks:
  * Hinged brace locked in full extension at all times for 6 weeks. Fifty percent weight bearing in brace with crutches to assist with ambulation, prone passive ROM with PT.
  * Remove the dressing on the second day after surgery, and replace it with gauze or self-adhesive bandages and an elastic compression (ACE) wrap.
  * Ice, elevation, and PRN pain medications are used for comfort.
  * A wound check, suture removal, and assessment of ROM and stability are performed at 10 to 14 days postoperatively.
* Postoperative 6 weeks to 3 months:
  * Obtain radiographs.
  * Assess ROM and stability at 3 months.
  * Wean the patient off crutches and discontinue the brace.
  * Advance PT.
* Postoperative 3+ months:
  * Assess ROM and stability.
  * The patient may begin treadmill running and continue to advance PT.
  * The patient may return to recreation activities or sports at 9 to 12 months.

Board Review
Isolated PCL injuries can most often be managed with conservative treatment options but combined ligamentous injuries often require surgical reconstruction.

SUGGESTED READINGS

Keller T, Miller MD: Posterior cruciate ligament reconstruction: posterior inlay technique. In Scott WM, editor: *Insall and Scott surgery of the knee*, ed 5, Philadelphia, 2012, Churchill Livingstone, pp 538–547.

Kim S, Kin T, Jo S, et al.: Comparison of the clinical results of three posterior cruciate ligament reconstruction techniques, *J Bone Joint Surg* 91(11):2543–2549, 2009.

Patel DV, Answorth AA, Warren RF, et al.: The nonoperative treatment of acute isolated (partial or complete) posterior cruciate ligament deficient knees: an intermediate-term follow-up study, *HSS J* 3:137–146, 2007.

Salata MJ, Wojtys EM, Sekiya JK: Posterior cruciate ligament injury. In Miller MD, Hart JA, MacKnight JM, editors: *Essential orthopaedics*, Philadelphia, 2010, Saunders, pp 616–619.

Voos JE, Mauro CS, Wente T, et al.: Posterior cruciate ligament: anatomy, biomechanics, and outcomes, *Am J Sports Med* 40:221–231, 2012.

MEDIAL COLLATERAL LIGAMENT INJURY

History
* Acute injury
  * The mechanism of injury is typically valgus stress to the knee. It can result from contact or noncontact injury.
  * Medial knee pain is present.
  * The patient is typically able to bear weight.
  * The patient may report a sensation of instability with pivoting.
  * Effusion may or may not be noted; localized swelling is more common.

Physical Examination
* **Observe:** Note effusion, ecchymosis, deformity, abrasion or contusion, and gait.
* **Palpate:** Palpate the entire course of the MCL, from proximal to distal. Tenderness typically indicates some degree of MCL injury. Joint line tenderness is indicative of concomitant meniscus tear. Lateral tenderness of the distal femur and proximal tibia may result from bony contusion.
* **ROM:** This may be limited by effusion.

Special Tests: Fig. 7.11
* Valgus stress testing with the knee in 30 degrees of flexion isolates the MCL and is the most sensitive test.
* Valgus stress testing should also be performed in full extension. Laxity in this position suggests grade III injury (complete rupture), as well as other ligamentous injury.
* The Slocum test is used to evaluate for posteromedial corner (PMC) laxity.

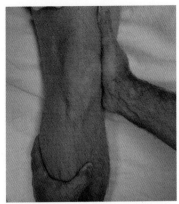

Fig. 7.11 Varus Stress Testing. A varus stress is applied across the knee. This examination is done in both 30 degrees of knee flexion and full extension. Opening in full extension implies concurrent injury to the cruciate ligament. (From Miller MD, Hart JA, MacKnight JM, editors: *Essential orthopaedics*, Philadelphia, 2010, Saunders.)

- Complete a through knee examination to rule out other ligamentous, meniscal, or patellar injury.

Imaging
- Radiographs
  - Standing flexion, lateral, and sunrise views are typically normal in acute injury unless bony avulsion is present. Stress radiographs may be helpful.
  - Pellegrini-Stieda lesion: MCL calcification is seen on plain radiographs in chronic MCL injury.
- MRI (Fig. 7.12)
  - MRI is not required to make the diagnosis, but it may be helpful to identify additional injuries.
  - Coronal sequences are best for identifying MCL injury.
  - Bone bruises of the lateral femoral condyle and lateral tibial plateau may be seen.
  - MRI allows for grading: grade I, periligamentous swelling and minor tearing; grade II, complete disruption of superficial layers, deep layers intact; grade III, complete disruption and fluid extravasation.

Classification
- Classification is based on the amount of opening noted with valgus stress test:
  - Grade I: 1 to 4 mm of laxity with end point
  - Grade II: 5 to 9 mm of laxity with end point

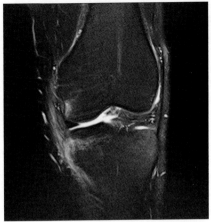

Fig. 7.12 Magnetic Resonance Imaging Demonstrating a Medial Collateral Ligament Tear.

  - Grade III: 10 to 15 mm of laxity with no firm end point
- MCL injury is also graded by MRI findings as previously described.

Differential Diagnoses
- Other ligamentous knee injury
- Meniscus tear

Initial Management
- Rest, ice, compression, elevation, NSAIDs
- **Patient Education.** The MCL is the most commonly injured ligament in the knee. Most MCL sprains will heal with bracing and activity modification. Persistent laxity may occur if the patient is noncompliant with brace wear.

Nonoperative Management
- Playmaker brace: worn during weight-bearing activities until physical examination reveals pain-free motion and stability, typically for 6 to 8 weeks
- Typical return to play: grade I, 10 days; grade II, 20 days; grade 3, at least 4 weeks (typically recommend the use of the brace with sports activities for an additional 6 weeks)

Operative Management
Codes
ICD-10 code: S83.419A Medial collateral ligament tear
CPT codes: 27427 Medial collateral ligament reconstruction

27405 Medial collateral ligament primary repair
Indications
- Surgical repair or reconstruction is indicated in patients with persistent laxity or rotatory instability following adequate bracing or in patients with acute multiligament injuries.

Informed consent and counseling
- Possible complications include loss of motion, bleeding, infection, DVT, neurovascular injury, residual laxity, instrument breakage, cartilage injury, hardware failure, and effusion. Anesthesia risks include cardiac arrest, paralysis, brain damage, and death.
- Postoperative PT is essential for full recovery and return to sports or physical activities.

Anesthesia
- General, with or without regional nerve block

Patient positioning
- Supine
- Tourniquet used if needed

Surgical Procedures
Primary Repair
- A medial incision is made between the medial epicondyle and the adductor tubercle. Various suturing techniques are used to re-tension and repair the MCL and surrounding structures such as the posterior oblique ligament and semimembranosus. Suture, suture anchor, or screw with washer is used to repair MCL avulsions from the origin or insertion.
- Wound closure: Multilayer closure is augmented with Steri-Strips; then a sterile dressing and an elastic compression (ACE) wrap are applied.

Reconstruction
- Diagnostic arthroscopy is performed to evaluate and treat concurrent meniscus tear and to determine whether the MCL is torn from the femoral or tibial side.
- A 10- to 15-cm medial hockey stick incision is made. Primary repair is typically completed as described earlier and is then combined or reinforced with MCL reconstruction using semitendinosus autograft or allograft. The graft tissue is used to reconstruct the superficial MCL anatomically. The graft is secured at the anatomic origin and insertion with screws and washers or sutures. The posteromedial capsule can be secured to the graft to eliminate laxity.

- Wound closure: Multilayer closure is augmented with Steri-Strips; then a sterile dressing and an elastic compression (ACE) wrap are applied

Estimated Postoperative Course
- Postoperative day 0 to 6 weeks:
  - An integrated ROM (IROM) brace locked in full extension is worn at all times for the first 2 weeks, then at 0 to 90 degrees for weeks 2 to 6. The patient has 50% weight bearing with crutches.
  - The patient may remove the dressing on the second day after surgery and replace it with gauze or self-adhesive bandages and an elastic compression (ACE) wrap.
  - Ice, elevation, and PRN pain medications are used for comfort.
  - A wound check, suture removal, and assessment of ROM and stability are performed at 10 to 14 days postoperatively.
  - Begin PT 10 to 14 days postoperatively.
- Postoperative 6 weeks to 3 months:
  - Full weight bearing is allowed as tolerated; the patient may be weaned off crutches. Discontinue the brace.
  - Obtain radiographs, evaluate healing of the surgical site, and assess ROM and stability of reconstruction.
  - PT: Advance to full ROM as soon as possible, facilitate gait normalization with treadmill walking, and continue quadriceps strengthening.
- Postoperative 3+ months:
  - Evaluate ROM and stability of reconstruction.
  - PT: The patient may begin jogging on a treadmill.
  - The patient may initiate sport-specific activities under supervision of a physical therapist or an ATC at 4 months, with full return to sports at 6 months.

SUGGESTED READINGS

Andrews K, Lu A, McKean L, Ebraheim N: Review: medial collateral ligament injuries, *J Orthop* 14(4):550–554, 2012.

Jacobson KE, Chi FS: Evaluation and treatment of medial collateral ligament and medial-sided injuries of the knee, *Sports Med Arthrosc Rev* 14:58–66, 2006.

Kurzweil RK, Kelley ST: Physical exam and imaging of the medial collateral ligament and posteromedial corner of the knee, *Sports Med Arthrosc Rev* 14:67–73, 2006.

Long JL, Carpenter JE: Medial collateral ligament injury. In Miller MD, Hart JA, MacKnight JM, editors: *Essential orthopaedics*, Philadelphia, 2010, Saunders, pp 620–623.

KNEE DISLOCATION

History

- The mechanism of injury is typically high-energy trauma such as a motor vehicle collision, but it can also occur in lower-velocity sports injuries. Knee dislocation can occur in obese patients with events that involve minimal trauma.
- Large effusion is noted.
- Pain is extreme.
- An obvious deformity may be present, but the knee may also spontaneously reduce before the patient seeks medical attention.

Physical Examination

- Observation
  - Effusion
  - Bruising and/or abrasions
  - Deformity

Special Tests

- Compartment syndrome evaluation
  - Remember the six Ps: pain, pressure, paresthesia, pulselessness, pallor, and paralysis.
  - Monitor compartment pressures.
  - Consider checking serum creatine kinase and urine myoglobin levels.
- Vascular examination
  - Serial examination must be performed.
  - Dorsalis pedis and posterior tibial pulses should be symmetric bilaterally.
  - Check the ankle-brachial index (ABI). An ABI greater than 0.9 is considered normal.
  - An abnormal ABI is an indication for an arteriogram with venous runoff.
  - Request a vascular surgery consultation if available.
- Neurologic examination
  - Evaluate motor function and sensation.
- Knee ligament examination (knee dislocation often causes multiligament injury)
  - ACL: Lachman, pivot shift, and anterior drawer tests.

- PCL: posterior drawer test.
- Collateral ligaments: valgus and varus stress tests.
- PLC: dial test.

Pearl

Many knee dislocations are obvious on clinical examination because of joint deformity, but the clinician should be cautious because some dislocations spontaneously reduce before medical examination. *Always* complete a thorough neurovascular examination on a patient who presents with an acute traumatic knee injury.

> **! CLINICAL ALERT**
>
> Neurovascular injury is exceedingly common with knee dislocation. Serial examination is key, and a high index of suspicion must be maintained when evaluating these injuries. Many centers recommend arteriograms and/or vascular consultations for all knee dislocations in the emergency department.

Imaging

- Radiographs (Fig. 7.13): Anteroposterior (AP) and lateral views help to identify associated osseous injuries such as tibial plateau fracture, proximal fibular fracture, avulsion of Gerdy tubercle, intercondylar spine fracture, fibular head avulsion, and Segond or PCL avulsion fragments. Stress views will help assess degree of laxity resulting from ligamentous injury.
- MRI is not needed on an emergency basis, but it is helpful for identifying the extent of ligament injury and preparing for surgical reconstruction.
- Arteriogram with venous runoff is used to assess for vascular injury.

Classification

- Open versus closed
- Reducible versus irreducible
- Types of dislocations also defined by the direction of displacement of the tibia in respect to the femoral condyles: posterior, anterior, medial, lateral, and rotator (Fig. 7.14)

Initial Management

- Closed reduction should be performed as soon as possible. Once the dislocation is reduced, repeat a neurovascular examination. Apply a long-leg splint or knee immobilizer; then repeat the radiographs to ensure that reduction is maintained.

- Rapid identification and repair of vascular injuries are essential. Delay of 6 to 8 hours is associated with a high amputation rate.

- **Patient Education.** Knee dislocation can result in multiligament injury. The peroneal nerve, which provides sensation to the dorsum of the foot and controls dorsiflexion of the ankle, is injured in up to 20% of knee dislocations. Popliteal artery injury occurs in approximately 19% of knee dislocations. The long-term risk of posttraumatic arthritis is approximately 50%.

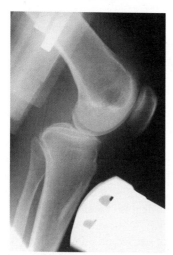

Fig. 7.13 Stress Radiograph Demonstrating Posterior Translation Secondary to Posterior Cruciate Ligament Rupture.

Nonoperative Management

- Nonoperative management is usually associated with significant instability and poor outcome.

Operative Management

- Emergency surgery may be necessary if the dislocation is not reducible or evidence indicates vascular injury.

- Surgical reconstruction will address multiligament injury. Timing often depends on the presence or absence of vascular injury. If vascular injury was previously repaired, consult a vascular surgeon for clearance before proceeding with ligament reconstruction.

- If initial surgery must be delayed because of other more urgent injuries, the use of an external fixator may be necessary until definitive treatment with ligament reconstruction can be safely performed.

- A combination of allograft and autograft is typically used for multiligament reconstruction.

- Ligament reconstruction is performed as described in previous sections.

- Later tendon transfer may be needed for patients with nerve injury to restore function.

Estimated Postoperative Course

- Postoperative day 0 to 6 weeks:
  - An IROM brace locked in full extension is worn at all times for the first 2 weeks and then at 0 to 90 degrees for weeks 2 to 6. The patient is 50% weight bearing with crutches for 6 weeks.

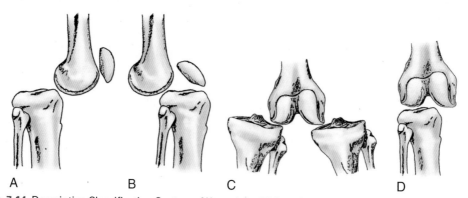

Fig. 7.14 Descriptive Classification System of Knee Joint Dislocations. **A,** Posterior. **B,** Anterior. **C,** Medial or lateral. **D,** Rotatory. (From Bryant BJ, Musahl V, Harner CD: The dislocated knee. In Scott WN, editor: *Insall and Scott surgery of the knee,* ed 5, Philadelphia, 2012, Churchill Livingstone.)

- Remove the dressing on the second day after surgery, and replace it with gauze or self-adhesive bandages and an elastic compression (ACE) wrap.
- Ice, elevation, and PRN pain medications are indicated.
- A wound check, suture removal, and assessment of ROM and stability are performed at 10 to 14 days postoperatively.
- PT: Straight leg raises with brace locked in extension, ROM exercises in the prone position, scar management, and modalities are used. The patient may begin using the stationary bike at 2 weeks.
- Postoperative 6 weeks to 3 months:
  - Full weight bearing is allowed as tolerated; the patient may be weaned off crutches. Discontinue the brace.
  - PT: Advance to full ROM as soon as possible, facilitate gait normalization with treadmill walking, and continue quadriceps strengthening.
- Postoperative 3+ months:
  - PT: The patient may begin jogging on a treadmill and doing isokinetic exercises.
  - The patient may initiate sport-specific activities under the supervision of a physical therapist or an ATC at 4 months, with full return to sports at 6 months.

Board Review

True knee dislocations require careful attention to the neurovascular examination due to their high associated with injury to these structures, especially to the popliteal artery and peroneal nerve.

SUGGESTED READINGS

Levy BA, Fanelli GC, Whelan DB, et al.: Controversies on the treatment of knee dislocation and multiligament reconstruction, *J Am Orthop Surg* 17:197–206, 2009.

Mook WR, Miller MD, Diduch DR, et al.: Multiple-ligament knee injuries: a systematic review of the timing of operative intervention and postoperative rehabilitation, *J Bone Joint Surg Am* 19, 2009. 2946–2857.

Salata MJ, Wojtys EM, Sekiya JK: Knee dislocation. In Miller MD, Hart JA, MacKnight JM, editors: *Essential orthopaedics*, Philadelphia, 2010, Saunders, pp 628–632.

PATELLA CHONDROMALACIA

History

- Patients complain of anterior knee pain that is aggravated by running, squatting, ascending or descending stairs, walking on inclines, sitting with the knee bent for a prolonged period, and rising from a seated position.
- Pain is typically described as "achy," but it may be sharp at times.
- Patients may complain that the knee gives way. This pseudoinstability is the result of pain, which inhibits proper contraction of the quadriceps (Fig. 7.15).
- "Popping" or "creaking" under the patella is a common complaint.
- The patient may complain of "catching" under the patella (pseudolocking); however, true locking is not typical of patellofemoral chondromalacia. Locking is an indication of other disorders such as a meniscus tear.

Physical Examination

- **Observe:** Gait, body habitus, knee alignment (valgus/varus), foot pronation, pes planus/cavus, quadriceps atrophy, and effusion are noted.
- **Palpate:** Note patellar tenderness, tenderness of quadriceps or patellar tendon, tight lateral retinaculum, and crepitus.

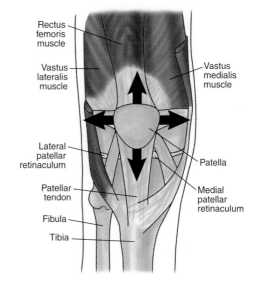

Fig. 7.15 The patella is stabilized by dynamic (muscles) and static (retinaculum and tendon) restraints. (From Miller MD, Hart JA, MacKnight JM, editors: *Essential orthopaedics*, Philadelphia, 2010, Saunders.)

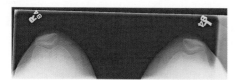

Fig. 7.16 Lateral patellar tilt is seen on a radiograph in a patient with patellofemoral pain.

- **ROM:** should be normal. There may be anterior knee pain with the full extension.
  - Assess patellar mobility.

Special Tests
- Patellar grind and patellar apprehension tests

Imaging
- Radiographs (Fig. 7.16)
  - Obtain standing flexion, lateral, and sunrise views.
  - Radiographs are helpful in ruling out other causes of pain such as loose body, degenerative changes, bipartite patella, and fracture.
  - Patellar tilt may be seen on the sunrise view.
- MRI
  - This is warranted only in refractory cases to rule out other pathologic processes.

Differential Diagnoses
- Patella chondral injury
- Patella tendinitis
- Meniscus tear

Initial Management
- Rest, ice, NSAIDs, PT
- **Patient Education.** Patellofemoral pain can almost always be managed nonoperatively with activity modification, PT, and a home exercise program. It may take an extended period for symptoms to improve; compliance with PT and a home exercise program is essential for recovery. Patients should be counseled on the importance of obtaining or maintaining a healthy body weight.

Nonoperative Management
- Initial treatment includes:
  - Activity modification: Patients must avoid activity that causes pain. Runners must decrease distance and frequency. Those with severe pain may have to stop running and cross train on a stationary bike or elliptical machine during the rehabilitation period.
  - NSAIDs: A short course (2 to 3 weeks) may help to decrease pain.
- PT for quadriceps strengthening with emphasis on the vastus medialis oblique (VMO), hip adductor strengthening, and stretching to increase quadriceps hamstring and iliotibial band (ITB) flexibility.
- Other modalities such as ice, electrical stimulation, iontophoresis, and ultrasound may be beneficial.
- Patellar taping or bracing can be used as adjunctive therapies.
- Orthotics may be used to address foot pronation and/or pes planus.
- Corticosteroid injection may be indicated when pain limits progress.

Operative Management
Codes
ICD-10 code: M22.40 Patellofemoral chondromalacia
CPT code: 29877 Arthroscopic débridement and shaving chondroplasty
Indications
- Arthroscopic débridement may be considered as a last resort when extensive conservative treatment has failed.
Informed consent and counseling
- Potential risks: bleeding, infection, DVT or pulmonary embolism (PE), loss of motion, cartilage injury, damage to nearby structures, and tourniquet complications
- Anesthesia complications: paralysis, cardiac arrest, brain damage, and death
Anesthesia
- General, and local anesthetic injected at portal sites after closure
Patient positioning
- Supine with a leg holder or post and a tourniquet

Surgical Procedures
Arthroscopic Débridement and Chondroplasty
- Two small incisions are made medial and lateral to the patella tendon slightly above the joint line. An arthroscope is used to explore the suprapatellar

pouch, patellofemoral joint, intercondylar notch, medial and lateral compartments, and medial and lateral gutters. A shaver is used to débride the patella and other areas of cartilage fraying.

Estimated Postoperative Course

- Postoperative day 0 to 6 weeks:
  - Full weight bearing is allowed as tolerated, and crutches or a cane may be used if needed.
  - Ice, elevation, and PRN pain medications are indicated for comfort.
  - Remove the dressing 2 days after surgery, and replace it with a self-adhesive bandage or gauze.
  - Patients may begin using a stationary bicycle 2 to 3 days after surgery. Start with low resistance for short periods and advance as tolerated. Swimming and use of an elliptical trainer may be started 1 week after surgery.
  - Sutures are removed 10 to 14 days after surgery.
  - Formal PT is indicated in patients with decreased ROM, persistent effusion, or quadriceps atrophy.
- Postoperative 6+ weeks:
  - Full recovery is likely by this time. If the patient is still experiencing pain; continued PT should be recommended.

Board Review

Patellofemoral pain is the most common cause of knee pain and typically presents with anterior knee pain which is worse with activities such as climbing stairs and standing up after prolonged knee flexion during sitting.

SUGGESTED READINGS

Collado H, Fredericson M: Patellofemoral pain syndrome, *Clin Sports Med* 29:379–398, 2010.

Fredericson M, Koon K: Physical examination and patellofemoral pain syndrome, *Am J Phys Med Rehabil* 85:234–243, 2006.

Parker RD: Patellofemoral pain syndrome. In Miller MD, Hart JA, MacKnight JM, editors: *Essential orthopaedics*, Philadelphia, 2010, Saunders, pp 660–662.

Prins MR, van der Wurff P: Females with patellofemoral pain syndrome have weak hip muscles: a systematic review, *Aust J Physiother* 55:5–15, 2009.

PATELLA AND QUADRICEPS TENDON DISORDERS

History

- Tendinitis
  - Typically, presentation is anterior knee pain at the superior (quadriceps) or inferior (patellar) poles of the patella.
  - The patient often reports a gradual onset, but symptoms may be aggravated by increasing or changing workouts.
  - This is most commonly seen in patients who participate in jumping, running, and kicking sports.
- Tendon rupture
  - Usually present after acute traumatic injury.
  - Inability to extend or lift the leg.
  - Severe pain.
  - Immediate effusion.
  - Possible history of knee pain or tendinitis before acute injury.
  - Possible history of steroid injection or anabolic steroid use.
  - Patella tendon ruptures more common in patients less than 40 years of age, whereas quadriceps tendon ruptures more common in patients more than 40 years of age.

Physical Examination

- Tendinitis
  - **Observe:** focal swelling of the affected tendon
  - **Palpate:** tenderness at the patellar poles and along the tendon
  - **ROM:** should be full; pain possible with the upper range of flexion

Tendon Rupture

- Observation: effusion, ecchymosis
- Palpation: palpable defect at the site of rupture
- ROM: complete loss of active extension
- Quadriceps tendon rupture: no movement of the patella with contraction of the quadriceps
- Patella tendon rupture: movement of the patella with contraction of the quadriceps

Imaging: Fig. 7.17

- Radiographs: AP, lateral, and sunrise views are used to rule out fracture (the patella may be "high" with patella tendon rupture and "low" with quadriceps tendon rupture).

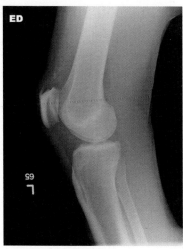

Fig. 7.17 A bony fragment avulsed from the patella can be seen on this lateral radiograph of a patient following quadriceps tendon rupture.

- MRI is not typically needed to evaluate acute tendon rupture, but it may be helpful in chronic tendinitis to evaluate degree of tendinopathy and other disorders.

Classification

- Patellar tendinitis can be classified using the system developed by Blazina in 1973:
  Phase I: pain only after activity
  Phase II: pain or discomfort during activity, but no interference with participation
  Phase III: pain both during and after participation that interferes with competition
  Phase IV: complete tendon disruption

Initial Management

- Tendinitis: rest, ice, NSAIDs
- Tendon rupture: immobilization in extension, ice, elevation
- **Patient Education.** Tendinitis is an overuse injury that can progress to tendon rupture. Activity modification and rest are the mainstays of treatment. Tendon rupture should be surgically repaired acutely to improve the chances of a good outcome.

Nonoperative Management

- Tendinitis
  - Rest for 4 to 6 weeks followed by gradual return to the previous level of activity

- PT: stretching (quadriceps, hamstring, and Achilles), core strengthening, endurance training
- Therapeutic modalities: ice, ultrasound, electrical stimulation
- Patella tendon strap or taping
- Tendon rupture
  - Rarely indicated as limits future knee function
  - Immobilization in extension and crutches pending surgical repair

Operative Management

Codes
ICD-10 codes: M76.50 Patellar tendinitis
  S86.819A Patella tendon rupture
  S76.11A Quadriceps tendon rupture
CPT codes: 27350 Tendon débridement
  27380 Patella tendon repair
  27385 Quadriceps tendon repair
Indications
- Tendinitis
  - Persistent symptoms after 3 to 6 months of extensive nonoperative measures
- Tendon rupture
  - Surgical repair: performed as soon as possible in all patients unless they are medically unstable
Informed consent and counseling
- Potential risks include rerupture, extensor mechanism dysfunction, loss of motion, failure to restore normal patella height, bleeding, infection, wound complications, and DVT or PE.
- Anesthesia risks include paralysis, cardiac arrest, brain damage, and death.
- Postoperative PT is essential to regain function, strength, and to return to sports or physical activity.
Anesthesia
- General, with or without regional block
Patient positioning
- Supine

Surgical Procedures
Tendon Débridement
- The surgical site is prepared and draped in standard sterile fashion. A midline incision is made to expose the tendon. The diseased portion of the tendon is excised and débrided. A rongeur or small drill bit may be used on the patellar pole to create marrow stimulation and promote healing. The tendon,

peritenon, and skin are closed in a multilayer fashion, and a sterile dressing is applied.

Tendon Repair

- Patellar tendon
  - The surgical site is prepared and draped in standard sterile fashion. A midline incision is made to expose the patella and ruptured tendon. Degenerated or inflammatory tissue is débrided. The distal pole of patella is dissected with a curette and rongeur; #5 Ethibond sutures are woven into the patellar tendon. Three longitudinal holes are drilled from the distal pole to the proximal pole of the patella. Ethibond sutures are passed through the drill holes with a suture passer. Sutures are tied to complete an anatomic reconstruction. The wound is irrigated and closed in a multilayer fashion, and then a sterile dressing is applied.
- Quadriceps tendon
  - The surgical site is prepared and draped in standard sterile fashion. A midline incision is made to expose the patella and ruptured tendon. The superior pole of the patella is dissected using a curette and rongeur. Using #5 FiberWire, three stitches are placed into the quadriceps tendon. Four longitudinal tunnels are drilled through the patella, and sutures are passed through the tunnels. Anatomic reconstruction is completed by securing knots at the distal end of the patella. The wound is irrigated and closed in a multilayer fashion, and then a sterile dressing is applied.

Estimated Postoperative Course

- Postoperative day 0 to 6 weeks:
  - A hinged knee brace locked in full extension is used for 4 weeks.
  - The patient is allowed full weight bearing in a brace.
  - Perform a wound check and suture removal at 10 to 14 days postoperatively.
  - Begin PT at 2 weeks postoperatively.
  - ROM can progress to 0 to 60 degrees at 4 weeks.
- Postoperative 6 weeks to 3 months:
  - Assess surgical site healing.
  - ROM is from 0 to 90 and advanced as tolerated.
  - Advance PT.
- Postoperative 3+ months:

- Assess the surgical site, extensor mechanism, and ROM.
- The patient may initiate jogging on a treadmill.

SUGGESTED READINGS

Blazina ME, Kerlan RK, Jobe FW, Carter VS, Carlson GJ. Jumper's knee. *Orthop Clin North Am.* 4(3):665–678.

Boublik M, Schlegel T, Koonce R, et al.: Patellar tendon rupture in national football league players, *Am J Sports Med* 39:2436–2442, 2011.

Parker RD: Extensor tendon rupture. In Miller MD, Hart JA, MacKnight JM, editors: *Essential orthopaedics*, Philadelphia, 2010, Saunders, p 677.

Parker RD: Quadriceps and patellar tendonitis. In Miller MD, Hart JA, MacKnight JM, editors: *Essential orthopaedics*, Philadelphia, 2010, Saunders, p 669.

Parr DM, Broe D, Cross M, Walsh WR: Biomechanics of the knee extensor mechanism and its relationship to patella tendinopathy: a review, *J Orthop Res* 36(12):3105–3112, 2018.

PATELLA INSTABILITY

History

- The patient may present with acute traumatic dislocation or with a complaint of chronic dislocation or subluxation.
- Acute patellar dislocation is a common cause of hemarthrosis.
- The patella may have to be manually reduced or may spontaneously reduce with knee extension.
- Patients with chronic instability often report anterior knee pain and a sensation that the knee is "giving way" or "going out."

Physical Examination

- **Observe:** gait, lower extremity alignment, effusion
- **Palpate:** tenderness along the medial border of the patella

Special Tests

- Patellar grind.
- Patella apprehension.
- J sign: The patella shifts laterally when the knee is extended (Fig. 7.18).
- Q angle: The angle is formed from a line drawn from the anterior superior iliac spine to the center of the

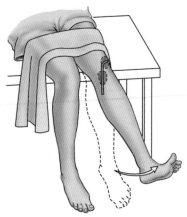

Fig. 7.18 The J sign is positive when the patella suddenly shifts laterally when the knee is extended. (From Miller MD, Hart JA, MacKnight JM, editors: *Essential orthopaedics*, Philadelphia, 2010, Saunders.)

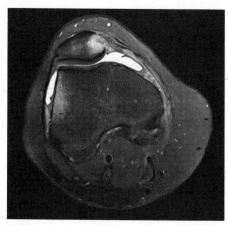

Fig. 7.19 Magnetic resonance imaging demonstrating subchondral edema of the medial patella and lateral femoral condyle following patella dislocation.

kneecap and from the center of the kneecap to the tibial tubercle. Measure that angle, and subtract from 180 degrees to determine Q angle.
- Thorough knee examination to rule out ligamentous and meniscal injury.

Imaging
- Radiographs: Standing flexion, lateral and sunrise views may show trochlear dysplasia, patella alta subluxation or tilt of the patella, and degenerative changes.
- MRI may show effusion, loose body, avulsion fracture, chondral injury, medial patellofemoral ligament (MPFL) tear, and subchondral edema (lateral femoral condyle and medial patella) (Fig. 7.19).
- Tibial tubercle-trochlear groove (TT-TG) is a valuable measurement of patella translation which can be calcular on a CT scan or MRI.

Classification
- A classification system was developed by Dejour et al.:
  - Major patellar instability: more than one documented dislocation
  - Objective patellar instability: one dislocation with associated anatomic abnormality
  - Potential patellar instability: patellar pain with associated radiographic abnormalities

- Patellar instability is also classified as congenital, traumatic, obligatory, subluxation, or dislocation.

Differential Diagnoses
- Collateral or cruciate ligament injury
- Meniscus tear
- Patella/quadriceps tendon rupture

Initial Management
- Reduction: Pain control and sedation may be required. Place the patient in the supine position with the hips flexed. Slowly extend the knee while applying medial pressure to the lateral aspect of the patella.
- **Patient Education.** The etiology of patellar instability is multifactorial. The following structural and functional factors can play a role in instability: patella alta, trochlear dysplasia or shallow groove, malalignment of the tibial tubercle, vastus medialis insufficiency, tight lateral structures, deficient MPFL, and joint laxity.
- The rate of recurrent dislocation can be as high as 60%.

Nonoperative Management
- Crutches may be needed initially to assist with ambulation.
- Rest, ice, elevation, and NSAIDs are indicated.
- Limit activities that cause pain.

- Aspiration may be indicated for a large effusion that interferes with ROM.
- PT is indicated for quadriceps strengthening with emphasis on the vastus medialis, strengthening of the hip abductors and flexors, edema control, and ROM.
- Patella taping or a patella stabilizing brace may provide symptomatic relief.
- Weight loss is recommended to reduce the patellofemoral load.

Operative Management

Codes
ICD-10 code: M25.369 Patella instability

    S83.006A Patella dislocation

CPT codes: 29873 Arthroscopic lateral release

    27427 Medial patellofemoral ligament reconstruction

    27418 Fulkerson osteotomy

Indications
- Recurrent instability despite adequate PT

Informed consent and counseling
- Potential risks: loss of motion, infection, DVT or PE, wound complications, neurovascular injury, recurrent dislocation, and nonunion (Fulkerson osteotomy)
- Anesthesia risks: paralysis, cardiac arrest, brain damage, and death

Anesthesia
- General, with or without regional block

Patient positioning
- Supine

Surgical Procedures

Proximal Repair and Realignment Procedures
- Primary repair of the MPFL: This procedure is indicated when instability is secondary to avulsion of the MPFL from the patellar or femoral attachment, rather than abnormal alignment. If the MPFL is disrupted at the patellar attachment, it is reattached to the patella with nonabsorbable sutures placed through drill holes in the patella. When the MPFL is torn from its femoral attachment, two suture anchors are placed into the femur at the MPFL origin, and mattress sutures are used to secure the MPFL.
- Reconstruction of the MPFL: This procedure is indicated when the MPFL is deficient or attenuated. Soft tissue autograft or allograft (semitendinosus tendon) is used. The graft can be fixed to the patella with an EndoButton fixation device, interference screw, or biotenodesis screw. A screw and washer are used for femoral fixation.
- Lateral retinaculum release: This procedure is most often performed in combination with the previously mentioned medial stabilization techniques. Lateral release is indicated only for patients with a tight retinaculum leading to patellar tilt. The lateral retinaculum is released proximal to the patellar pole; the vastus lateralis is left intact to reduce medial patellar subluxation.

Distal Realignment Procedure
- This procedure is performed when instability results from malalignment.

Anterior Tibial Tubercle Transfer (Fulkerson Osteotomy): Fig. 7.20
- This procedure is indicated when the patella does not track properly because of an abnormal trochlea or high patella. The tibial tubercle is detached and then anteriorized, medialized, and secured with cortical screws. This procedure unloads the patellofemoral joint and corrects the Q angle.
- Proximal and distal realignment procedures are often used in combination.

Estimated Postoperative Course
- Postoperative day 0 to 6 weeks:
  - Hinged brace locked in full extension.
  - Crutches and toe touch weight bearing for 2 weeks for MPFL reconstruction and 6 weeks for Fulkerson osteotomy.

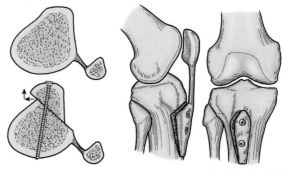

Fig. 7.20 Fulkerson Osteotomy. (From Aglietti P, Buzzi R, Insall J: Disorders of the femoral joint. In Scott WN, editor: *Insall and Scott surgery of the knee,* ed 4, Philadelphia, 2006, Churchill Livingstone.)

- Removal by the patient of the surgical dressing the third day after surgery and replacement with gauze or self-adhesive bandages.
- Wound check and suture removal 10 to 14 days postoperatively.
- Passive ROM 0 to 90 degrees for the first 6 weeks.
- Postoperative 6 weeks to 3 months:
  - Discontinuation of brace.
  - Radiographs after Fulkerson osteotomy; partial weight bearing and gait training begun for patients with adequate healing.
  - ROM: 0 degrees to full.
  - Exercise bicycle, closed chain kinetic exercises, and hamstring, adductor, abductor, quadriceps, and Achilles stretching begun.
- Postoperative 3+ months:
  - Radiographs to assess bony union after Fulkerson osteotomy at 3 months.
  - Progressive quadriceps strengthening exercises; return to sports typically 3 to 5 months after MPFL repair and reconstruction and 8 to 12 months after Fulkerson osteotomy.

Board Review

Patella dislocations are the second most common cause of almost immediate knee effusion after injury.

SUGGESTED READINGS

Dejour H, Walch G, Nove-Josserand L, et al.: Factors of patella instability: an anatomic radiographic study, *Knee Surg Sports Traumatol Arthrosc* 2:19–26, 1994.

Farr J, Schepsis AA: Reconstruction of the medial patellofemoral ligament for recurrent patellar instability, *J Knee Surg* 19:307–316, 2008.

Hiemstra LA, Page JL, Kerslake S: Patient reported outcome measures for patellofemoral instability: a critical review, *Curr Rev Musculoskelet Med* 12(2):124–137, 2019.

Moiz M, Smith N, Smith TO, Chawla A, Thompson P, Metcalfe A: Clinical outcomes after the nonoperative management of lateral patella dislocations: a systemic review, *Orthop J Sports Med* 6(6), 2018.

Parker RD: Patellar instability. In Miller MD, Hart JA, MacKnight JM, editors: *Essential orthopaedics*, Philadelphia, 2010, Saunders, pp 663–665.

Redziniak DE, Diduch DR, Mihalko WM, et al.: Patellar instability, *J Bone Joint Surg Am* 91:2264–2265, 2009.

CARTILAGE INJURIES

History

- These injuries may occur along with acute injury to ACL, meniscus, collateral ligaments or patella dislocation.
- These injuries can occur secondary to high-energy trauma or dashboard injury when the patella is forced into the trochlea.
- Acute pain with or without effusion (possible hemarthrosis if subchondral bone is fractured) is noted.
- Pain is aggravated by weight bearing.
- Mechanical symptoms such as locking or catching may occur if there is a cartilage flap or loose body (cartilage displaced into the joint).
- Osteochondritis dissecans (OCD) is a condition that typically affects the pediatric population. This condition is characterized by separation of an osteochondral fragment with or without articular cartilage involvement. It manifests with the foregoing symptoms. The origin appears to be idiopathic.

Physical Examination

- **Observe:** gait, effusion, ecchymosis or abrasion, quadriceps atrophy
- **Palpate:**
  - Tenderness of the femoral condyles or undersurface of the patella
  - Ballotable effusion
  - Palpable "clunk" with ROM an indication of a displaced cartilage flap
- **ROM:**
  - Possibly decreased secondary to effusion
  - Possible blockage by loose body of full extension and/or flexion
  - Crepitus possible with large lesions

Special Tests

- No special test for cartilage injury is available, but a thorough examination should be completed to rule out ligamentous or meniscal injury.

Imaging

- Radiographs
  - Standing flexion, lateral, and sunrise views to rule out osteoarthritis (OA), fracture, or OCD
- MRI (Fig. 7.21)
  - Helps to identify location and size of lesion

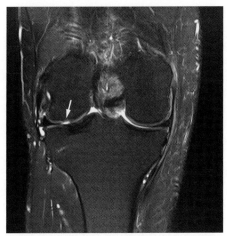

Fig. 7.21 Magnetic resonance imaging demonstrating a chondral defect *(arrow)*.

TABLE 7.7	Clanton and DeLee Classification System for Osteochondritis Dissecans Lesions
Type I	Depressed chondral fracture
Type II	Fragment attached by osseous bridge
Type III	Detached nondisplaced fragment
Type IV	Displaced fragment

Data from Clanton TO, DeLee JC: Osteochondritis dissecans. History, pathophysiology, and current treatment concepts, *Clin Orthop Relat Res* 167:50-64, 1982.

TABLE 7.8	Outerbridge Arthroscopic Grading System
Grade 0	Normal cartilage
Grade I	Softening and swelling
Grade II	Partial thickness defect, fissures <1.5 cm diameter
Grade III	Fissures down to subchondral bone, diameter >1.5 cm
Grade IV	Exposed subchondral bone

Data from Spahn G, Klinger HM, Hofmann GO: How valid is the arthroscopic diagnosis of cartilage lesions? Results of an opinion survey among highly experienced arthroscopic surgeons, *Arch Orthop Trauma Surg* 129:1117-1121, 2010.

TABLE 7.9	International Cartilage Repair Society Grading System
Grade 0	Normal
Grade 1	Nearly normal, superficial lesions
Grade 2	Abnormal, lesions extend <50% of cartilage depth
Grade 3	Severely abnormal, lesions extend >50% of cartilage depth
Grade 4	Lesions extend to subchondral bone

Data from Spahn G, Klinger HM, Hofmann GO: How valid is the arthroscopic diagnosis of cartilage lesions? Results of an opinion survey among highly experienced arthroscopic surgeons, *Arch Orthop Trauma Surg* 129:1117-1121, 2010.

- May show bone edema indicating overloading of the affected area
- Can identify or rule out other disorders
- Computed tomography (CT)
- Identifies fractures and size of bone fragments

Classification: Tables 7.7 through 7.9

- Classification systems for articular cartilage defects are shown in Tables 7.8 and 7.9.

Differential Diagnoses

- Meniscus tear
- Patella instability

Initial Management

- Rest, ice, compression, elevation, NSAIDs
- **Patient Education.** Articular cartilage lesions have limited healing potential, and persistent defects may progress to secondary OA. The goal of surgical intervention is to repair the defect or promote the formation of tissue with structure and durability similar to those of normal articular cartilage, thus leading to pain-free joint function.

Nonoperative Management

- Rest, ice, elevation, NSAIDs, and compression for symptom management
- PT for quadriceps strengthening and to restore ROM
- An unloader brace possibly helpful if there is overloading in a single compartment
- Surgical intervention possibly required if no response to conservative measures
- Surgical options: arthroscopic chondroplasty and loose body removal, microfracture, cartilage transfer (autograft versus allograft)

Operative Management

Codes

ICD-10 code: M23.90 Articular cartilage disorder of the knee

CPT codes: 29879 Microfracture

29877 Chondroplasty/débridement

29866 Osteochondral autograft, knee arthroscopic

27415 Osteochondral allograft, knee open

Indications

- Operative management is indicated in symptomatic focal full-thickness cartilage lesions, without significant concomitant arthritis, that have not responded to nonoperative measures.

Informed consent and counseling

- Potential risks: bleeding, infection, wound complications, loss of motion, DVT or PE, and failure of the procedure to hold up over time
- Anesthesia complications: paralysis, cardiac arrest, brain damage, and death
- Postoperative PT and compliance with weight-bearing restrictions essential for full recovery

Anesthesia

- General, with or without regional block

Patient positioning

- Supine, with tourniquet use

Surgical Procedures

Chondroplasty/Débridement

- Two small incisions are made medial and lateral to the patella tendon slightly above the joint line. An arthroscope is used to explore the suprapatellar pouch, patellofemoral joint, intercondylar notch, medial and lateral compartments, and medial and lateral gutters. A shaver is used to débride identified cartilage defects.

Fixation of Unstable Fragments

- This procedure can be performed if there is an osteochondral fragment and adequate subchondral bone. The defect is identified arthroscopically, and then underlying nonviable tissue is débrided with a shaver. Subchondral bone may be drilled or supplemented with bone graft, after which the osteochondral fragment is fixed with absorbable or nonabsorbable screws.

Microfracture

- This procedure is performed arthroscopically. The defect is identified and débrided to subchondral bone. An awl is used to make holes in the bone. This procedure stimulates the production of fibrocartilage, which will eventually fill the defect (Fig. 7.22).

Osteochondral Autograft Transfer System (OATS)

- This procedure may be performed openly or arthroscopically. A cylindrical instrument is used to harvest plugs of cartilage and bone from a non–weight-bearing area. The cartilage defect is débrided and prepared, and then the plug is placed into the defect.

Osteochondral Allograft

- Two different techniques using osteochondral allograft exist. Very large defects can be "filled" using large osteochondral allograft plugs ("megaOATS") that are cut to size and press fit into the defect. Minced juvenile allograft cartilage has also gained popularity to fill smaller defects and is particularly useful for patella defects, in which traditional OATS procedures have been difficult. The cartilage defect is débrided and filled with juvenile cartilage cells and is then sealed

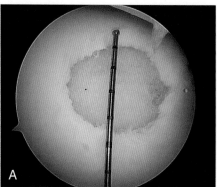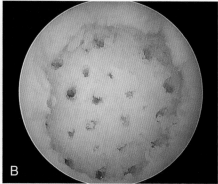

Fig. 7.22 Arthroscopic Images of a Cartilage Defect. **A,** Defect after débridement. **B,** Microfracture of the defect.

with fibrin glue. Hyaline cartilage fills the defect and functions similar to normal articular cartilage.

Estimated Postoperative Course

- Postoperative day 0 to 6 weeks:
  - The surgical dressing can be removed on the second day after surgery and replaced with adhesive bandages or gauze.
  - A wound check and suture removal are performed at 10 to 14 days postoperatively.
  - Microfracture: Crutches and 25% weight bearing are indicated for 6 weeks. No limits on ROM are necessary; advance as tolerated.
  - OATS: A brace and 50% weight bearing are indicated for 6 weeks.
  - Ice, elevation, and PRN pain medication indicated for comfort.
  - Begin PT at 10 to 14 days postoperatively.
  - Arthroscopic débridement and chondroplasty: Only one postoperative visit is typically needed. The patient may bear weight and progress activity as tolerated.
- Postoperative 6 weeks to 3 months:
  - Assess surgical site healing and ROM.
  - Discontinue the brace and advance to full weight bearing.
  - Normalize gait mechanics and progress open and closed chain exercises as tolerated.
- Postoperative 3+ months:
  - Begin sport-specific drills and plyometrics.
  - Return to sports typically occurs 5 to 6 months after microfracture or OATS; however, some surgeons may allow earlier return.

SUGGESTED READINGS

Magnussen RA, Dunn WR, Carey JL, et al.: Treatment of focal articular cartilage defects in the knee: a systematic review, *Clin Orthop Relat Res* 466(4):952–962, 2008.

Marcu DM, Baer GS: Chondral injuries of the knee. In Miller MD, Hart JA, MacKnight JM, editors: *Essential orthopaedics*, Philadelphia, 2010, Saunders, pp 642–646.

Redondo ML, Beer AJ, Yanke AB: Cartilage restoration: microfracture and osteochondral autograft transplantation, *J Knee Surg* 31(3):231–238, 2018.

Salzmann GM, Niemeyer P, Hochrein A, Stoddart MJ, Angele P: Articular cartilage repair in the knee in children and adolescents, *Orthop J Sports Med* 6(3), 2018.

KNEE OSTEOARTHRITIS

History

- Joint swelling
- Pain aggravated by weight bearing and relieved by rest
- Stiffness
- Periodic flares
- Night pain and pain at rest with severe OA
- Mechanical symptoms such as catching and locking possible secondary to loose bodies, cartilage flap, and concurrent meniscus tears
- Most common in older obese patients

Physical Examination

- **Observe:**
  - Gait and use of assistive device
  - Alignment: valgus (medial compartment OA), varus (lateral compartment OA)
  - Quadriceps atrophy
  - Effusion
- **Palpate:**
  - Effusion
  - Crepitus
  - Tenderness
- **ROM:**
  - Often decreased; may lack full extension

Imaging

- Radiographs
  - Standing flexion weight-bearing, AP lateral, and sunrise views are obtained. Bilateral films are often helpful for comparison.
  - Common radiographic changes seen in OA include decreased joint space, osteophyte formation, subchondral sclerosis, cyst formation, and flattening of the femoral condyles (Fig. 7.23).
  - Full-length hip to ankle films are helpful to assess alignment if surgical intervention is indicated.

Classification

- Primary: Arthritis is not associated with a specific trauma, inflammatory, or metabolic condition.
- Secondary: Arthritis develops secondary to injury of the articular cartilage or other structures in the knee, such as intraarticular fracture, chondral defect, meniscus tear, or ligament rupture.

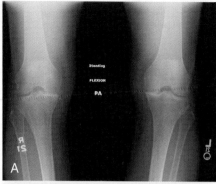

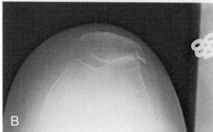

Fig. 7.23 Radiographs Demonstrating Osteoarthritis (OA). **A**, Medial compartment OA. **B**, Patellofemoral OA. *PA*, Posteroanterior.

Differential Diagnoses

- Meniscus tear
- Patellofemoral pain
- Pes anserine bursitis
- Hip osteoarthritis (pain can radiate to the knee)

Initial Management

- Activity modification, ice or heat, acetaminophen or NSAIDs
- **Patient Education.** OA is a common joint disease that can cause significant disability. It is caused by cartilage breakdown and subsequent changes to the underlying bone. Joint changes are irreversible, but lifestyle modification, such as weight loss, can help slow the progression.

Nonoperative Management

- Lifestyle modification includes low-impact exercise (stationary bicycle, elliptical trainer, swimming) and weight loss.
- PT may help patients to develop an appropriate exercise routine.

- Medications: Acetaminophen and NSAIDs are indicated. Narcotics are not recommended for long-term symptom management.
- Topical NSAIDs can be used in cases when oral NSAIDs are contraindicated.
- Dietary supplements: Glucosamine (1500 mg) and chondroitin sulfate (1200 mg) are recommended.
- Orthotics and/or unloader brace (if OA is isolated to a single compartment).
- Intraarticular injections: Corticosteroid injections can be administered up to three times per year. Hyaluronic acid (HA) injections act as a lubricant, have few side effects, and may be helpful in patients in whom corticosteroid injection has failed. However, HA injections are expensive and often require insurance preauthorization.

Operative Management

Codes

ICD-10 code: M17.10 Knee osteoarthritis
CPT codes: 29877 Arthroscopic débridement and chondroplasty

- 27457 High tibial osteotomy
- 27446 Unicondylar arthroplasty
- 27447 Total knee arthroplasty

Indications

- Surgical intervention is indicated in patients in whom extensive conservative measures fail and who have significant disability or decreased quality of life.
- Arthroscopic débridement is typically used in patients with loose bodies or meniscus tears along with OA. It may help relieve mechanical symptoms (catching, locking).
- High tibial osteotomy is indicated for young to middle-aged active patients with degenerative changes that are isolated to the medial or lateral compartment.
- Unicondylar arthroplasty is indicated for isolated medial or lateral compartment OA in older, low-demand patients.
- Total knee arthroplasty is indicated for older, low-demand patients with multicompartment OA.

Informed consent and counseling

- Potential risks include DVT or PE, patella fracture, component loosening, peroneal nerve palsy, periprosthetic fracture, wound complications, infection, instability, popliteal artery injury, quadriceps and patellar tendon rupture, stiffness, fat embolism, collateral ligament injury, and need for revision.

- Anesthesia complications include paralysis, cardiac arrest, brain damage, and death.
- Research indicates that 10-year survivorship for unicompartmental arthroplasty is approximately 90%, and it drops to 85% at greater than 10 years.
- Research indicates that 5-year success rates for high tibial osteotomy range from 80% to 96%; the 10-year success rate ranges from 53% to 85%.
- Research indicates that 15-year survivorship for total knee arthroplasty may be as high as 94%.
  Anesthesia
- General, with or without regional block
  Patient positioning
- Supine

Surgical Procedures
Arthroscopic Débridement
- The extremity is prepared and draped in standard sterile fashion. Two small incisions are made medial and lateral to the patella tendon slightly above the joint line. An arthroscope is used to explore the suprapatellar pouch, patellofemoral joint, intercondylar notch, medial and lateral compartments, and medial and lateral gutters. A shaver is used to débride identified cartilage defects. Loose bodies are identified and removed, and meniscus tears are débrided. Portals are closed, and a sterile dressing is applied.

High Tibial Osteotomy
- The extremity is prepared and draped in standard sterile fashion. A midline or lateral incision is made to expose the proximal tibia. An opening wedge or closing wedge osteotomy is performed to correct alignment and unload the affected compartment. During opening wedge osteotomy, a bone wedge is removed from the tibia, and a plate is applied and tensioned; bone graft is often used to fill the defect. During closing wedge osteotomy, a wedge of bone is removed from the tibia, and plate systems or staples are used for compression. Incisions are closed in a multilayer fashion, and a sterile dressing is applied.

Unicondylar Replacement
- The extremity is prepared and draped in standard sterile fashion. A short vertical incision is made from the top of the patella to the tibial tubercle. The knee is positioned in 90 degrees of flexion. The collateral ligaments are retracted and protected throughout the case. Osteophytes are removed. Tibial resection is then performed with a saw, and tibial trial components are used to determine the appropriate component size. The flexion gap is measured and balanced using spacer blocks. A cutting block is used to prepare the femoral side, and the trial components are again used to determine the appropriate component size. Components are cemented in place, the wound is irrigated and closed in a multilayer fashion, and a sterile dressing is then applied.

Total Knee Replacement
- Various prostheses and surgical techniques are available. The extremity is prepared and draped in standard sterile fashion. A midline incision is made over the patella, and then subcutaneous tissue and peritenon are dissected. The patella is everted, and osteophytes are excised from all three compartments. Using a tibial intramedullary (IM) guide, a hole is drilled in line with tibial shaft, usually just lateral to insertion of the ACL. The MCL and LCL are retracted and protected. A transverse osteotomy of the proximal tibia is then performed. The femoral component is sized, and the distal femoral cut is made with the assistance of an IM guide and cutting block. Next, the patella is measured, and holes are drilled for placement of the patellar component. All components are secured with cement. Multilayer closure is performed, and a sterile dressing is applied (Fig. 7.24).

Estimated Postoperative Course
Postoperative day 0 to 6 weeks:
- High tibial osteotomy
  - Surgical dressing removal by the patient 2 to 3 days after the procedure
  - Ice, elevation, and PRN pain medication for comfort
  - No weight bearing, and use of a hinged brace for 6 to 8 weeks
  - Wound check and suture removal at 10 to 14 days
  - PT begun at 10 to 14 days postoperatively, with flexion limited to 120 degrees for 15 days and then gradually advanced
- Unicondylar arthroplasty
  - 1- to 2-day hospital stay
  - Ice, elevation, and PRN pain medication for comfort

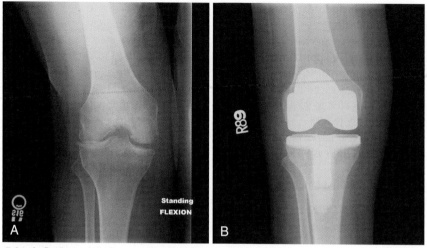

Fig. 7.24 A, Radiograph before total knee replacement. B, Radiograph after total knee replacement.

- Removal of the surgical dressing by the patient 2 to 3 days after the procedure
- Weight bearing as tolerated and walking with an assistive device shortly after surgery
- PT begun in the hospital, with transition to home health or outpatient therapy
- Wound check and suture or staple removal at 10 to 14 days
- Total knee arthroplasty
  - 2- to 3-day hospital stay
  - CPM begun shortly after surgery 0 to 90 degrees initially and then advanced as tolerated; used for 8 hours daily
  - Ice, elevation, and PRN pain medication for comfort
  - Weight bearing as tolerated and ambulation with an assistive device
  - PT begun in the hospital, with transition to home health or outpatient therapy

Postoperative 6 weeks to 3 months:
- High tibial osteotomy
  - Brace discontinued
  - Evaluation of surgical site healing and ROM
  - PT advanced
  - Radiographs obtained and reviewed
- Unicondylar arthroplasty
  - Evaluation of surgical site healing and ROM
  - PT advanced
  - Radiographs obtained and reviewed
- Total knee arthroplasty

- Goal: full ROM at this point
- Ambulation indoors possible without an assistive device

Postoperative 3+ months:
- High tibial osteotomy
  - Return to strenuous work at 3 months and sports at 6 months
- Unicondylar arthroplasty
  - Evaluation of ROM; repeat radiographs considered at 6 or 12 months
- Total knee arthroplasty
  - Ambulation with no assistive device
  - Radiographs obtained and reviewed

SUGGESTED READINGS

Fitz W, Scott RD: Unicompartmental knee arthroplasty. In Scott WM, editor: *Insall and Scott surgery of the knee*, ed 5, Philadelphia, 2012, Churchill Livingstone, pp 988–995.

Leone JM, Hanssen AD: Osteotomy about the knee: American perspective. In Scott WM, editor: *Insall and Scott surgery of the knee*, ed 5, Philadelphia, 2012, Churchill Livingstone, pp 910–925.

Marcu DM, Baer GS: Osteoarthritis of the knee. In Miller MD, Hart JA, MacKnight JM, editors: *Essential orthopaedics*, Philadelphia, 2010, Saunders, pp 651–656.

Micheal JW, Schuluter-Brust KU, Eysel P: The epidemiology, etiology, diagnosis and treatment of osteoarthritis of the knee, *Dtsch Arztebl Int* 107(9):152–162, 2010.

KNEE BURSITIS

History

- Prepatellar bursitis (Fig. 7.25)
  - Anterior knee pain and swelling
  - Difficulty kneeling
  - Possible occupation requiring excessive kneeling
  - Possible history of trauma to the anterior knee
- Pes anserine bursitis (Fig. 7.26)
  - Common causes: athletic overuse, medial knee acute trauma, and chronic mechanical or degenerative processes
  - Pain in the medial knee, over the proximal tibia
  - Pain possibly particularly severe at night
  - Pain possibly aggravated by ascending or descending stairs and rising from a seated position

Physical Examination

- Prepatellar bursitis
  - A ballotable collection of fluid is located just over the patella, with or without erythema and warmth.
  - Tenderness over the bursal sac is noted.
  - Crepitus may or may not be present.
  - Chronic bursitis is characterized by palpable subcutaneous cobblestone-like roughness.
- Pes anserine bursitis
  - Examination should include observation and analysis of gait.
  - Palpate the tibial plateau to localize tenderness, and differentiate between tenderness of the MCL and that of the pes anserine bursa.
  - The patient may have pain with valgus stress, resisted internal rotation, and resisted flexion.

Imaging

- Radiographs: Standing flexion, lateral, and sunrise views are obtained. Radiographs are not needed to make the diagnosis of bursitis, but they can rule out underlying fracture if the patient has a history of trauma and assess for concurrent arthritis. Typically, radiographs are unremarkable, except for soft tissue swelling of the anterior knee in prepatellar bursitis.
- MRI is not necessary, but it rules out other disorders. Fluid may be seen in the bursa.

Differential Diagnoses

- Patellofemoral pain
- Tendinitis
- Meniscus tear

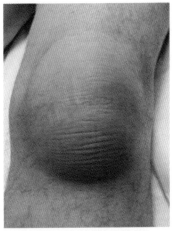

Fig. 7.25 Patient with Acute Prepatellar Bursitis. (From Miller MD, Hart JA, MacKnight JM, editors: *Essential orthopaedics*, Philadelphia, 2010, Saunders.)

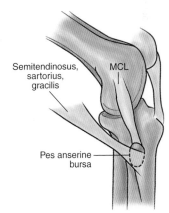

Fig. 7.26 Location of the Pes Anserine Bursa on the Medial Side of the Knee. *MCL,* Medial collateral ligament. (From Miller MD, Hart JA, MacKnight JM, editors: *Essential orthopaedics*, Philadelphia, 2010, Saunders.)

Initial Management

Patient Education

- Prepatellar bursitis
  - It is most commonly caused by trauma, such as a fall onto the anterior knee, or direct pressure and friction caused by repetitive kneeling ("housemaid's knee").
  - It may become chronic in a small percentage of patients.
  - The prepatellar bursa may become infected (typically by *Staphylococcus aureus*) and can also be inflamed secondary to gout.

- Pes anserine bursitis
  - It commonly occurs along with medial compartment OA or results from overuse.
  - It can result from trauma, but abnormal gait is a more common cause. Increased friction on the bursa secondary to loss of normal mechanical relationships leads to inflammation.
- Knee bursitis typically responds well to nonoperative treatment.

Nonoperative Management

- Prepatellar bursitis
  - Avoid activities that put direct pressure on the bursa, such as squatting and crossing the legs.
  - Use knee pads.
  - Limit repetitious bending.
  - If infection of the prepatellar bursa is suspected, aspiration is recommended. Send fluid for cell counts, Gram stain, culture and sensitivity, and crystal analysis. Serum erythrocyte sedimentation rate and C-reactive protein determinations may be helpful as well. Treat septic bursitis with appropriate antibiotics.
  - PT is indicated for stretching and strengthening, as well as treatment modalities such as ultrasound and electrical stimulation.
  - If symptoms persist despite conservative measures, corticosteroid injection is indicated.
- Pes anserine bursitis
  - Activity modification, rest, and NSAIDs are recommended.
  - PT is indicated for stretching and strengthening, as well as treatment modalities such as ultrasound and electrical stimulation.
  - If symptoms persist despite conservative measures, corticosteroid injection is indicated.
  - It may be helpful to place a small cushion between the thighs while sleeping.

Operative Management

Codes
ICD-10 codes: M70.40 Prepatellar bursitis
M70.50 Pes anserine bursitis

CPT codes: 27340 Prepatellar bursectomy
27599 Pes anserine bursectomy
Indications
- Surgical bursectomy is rarely needed, but it is indicated for severe intractable bursitis.
Informed consent and counseling
- Possible complications: bleeding, infection, wound complication, loss of motion, and damage to nearby tissues, vessels, and nerves
- Anesthesia risks: paralysis, cardiac arrest, brain damage, and death
Anesthesia
- General, and local at portal site after closure
Patient positioning
- Supine, with tourniquet

Surgical Procedures
Arthroscopic Prepatellar Bursectomy
- The surgical site is prepared and draped in standard sterile fashion. An anteromedial portal and an anterolateral portal are routinely used. The bursal cavity and synovial thickening are visualized with the arthroscope. A motorized shaver is inserted, and total synovectomy (including the bursa) is performed. Portals are closed, and a sterile dressing is applied.

Pes Anserine Bursectomy
- The surgical site is prepared and draped in standard sterile fashion. A small incision is made over the pes anserine. Soft tissues are dissected so that the bursa can be visualized. The bursa and any bony exostosis are excised. The wound is irrigated and closed in a multilayer fashion.

Estimated Postoperative Course
- The surgical dressing can be removed on the second postoperative day.
- Sutures are removed at 10 to 14 days postoperatively.
- Prepatellar bursectomy: No vigorous physical activity is allowed for 2 weeks after surgery; return to normal physical activity occurs at 3 weeks postoperatively.
- Pes anserine bursectomy: The knee should be braced in extension or slight flexion for 2 weeks; then advance ROM as tolerated.
- PRN follow-up occurs after the initial postoperative clinic appointment.

SUGGESTED READINGS

Huang Y, Yeh W: Endoscopic treatment of prepatellar bursitis, *Int Orthop* 35(3):355–358, 2011.

Parker RD: Pes anserine bursitis. In Miller MD, Hart JA, MacKnight JM, editors: *Essential orthopaedics*, Philadelphia, 2010, Saunders, pp 674–676.

Parker RD: Prepatellar bursitis. In Miller MD, Hart JA, MacKnight JM, editors: *Essential orthopaedics*, Philadelphia, 2010, Saunders, pp 671–673.

Rennie WJ, Saiffuddin A: Pes anserine bursitis: incidence in symptomatic knees and clinical presentation, *Skeletal Radiol* 34:395–398, 2005.

MENISCUS INJURY

History

- Acute injury
  - The mechanism of injury is typically twisting or hyperflexion.
  - Acute pain is present, with or without effusion.
  - Pain is aggravated by squatting or pivoting.
  - Mechanical symptoms such as locking and catching may be present.
  - Root tears may present as a sudden painful pop in the back of the knee.
- Chronic (degenerative) injury
  - This often occurs in older patients with OA.
  - It is frequently caused by an atraumatic mechanism.

Physical Examination

- **Observe:**
  - Effusion
  - Antalgic gait
  - Ecchymosis or abrasion
- **Palpate:**
  - Joint line tenderness: Assess the medial and lateral joint lines with the knee flexed.
  - Perform patella ballottement to evaluate for effusion.
  - Palpate the popliteal fossa for a Baker cyst.
- **ROM:**
  - Lack of full extension, which is referred to as a locked knee, may be caused by a displaced bucket handle tear.
  - Decreased flexion may occur secondary to effusion.

Special Tests

- **McMurray test:** Pain with McMurray test is more common and is often considered a positive test result, but pain is less sensitive for a meniscus tear than a palpable click.
- The patella apprehension, Lachman, pivot shift, posterior drawer, and valgus and varus stress tests should also be performed to rule out concurrent injury.

Imaging

- Radiographs
  - Order standing flexion, lateral, and sunrise views.
  - Radiographs are often unremarkable in younger patients with acute tear; they may show effusion if present. Joint space narrowing is seen in patients with degenerative meniscus tears secondary to OA.
- MRI
  - No contrast is needed to evaluate for meniscus tears, but arthrogram MRI is useful to evaluate healing or recurrent tear at the site of previous meniscal repair.
  - MRI can determine location of the tear, tear pattern, and displacement.

Classification

- Meniscus tears are classified by location and tear pattern (Fig. 7.27).

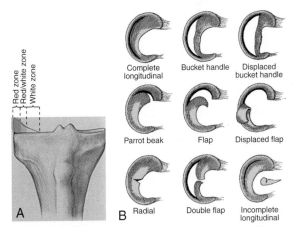

Fig. 7.27 Classification of Meniscal Tears. A, Classification based on location. **B,** Classification based on appearance and orientation. (From Miller MD: *Review of orthopaedics*, ed 5, Philadelphia, 2008, Saunders.)

- Discoid meniscus: Typically, this is a normal anatomic variant in which the meniscus is abnormally shaped, covering a larger portion of the tibial plateau than the normally shaped meniscus. This condition is classified into three types: incomplete, complete, and Wrisberg variant. Discoid meniscus is typically asymptomatic, but it may require meniscectomy or repair if it is torn or if snapping and popping develop.

Differential Diagnoses

- Ligament injury
- Knee osteoarthritis
- Chondral injury

Initial Management

- Initial treatment is symptom based: rest, ice, compression, and elevation are helpful to relieve pain and swelling.
- **Patient Education.** Meniscus tears may become less symptomatic over time, or symptoms may be intermittent and aggravated by physical activity. Peripheral meniscus tears can be repaired, but tears that involve the inner portion of the meniscus are débrided.

Nonoperative Management

- Observation is indicated for small tears or in arthritic patients with no mechanical symptoms.
- PT may be beneficial to restore motion, reduce swelling, and increase quadriceps strength.

Operative Management

Codes

ICD-10 code:
  S83.289A Lateral meniscus tear
  S83.249A Medial meniscus tear
CPT codes: 29881 Arthroscopic partial medial or lateral meniscectomy
  29880 Arthroscopic partial medial and lateral meniscectomy
  29882 Medial or lateral meniscus repair
  29883 Medial and lateral meniscus repairs

Indications

- Failure of nonoperative management, mechanical symptoms (catching, clicking, locking), and persistent pain or swelling that interferes with activity are operative indications.
- Vertical and longitudinal tears in the periphery of the meniscus (red-red/white zone) can be repaired. Meniscus tears that occur in the avascular region of the meniscus are treated with partial meniscectomy.
- Meniscus transplant is an option for younger patients with near total meniscectomy, particularly in the lateral meniscus.

Informed consent and counseling

- Potential complications: damage to articular cartilage, hemarthrosis, neurovascular injury, tourniquet complications, fluid extravasation, DVT, loss of motion, and infection
- Anesthesia risks: paralysis, cardiac arrest, brain damage, and death

Anesthesia

- General, and local at portal sites after closure

Patient positioning

- Supine with a leg holder or post, with a tourniquet

Surgical Procedures

Arthroscopic Partial Meniscectomy

- The extremity is prepared and draped in a sterile fashion. Two small incisions are made medial and lateral to the patella tendon slightly above the joint line. An arthroscope is used to explore the suprapatellar pouch, patellofemoral joint, intercondylar notch, medial and lateral compartments, and medial and lateral gutters. Shavers and biters are used to débride the meniscus tear back to a stable border. Any visualized loose bodies are removed, and areas of cartilage fraying can be débrided with a shaver. Portals are closed, and local anesthetic is injected. A sterile dressing and an elastic compression (ACE) wrap are applied.

Meniscus Repair: Fig. 7.28

- The extremity is prepared and draped in a sterile fashion. Diagnostic arthroscopy is used to identify the meniscus tear, after which a 2- to 3-cm vertical incision (medial or lateral) is made to allow for tying of the sutures. Various techniques are available for meniscus repair. Placement of inside-out vertical

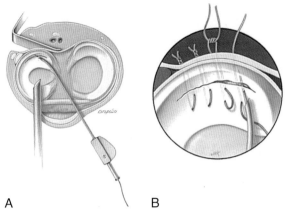

Fig. 7.28 Inside-Out Meniscal Repair Technique. **A,** Passing the suture. **B,** Tying the knots and completing the repair. (From Miller MD: *Review of orthopaedics*, ed 5, Philadelphia, 2008, Saunders.)

mattress sutures is a commonly used technique and remains the gold standard. Tensionable all-inside devices have been developed and are most commonly used with concomitant ACL reconstruction, which provides the best environment for meniscal healing. Neurovascular structures must be identified and protected: the saphenous nerve and vein medially and the common peroneal nerve laterally. The incision is closed in a multilayer fashion. A sterile dressing and an elastic compression (ACE) wrap are applied.

Estimated Postoperative Course
Postoperative day 0 to 6 weeks:
- Partial meniscectomy
  - The wound dressing can be removed and replaced with self-adhesive bandages after 2 days.
  - Sutures are removed at 10 to 14 days postoperatively.
  - Weight bearing is allowed as tolerated, with crutches for assistance if needed.
  - Use of a stationary bicycle and quadriceps strengthening exercise can be started several days after surgery, and activity is advanced as tolerated.
  - Formal PT is not typically needed, but it may be beneficial for patients who have decreased ROM, quadriceps atrophy, or persistent edema.
  - Return to sports typically occurs 3 to 4 weeks postoperatively.
  - Follow-up PRN occurs after the initial postoperative visit.

- Meniscus repair
  - The wound dressing can be removed and replaced with self-adhesive bandages after 2 days.
  - Sutures are removed at 10 to 14 days postoperatively.
  - Toe touch weight bearing with crutches is allowed for 4 weeks, followed by 50% weight bearing.
  - ROM is from 0 to 90 degrees.
  - Begin PT at 10 to 14 days postoperatively.

Postoperative 6 weeks to 3 months:
- Meniscus repair
  - Assess ROM and surgical site healing at the clinic visit.
  - Progress ROM as tolerated.
  - Continue to advance PT.

Postoperative 3+ months:
- Meniscus repair
  - The patient begins running on a treadmill and plyometrics at 3 months.
  - The patient returns to full sport at 5 months.

Board Review
Meniscus tears can be acute or chronic and typically present with swelling and mechanical symptoms such as catching, locking, and giving way.

SUGGESTED READINGS

Kalliakmanis A, Zourntos S, Bousgas D, et al.: Comparison of arthroscopic meniscus repair results using 3 different devices in anterior cruciate ligament reconstruction patients, *Arthroscopy* 24:810–816, 2008.

Marcu DM, Baer GS: Meniscus tears. In Miller MD, Hart JA, MacKnight JM, editors: *Essential orthopaedics*, Philadelphia, 2010, Saunders, pp 671–673.

Miller MD, Howard RF, Plancher KD: *Surgical atlas of sports medicine*, Philadelphia, 2003, Elsevier Science.

Noyes FR, Chen RC, Barber-Westin SD, et al.: Greater than 10-year results of red-white longitudinal meniscal repairs in patients 20 years of age or younger, *Am J Sports Med* 39(5):1008–1016, 2011.

ILIOTIBIAL BAND SYNDROME

History
- Lateral knee pain worsens with activity (Fig. 7.29).
- Typically, the syndrome has an insidious onset.
- Patients can typically point to the exact area of involvement.

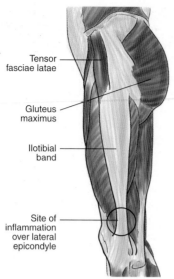

Fig. 7.29 Anatomy of Iliotibial Band Syndrome. Note the area of involvement over the lateral femoral epicondyle. (From Miller MD, Hart JA, MacKnight JM, editors: *Essential orthopaedics*, Philadelphia, 2010, Saunders.)

Physical Examination
- **Observe:** There may be swelling at the insertion of the ITB.
- **Palpate:** Minimal to no effusion is noted; tenderness to palpation at the insertion of the ITB is evident.
- **ROM:** Typically, full ROM may cause pain.

Special Tests
- **Ober test:** Have the patent lie on the unaffected side with the involved extremity up. Extend and adduct the hip, and then flex and extend the knee. An inability to adduct the leg and pain with flexion or extension indicate a positive test result.
- Complete McMurray test, special tests for ligamentous injury, and patella examination to rule out other injury.
- Other tests: Injection of a local anesthetic (lidocaine or bupivacaine) may be diagnostic and therapeutic.

Imaging
- Radiographs and MRI are not indicated.

Differential Diagnoses
- Meniscus tear
- Bursitis

Initial Management
- **Patient Education.** The ITB is a superficial thickening of tissue that runs from the hip to just below the knee. The ITB rubs the lateral femoral epicondyle with flexion and extension. ITB syndrome primarily occurs secondary to overuse, particularly in cyclists, runners, and skiers.

Nonoperative Management
- Initial treatment involves the following conservative measures: rest, ice, PT (stretching and strengthening), orthotics, and cross training.
- Corticosteroid injection is performed at the point of maximal tenderness.

Operative Management
- If conservative measures fail and the patient is unwilling to change activity level, surgical interventions may be considered.
- Surgery typically involves open exploration of the area, débridement of the bursa, shaving of bony prominences, and excision or fenestration of the ITB over the lateral femoral condyle.
  #### Codes
  ICD-10 code: M76.30 Iliotibial band syndrome
  CPT code: 27305 Open ITB fasciotomy/débridement
  #### Indications
- Intractable symptoms following extensive conservative treatment
  #### Informed consent and counseling
- Possible complications: bleeding, infection, wound complication, stiffness and damage to nearby structures, loss of motion, and DVT or PE.
- Anesthesia risks: paralysis, cardiac arrest, brain damage and death
  #### Anesthesia
- General
  #### Patient positioning
- Supine

Surgical Procedures
Iliotibial Band
- Prepare and drape the extremity in standard sterile fashion. A diagnostic arthroscopy may be performed to rule out concomitant meniscus tear or cartilage defect. A short longitudinal incision

is made laterally over the later femoral condyle. Soft tissue is dissected. The synovium or bursa is débrided, and a small triangular piece of the ITB that contacts the lateral femoral epicondyle when the knee is flexed to 30 degrees is excised. The incision is closed in a multilayer fashion, and a sterile dressing is applied.

Estimated Postoperative Course

- A wound check and suture removal are performed at 10 to 14 days postoperatively.
- PT focuses on stretching, strengthening, and slow return to sports.
- The patient may return at 3 months for reevaluation or on a PRN basis.

SUGGESTED READINGS

Drogset JO, Rossvoli I, Grontvedt T: Surgical treatment of iliotibial band friction syndrome: a retrospective study of 49 patients, *Scand J Med Sci Sports* 9:296–298, 1999.

Hariri S, Savidge ET, Reinold MM, et al.: Treatment of recalcitrant iliotibial band syndrome with open iliotibial band bursectomy: indications, technique, and clinical outcomes, *Am J Sports Med* 37:1417–1424, 2009.

Parker RD: Iliotibial band syndrome. In Miller MD, Hart JA, MacKnight JM, editors: *Essential orthopaedics*, Philadelphia, 2010, Saunders, pp 666–678.

CHRONIC EXERTIONAL COMPARTMENT SYNDROME

History

- Gradually increasing pain is noted in a specific muscle region during exertion.
- Symptoms typically occur at a specific and reproducible point of exercise, such as a particular distance or length of time.
- Pain is described as tightness, aching, squeezing, or cramping.
- The syndrome often occurs bilaterally.
- Neurologic symptoms such as paresthesia, weakness, and foot drop may be present.
- Pain typically resolves with rest, but some patients may report pain with daily activities and at rest.

TABLE 7.10 Physical Examination Findings Vary Based on Which Compartments Are Affected	
Anterior compartment	Numbness of the first web space or dorsum of foot, weakness of ankle dorsiflexion and toe extension, and possible foot drop
Deep posterior compartment	Weak toe flexion and foot inversion, as well as sensory changes on the plantar surface of the foot
Lateral compartment	Weak ankle eversion and numbness of the anterolateral leg
Superficial posterior compartment	Weak foot plantar flexion and numbness of the lateral foot

Physical Examination: Table 7.10

- Findings are often unremarkable at rest; it may be helpful to examine the patient after exercise that is sufficient to elicit symptoms.
- **Observe:** Swelling may be noted.
- **Palpate:** Palpable fascial hernia may be present. Involved compartments may be tight and tender.

Imaging

- Radiographs, MRI, or CT may be used to identify concurrent stress fractures or to rule out other possible causes.

Compartment Pressure Measurement

- The definitive diagnosis of chronic exertional compartment syndrome (CECS) is made by measuring compartment pressures.
- Pressure measurements are obtained at rest and after exercise challenge.
- The diagnosis is made based on the presence of one or more of the following criteria:
  - Pre-exercise pressure 15 mm Hg or greater
  - 1-minute postexercise pressure 30 mm Hg or greater
  - 5-minute postexercise pressure 20 mm Hg or greater

Differential Diagnoses

- Tibial stress fracture
- Medial tibial stress syndrome
- Gastrocnemius strain

Initial Management

- **Patient Education.** CECS is an overuse condition that most commonly occurs in young endurance athletes, particularly distance runners. Reversible ischemia is caused by increased pressure within the noncompliant fascial planes of a muscle compartment. It occurs during exercise as muscle volume expands in response to increased blood flow and edema. CECS occurs most commonly in the anterior compartment of the lower leg, followed by the deep posterior, lateral, and superficial posterior compartments. It may also occur in the foot, thigh, forearm, and hand.

Nonoperative Management

- Limitation on or cessation of the activity that causes symptoms
- Cross training
- NSAIDs
- Orthotics
- PT: massage, soft tissue mobilization, muscle stretching and strengthening

Operative Management

Codes

ICD-10 code: M79.A29 Exertional compartment syndrome of the lower extremity

CPT codes: 27600 Anterior and lateral compartment release/fasciotomy

27603 Four compartment release/fasciotomy

Indications

- Operative management is indicated in patients with intractable symptoms despite extensive conservative measures and documented increased compartment pressures.

Informed consent and counseling

- Possible complications: bleeding, wound infection, wound healing complications, nerve entrapment, nerve injury, swelling, arterial injury, hematoma, and DVT or PE
- Anesthesia risks: cardiac arrest, brain damage, paralysis, and death

Anesthesia

- General

Patient positioning

- Supine, with or without a tourniquet

Surgical Procedures: Fig. 7.30

Anterior and Lateral Compartment Release

- The lower extremity is prepared and draped in a sterile fashion. A 4- to 5-cm incision is made halfway between the fibular shaft and the tibia crest. A second more proximal incision may be made as needed. Skin edges are undermined, and a transverse incision is made in the fascia. The anterior intermuscular septum is identified; then Metzenbaum scissors and a fasciotome are used to release the fascia proximal and distal to the incision. Make sure the superficial peroneal nerve is identified and protected during the release.

Superficial Posterior and Deep Posterior Compartment Release

- The lower extremity is prepared and draped in a sterile fashion. A 4- to 5-cm incision is made 2 cm posterior to the posterior tibial margin. The saphenous nerve and vein are identified and protected. A transverse incision is made in the fascia, and the septum between the two compartments is identified; the superficial compartment is released first. The deep compartment is released distally and then proximally.

Wound Closure

- Deep tissues are closed with #3-0 Monocryl suture in an interrupted fashion, followed by #3-0 suture in a running fashion. Incisions are reinforced with Steri-Strips, and sterile dressings are applied. Posterior left splints are placed with the foot in neutral position.

Estimated Postoperative Course

- Postoperative day 0 to 6 weeks:
  - At 10 to 14 days after surgery, splint removal, wound check, and suture removal are performed, and PT is begun.
  - Crutches and no weight bearing are indicated for the first 2 weeks, with gradual progression as tolerated.
  - Early PT focuses on edema control, scar management, and ROM (ankle and knee). PT may

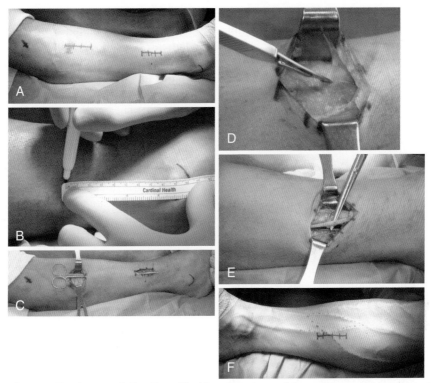

Fig. 7.30 Surgical Fasciotomy. A, Dual lateral incisions for release of the anterior and lateral compartments. **B,** The distal lateral incision is centered 10 to 12 cm proximal to the tip of the distal fibula, at the site where the superficial peroneal nerve penetrates the fascia. **C,** Blunt dissection produces subcutaneous connection of the incisions to allow adequate release of the compartments throughout their lengths. **D,** Anterior compartment fascial incision. The fascial incision is then extended proximally and distally under direct visualization. **E,** Superficial peroneal nerve after release of the anterior and lateral compartments. It is important to mobilize the nerve freely. **F,** Medial incision for release of the superficial and deep posterior compartments. (From Miller MD, Hart JA, MacKnight JM, editors: *Essential orthopaedics*, Philadelphia, 2010, Saunders.)

progress at approximately 4 weeks to include gentle stretching, ankle strengthening, balance and proprioception exercises, and gait training.

- Postoperative 6 weeks to 3 months:
  - Check wound healing at the office visit.
  - PT: Progress from water walking (if wounds are well healed) to the elliptical trainer and then to light jogging at 6 to 8 weeks.
- Postoperative 3+ months:
  - The patient may begin sport-specific training.

SUGGESTED READINGS

Buerba RA, Fretes NF, Devana SK, Beck JJ: Chronic exertional compartment syndrome: current management strategies, *Open Access J Sports Med* 10:71–79, 2019.

Campano D, Robaina JA, Kusnezov N, Dunn JC, Waterman BR: Surgical management for chronic exertional compartment syndrome of the leg: a systematic review of the literature, *Arthroscopy* 32(7):1478–1486, 2016.

Schubert AG: Exertional compartment syndrome: review of the literature and proposed rehabilitation guidelines following surgical release, *Int J Sports Phys Ther* 6(2):126–141, 2011.

Wilder RP: Exertional compartment syndrome. In Miller MD, Hart JA, MacKnight JM, editors: *Essential orthopaedics*, Philadelphia, 2010, Saunders, pp 684–686.

MEDIAL TIBIAL STRESS SYNDROME (SHIN SPLINTS)

History

- Vague diffuse pain occurs over the middle and/or distal tibia.

- Initially, pain is worse at the beginning of exercise, but it gradually resolves during exercise or shortly after cessation of activity.
- As the condition progresses, pain is more intense, persists throughout exercise, and may be present at rest and with ambulation.
- The patient has often had a change in a recent training regimen, such as increased activity, intensity, or duration.

Physical Examination

- **Observe:**
  - Evaluation for biomechanical abnormalities: genu varus or valgus, pes planus or pes cavus, hindfoot valgus, foot pronation, tibial torsion, femoral anteversion, and leg length discrepancy
  - Muscle imbalance, tightness, or weakness of the gastrocnemius, soleus, and plantaris
  - Shoe wear patterns
- **Palpate:**
  - Diffuse tenderness over the medial ridge of the distal and middle tibia
  - Tenderness possibly extending proximally with increasing severity
- **ROM:**
  - Pain with passive ankle dorsiflexion, resisted plantar flexion, standing toe raises, or jumping

Imaging

- Radiographs are usually not necessary for diagnosis, but they may show periosteal exostoses.
- Bone scan can help determine whether medial tibial stress syndrome (MTSS) has progressed to stress fracture although MRI has largely replaced this as a preferred imaging modality. Scans show diffuse uptake with MTSS; uptake is more focal in stress fracture.
- MRI may help differentiate MTSS, stress fracture, and stress reaction. Scans can show periosteal edema, marrow involvement, and cortical stress fracture.

Differential Diagnoses

- Tibial stress fracture
- Exertional compartment syndrome
- Gastrocnemius strain

Initial Management

- Rest, ice, activity modification
- **Patient Education.** Shin splints are a common cause of exertional leg pain and most often occur in patients who run or participate in activities that require repetitive jumping. Symptoms can worsen with continued activity; shin splints can progress to stress fracture without adequate rest and activity modification.

Nonoperative Management

- Acute phase: rest and ice
- Activity modification: decreased intensity, frequency, and duration
- Low-impact cross training
- Gradual return to sport when pain free
- Regular stretching and strengthening exercises of the gastrocnemius, soleus, ankle dorsiflexors and planter flexors, and foot invertors and evertors
- Change of shoes in runners every 250 to 500 miles
- Orthotics if indicated
- Absolute rest possibly indicated if no response to conservative measures

Operative Management

Indications

- Failure of 6 to 12 months of conservative treatment is an indication for fasciotomy of the deep posterior compartment and periosteal stripping.

  Surgical procedure and postoperative course. The surgical procedure and postoperative course for fasciotomy are discussed in the CECS section earlier in this chapter.

SUGGESTED READINGS

Blackham J, Amendola N: Medial tibial stress syndrome (shin splints). In Miller MD, Hart JA, MacKnight JM, editors: *Essential orthopaedics*, Philadelphia, 2010, Saunders, pp 680–683.

Couture C, Karlson K: Tibial stress injuries: decisive diagnosis and treatment of "shin splints," *Phys Sportsmed* 30(6):29–36, 2002.

Galbraith RM, Lavallee ME: Medial tibial stress syndrome: conservative treatment options, *Curr Rev Musculoskelet Med* 2:127–133, 2009.

Wilder RP, Sethi S: Overuse injuries: tendinopathies, stress fractures, compartment syndrome, and shin splints, *Clin Sports Med* 23:55–81, 2004.

STRESS FRACTURE

History

- Typically, patients present with progressively worsening activity-related pain. Pain may occur at rest as the injury progresses.
- On occasion, the patient may present with a sudden increase in pain at a site where there has been a chronic low-level discomfort; this finding indicates that a stressed bone has fractured.
- This injury is common in athletes and military recruits.
- It is more common in women than in men.
- Female patients with eating disorders and amenorrhea are at increased risk.

Physical Examination

- **Observe:**
  - Antalgic gait with walking or running
  - Localized swelling over the fracture site
- **Palpate:**
  - Tenderness localized to a discrete area
  - Palpable bump resulting from periosteal edema

Special Tests

- **Hop test:** The result is positive if the patient is unable to hop on the affected leg for 10 repetitions.
- **Tuning fork test:** The result is positive if pain is elicited by placing a vibrating tuning fork over the fracture site.
- **Percussion test:** The result is positive if percussion of the bone at a site other than the fracture site causes pain.
- Neurovascular examination should be normal.

Imaging

- Radiographs: Obtain AP and lateral views of the tibia and fibula. Periosteal elevation, cortical thickening, sclerosis, and true fracture are positive findings. These findings are seen only in 20% to 30% of initial radiographs. Radiographs taken 3 to 4 weeks after diagnosis are more likely to show the previously

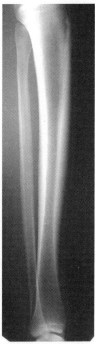

Fig. 7.31 Radiograph showing the "dreaded black line" of an anterior tibia stress fracture with a thickened anterior cortex and a lucent line. (From Miller MD, Hart JA, MacKnight JM, editors: *Essential orthopaedics*, Philadelphia, 2010, Saunders.)

mentioned changes. The "dreaded black line" seen on the lateral radiograph is a stress fracture of the midshaft anterior tibia, which is at high risk for delayed healing and nonunion (Fig. 7.31).

- Bone scan shows a focal area of uptake in stress fracture that helps differentiate stress fracture from MTSS, which has diffuse linear uptake. Bone scans have become less commonly used than MRI as an imaging modality for stress fractures.
- MRI can be particularly helpful in differentiating stress fracture from shin splints. MRI is also useful to differentiate intraarticular stress fracture from ligament, cartilage, or meniscal injury.
- CT may be helpful to determine whether the fracture has extended or developed into nonunion. It also defines fracture lines and shows evidence of healing with resolution of lucency and development of sclerosis.
- Repeat imaging is not needed unless the patient fails to respond to treatment. Radiographic healing typically lags behind clinical healing; bone scan and MRI may remain positive for up to 1 year after the initial injury.

Differential Diagnoses

- Medial tibial stress syndrome
- Exertional compartment syndrome
- Gastrocnemius strain

Initial Management

- Rest and activity modification
- The most common site of stress fracture is the tibia.
- Stress fractures are common in athletes, particularly runners. They also commonly occur in non-athletes who suddenly increase their activity level. Prolonged walking and jumping also increase the risk.
- **Patient Education.** Risk factors include excessive training, training on irregular or hard terrain, poor foot wear, weak and inflexible calf muscles, leg length discrepancy, pes planus or pes cavus, and hormonal or nutritional imbalances that lead to bone demineralization.

Nonoperative Management

- Diagnosis and treatment are often presumptive, based on history and physical examination because initial radiographic findings are often negative.
- NSAIDs, ice, and PT modalities can help alleviate pain.
- Vitamin D levels should be checked as vitamin D supplementation may be helpful if levels are below normal.
- Treatment depends on the site of injury and the risk for delayed healing or nonunion.

  High risk: anterior tibia

- Avoidance of weight bearing: Use of crutches, casting, or bracing is indicated for 3 to 12 weeks; discontinue as symptoms allow.
- Activity can be gradually progressed as long as the patient is pain free.

  Low risk: posteromedial tibia or fibula

- Treatment depends on the patient's goals and on whether pain interferes with performance.
- For athletes, if performance is not affected by pain and pain is not progressing, activity level may be continued without significant limitations.
- If performance is limited by pain, relative rest and cross training are recommended.

- If pain is present with walking, bracing or crutches and cross training should be implemented until the patient is pain free.

Operative Management

Indications

- Operative management is indicated if there is a clear fracture line or conservative treatment has failed.

  Codes

  ICD-10 code: M84.369A Stress fracture of the tibia
  CPT code: 27759 Tibial intramedullary nail

  Surgical procedure and postoperative course. The surgical procedure for tibial IM nail fixation and postoperative recovery are discussed in the tibial shaft fracture section later in this chapter.

SUGGESTED READINGS

Blackham J, Amendola N: Stress fractures of the tibia and fibula. In Miller MD, Hart JA, MacKnight JM, editors: *Essential orthopaedics*, Philadelphia, 2010, Saunders, pp 690–693.

Iwamoto J, Takeda T: Stress fractures in athletes: review of 196 cases, *J Orthop Sci* 8:273–278, 2008.

Kaeding CC, Yu JR, Wright R, et al.: Management and return to play of stress fractures, *Clin J Sport Med* 15:442–447, 2005.

Ohta-Fukushima M, Mutoh Y, Takasugi S: Characteristics of stress fractures in young athletes under 20 years, *J Sports Med Phys Fitness* 42(2):198–206, 2002.

FRACTURES OF THE KNEE (PATELLA, DISTAL FEMUR, PROXIMAL TIBIA)

History

Patella Fracture

- Trauma: direct or indirect
- Pain and swelling
- Diminished or absent knee extension
- Difficulty bearing weight and ambulating

Distal Femur and Proximal Tibia Fractures

- Trauma: high or low energy
- Pain and swelling
- Inability to bear weight

Physical Examination

Patella Fracture

- **Observe:** effusion, visible patella deformity, skin abrasions or lacerations

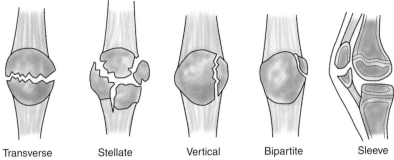

| Transverse | Stellate | Vertical | Bipartite | Sleeve |

Fig. 7.32 Patella Fracture Classification. Adult fracture patterns include transverse, stellate or comminuted, and vertical. The bipartite patella is frequently confused with a patella fracture. (From Miller MD, Hart JA, MacKnight JM, editors: *Essential orthopaedics*, Philadelphia, 2010, Saunders.)

- **Palpate:** palpable defect, effusion, tenderness
- **ROM:** active extension (intact, absent, extensors lag); flexion likely limited by effusion and pain
- Special tests:
  - **Saline load test:** Sterile arthrocentesis is performed; then 60 mL of sterile saline with or without methylene blue is injected into the joint. Extravasation confirms open fracture. The remaining fluid is aspirated.

Distal Femur and Proximal Tibia Fractures
- Observation: effusion, deformity, abrasion, laceration, fracture blisters
- Palpation: tenderness over fracture site, crepitus
- Neurovascular examination: assessment of sensory and motor function of the lower extremity and palpation of pulses
- Special tests:
  - Complete a thorough knee examination to evaluate for ligamentous and/or meniscal injury.
  - Measure compartment pressures if indicated.
  - If vascular injury is suspected, measure the ABI.

Imaging
Patella Fracture
- Radiographs: AP, lateral, and sunrise (if patient is able to flex the knee) views are obtained. They help evaluate the fracture pattern and displacement.
- MRI is not typically needed to diagnose patella fracture, but it may identify osteochondral or ligament injuries.

Distal Femur and Proximal Tibia Fractures
- Radiographs: AP, lateral, and 45-degree oblique views are indicated. Obtain radiographs of the joint above and the joint below.

- CT characterizes intraarticular extension and depression and is helpful for surgical planning.
- MRI may be ordered to evaluate for ligamentous or meniscal disorders.

Classification
Patella Fracture
- Classified as open or closed and by fracture pattern (Fig. 7.32)

Distal Femur Fracture
- Open versus closed
- Supracondylar versus intercondylar
- Type A, extraarticular; type B, unicondylar (partial articular, portion of articular surface remains in continuity with shaft); type C, intraarticular (articular fragment separated from shaft)

Proximal Tibia Fracture
- Classified by the Schatzker grading system (Fig. 7.33)

Initial Management
- **Patient Education.** Counsel patients on weight-bearing and ROM restrictions. Patients should be informed to call or return to the clinic or emergency department if they experience the following symptoms: increased pain, swelling, or neurovascular changes.

Patella Fracture
- A long-leg splint, immobilizer, or IROM brace locked in extension is used.

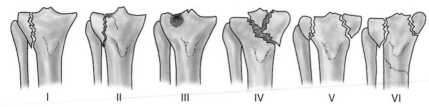

Fig. 7.33 Schatzker Classification of the Tibial Plateau Fractures. *I*, Lateral split; *II*, lateral split depression; *III*, lateral isolated depression; *IV*, medial; *V*, bicondylar; *VI*, bicondylar with metadiaphyseal dissociation. (From Miller MD, Hart JA, MacKnight JM, editors: *Essential orthopaedics*, Philadelphia, 2010, Saunders.)

- For open fracture, apply a sterile dressing, and administer appropriate antibiotics and tetanus prophylaxis.

Distal Femur and Proximal Tibia Fractures
- Reduce the fracture, and apply a long-leg splint for closed fractures.
- For open fracture, apply a sterile dressing, and administer appropriate antibiotics and tetanus prophylaxis.

Nonoperative Management
Patella Fracture
- Conservative management is indicated for minimally or nondisplaced fractures with an extensor mechanism that is intact.
- Immobilize the joint in full extension as discussed earlier.
- Patient may bear weight as tolerated with crutches or a walker.

Distal Femur and Proximal Tibia Fractures
- Nonoperative treatment is indicated in the following situations:
  - Isolated lateral tibial plateau fracture with less than 3 mm of articular step off and less than 10 degrees of valgus or varus instability
  - Isolated, nondisplaced, extraarticular distal femur fracture
- Place a locked hinged knee brace for 6 to 12 weeks.
- Begin gentle knee ROM under the guidance of a physical therapist at 2 to 4 weeks.
- Obtain serial radiographs to ensure proper alignment.

Operative Management
Codes
ICD-10 codes:
    S72.453A Supracondylar fracture of the femur
    S82.143A Tibial plateau fracture
    S82.009A Patella fracture

CPT codes:
    27524 Patella open reduction, internal fixation (ORIF)
    27535 ORIF of unicondylar tibial plateau fracture
    27536 ORIF of bicondylar tibial plateau fracture
    27506 Open treatment of femoral fracture
Indications
- Patella fracture: Fixation is recommended for fractures that disrupt the extensor mechanism or demonstrate more than 2 to 3 mm of step-off and more than 1 to 4 mm of displacement.
- Distal femur fracture: Surgical fixation is indicated for any distal femur fracture other than isolated, nondisplaced, or extraarticular fractures.
- Proximal tibia fracture: Surgical fixation is indicated for open fracture, compartment syndrome, vascular injury, displaced bicondylar fracture, displaced medial condyle fracture, lateral plateau fracture with joint instability, more than 2 mm of articular depression, and more than 10 degrees of varus or valgus instability.
Informed consent and counseling
- Possible risks: infection, nonunion, malunion, loss of fixation, painful hardware, DVT or PE, incomplete relief of pain, and incomplete return of function
- Anesthesia risks: cardiac arrest, brain damage, paralysis, and death
Anesthesia
- General, with or without regional block
Patient positioning
- Supine, with all bony prominences well padded
- Tourniquet on thigh

Surgical Procedures
Patella Open Reduction, Internal Fixation
- The extremity is prepared and draped in standard sterile fashion. A vertical midline incision is made to expose the fracture site, as well as the medial and lateral retinaculum. The fracture is reduced

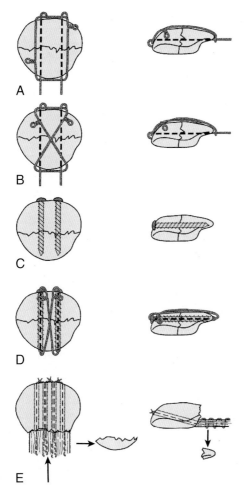

Fig. 7.34 Techniques of Patellar Fracture Fixation. **A,** Modified tension band with circular wire. **B,** Modified tension wire with figure-of-eight technique. **C,** Lag screw fixation. **D,** Combined cannulated lag screw and tension band wiring. **E,** Partial patellectomy. (From Brinker MR: *Review of orthopaedic trauma*, Philadelphia, 2001, Saunders.)

with reduction forceps; reduction is confirmed by palpation of articular surface and/or C-arm images. Fixation can be obtained with a variety of methods, depending on the fracture pattern and the surgeon's preference (Fig. 7.34). The medial retinaculum and lateral retinaculum are repaired if indicated. Irrigate the wound, and close it in a multilayer fashion.

Tibial Plateau Open Reduction, Internal Fixation

- The extremity is prepared and draped in standard sterile fashion. Arthroscopy is performed to evacuate hematoma and evaluate the articular surface and for associated injury. Arthroscopy is not useful for type IV to VI fractures because of the loss of capsular integrity leading to extravasation. The fracture is reduced; reduction is maintained with Kirschner wires (K-wires), which can be exchanged for cannulated screws. Fluoroscopy is used to verify anatomic reduction (length, rotation, varus, valgus, and recurvatum). An appropriate plate is inserted, and proper alignment is verified in the AP and lateral planes. Locking screws are inserted in each fragment. Voids may be filled with bone graft. The wound is irrigated and then closed in a multilayer fashion, and a sterile dressing is applied.

Distal Femur Retrograde Intramedullary Nail Fixation

- The extremity is prepared and draped in standard sterile fashion. A midline incision from the patella to the tibial tubercle is made. Then the patellar tendon is split, and the fat pad is excised as needed. A guide pin is placed 1 cm anterior to the PCL origin; placement is verified with fluoroscopy. An entry hole is drilled. Longitudinal traction is used to reduce the fracture. A guidewire is passed across the fracture site under fluoroscopic guidance. The site is reamed and measured to determine nail length width. The nail is placed and locked distally, and then leg length and alignment are evaluated. After necessary adjustments are made, the nail is locked proximally. The wound is irrigated and then closed is a multilayer fashion, and a sterile dressing is applied.

Distal Femur Open Reduction, Internal Fixation

- The extremity is prepared and draped in standard sterile fashion. A medial or lateral incision is made; skin and soft tissues are dissected so the fracture site can be visualized. The fracture is reduced, and then reduction is maintained with K-wires, which can be exchanged for cannulated screws. Fluoroscopy is used to verify anatomic reduction (length, rotation, varus, valgus, and recurvatum). An appropriate plate is inserted, and alignment is verified in the AP and lateral planes. Locking screws are inserted in each fragment. Voids may be filled with bone graft. The wound is irrigated, the incision is closed in a multilayer fashion, and a sterile dressing is applied.

Estimated Postoperative Course

Postoperative day 0 to 6 weeks:

- Patella ORIF
  - The knee brace is locked in extension, and weight bearing is allowed as tolerated in the brace.
  - Confirm reduction on radiographs at the initial postoperative visit.
  - Perform a wound check and suture removal at 10 to 14 days postoperatively.
  - Consider allowing knee ROM to some degree based on the stability of fixation at surgery.
- Tibial plateau ORIF and distal femur ORIF
  - Place a hinged knee brace; the patient is non–weight bearing for 6 weeks.
  - Confirm reduction on radiographs at the initial postoperative visit.
  - Perform a wound check and suture removal at 10 to 14 days postoperatively.
- Distal femur retrograde nail
  - Toe touch weight bearing is allowed, depending on the fracture configuration. Consider weight bearing as tolerated for short oblique or transverse fractures with 100% cortical contact.
  - Confirm reduction on radiographs at the initial postoperative visit.
  - Perform a wound check and suture removal at 10 to 14 days postoperatively.

Postoperative 6 weeks to 3 months:

- Patella ORIF
  - Obtain radiographs to evaluate for union.
  - Advance ROM.
- Tibial plateau ORIF and distal femur ORIF
  - Obtain radiographs at 6 weeks; the patient may progress to toe touch weight bearing if adequate callus formation is seen.
- Distal femur retrograde nail
  - Obtain radiographs at 6 weeks; the patient may advance to full weight bearing when bridging callus is visible on radiographs.
  - Evaluate knee ROM.

Postoperative 3+ months:

- Patella ORIF
  - Progress with ROM and strengthening.
  - Permit full sport and activity at 5 to 6 months.
- Tibial plateau ORIF and distal femur ORIF
  - Obtain radiographs at 12 weeks; the patient may progress to full weight bearing if adequate callus formation is seen.

SUGGESTED READINGS

Gurkan V, Orhun H, Doganay M: Retrograde intramedullary interlocking nailing in fractures of the distal femur, *Acta Orthop Traumatol Turc* 43(3):199–205, 2009.

Melvin JS, Mehta S: Patellar fractures in adults, *J Am Acad Orthop Surg* 19:198–207, 2011.

Okike K, Bhattacharyya T: Trends in the management of open fractures: a critical analysis, *J Bone Joint Surg Am* 88:2739–2748, 2006.

Shuler FD, Beimesch CF: Distal femur and proximal tibia fractures. In Miller MD, Hart JA, MacKnight JM, editors: *Essential orthopaedics*, Philadelphia, 2010, Saunders, pp 694–698.

Shuler FD, Davis BC: Patella fractures. In Miller MD, Hart JA, MacKnight JM, editors: *Essential orthopaedics*, Philadelphia, 2010, Saunders, pp 699–702.

Zlowodzki M, Bhandari M, Marek DJ, et al.: Operative treatment of acute distal femur fractures: systematic review of 2 comparative studies and 45 case series, *J Orthop Trauma* 5:366–371, 2006.

TIBIAL AND FIBULAR SHAFT FRACTURES

History

- Typically, patients present after acute injury; fractures may result from low- or high-energy trauma or penetrating injury such as a gunshot wound.
- The patient has leg pain and an inability to bear weight.

Physical Examination

- **Observe:** deformity, abrasion, laceration, fracture blisters, skin discoloration, capillary refill
- **Palpate:** crepitus, tenderness
- **ROM:** assessment of knee and ankle ROM after the fracture is stabilized
- **Neurovascular examination:**
  - Vascular examination: palpation of dorsalis pedis and posterior tibial pulses to ensure that they are present and equal to those in the uninjured extremity
  - Neurologic examination: evaluation of motor and sensory function
- **Compartment syndrome evaluation:**
  - Manual compression of compartments to assessed firmness compared with the unaffected extremity
  - Compartment pressures obtained if indicated

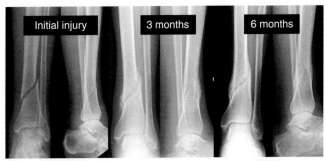

Fig. 7.35 Nonoperative Management: Anteroposterior and Lateral Radiographs. Callus formation is noted in the 3-month radiograph, with healed fracture and acceptable alignment demonstrated 6 months after injury. (From Miller MD, Hart JA, MacKnight JM, editors: *Essential orthopaedics*, Philadelphia, 2010, Saunders.)

Imaging

- Radiographs: AP and lateral views of the tibia and fibula identify fracture and help characterize the fracture pattern. Repeat radiography after reduction. Obtain radiographs of the knee and ankle as well, to assess for concomitant injuries.

Classification

- Open versus closed. Open fractures are further classified as follows:
  Grade I: less than 1 cm skin opening
  Grade II: 1 to 10 cm skin opening
  Grade III: A, 10 cm; B, 10 cm requiring soft tissue coverage; C, vascular injury requiring repair
- Location: proximal, middle, distal
- Pattern: transverse, oblique, spiral, segmental, comminuted
- Amount of shortening (cm) and degree of angulation and rotation

Initial Management

- Tibial shaft: Reduce closed fractures and apply a long-leg splint. Apply a sterile dressing to an open fracture, and administer antibiotics and tetanus prophylaxis.
- Fibular shaft: Immobilize the leg in a short-leg splint.
- **Patient Education.** Counsel patients on weight-bearing and ROM restrictions. Patients should be informed to call or return to the clinic or emergency department if they experience the following symptoms: increased pain, swelling, or neurovascular changes.

Nonoperative Management: Fig. 7.35

- Tibial shaft fracture with less than 1 cm of shortening, less than 5 degrees of angulation, less than 5 degrees of rotation, and competent soft tissues
  - A long-leg splint is placed until swelling resolves (1 to 2 weeks); then it is converted to a long-leg cast.
  - Non–weight bearing is indicated for 6 weeks. Begin protected weight bearing in a brace or cast if radiographs look favorable at 6 weeks.

Operative Management

Codes
ICD-10 code:
  S82.209A Fracture of tibial shaft, closed
  S82.209B Fracture of tibial shaft, open
CPT codes: 27759 Intramedullary nail fixation of the tibia
  20690 Tibial shaft fracture external fixation

Indications
- Tibial shaft
  - IM nail: unstable pattern (>1 cm of shortening, >5 degrees of angulation, >5 degrees of rotation) and incompetent soft tissues
  - External fixation: severe soft tissue injury and an unstable patient

Informed consent and counseling
- Possible complications: nonunion, infection, neurovascular injury, painful hardware, compartment syndrome, and DVT or PE
- Anesthesia risks: cardiac arrest, brain damage, paralysis, and death

Anesthesia
- General, with or without regional block

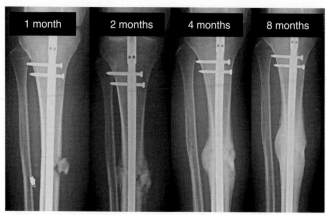

Fig. 7.36 Operative Management with Intramedullary Fixation: Anteroposterior Radiographs. Callus formation is noted in the 2-month postoperative radiograph. Note that surgery does not change the overall time required for fracture healing. (From Miller MD, Hart JA, MacKnight JM, editors: *Essential orthopaedics*, Philadelphia, 2010, Saunders.)

Patient positioning

- Supine on a fracture table with all bony prominences well padded

Surgical Procedures

Tibial Shaft Fracture

- IM nail fixation (Fig. 7.36): The extremity is prepared and draped in standard sterile fashion. The fracture is reduced. A 2- to 3-cm longitudinal or transverse incision is made. The soft tissues medial to the patellar tendon are dissected. An awl is used to make a starting point, and then a guidewire is placed across the fracture site. The site is reamed in 0.5-cm increments to 1.5 mm greater than the selected nail size. Nail length is measured off the guidewire. The nail and distal locking screws are placed. The fracture site is compressed to eliminate any distraction that occurred during nail placement. Proximal locking screws are placed. Proximal and distal nail placement is evaluated using a C-arm. The wound is irrigated. The incision is closed in a multilayer fashion, and a sterile dressing is applied.
- External fixation: The extremity is prepared and draped in standard sterile fashion. A 1-cm incision is made over the preplanned pin site on the anteromedial border of tibia. Soft tissue is incised to bone. A tissue protector is used to predrill, and then half-pins are placed. Fluoroscopy is used to ensure proper pin placement. A frame is applied according to the manufacturer's recommendations or the preoperative plan. Skin encroachment around the fixator pins

is released, and pins are dressed with petrolatum gauze (Xeroform) and 4 × 4 gauze pads.

Estimated Postoperative Course

Postoperative day 0 to 6 weeks:

- Tibial IM nail
  - At 10 to 14 days postoperatively, remove the splint and sutures, and obtain radiographs to evaluate alignment.
  - Allow weight bearing as tolerated.
  - Begin PT of knee and ankle mobilization if the fracture is stable.
- Tibial external fixator
  - At 10 to 14 days postoperatively, evaluate for pin site infection, and obtain radiographs to evaluate alignment.
  - Continue pin site care.
  - Convert to an IM nail at 2 weeks, if possible, to decrease the infection risk.

Postoperative 6 weeks to 3 months:

- Tibial IM nail
  - Check radiographs at 6 weeks, and advance PT.
- Tibial external fixator
  - Evaluate for pin site infection and continue pin care.
  - Obtain radiographs at 6 weeks to evaluate alignment. Advance weight bearing when callus is seen on radiographs.
  - The frame may be removed, and a straight-leg cast may be placed at 8 weeks if adequate callous formation is seen.

Postoperative 3+ months:

- Tibial IM nail
  - Check radiographs. Begin sport-specific PT. The patient returns to full activity at 6 months.
- Tibial external fixator
  - Review radiographs.
  - Transition to a controlled ankle motion (CAM) walker or a fracture brace.
  - The patient returns to full activity at 6 months.

SUGGESTED READINGS

Beardi J, Hessman M, Hansen M, et al.: Operative treatment of tibial shaft fractures: a comparison of different methods for primary stabilization, *Arch Orthop Trauma Surg* 128:709–715, 2008.

Dell Rocca GJ, Crist B: External fixation versus conversion to intramedullary nailing for definitive management of closed fractures of the femoral and tibial shaft, *J Am Acad Orthop Surg* 14:S131–S135, 2006.

Melvin JS, Domdroski DG, Torbert JT, et al.: Open tibial shaft fractures: I. Evaluation and initial wound management, *J Am Acad Orthop Surg* 18:10–19, 2010.

Shuler FD, Dietz MJ: Tibial and fibular shaft fractures. In Miller MD, Hart JA, MacKnight JM, editors: *Essential orthopaedics*, Philadelphia, 2010, Saunders, pp 703–707.

White TO, Howell GE, Will EM, et al.: Elevated intramuscular compartment pressures do not influence outcomes after tibial fracture, *J Trauma* 55:1133–1138, 2003.

ORTHOPAEDIC PROCEDURES

Knee Aspiration and/or Injection

Code
CPT code: 20610 Arthrocentesis, aspiration and/or injection; major joint or bursa

Indications
- Aspiration
  - Knee effusion or hemarthrosis
  - Suspected joint infection
- Injection with or without aspiration
  - OA of the knee
  - Gout or pseudogout of the knee
  - Rheumatoid arthritis of the knee
  - Patella chondromalacia

Contraindications
- Coagulopathy: severe or uncontrolled
- Suspected joint infection (may aspirate, do not inject steroid)
- Cellulitis or dermatitis of the overlying skin
- Adjacent osteomyelitis
- Impending knee surgery
- Bacteremia

Equipment and Supplies Needed
- Ethyl chloride
- Topical cleansing agent (e.g., povidone-iodine [Betadine])
- Sterile gloves and tray
- Needles: 25-gauge for injection of local anesthetic, 16- to 18-gauge for aspiration, 21-gauge for injection of steroid
- Hemostat
- Syringes: injection syringe (5- to 10-mL), aspiration syringe (30-mL)
- Sterile cup and appropriate laboratory tubes if fluid will be sent for analysis
- Injectate: steroid (1 mL) or other agent (e.g., triamcinolone [Kenalog], 40 mg/mL, hyaluronic acid) and 3 mL lidocaine, 1% without epinephrine
- Aspiration: 5 mL lidocaine, 1% without epinephrine anesthetize before aspiration
- Elastic compression (ACE) wrap, sterile dressing, or self-adhesive bandage

Procedure
1. Place the patient in the supine position on the examination table with the knee extended.
2. Palpate the superior pole of the patella, and locate the "soft spot," which is typically one fingerbreadth above and one fingerbreadth lateral to the superior pole. Mark this site with a pen or marker.
3. Apply ethyl chloride to the injection site. Put on sterile gloves. Prepare the skin with topical cleansing solution (Figs. 7.37 and 7.38).
4. If aspiration is planned:
   - Use a 25-gauge needle attached to a 5- to 10-mL syringe to infiltrate the skin with local anesthetic before inserting the larger aspiration needle (Fig. 7.39).
   - Insert the larger-bore needle tilted at a 45-degree angle into the injection site (Fig. 7.40).

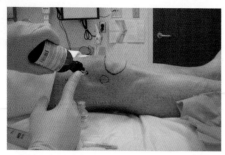

Fig. 7.37 Ethyl chloride is applied to the injection site. (From Miller MD, Hart JA, MacKnight JM, editors: *Essential orthopaedics*, Philadelphia, 2010, Saunders.)

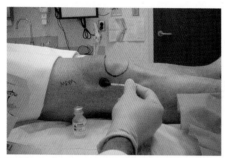

Fig. 7.38 The skin is sterilized. (From Miller MD, Hart JA, MacKnight JM, editors: *Essential orthopaedics*, Philadelphia, 2010, Saunders.)

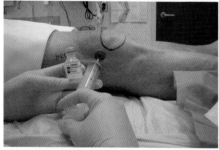

Fig. 7.39 Local anesthetic is injected. (From Miller MD, Hart JA, MacKnight JM, editors: *Essential orthopaedics*, Philadelphia, 2010, Saunders.)

- Once the needle has been inserted, apply gentle pressure to the plunger to aspirate the fluid. Using the nondominant hand to compress the opposite side of the joint or the patella may be helpful (Fig. 7.41).
- When the syringe is full, place a hemostat on the hub of the needle to stabilize it; then the syringe can be disconnected and emptied into the sterile cup or

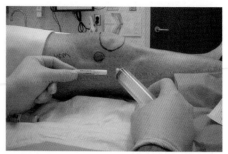

Fig. 7.40 A large-bore needle tilted at a 45-degree angle is injected into the injection site. (From Miller MD, Hart JA, MacKnight JM, editors: *Essential orthopaedics*, Philadelphia, 2010, Saunders.)

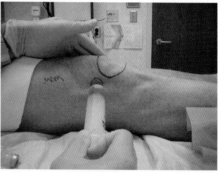

Fig. 7.41 Gentle pressure is applied to the plunger to aspirate the fluid. Use of the nondominant hand to compress the opposite side of the joint or the patella may be helpful. (From Miller MD, Hart JA, MacKnight JM, editors: *Essential orthopaedics*, Philadelphia, 2010, Saunders.)

tubes for laboratory studies. Reconnect the syringe, and continue aspiration if more fluid remains. If corticosteroid injection is indicated, attach the syringe with corticosteroid mixed with local anesthetic and then inject it into the joint. Hyaluronic acid injection can be performed in a similar manner.

5. Injection only: Identify the "soft spot," and prepare the injection site as described earlier. Insert the needle at a 45-degree angle, and inject the steroid-local anesthetic mixture or hyaluronic acid (Fig. 7.42).
6. Apply a sterile dressing or self-adhesive bandage to the injection site, and apply an elastic compression (ACE) wrap for compression.

Aftercare Instructions

1. Remove the dressing the day following the injection.
2. Use ice for local discomfort at the injection site.

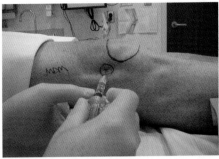

Fig. 7.42 A steroid-local anesthetic mixture or hyaluronic acid is injected. (From Miller MD, Hart JA, MacKnight JM, editors: *Essential orthopaedics*, Philadelphia, 2010, Saunders.)

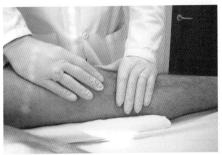

Fig. 7.43 The patient is in the supine position. A small pillow may be placed under the knee for comfort. (From Miller MD, Hart JA, MacKnight JM, editors: *Essential orthopaedics*, Philadelphia, 2010, Saunders.)

3. Diabetic patients may need to monitor blood glucose more closely because of the risk for transient increase in blood glucose level.
4. Possible side effects after the injection:
   • Pain or discomfort at the injection site may occur, but it typically subsides within 24 to 48 hours. This pain can be treated with ice and NSAIDs.
5. Contact your medical provider if any of the following symptoms develop: difficulty breathing, fever, chills, rash, or erythema and warmth at the injection site because they may be a sign of an adverse or allergic reaction.

Prepatellar Bursa Aspiration and/or Injection
Code
CPT code: 20610 (Arthrocentesis, aspiration and/or injection; major joint or bursa)

Indications
• Acute or chronic prepatellar bursitis

Contraindications
• Cellulitis or dermatitis of the skin overlying the injection site is a contraindication
• Do not inject steroid if septic bursitis is suspected

Equipment and Supplies Needed
• Ethyl chloride
• Topical cleansing agent (e.g., povidone-iodine [Betadine])
• Sterile gloves and tray
• Needles (1- to 1.5-inch): 21-gauge needle for injection of local anesthetic, 16- to 18-gauge needle for aspiration

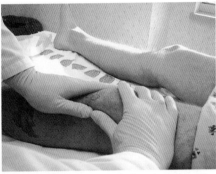

Fig. 7.44 The area over the patella is palpated for fluctuance. (From Miller MD, Hart JA, MacKnight JM, editors: *Essential orthopaedics*, Philadelphia, 2010, Saunders.)

• Syringes: injection syringe (5- to 10-mL), aspiration syringe (30-mL)
• Injectate: 1 mL steroid (e.g., triamcinolone [Kenalog], 40 mg/mL) and 1 mL 1% lidocaine without epinephrine
• Local anesthetic: lidocaine (1% without epinephrine) 5 mL to anesthetize the skin
• Elastic compression (ACE) wrap and sterile dressing or self-adhesive bandage

Procedure
1. The patient should be in the supine position. A small pillow may be placed under the knee for comfort (Fig. 7.43).
2. Palpate the area over the patella for fluctuance (Fig. 7.44).
3. Use ethyl chloride to anesthetize the skin, and then prepare it with a topical cleansing agent (Figs. 7.45 and 7.46).

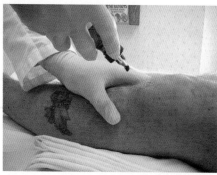

Fig. 7.45 Ethyl chloride is used to anesthetize the skin site. (From Miller MD, Hart JA, MacKnight JM, editors: *Essential orthopaedics*, Philadelphia, 2010, Saunders.)

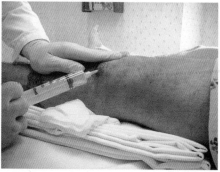

Fig. 7.47 A 25-gauge needle and a 30-mL syringe are used to aspirate the bursa. (From Miller MD, Hart JA, MacKnight JM, editors: *Essential orthopaedics*, Philadelphia, 2010, Saunders.)

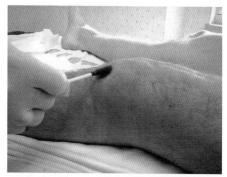

Fig. 7.46 The skin site is prepared with a topical cleansing agent. (From Miller MD, Hart JA, MacKnight JM, editors: *Essential orthopaedics*, Philadelphia, 2010, Saunders.)

4. If aspirating the bursa, use the 21-gauge needle to inject local anesthetic before inserting the larger aspiration needle. From the lateral side, place the needle directly into the fluid-filled bursa.
5. Use the 25-gauge needle and the 30-mL syringe to aspirate the bursa (Fig. 7.47).
6. If steroid injection is planned, leave the needle in place. Use a hemostat to hold the needle while removing the aspiration syringe, and then connect the injection syringe and inject the steroid.
7. Apply a self-adhesive bandage or gauze and an elastic compression (ACE) wrap for compression.

Aftercare Instructions
1. Remove the dressing the day after the injection.
2. Possible side effects after the injection:
   - Pain or discomfort at the injection site may occur, but it typically subsides within 24 to 48 hours. This pain can be treated with ice and NSAIDs.

3. Contact your medical provider if any of the following symptoms develop: difficulty breathing, fever, chills, rash, or erythema and warmth at the injection site because they may be a sign of an adverse or allergic reaction.

Pes Anserine Bursa Injection
Code
CPT code: 20610

Indications
- Pes anserine bursitis

Contraindications
- Cellulitis/dermatitis of the skin overlying the injection site

Equipment and Supplies Needed
- Ethyl chloride
- Topical cleansing agent (e.g., povidone-iodine [Betadine])
- Sterile gloves and tray
- 21-gauge needle
- 5- to 10-mL syringe
- Injectate: 1 mL steroid (e.g., triamcinolone [Kenalog], 40 mg/mL) and 1 mL local anesthetic (e.g., lidocaine 1% without epinephrine)
- Elastic compression (ACE) wrap, sterile dressing, or self-adhesive bandage

Procedure
1. Place the patient in the supine position, and slightly flex the knee.

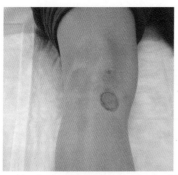

Fig. 7.48 The skin site has been anesthetized with ethyl chloride and prepared with a topical cleansing agent. (From Miller MD, Hart JA, MacKnight JM, editors: *Essential orthopaedics*, Philadelphia, 2010, Saunders.)

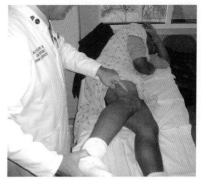

Fig. 7.50 The patient is placed in the lateral decubitus position with the affected extremity up and the knee flexed 20 to 30 degrees. (From Miller MD, Hart JA, MacKnight JM, editors: *Essential orthopaedics*, Philadelphia, 2010, Saunders.)

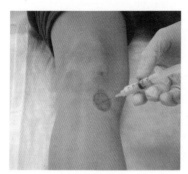

Fig. 7.49 A mixture of a local anesthetic and steroid is injected. (From Miller MD, Hart JA, MacKnight JM, editors: *Essential orthopaedics*, Philadelphia, 2010, Saunders.)

2. Identify the pes anserine bursa; it is located along the medial aspect of the knee approximately 2 cm below the joint line.
3. Apply ethyl chloride to the injection site, put on sterile gloves, and then prepare the skin with the topical cleansing agent (Fig. 7.48).
4. Insert the needle into the point of maximal tenderness, and gently advance it to bone. Retract the needle 2 to 3 mm, and then inject the mixture of the local anesthetic and steroid (Fig. 7.49).
5. Apply an elastic compression (ACE) wrap, sterile dressing, or self-adhesive bandage.

Aftercare Instructions
1. Remove the dressing the day after the injection.
2. Possible side effects after the injection:
   - Pain or discomfort at the injection site may occur, but it typically subsides within 24 to 48 hours. This pain can be treated with ice and NSAIDs.

3. Contact your medical provider if any of the following symptoms develop: difficulty breathing, fever, chills, rash, or erythema and warmth at the injection site because they may be a sign of an adverse or allergic reaction.

Iliotibial Band Injection
Code
CPT code: 20610

Indications
- ITB syndrome

Contraindications
- Cellulitis or dermatitis of the skin overlying the injection site

Equipment and Supplies Needed
- Ethyl chloride
- Topical cleansing agent for sterile preparation (e.g., povidone-iodine [Betadine])
- Sterile gloves and tray
- Injectate: 1 mL steroid (e.g., triamcinolone [Kenalog], 40 mg/mL) and 1 mL lidocaine (1% without epinephrine)
- 21-gauge needle
- 5- to 10-mL syringe
- Sterile dressing or self-adhesive bandage

Procedure
1. Place the patient in the lateral decubitus position with the affected extremity up. Flex the knee 20 to 30 degrees (Fig. 7.50).

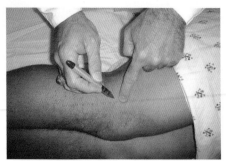

Fig. 7.51 The point of maximal tenderness is identified. (From Miller MD, Hart JA, MacKnight JM, editors: *Essential orthopaedics*, Philadelphia, 2010, Saunders.)

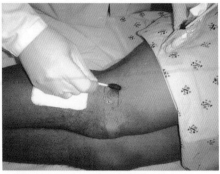

Fig. 7.53 The skin is prepared with a topical cleansing agent. (From Miller MD, Hart JA, MacKnight JM, editors: *Essential orthopaedics*, Philadelphia, 2010, Saunders.)

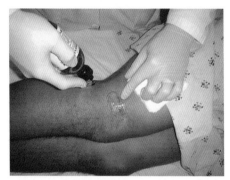

Fig. 7.52 Ethyl chloride is applied to the injection site. (From Miller MD, Hart JA, MacKnight JM, editors: *Essential orthopaedics*, Philadelphia, 2010, Saunders.)

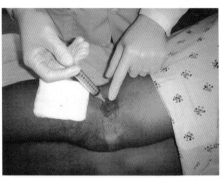

Fig. 7.54 The needle is inserted into the point of maximal tenderness, and a combination of steroid and lidocaine is injected. (From Miller MD, Hart JA, MacKnight JM, editors: *Essential orthopaedics*, Philadelphia, 2010, Saunders.)

2. Palpate the ITB, and identify its insertion site on the proximal tibia (Gerdy tubercle), and then identify the point of maximal tenderness (Fig. 7.51).
3. Apply ethyl chloride to the injection site, put on sterile gloves, and prepare the skin with the topical cleansing agent (Figs. 7.52 and 7.53).
4. Insert the needle into the point of maximal tenderness, and inject the combined steroid and lidocaine (Fig. 7.54).
5. Apply an elastic compression (ACE) wrap, sterile dressing, or self-adhesive bandage.

Aftercare Instructions
1. Remove the dressing the day after the injection.
2. Possible side effects after the injection:

- Pain or discomfort at the injection site may occur, but it typically subsides within 24 to 48 hours. This pain can be treated with ice and NSAIDs.
3. Contact your medical provider if any of the following symptoms develop: difficulty breathing, fever, chills, rash, or erythema and warmth at the injection site because they may be a sign of an adverse or allergic reaction.

ACKNOWLEDGMENTS

The authors would like to acknowledge the contribution of the previous edition author, Cara Garrett.

8

Foot and Ankle

Michael Noordsy

ANATOMY

Bones: Fig. 8.1

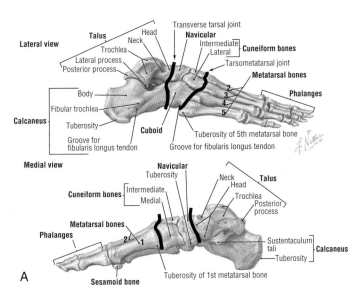

Lateral view

Talus — Head

Transverse tarsal joint

Navicular

Intermediate

Lateral

Trochlea

Neck

Cuneiform bones

Lateral process

Posterior process

Tarsometatarsal joint

Metatarsal bones

Body

Phalanges

Fibular trochlea

2

3

Calcaneus

4

Tuberosity

5

Cuboid

Groove for
fibularis longus tendon

Tuberosity of 5th metatarsal bone

Groove for fibularis longus tendon

Medial view

Navicular

Tuberosity

Neck

Talus

Head

Cuneiform bones — Intermediate

Trochlea

Medial

Posterior
process

Metatarsal bones

Phalanges

2

1

Sustentaculum
tali

Calcaneus

Tuberosity

A

Sesamoid bone

Tuberosity of 1st metatarsal bone

Fig. 8.1A Bones of the Foot. (From Netter illustration from www.netterimages.com. Copyright Elsevier Inc. All rights reserved.)

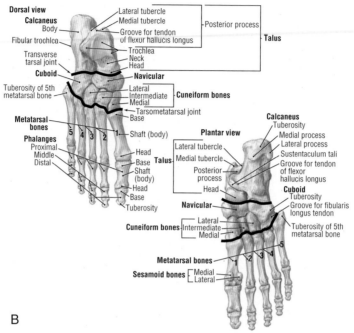

Fig. 8.1B **Bones of the Foot.** (From Netter illustration from www.netterimages.com. Copyright Elsevier Inc. All rights reserved.)

Ligaments: Fig. 8.2

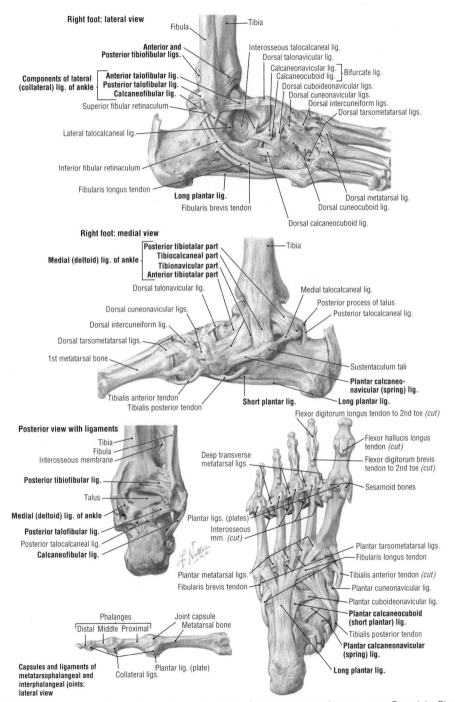

Right foot: lateral view

Fibula — Tibia

Anterior and
Posterior tibiofibular ligs.

Interosseous talocalcaneal lig.
Dorsal talonavicular lig.
Calcaneonavicular lig.
Calcaneocuboid lig. — Bifurcate lig.

Components of lateral
(collateral) lig. of ankle
Anterior talofibular lig.
Posterior talofibular lig.
Calcaneofibular lig.

Dorsal cuboideonavicular ligs.
Dorsal cuneonavicular ligs.
Dorsal intercuneiform ligs.
Dorsal tarsometatarsal ligs.

Superior fibular retinaculum

Lateral talocalcaneal lig.

Inferior fibular retinaculum

Fibularis longus tendon

Long plantar lig.
Fibularis brevis tendon

Dorsal metatarsal lig.
Dorsal cuneocuboid lig.

Dorsal calcaneocuboid lig.

Right foot: medial view

Tibia

Medial (deltoid) lig. of ankle
Posterior tibiotalar part
Tibiocalcaneal part
Tibionavicular part
Anterior tibiotalar part

Dorsal talonavicular lig.

Medial talocalcaneal lig.
Posterior process of talus
Posterior talocalcaneal lig.

Dorsal cuneonavicular ligs.

Dorsal intercuneiform lig.

Dorsal tarsometatarsal ligs.

1st metatarsal bone

Sustentaculum tali

Plantar calcaneo-
navicular (spring) lig.

Tibialis anterior tendon
Tibialis posterior tendon

Short plantar lig.
Long plantar lig.

Posterior view with ligaments

Tibia
Fibula
Interosseous membrane

Flexor digitorum longus tendon to 2nd toe (cut)

Deep transverse
metatarsal ligs.

Flexor hallucis longus
tendon (cut)

Flexor digitorum brevis
tendon to 2nd toe (cut)

Posterior tibiofibular lig.

Talus

Sesamoid bones

Medial (deltoid) lig. of ankle

Posterior talofibular lig.
Posterior talocalcaneal lig.
Calcaneofibular lig.

Plantar ligs. (plates)
Interosseous
mm. (cut)

Plantar tarsometatarsal ligs.
Fibularis longus tendon

Plantar metatarsal ligs.
Fibularis brevis tendon

Tibialis anterior tendon (cut)
Plantar cuneonavicular lig.

Plantar cuboideonavicular lig.

Plantar calcaneocuboid
(short plantar) lig.

Tibialis posterior tendon

Plantar calcaneonavicular
(spring) lig.

Long plantar lig.

Phalanges
Distal Middle Proximal
Joint capsule
Metatarsal bone

Capsules and ligaments of
metatarsophalangeal and
interphalangeal joints:
lateral view

Collateral ligs.
Plantar lig. (plate)

Fig. 8.2 Ligaments of the Foot. (From Netter illustration from www.netterimages.com. Copyright Elsevier Inc. All rights reserved.)

Muscles, Nerves, and Arteries: Figs. 8.3 through 8.5

Superficial dissection

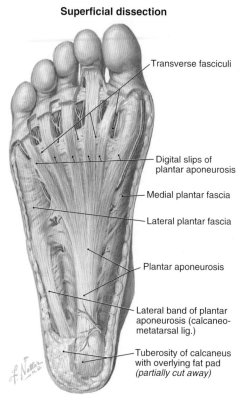

Transverse fasciculi

Digital slips of
plantar aponeurosis

Medial plantar fascia

Lateral plantar fascia

Plantar aponeurosis

Lateral band of plantar
aponeurosis (calcaneo-
metatarsal lig.)

Tuberosity of calcaneus
with overlying fat pad
(partially cut away)

Fig. 8.3 Dorsal View of the Foot Sole. (From Netter illustration from www.netterimages.com. Copyright Elsevier Inc. All rights reserved.)

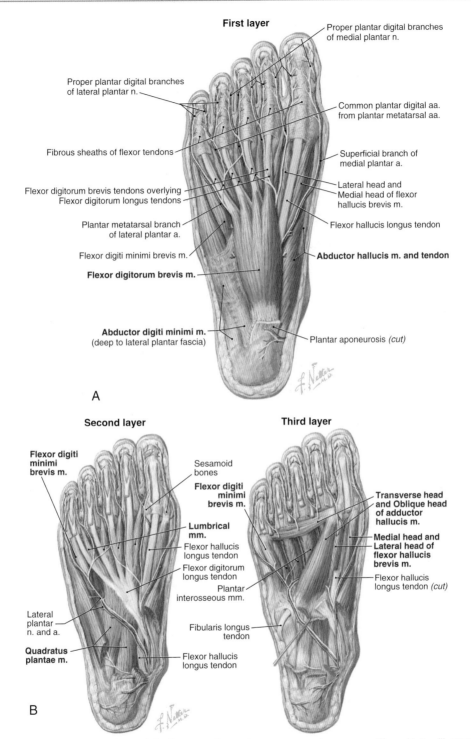

First layer

Proper plantar digital branches
of medial plantar n.

Proper plantar digital branches
of lateral plantar n.

Common plantar digital aa.
from plantar metatarsal aa.

Fibrous sheaths of flexor tendons

Superficial branch of
medial plantar a.

Flexor digitorum brevis tendons overlying
Flexor digitorum longus tendons

Lateral head and
Medial head of flexor
hallucis brevis m.

Plantar metatarsal branch
of lateral plantar a.

Flexor hallucis longus tendon

Flexor digiti minimi brevis m.

Abductor hallucis m. and tendon

Flexor digitorum brevis m.

Abductor digiti minimi m.
(deep to lateral plantar fascia)

Plantar aponeurosis *(cut)*

A

Second layer

**Flexor digiti
minimi
brevis m.**

Sesamoid
bones

**Flexor digiti
minimi
brevis m.**

**Lumbrical
mm.**

Flexor hallucis
longus tendon

Flexor digitorum
longus tendon

Plantar
interosseous mm.

Lateral
plantar
n. and a.

**Quadratus
plantae m.**

Flexor hallucis
longus tendon

Third layer

**Transverse head
and Oblique head
of adductor
hallucis m.**

**Medial head and
Lateral head of
flexor hallucis
brevis m.**

Flexor hallucis
longus tendon *(cut)*

Fibularis longus
tendon

B

Fig. 8.4 A and B, Plantar views of the foot muscles. *a,* Artery; *m,* muscle; *n,* nerve. (From Netter illustration
from www.netterimages.com. Copyright Elsevier Inc. All rights reserved.)

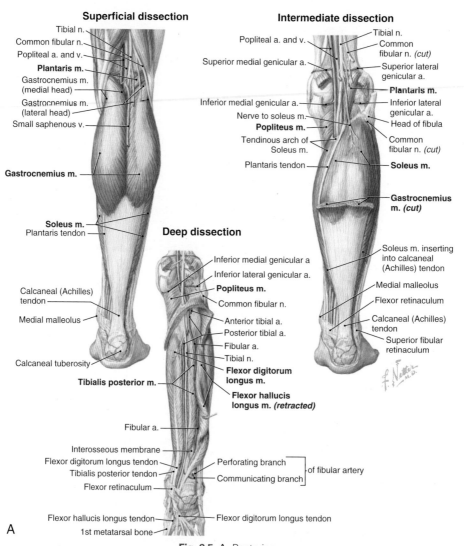

Superficial dissection

Tibial n.
Common fibular n.
Popliteal a. and v.
Plantaris m.
Gastrocnemius m.
(medial head)
Gastrocnemius m.
(lateral head)
Small saphenous v.

Gastrocnemius m.

Soleus m.
Plantaris tendon

Calcaneal (Achilles)
tendon

Medial malleolus

Calcaneal tuberosity

Intermediate dissection

Popliteal a. and v.
Superior medial genicular a.

Inferior medial genicular a.
Nerve to soleus m.
Popliteus m.
Tendinous arch of
Soleus m.
Plantaris tendon

Tibial n.
Common
fibular n. (cut)
Superior lateral
genicular a.
Plantaris m.
Inferior lateral
genicular a.
Head of fibula
Common
fibular n. (cut)
Soleus m.

**Gastrocnemius
m. (cut)**

Soleus m. inserting
into calcaneal
(Achilles) tendon
Medial malleolus
Flexor retinaculum
Calcaneal (Achilles)
tendon
Superior fibular
retinaculum

Deep dissection

Inferior medial genicular a
Inferior lateral genicular a.
Popliteus m.
Common fibular n.
Anterior tibial a.
Posterior tibial a.
Fibular a.
Tibial n.
**Flexor digitorum
longus m.**
**Flexor hallucis
longus m. (retracted)**

Tibialis posterior m.

Fibular a.

Interosseous membrane
Flexor digitorum longus tendon
Tibialis posterior tendon
Flexor retinaculum

Perforating branch
Communicating branch

of fibular artery

Flexor hallucis longus tendon
1st metatarsal bone

Flexor digitorum longus tendon

A

Fig. 8.5 A, Posterior,

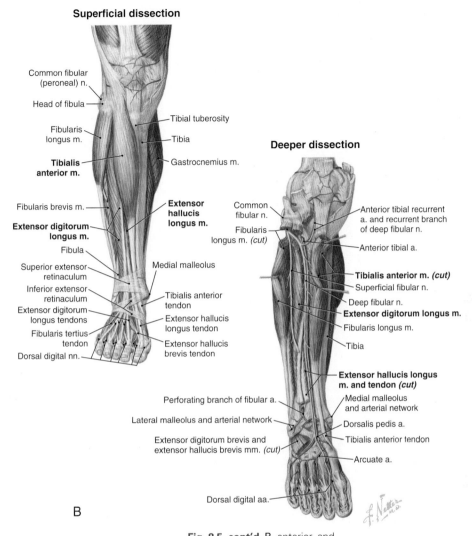

Superficial dissection

Common fibular (peroneal) n.

Head of fibula

Fibularis longus m.

Tibialis anterior m.

Fibularis brevis m.

Extensor digitorum longus m.

Fibula

Superior extensor retinaculum

Inferior extensor retinaculum

Extensor digitorum longus tendons

Fibularis tertius tendon

Dorsal digital nn.

Tibial tuberosity

Tibia

Gastrocnemius m.

Extensor hallucis longus m.

Medial malleolus

Tibialis anterior tendon

Extensor hallucis longus tendon

Extensor hallucis brevis tendon

Deeper dissection

Common fibular n.

Fibularis longus m. *(cut)*

Anterior tibial recurrent a. and recurrent branch of deep fibular n.

Anterior tibial a.

Tibialis anterior m. *(cut)*

Superficial fibular n.

Deep fibular n.

Extensor digitorum longus m.

Fibularis longus m.

Tibia

Extensor hallucis longus m. and tendon *(cut)*

Medial malleolus and arterial network

Dorsalis pedis a.

Tibialis anterior tendon

Arcuate a.

Perforating branch of fibular a.

Lateral malleolus and arterial network

Extensor digitorum brevis and extensor hallucis brevis mm. *(cut)*

Dorsal digital aa.

B

Fig. 8.5, cont'd B, anterior, and

Continued

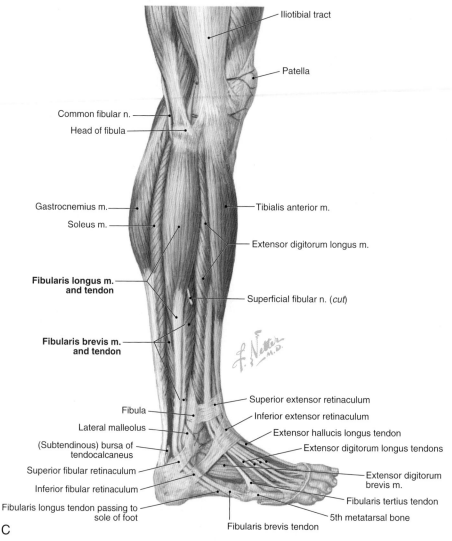

Iliotibial tract

Patella

Common fibular n.

Head of fibula

Gastrocnemius m.

Soleus m.

Tibialis anterior m.

Extensor digitorum longus m.

Fibularis longus m. and tendon

Superficial fibular n. (*cut*)

Fibularis brevis m. and tendon

Fibula

Lateral malleolus

(Subtendinous) bursa of tendocalcaneus

Superior fibular retinaculum

Inferior fibular retinaculum

Fibularis longus tendon passing to sole of foot

Superior extensor retinaculum

Inferior extensor retinaculum

Extensor hallucis longus tendon

Extensor digitorum longus tendons

Extensor digitorum brevis m.

Fibularis tertius tendon

5th metatarsal bone

Fibularis brevis tendon

C

Fig. 8.5, cont'd C, lateral views of the lower leg and ankle muscles. *a,* Artery; *m,* muscle; *n,* nerve; *v,* vein. (From Netter illustration from www.netterimages.com. Copyright Elsevier Inc. All rights reserved.)

Nerve Function: Table 8.1

TABLE 8.1	**Nerve Function**			
Nerve	**Branches**	**Motor**	**Testing**	**Sensory**
Fibular (Peroneal)	Deep	Tibialis anterior, EHL, EDL, EDB, EHB	Ankle and great toe dorsiflexion, toe extension	Webspace between great toe and second toe
	Superficial	Peroneus longus and brevis	Ankle/subtalar eversion	Distal one-third of anterior lower leg, dorsum of foot (except webspace between great toe and second toe and distal portion toes)
Saphenous		None		Medial portion of lower leg, medial foot
Sural		None		Posterior lower leg, lateral foot
Tibial		Gastrocnemius, soleus, plantaris, tibialis posterior, FHL, FDL	Ankle and great toe plantarflexion, Achilles reflex	Plantar surface of foot and toes, dorsal aspect of distal portion of toes

EDB, Extensor digitorum brevis; *EDL,* extensor digitorum longus; *EHL,* extensor hallucis longus; *FDL,* flexor digitorum longus; *FHL,* flexor hallicus longus.

Surface Anatomy: Fig. 8.6

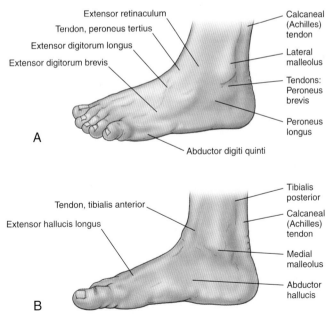

Fig. 8.6 Surface anatomy of (**A**) lateral and (**B**) medial aspects of the foot. (From O'Neal LW: Surgical pathology of the foot and clinicopathologic correlations. In Bowker JH, Pfeifer M, editors: *Levin and O'Neal's the diabetic foot,* ed 7, Philadelphia, 2008, Mosby.)

PHYSICAL EXAMINATION

- **Inspect** for edema, erythema, ecchymosis, deformity, callus formation, ulceration, and hairlessness. On standing examination, note hindfoot alignment. Assess gait pattern.
- **Palpate** to evaluate clinical complaint:
  - Anterior ankle joint line
  - Fibula, both distally and proximally
  - Medial malleolus
  - Peroneal tendons
  - Posterior tibial tendon
  - Sinus tarsi
  - Achilles tendon
  - Anterior tibial tendon
  - Metatarsals
  - Insertion of plantar fascia

Normal Range of Motion: Table 8.2

Neurovascular Examination: Table 8.3

Differential Diagnosis: Table 8.4

TABLE 8.2　Normal Ankle/Foot Range of Motion

Ankle dorsiflexion	10–23 degrees
Ankle plantarflexion	23–48 degrees
Inversion	5–35 degrees
Eversion	5–25 degrees
First metatarsophalangeal dorsiflexion	45–90 degrees
First metatarsophalangeal plantarflexion	10–40 degrees

TABLE 8.3　Neurovascular Examination

Nerve	Location of Test	Tests
SPN	Dorsum of foot	Tinel
DPN	1st/2nd MTP webspace	Tinel
Sural	Lateral border foot	Tinel
Saphenous	Medial border foot	Tinel
Tibial	Plantar foot	Tinel
Post tibialis artery	Posterior to medial malleolus	
Dorsalis pedis artery	Dorsum of midfoot	

DPN, Deep peroneal nerve; *SPN*, superficial peroneal nerve; *MTP*, metatarsal-phalangeal.

TABLE 8.4　Differential Diagnosis

Anterior ankle pain	Ankle arthritis, osteochondral dessicans talus
Medial ankle pain	Posterior tibial tendinopathy, medial malleolar injury
Lateral ankle pain	Peroneal tendinopathy, ankle sprain
Posterior ankle pain	Achilles tendinopathy or rupture, os trigonum, posterior impingement
Midfoot	Lisfranc injury, midfoot arthritis
Forefoot	Metatarsal fracture, stress fracture, metatarsalgia
Heel pain	Plantar fasciitis, calcaneal stress fracture, insertional Achilles tendinopathy
Great toe	Hallux rigidus, hallux valgus
Lesser toes	Toe fracture, hammertoe deformity, Morton's neuroma

ANKLE ARTHRITIS

Arthritis of the tibiotalar joint, commonly referred to as ankle arthritis, is where cartilage, joint space, and range of motion (ROM) of the ankle are diminished over the course of time. Ankle arthritis can be a debilitating condition that causes pain along with decreased function and decreased quality of life. While there is no cure, there are several treatment options. Advancement in care, including total ankle replacement, has patients facing a brighter future in terms of treatment modalities for ankle arthritis.

History

- Ankle arthritis may affect tibiotalar or subtalar joints.
- Usually, the patient has unilateral ankle pain, stiffness, swelling, with or without a history of injury. Pain worsens with weight-bearing activity.
- Posttraumatic arthritis is the most common etiology. Other causes include inflammatory arthritis, neuropathic arthropathy, and primary osteoarthritis (rare).

Physical Examination

- Standing evaluation may reveal varus/valgus deformity.
- Patient often experiences decreased motion in plantarflexion, dorsiflexion, or both.
- Tenderness occurs on palpation of the anterior tibiotalar joint line.

Imaging

- Radiographs: weight-bearing anteroposterior (AP), mortise, lateral

- May reveal joint space narrowing of the tibiotalar joint, osteophytes, subchondral sclerosis and cysts, flattening of talus, loose bodies. Erosive changes are noted in inflammatory arthropathy. Neuropathic arthropathy joint collapse and significant bony deformity (Fig. 8.7)

Initial Management
Nonoperative Management
- First treatment steps include activity modification, weight loss if indicated, lace-up ankle brace, and nonsteroidal antiinflammatory drugs (NSAIDs).
- Intraarticular corticosteroid injection (see ankle injection procedure, p. 314). Risks include local skin reaction (depigmentation or subcutaneous fat atrophy) and infection.
- Bracing/shoe modification options are a lace-up ankle brace, an ankle-foot orthotic (AFO), an Arizona brace, and a rocker-bottom sole.

Operative Management
ICD-10 code:

   M19.079 ankle arthritis

CPT code:

   27625 Ankle arthrotomy with débridement/loose body removal

   27870 Ankle arthrodesis

   27702 Total ankle arthroplasty

Indications
- Ankle arthrotomy with débridement/loose body removal:

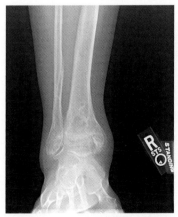

Fig. 8.7 Severe Posttraumatic Ankle Arthritis with Complete Loss of Tibiotalar Joint Space.

- Generally has limited value and indicated only in mild arthritis without significant joint space narrowing
- Ankle arthrodesis:
  - Indications: painful tibiotalar arthritis not responsive to nonoperative treatment, failed arthroplasty
  - Contraindications: acute infection, acute neuropathic arthropathy, severe vascular disease
- Total ankle arthroplasty:
  - Indications: tibiotalar arthritis not responsive to nonoperative management, low demand patients older than age 50 to 55 years, weight less than 200 lbs., maintained ROM, normal/near normal alignment, no preexisting subtalar arthritis.
  - Contraindications: acute infection, significantly diminished bone stock, neuropathy, severe vascular disease. Relative contraindications include deformity greater than 5 degrees and talar avascular necrosis.

Informed consent and counseling
- Arthrodesis:
  - Major risks include nonunion (<10%), wound complications, nerve injury, infection, deep vein thrombosis (DVT), hardware loosening/failure, and progression of arthritis in hindfoot/subtalar joint. A risk of amputation exists in cases of severe complication (≤5%).[1]
  - The complication rate increases with nicotine use, neuropathy, and vascular disease.
- Total ankle arthroplasty:
  - Informed consent and counseling: Risks are similar to arthrodesis (infection, wound complications, DVT, hardware loosening). Recent studies report 10% to 30% reoperation rate and survival rates of 77% to 90% at 5- and 10-year follow-up. If surgery fails, consider conversion to arthrodesis (contraindicated in infection).[2] Limited revision options are available.

Anesthesia
- General anesthesia with or without peripheral nerve block

Patient positioning
- Positioning: supine with toes pointing directly toward ceiling. A small bump can be placed under the ipsilateral hip to internally rotate leg. A thigh tourniquet should be placed.

Surgical Procedures

Ankle Arthrodesis: Fig. 8.8

There are several fixation/implant options for ankle arthrodesis. The more common option is an anterior plate with cross screws. The open anterior ankle incision is made equidistant between the medial malleolus and lateral malleolus. Dissection is taken down to the interval between the extensor hallicus longus (EHL) and the extensor digitorum longus (EDL). Care is taken to avoid the superficial peroneal nerve and the neurovascular bundle, which are found posterior to the EHL. The neurovascular bundle is mobilized and the tibial osteophytes are removed to visualize the joint. The tibiotalar joint is prepared by removing any remaining articular cartilage, and microfracturing and/or drilling the subchondral bone. A lamina spreader (with teeth) can be helpful for visualization. After joint preparation, align the tibiotalar joint into neutral dorsiflexion/plantarflexion, 0 to 5 degrees of hindfoot valgus, 5 degrees external rotation. Intraoperative radiography is used to determine correct alignment for fixation. Careful wound closure is performed, making sure to reapproximate the extensor retinaculum. A Robert Jones dressing/splint (posterior short leg splint with additional sugar tong application) is applied in the operating room after closure. The patient will likely be non–weight bearing for at least 6 to 8 weeks postoperatively.

Estimated Postoperative Course

Postoperative 2 weeks:
- Sutures are removed and radiographs are obtained. A non–weight-bearing cast is applied for 4 weeks.

Postoperative 6 weeks:
- Radiographs reviewed. The patient is transitioned to a weight-bearing cast or boot for an additional 6 weeks.

Postoperative 3 months:
- Remove cast. Obtain radiographs to evaluate for healing.
- Physical therapy is generally not indicated, but some patients may need some therapy for gait training. Consider rocker bottom shoe to facilitate improved gait with loss of ankle motion.

Total Ankle Arthroplasty: Fig. 8.9

Total ankle arthroplasty is another treatment option for patients with end-stage tibiotalar arthritis. First-generation implants have a history of a high failure rate. Second- and third-generation implants are now available with early results indicating improved longevity and decreased complication rate. An open anterior ankle approach is used, as described in ankle arthrodesis. Major structures at risk include the superficial **peroneal nerve and neurovascular bundle**.

Estimated Postoperative Course

Postoperative 2 weeks:
- Non–weight-bearing splint for 1 to 2 weeks. Remove sutures about 2 weeks after surgery and apply a non–weight-bearing cast or boot.

Postoperative 4 to 6 weeks:
- Transition to weight bearing in a boot. Remove boot multiple times daily for gentle ROM in plantarflexion and dorsiflexion.

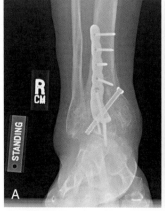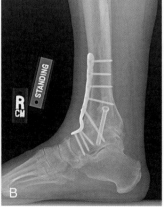

Fig. 8.8 Postoperative anteroposterior (**A**) and lateral (**B**) views following ankle arthrodesis using anterior plate.

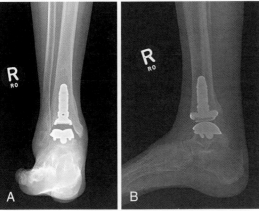

Fig. 8.9 Postoperative anteroposterior (**A**) and lateral (**B**) views following ankle arthroplasty using Wright Medical INBONE prosthesis.

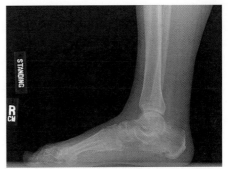

Fig. 8.10 Posttraumatic subtalar arthritis on lateral radiograph. There is evidence of prior calcaneal fracture with collapse of subtalar joint.

Postoperative 3 months:

- Formal physical therapy may be initiated about 3 months postoperatively if the patient has significant stiffness or weakness.
- After recovery, radiographs may be obtained every 1 to 2 years.

SUBTALAR ARTHRITIS

Subtalar arthritis refers to a degenerative condition of the articular cartilage in the joint that accounts for a large portion of the inversion and eversion of the hindfoot. There is no current treatment option for restoration of the subtalar cartilage loss. However, there are multiple conservative and surgical treatment options for this condition that alleviate pain and associated swelling that accompany the condition.

History

- Posttraumatic arthritic changes are the most common etiology (calcaneal fracture or subtalar dislocation). The subtalar joint is also a common site for rheumatoid arthritis and Charcot arthropathy.
- Pain lateral aspect hindfoot, worse with walking on uneven ground.

Physical Examination

- Tenderness over sinus tarsi, limited subtalar motion (inversion/eversion), pain and possible crepitus with subtalar motion

Imaging

- Radiographs: weight-bearing foot AP, lateral, oblique and weight-bearing ankle AP, mortise, lateral
  - Lateral views are best to evaluate subtalar joint (Fig. 8.10)

Additional Imaging

- Magnetic resonance imaging/computed tomography (MRI/CT) scan: not necessary for diagnosis. CT will show joint in more detail (osteophytes, subchondral cysts, and loose bodies)

Initial Management
Nonoperative Management

Initial treatment should be nonoperative. NSAIDs, lace-up ankle brace, weight loss if indicated, activity modification (limit uneven surfaces), and corticosteroid injections.

Operative Management
ICD-10 code

   M19.079 Subtalar arthritis

CPT code

   29904 Arthroscopic subtalar joint débridement
   28725 Subtalar arthrodesis

Indications

- Arthroscopic subtalar joint débridement:
  - Arthroscopy difficult due to joint space narrowing. Open débridement of osteophytes. Synovectomy is occasionally performed in mild/moderate arthritis not responsive to nonoperative treatment. Generally limited value for long-term pain relief.

- Subtalar arthrodesis:
  - Indication: Isolated subtalar degenerative disease unresponsive to nonoperative treatment.
  - Contraindications: same as ankle arthrodesis.
  - There is an increased nonunion rate in patients with previous history of tibiotalar arthrodesis and/or smoking.

  Informed consent and counseling
- Risks include infection, wound complications, arthritis in surrounding joints, nonunion (reported rates 0.5%), DVT, symptomatic hardware (especially if screw heads are prominent posteriorly).[3] Some patients feel instability on uneven ground. At-risk structures: superficial peroneal and sural nerves, peroneal tendons.

  Anesthesia
- General anesthesia with or without peripheral nerve block

  Patient positioning
- Positioning for arthrodesis: supine with toes pointing directly toward ceiling. A small bump can be placed under ipsilateral hip to internally rotate leg. Thigh tourniquet placed.

Surgical Procedure
Subtalar Arthrodesis

The surgical approach to the subtalar joint is made via a lateral incision approximately 2 cm distal to lateral malleolus, extending to the base of the fourth metatarsal (MT). The extensor digitorum brevis is reflected to expose the subtalar joint. Peroneal tendons are elevated from the lateral calcaneus and retracted to facilitate the exposure of the joint. Any remaining articular cartilage is removed, and the joint is débrided to cancellous bone. Microfracture and/or drilling is performed. Allograft materials may be placed at this time, to augment fixation. Bone block may be needed if bone loss is present from previous trauma/calcaneal fracture. Fusion is performed at 5 degrees valgus. Commonly, two cannulated screws are placed across the subtalar joint to provide fixation. Fixation screws are placed from the non–weight-bearing portion of the calcaneus toward the anterior margin of the posterior facet into the talus. Divergent screws have improved compression forces compared with parallel screw or single screw fixation. Intraoperative radiographs and guide wires are used to ensure appropriate placement of screws (Fig. 8.11). A Robert Jones dressing/splint is applied and the patient will likely be non–weight bearing for at least 6 to 8 weeks.

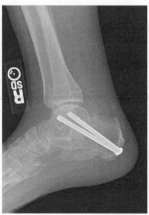

Fig. 8.11 Lateral radiograph status post subtalar arthrodesis using two divergent cannulated screws.

Estimated Postoperative Course

Postoperative 2 weeks:

- Sutures removed. Non–weight bearing in a boot. Remove boot multiple times daily for ankle motion to prevent stiffness.

Postoperative 6 weeks:

- Radiograph reviewed. Start weight bearing in boot from weeks 6 to 12.

Postoperative 3 months:

- Transition to regular shoes at 12 weeks if fusion is radiographically healed.

SUGGESTED READINGS

Coughlin MJ: In *Mann's surgery of the foot and ankle*, ed 9, Philadelphia, 2014, Mosby.

DeOrio JK, Parekh SG: In *Total ankle replacement*, ed 1, Lippincott Williams and Wilkens, 2014.

Greisberg J, Vossellar J: *Foot and ankle: core knowledge in orthopaedics*, Philadelphia, 2019, Elsevier.

Kitaoka Harold B: In *Master techniques in orthopaedic surgery: the foot and ankle*, ed 3, Lippincott Williams and Wilkens, 2013.

Levine David: *Hospital for Special Surgery's illustrated tips and tricks in foot and ankle surgery*, Lippincott Williams and Wilkens, 2019.

Miller MD, editor: *Review of orthopedics*, ed 7, Philadelphia, PA, 2015, Saunders.

Murphy GA, editor: *Campbell's operative orthopaedics*, ed 12, Philadelphia, 2017, PA Elsevier.

Park JS, Mroczek KJ: Total ankle arthroplasty, *Bull NYU Hosp Jt Dis* 69(1):27–35, 2011.

REFERENCES

1. Yasui Y, Hannon CP, Seow D, Kennedy JG: Ankle arthrodesis: a systematic approach and review of the literature, *World J Orthop* 7(11):700–708, 2016.
2. Lawton CD, Butler BA, Dekker 2nd RG, Prescott A, Kadakia AR: Total ankle arthroplasty versus ankle arthrodesis-a comparison of outcomes over the last decade, *J Orthop Surg Res* 12(1):76, 2017.
3. Easley ME, Trnka HJ, Schon LC, Myerson MS: Isolated subtalar arthrodesis, *J Bone Joint Surg-Am.* 82(5):613–624, 2000.

ANKLE FRACTURES

Ankle fractures are one of the more common injuries encountered by orthopaedic surgeons and can represent a significant burden in terms of patient morbidity. One of the primary concerns regarding ankle fractures is the long-term risk of posttraumatic arthritis. Although there is some controversy regarding both the diagnosis and treatment for ankle fractures, the mainstay of treatment continues to be maintenance or restoration of normal anatomy to help minimize the risk of arthritis.

History

- Trauma, low-energy twisting injuries to high-energy injuries (motor vehicle accidents or fall from height)
- Pain (worse with weight bearing), swelling, ecchymosis, with or without deformity. Patient may report "pop" at the time of injury

Physical Examination

- Edema, ecchymosis, tenderness over fracture site. Medial tenderness without medial malleolus fracture suggests deltoid ligament injury; does not necessarily signify unstable ankle joint
- Fracture blisters with severe edema and soft tissue trauma
- Visual deformity present if ankle dislocated or severe displacement of fracture
- Complete neurovascular examination required. If ankle reduction performed, neurovascular examination should be repeated after reduction
- Evaluation for syndesmotic injury: palpation of proximal fibula (tenderness suggests syndesmotic injury), calf compression test, external rotation test:

- **Calf compression test:** medial-lateral compression at mid-calf. Pain at ankle joint suggests syndesmotic injury
- **External rotation test:** external rotation of the ankle with the knee at 90 degrees of flexion. Pain at syndesmosis suggests injury

Imaging

- Radiographs:
  - Weight-bearing ankle AP, mortise, lateral. Assess fracture, alignment, displacement.
  - Weight-bearing foot AP, oblique, lateral. Assess for fracture or malalignment.
  - Stress radiographs of the ankle should be performed for isolated fibular fractures at the level of the ankle joint. To perform, gravity stress or external rotation and/or abduction stress is applied in a non–weight-bearing mortise view. Medial clear space greater than 4 to 5 mm indicates deltoid ligament injury and ankle instability (Fig. 8.12).
  - Compare with contralateral ankle (mortise view is best). A 2-mm side-to-side difference in medial clear space indicates instability.

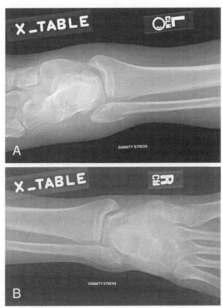

Fig. 8.12 Gravity stress views of the injured (**A**) and uninjured (**B**) ankles. Medial clear space widening is obvious, and operative intervention is recommended for this fracture.

Additional Imaging

- CT scans are helpful to evaluate comminution and subtle displacement. Scan should be performed of bilateral ankles to compare syndesmosis and medial clear space.
- MRIs are usually not necessary but can be useful to evaluate the deltoid ligament and help determine ankle stability.

Classification Systems

- Danis-Weber classification is based on the location of the fibular fracture and does not address the medial structures.
  - Type A: Transverse fracture at the level of or distal to the tibial plafond
  - Type B: Spiral, oblique fracture at the level of distal tibiofibular joint and extends proximally. Associated with possible disruption of syndesmosis (Fig. 8.13)
  - Type C: Fracture proximal to distal tibiofibular joint. Syndesmosis completely disrupted; anterior and posterior tibiofibular ligaments and interosseous membrane ruptured (Fig. 8.14)
- Lauge-Hansen classification: Fracture types are described by two terms that describe the fracture mechanism. The first term is supination or pronation, and the second term is adduction or external rotation. Additional subtypes exist within each classification.

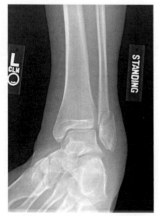

Fig. 8.13 Mortise View of Weber B Fracture. The fracture line is at the level of the ankle joint.

Initial Management

- Immobilization in Robert Jones splint, non–weight bearing, and elevation. Refer to an orthopaedic surgeon to be seen within 7 to 10 days.
- **Patient Education.** Unstable fractures require surgical fixation. Fractures that heal in nonanatomic alignment result in pain and increased risk of post-traumatic arthritis.

Nonoperative Management

- Weber A fractures: Nearly all can be treated nonoperatively, even with mild displacement.
  - Immobilization in cast or walking boot, weight bearing as tolerated. Most fractures heal in 6 weeks.
- Weber B: Isolated Weber B fractures require thorough evaluation to determine stability. If stable, consider nonoperative treatment. Unstable fractures require open reduction, internal fixation (ORIF).
  - Consider nonoperative management when medial clear space is less than 4 to 5 mm and less than 2 mm greater than contralateral side on stress and static radiographs.
  - Immobilization in cast or walking boot for 6 weeks. Weight bearing is progressed as tolerated.
  - Frequent follow-up with radiographs (weekly for first 2 to 3 weeks). Surgical fixation is recommended if there is a change in stability or alignment.
  - After 6 weeks of immobilization, transition to brace. Physical therapy may be helpful to regain motion and strength.
- Weber C: Nonoperative management is not recommended.
  - Medial malleolus fractures: Only small avulsion fractures can be treated nonoperatively if isolated and minimally displaced. Treatment includes short leg cast or cast boot for 6 weeks.

Operative Management

ICD-10

    S82.53XA Closed medial malleolus fracture

    S82.63XA Closed lateral malleolus fracture

    S82.843A Closed bimalleolar ankle fracture

    S82.853A Closed trimalleolar fracture

    S82.873A Closed tibial pilon fracture

CPT

    27792 ORIF lateral malleolus

    27814 ORIF bimalleolar fracture

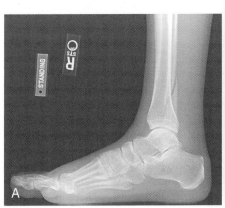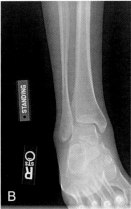

Fig. 8.14 Lateral (**A**) and mortise (**B**) views of Weber C fracture. Medial clear space widening noted with fracture line above the ankle joint line.

27823 ORIF trimalleolar fracture (with posterior malleolus ORIF)

Indications

- Instability of ankle or syndesmosis, significant fracture displacement
- Open fractures require immediate surgical débridement and antibiotic therapy. Staged treatment is often used in open fractures. External fixator is initially placed to stabilize the fracture/joint followed by delayed ORIF once soft tissues allow.
- Bimalleolar and trimalleolar fractures result in instability of mortise and surgical fixation necessary to stabilize ankle.
- Medial malleolar fractures are often associated with injury to the deltoid ligament and most require ORIF.

Informed consent and counseling

- Risks include wound complications, infection, nonunion, and DVT. The rate of complication is significantly higher in diabetics, nicotine users, and patients with peripheral vascular disease.[1] Posttraumatic arthritis may still occur despite proper stabilization. Major structures at risk are the superficial peroneal nerve (crosses fibula approximately 4 to 5 cm proximal to joint) and saphenous vein (for medial incisions).

Anesthesia

- General anesthesia with ankle or popliteal block

Patient positioning

- Supine with toes pointing directly toward ceiling. A small bump can be placed under the ipsilateral hip to internally rotate the leg. Place a thigh tourniquet.

Surgical Procedure
Open Reduction, Internal Fixation

There are multiple hardware options available for fixation of ankle fractures. Distal fibular fractures often require fixation with locking plate and screws. Locking plates should be used when bone quality is poor where the patient is at high risk for nonunion (diabetes, osteoporosis). Medial malleolar fractures often require fixation devices including lag, partially threaded, or cannulated screw placement. A buttress plate may be necessary for fixation for vertical sheer fractures to prevent proximal migration of fracture fragment. Use the lateral approach to the ankle for fixation of the distal fibula, syndesmosis, and possibly posterior malleolus. Longitudinal incision is made directly over the distal fibula. The fibular fracture is reduced and stabilized, restoring proper length and rotation. Intraoperative radiographs are obtained to confirm reduction, proper screw placement, as well as determine stability. After ORIF of the fibula, a radiograph is taken to evaluate for stability/medial clear space. If widening of the medial clear space is evident after ORIF of the fibula, syndesmotic fixation is required via screw or suture button fixation (Fig. 8.15).

Use the medial approach to the ankle for fixation of medial malleolus fractures or possible deltoid ligament repair. A longitudinal incision is made over the medial malleolus. The saphenous vein is identified and carefully retracted. Many fractures require both medial and lateral surgical approaches/fixation. A Robert Jones dressing/short leg splint is applied before leaving the operating room and the patient remains non-weight bearing on the affected extremity.

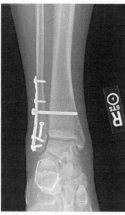

Fig. 8.15 Status post-open reduction, internal fixation distal fibular fracture (Weber B) requiring syndesmotic screw.

Estimated Postoperative Course

Postoperative 2 to 3 weeks:

- Sutures removed. Radiographs are obtained at each postoperative visit until complete healing is noted.
- In general, the patient should be non–weight bearing with immobilization in a sugar tong splint, cast, or boot for 6 weeks postoperative. Gentle ROM and partial weight bearing can begin 2 to 4 weeks postoperative when there is good bone quality and stable fixation. Strict immobilization and no weight bearing should be followed for a full 6 weeks if there is poor bone quality, ligamentous instability, or less stable fixation

Postoperative 6 weeks:

- Progress to full weight bearing in boot. Remove boot daily for ROM.

Postoperative 8 to 10 weeks:

- Discontinue boot and progress to shoe with ankle brace.
- Syndesmotic screw removal should be performed no sooner than 3 to 4 months postoperative. No definitive evidence exists to show a difference in clinical outcome whether a syndesmotic screw is removed or left in place.

Board Review

Ankle fractures are typically low-energy injuries, rotational as opposed to axial loading. Always evaluate for deltoid ligament or syndesmosis injury. Medial clear space widening of the ankle mortise indicates an unstable fracture pattern. Be sure to closely assess the medial and posterior malleolus for injuries/fractures to define bimalleolar or trimalleolar fracture patterns respectively.

SUGGESTED READINGS

Clare MP: A rational approach to ankle fractures, *Foot Ankle Clin* 13:593–610, 2008.

Jones CB, Wenke JC: *Skeletal trauma: basic science, management, and reconstruction*, Philadelphia, 2015, Elsevier.

Kitaoka Harold B: In *Master techniques in orthopaedic surgery: the foot and ankle*, ed 3, Philadelphia, 2013, Lippincott Williams and Wilkins.

Levine David: *Hospital for Special Surgery's illustrated tips and tricks in foot and ankle surgery*, Philadelphia, 2019, Lippincott Williams and Wilkins.

Michel P, van den Bekeron J, Lamme B, et al.: Which ankle fractures require syndesmotic stabilization? *J Foot Ankle Surg* 46(6):456–463, 2007.

Miller MD, editor: *Review of orthopedics*, ed 7, Philadelphia, PA, 2015, Saunders.

Rudloff MI: Fractures of the lower extremity, Chapter 54, e 17. In Beaty JH, Azar FM, Canale ST, Authors. *Campbell's operative orthopaedics*, Elsevier, pp 2812–2908, 2020.

Scott AM: Diagnosis and treatment of ankle fractures, *Radiol Technol* 81(5):457–475, 2010.

REFERENCE

1. Manway JM, Blazek CD, Burns PR: Special considerations in the management of diabetic ankle fractures, *Curr Rev Musculoskelet Med* 11(3):445–455, 2018, https://doi.org/10.1007/s12178-018-9508-x.

PLANTAR FASCIITIS

Plantar fasciitis (PF) is a regularly encountered clinical issue with nearly two million outpatient visits per year. It effects both sedentary and active patient populations, most commonly in the 40- to 60-year-old patient demographic. The diagnosis of PF is often one of patient history and clinical examination. Atypical presentations may warrant a more thorough diagnostic workup. Knowledge of the diagnosis and optimization of treatment plans may yield positive outcomes with noninvasive procedures in up to 90% to 95% of patients.

History

- PF is the most common cause of plantar heel pain.
- Plantar heel pain at the distal plantar fascia (medial calcaneal tuberosity) may extend into midsubstance plantar fascia.

- Start-up pain is characteristic of plantar fasciitis. Pain is greatest with the first steps in the morning or after prolonged sitting. Symptoms improve or resolve with non–weight bearing.

Physical Examination

- Tenderness occurs on palpation of plantar fascia, most pronounced at insertion on plantar medial calcaneus.
- Patients often have a tight gastrocnemius and/or Achilles tendon.
- Edema and ecchymosis are not present.

Imaging

- Radiograph: Weight-bearing foot AP, lateral, oblique. Presence of plantar calcaneal enthesophyte has no clinical relevance to PF.

Additional Imaging

- MRI/Ultrasound: Usually not necessary, may reveal thickening of plantar fascia.

Initial Management

- Stretching program to include Achilles, gastrocnemius, and plantar fascia–specific stretches; ice, massage, heel cups
- **Patient Education.** PF is a self-limiting process with 80% to 90% resolution within 10 months.[1]

Nonoperative Management

- Stretching should be done at minimum three times per day.
- Dorsiflexion splints worn at night keep the ankle at neutral position to prevent calf and plantar fascia contracture. Most improvement is noted in morning symptoms.
- Silicone heel cups, arch supports, custom orthotics, or over-the-counter (OTC) orthotics may be helpful. Custom inserts have no proven advantage over prefabricated inserts.
- Physical therapy and iontophoresis may provide symptomatic improvement, but symptoms return within 1 month of discontinuing treatment.
- Corticosteroid injections (see Orthopaedic Procedures, plantar fascia injection, p. 314) provide focused delivery of antiinflammatory medication. Risks include fascial rupture and fat pad atrophy. Improvement of symptoms generally lasts less than 3 months.

Operative Management

ICD-10:

  M72.2 Plantar fasciitis

CPT:

  28060 Partial plantar fascia fasciectomy

  Direct surgical interventions for partial plantar fascia fasciectomy are rarely performed. May consider gastrocnemius recession and/or orthotripsy (extracorporeal shock waves) treatment/surgical options.

Board Review

Plantar fasciitis is very common in runners and overweight patients. Generally, it is caused by microscopic tears in in the plantar fascia at the calcaneal origin. Patients will often complain of heel pain with the first few steps in the morning and possibly at night. Examination with reveal pain at the calcaneal origin and an inflexible Achilles/gastrocnemius contracture. Treatment is largely conservative with physical therapy, stretching of Achilles/gastrocnemius, arch supports, and massage.

SUGGESTED READINGS

DiGiovanni B, Nawoczenski D, Malay D, et al.: Plantar fascia-specific stretching exercise improves outcomes in patients with chronic plantar fasciitis, *J Bone Joint Surg Am* 88(8):1775–1781, 2006.

League A: Current concepts review: plantar fasciitis, *Foot Ankle Int* 29(3):358–366, 2008.

Miller MD, editor: *Review of orthopedics*, ed 7, Philadelphia, PA, 2015, Saunders.

Thomas JL, Christensen JC, Kravitz SR, et al.: The diagnosis and treatment of heel pain: a clinical practice guideline revision 2010, *J Foot Ankle Surg* 49(3 Suppl):S1–S19, 2010.

REFERENCE

1. Schwartz EN, Su J: Plantar fasciitis: a concise review, *Perm J* 18(1):e105–e107, 2014, https://doi.org/10.7812/TPP/13-113.

MORTON'S (INTERMETATARSAL) NEUROMA

Morton's neuroma, or interdigital neuritis, is a compressive neuropathy of the interdigital nerve that usually occurs between the third and fourth metatarsals.

It is a frequent cause of forefoot pain and disability. It more commonly occurs in women than men, possibly attributed to narrow footwear. Morton's neuroma is a paroxysmal neuralgia with associated sharp, burning pain. It is not a neuroma by formal definition, but rather a perineural fibrosis. Treatment may include surgical incision of the transverse intermetatarsal ligament with associated resection of a portion of the nerve itself.

History

- Compression neuropathy of common digital nerve: most common is third intermetatarsal space. Others are less common.
- Incidence in females is greater than males.
- Burning and/or radiating pain, and numbness/tingling exist, usually in plantar aspect of intermetatarsal space but can radiate to toes.
- Symptoms improve when barefoot.

Physical Examination

- Tenderness to palpation of intermetatarsal space. Pain is not reproduced with palpation of metatarsal heads or metatarsal-phalangeal (MTP) joints.
- **Mulder's sign:** Squeeze forefoot medial to lateral and apply dorsal pressure over affected web space. A positive test is audible or palpable click that causes pain.
- Edema, erythema, and ecchymosis are not present, and there is ± sensory deficit at affected web space/toes and ± divergence of toes.

Imaging

- Radiographs: Weight-bearing foot AP, lateral, oblique. Neuromas are not visible on x-rays.

Additional Imaging

- Ultrasound and MRI: Can be used for atypical presentations, but usually not necessary. Neuroma appears as an ovoid/dumbbell-shaped plantar mass between metatarsal heads.
- Ultrasound: A hypoechoic signal is present, but not all neuromas are visible.
- MRI: Best identified on T1 images, low intensity signal. Contrast MRI can differentiate from other masses.
- The gold standard for diagnosis is surgical visualization.

Nonoperative Management

- The goals are to alleviate pressure and decrease irritation of the nerve.
- Shoes with wide toe boxes are best. Avoid high heels.
- Metatarsal pads placed proximal to metatarsal heads spread apart the metatarsal heads and decrease pressure on nerve.
- Corticosteroid injections (see Orthopaedic Procedures, Morton's neuroma injection, p. 315) have variable results. Multiple injections have higher success rates (reported resolution of symptoms 11% to 47%). Risks of injections include atrophy of plantar fat pad and MTP joint subluxation.[1]

Operative Management

ICD-10:

G57.60 Lesion of plantar nerve

CPT code:

28080 Excision of interdigital neuroma

Indications

- Persistent symptoms following nonoperative treatment

Informed consent and counseling

- Risks include infection, wound complication (greater for plantar approach), hematoma, stump neuroma formation, and chronic pain. Recurrent neuromas may require additional surgery. Major structures at risk are the digital artery and vein.

Anesthesia

- Ankle block with or without sedation or general anesthesia; ankle tourniquet

Patient positioning

- Supine, toes toward ceiling; ipsilateral bump under the hip if necessary

Surgical Procedure
Interdigital Neuroma Excision

Excision of an interdigital neuroma occurs via a dorsal approach/dorsal incision made over the involved web space/intermetatarsal space. The dorsal interosseous fascia is split and retracted. The interosseous muscle is partially detached, metatarsal heads are retracted, and the intermetatarsal ligament is cut. The neuroma is exposed by retracting the digital artery and lumbrical muscle. Once the neuroma is exposed, it is dissected proximally and it is sharply cut. The proximal stump of the interdigital nerve retracts into the intrinsic muscles. Evaluate vascular status after excision to ensure digital artery is intact and functioning. Closure as indicated and weight bearing as tolerated in postoperative rigid soled shoe.

A plantar approach may be used, but is generally reserved for revision procedures. A longitudinal incision is made between the metatarsal heads. The planter fascia is split and retracted to expose the neuroma. Closure as indicated with the patient non–weight bearing for several weeks postoperatively to maintain wound/incision integrity.

Estimated Postoperative Course

- Dorsal approach: weight bearing as tolerated in hard-soled postoperative shoe. Progress to normal shoe wear and activities as tolerated once incision healed, usually between 2 and 3 weeks postoperative.
- The plantar approach requires greater protection with a splint or cast boot and more limited weight bearing to prevent wound complications. Sutures are removed 2 to 3 weeks postoperative. Progress to normal shoe wear and activities as tolerated once the wound has completely healed. This may be 3 to 4 weeks postoperative.

Board Review

Morton's neuroma is a result of traction of the interdigital nerve against the transverse metatarsal ligament, causing degeneration of the nerve and chronic inflammation. It most commonly occurs in the third web space and is more common in women than men. Patients complain of pain and numbness in the affected area with weight bearing, relieved by rest. A mass is sometimes palpable in the web space. Squeezing/compression of the metatarsals will often reproduce the symptoms. Treatment consists of conservative measures like metatarsal pads, shoes with a wide toe box, steroid injections into the web space, and possible surgical excision.

SUGGESTED READINGS

Miller MD, editor: *Review of orthopedics*, ed 7, Philadelphia, PA, 2015, Saunders.

Grear BJ: Neurogenic disorders, Chapter 87, e 2. In Beaty JH, Azar FM, Canale ST, Authors. *Campbell's operative orthopaedics*, Elsevier, pp 4345–4381, 2020.

Thomas J, Blitch E, Martin Chaney D, et al.: Diagnosis and treatment of forefoot disorders. Section 3. Morton's intermetatarsal neuroma, *J Foot Ankle Surg* 48(2):251–256, 2009.

Womack J, Richardson D, Murphy A, et al.: Long-term evaluation of interdigital neuroma treated by surgical excision, *Foot Ankle Int* 29(6):574–577, 2008.

REFERENCE

1. Wu K: Morton's interdigital neuroma: a clinical review of its etiology, treatment, and results, *J Foot Ankle Surg* 35(2):112–119, 1996.

DIABETIC FOOT AND CHARCOT ARTHROPATHY

Management and treatment of diabetes as well as its multiple possible complications can be a sizable undertaking. Diabetic patients with peripheral neuropathy can develop significant foot and ankle issues, including ulceration and Charcot arthropathy. Ulceration development in a diabetic foot is quite common, occurring in up to 12% of the diabetic population.[1] The plantar surface of the foot, particularly areas of bony prominence, is the most common site of ulceration. Complications of diabetic foot ulcerations are responsible for up to 85% of lower extremity amputations.[1] Charcot arthropathy is the progressive destruction of bony morphology of the foot in patients with peripheral neuropathy. Although diabetic neuropathy is the most frequent cause of Charcot deformity, other causes may include syringomyelia, alcoholism, chemotherapy-induced neuropathy, syphilis, and multiple sclerosis. Charcot arthropathy is a result of an inflammatory response that leads to bony resorption and potential deformity of the foot and ankle.

History

- Diabetic patients with neuropathy are at high risk for developing ulcers and infections.
- Symptoms of neuropathy are numbness, paresthesias or dysesthesias, slow wound healing, and no pain after injury.
- Charcot arthropathy is a destructive disease of bones and joints that occurs in sensory neuropathy. It is noninfectious and progressive. Unilateral involvement occurs at initial presentation.
- Charcot arthropathy can develop in patients with diabetic neuropathy. The average duration of diabetes at onset is 20 to 24 years for type I and 5 to 9 years for type II.[1]

- Risk factors for ulcers are peripheral neuropathy; absent pedal pulses; claudication; trophic skin changes (decreased hair growth, skin discoloration or atrophy); history of ulcer; and hospitalization for foot infection, bony deformity, or peripheral edema.
- The risk of osteomyelitis is high.

Physical Examination

- Visual deformities: Claw-toe deformities are common from loss of intrinsic muscle tone. Rocker-bottom midfoot deformity is often present in Charcot arthropathy of midfoot.
- Skin:
  - Inspect for presence of corns or calluses, open wounds, swelling, trophic changes, dependent rubor (arterial insufficiency), and bony prominences.
  - Ulcers often develop at sites of callus formation or as a result of microtrauma.
  - Increased warmth compared with the contralateral side can indicate Charcot arthropathy, venous insufficiency, or infection.
- Sensory examination: Conduct monofilament testing (Semmes-Weinstein) for loss of protective sensation. The threshold for peripheral neuropathy is 10 g. Generalized neuropathy with diminished sensation in "stocking" distribution is characteristic of diabetic neuropathy.
- Vascular: Decreased or absent pedal pulses indicate peripheral vascular disease. Delayed capillary refill indicates ischemic disease.

Imaging

- Radiograph: weight-bearing AP, lateral, oblique of foot and AP, lateral, mortise of ankle
  - May be normal in early disease processes
  - Difficult to differentiate Charcot arthropathy from osteomyelitis
  - Charcot arthropathy: disorganization of bony structure, bony erosion, intraarticular loose bodies, may have subluxation or dislocation of joints (Fig. 8.16)

Additional Imaging

- Nuclear medicine: Bone scan with indium-labeled leukocyte scintigraphy useful to diagnosis osteomyelitis; 93% to 100% sensitivity, 80% specificity[1]

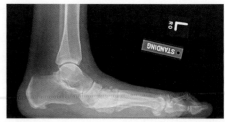

Fig. 8.16 Charcot Arthropathy of the Midfoot. Joint debris and collapse of the midfoot are noted.

- MRI:
  - Less specific than indium-labeled scintigraphy. Difficult to differentiate acute Charcot arthropathy from osteomyelitis
  - Presence of sinus tract or abscess helpful in confirming osteomyelitis
  - Subchondral cysts and intraarticular loose bodies/debris suggest Charcot

Classification Systems

- Multiple classification systems for diabetic foot ulcers, and Charcot arthropathy
- **Pinzur "risk factor" system to guide treatment of diabetic patients**
  - Risk Category 0: Normal appearance and sensation, mild to no deformity
  - Risk Category 1: Normal appearance, insensate, no deformity
  - Risk Category 2: Insensate foot with deformity, no history of prior ulcer
  - Risk Category 3: Insensate foot with deformity and history of prior ulcer
- **Classification system of Charcot arthropathy:**
  - Stage 0: Clinical examination findings of erythema and edema. Radiographs are normal.
  - Stage I: Fragmentation or dissolution phase. Radiographs demonstrate periarticular fragmentation, subluxation, or dislocation of joint. On examination, foot is warm, edematous, and erythematous.
  - Stage II: Coalescence period, early healing phase. Radiographs show early sclerosis, fusion of bony fragments, and absorption of debris. On examination, there is less erythema and warmth than stage I.
  - Stage III: Reconstruction phase. Radiographs reveal subchondral sclerosis, osteophytes, and narrow or absent joint spaces. On examination, visual deformity is present and there is no acute inflammation.

Initial Management

- Patients with neuropathy should not walk around barefoot or use corn or callous removers. Inspect feet daily and notify clinician if redness, ulceration, or blistering is present.
- **Patient Education** is especially important for diabetic patients. Stress importance of regular foot examinations and proper shoe wear (wide and tall toe box, supportive insoles).

Nonoperative Management

Indications

- **At-risk patients without Charcot arthropathy: based on Pinzur classification**
  - Risk Category 0: education, normal footwear, yearly clinical examination
  - Risk Category 1: education, daily foot self-examination, protective OTC insoles, appropriate footwear, biannual clinical examination
  - Risk Category 2: education, daily foot self-examination, custom pressure-dissipating accommodative orthoses, inlay depth soft-leather shoes, clinical examination every 4 months
  - Risk Category 3: education, daily foot self-examination, custom pressure-dissipating orthoses, inlay depth soft-leather shoes, clinical examination every 2 months
- **Charcot arthropathy: based on stage**
  - Stage I: immobilization using total contact casting, which reduces total load on the foot by one-third. Length of immobilization depends on progression of disease/collapse, often 2 to 4 months.
  - Stage II: ankle-foot orthosis or Charcot restraint orthotic walker (CROW) boot.
  - Stage III: accommodative shoe and custom insole to decrease pressure on bony prominences.

Operative Management

ICD-10 code
  M14.60 Charcot foot
CPT code
  28124 Exostectomy CPT for ostectomy of toe. Multiple CPT codes exist and vary depending on which bone is involved. Options also include amputation or arthrodesis.

Indications

- Exostectomy: Significant bony deformity not controlled by orthosis. May have osteomyelitis.

Informed consent and counseling

- Exostectomy: Recurrence requiring revision surgery is common (up to 25%). Patients are at high risk of wound complications. Due to decreased vascular and immune function, diabetics may require prolonged antibiotic use postoperatively.[2]

Anesthesia

- General anesthesia. Blocks are often not necessary in diabetics with peripheral neuropathy.

Patient positioning

- Supine, toes toward the ceiling (ipsilateral bump under the hip may be necessary)

Surgical Procedures

There are multiple surgical options and considerations for treatment of the diabetic foot and Charcot arthropathy. May consider exostectomy of bony prominences to minimize risk of skin breakdown/ulceration. Exostectomy occurs via a longitudinal incision made at the border of the plantar and dorsal skin. Careful dissection is made to prominent exostosis and prominent bone is excised using an osteotome or saw. The edges of the bone are then smoothed; imprecise closure is completed. May also consider arthrodesis of affected joints, as described in other sections of the chapter. Lastly, may consider amputation of affected extremity if salvage of the limb is not possible. The level of amputation and surgical techniques vary, depending upon disease involvement and affected extremity.

Estimated Postoperative Course

- A well-padded sugar tong splint/Robert Jones splint is applied in the operating room, and the patient must not bear weight for 2 weeks. At 2 weeks, the patient is transitioned to a diabetic shoe if no ulcer is present. If an ulcer is present, a total contact cast or CROW boot is used until the ulcer heals.

SUGGESTED READINGS

Besse J, Leemrijse T, Deleu P: Diabetic foot: the orthopedic surgery angle, *Orthop Traumatol Surg Res* 97:314–329, 2011.

Kolker D, Weinfeld S: Diabetic foot disorders. In DiGiovanni C, Greisberg J, editors: *First edition core knowledge in orthopaedics—foot and ankle*, Philadelphia, 2007, Elsevier.

Miller MD, editor: *Review of orthopedics*, ed 7, Philadelphia, PA, 2015, Saunders.

Bettin CC: Diabetic foot, Chapter 86, e3. In Beaty JH, Azar FM, Canale ST, Authors. *Campbell's operative orthopedics*, Elsevier, pp 4314–4344, 2020.

Pinzur M, Slovenkai M, Trepman E, Shields N: Guidelines for diabetic foot care: recommendations endorsed by the Diabetes Committee of the American Orthopaedic Foot and Ankle Society, *Foot Ankle Int* 26:113–118, 2005.

REFERENCES

1. Van der Ven A, Chapman C, Bowker J: Charcot neuroarthropathy of the foot and ankle, *J Am Acad Orthop Surg* 17:562–571, 2009.
2. Zgonis T: *Surgical reconstruction of the diabetic foot and ankle*, Philadelphia, 2009, Lippincott Williams & Wilkins.

METATARSAL FRACTURES (INCLUDING JONES FRACTURE)

The metatarsals are the most important weight-bearing structure of the forefoot. Complex relationships between the metatarsals exist, working in conjunction, for ideal biomechanical foot function. The fifth MT is the most common metatarsal fractured. First metatarsal fractures warrant careful evaluation as it has unique biomechanical and anatomic relationships that make it vital to the stability of the transverse and sagittal planes of the foot. Stress fractures commonly occur in the second metatarsal, classically described in amenorrheal dancers. Multiple metatarsal fractures commonly occur with trauma.

History

- One of the most common foot injuries. Most have minimal or no displacement.
- Common mechanisms are inversion injuries or falls from heights. Symptoms include pain with weight bearing, swelling, and bruising.
- Multiple metatarsal (MT) fractures are common.[1]

Physical Examination

- Edema, ecchymosis, and tenderness at fracture site(s) can exist.
- Inspect skin for evidence of open fracture.
- Displaced fractures may result in visual deformity or abnormal angulation of metatarsal.

Imaging

- Radiograph: weight-bearing AP, lateral, oblique foot (Fig. 8.17).

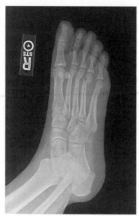

Fig. 8.17 Second, Third, and Fourth Metatarsal Fractures. The fourth metatarsal fracture is displaced greater than 3 to 4 mm, so open reduction, internal fixation should be considered.

Additional Imaging

- MRI is generally not indicated but can be used to evaluate ligamentous structures if there is concern for injury.
- CT is often used when there is concern for occult fracture or to evaluate Lisfranc injury.

Classification System

- Fifth metatarsal fractures are classified on the basis of location. Treatment recommendations are based on this classification system.
  - Zone 1 (avulsion): Fifth metatarsal tuberosity fracture. Most common type (>90%). Often extends from insertion of peroneal brevis to involve the tarsometatarsal joint.
  - Zone 2 (Jones fracture): Distal to the tuberosity at metaphyseal-diaphyseal junction. Fracture extends to fourth to fifth intermetatarsal joint. Mechanism is adduction or inversion of the forefoot (Fig. 8.18).
  - Zone 3: Proximal diaphyseal shaft fracture. Rare, less than 3% of fifth MT fractures. Frequently a stress injury and patients may report prodromal pain.[2]

Initial Management

- Immobilization in a sugar tong splint, short leg cast, or cast boot, non–weight bearing.
- Treatment is determined by fracture location and level of displacement.

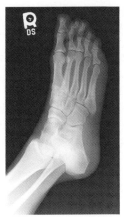

Fig. 8.18 Jones Fracture of the Fifth Metatarsal.

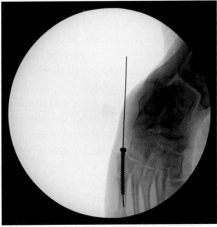

Fig. 8.19 Intraoperative radiograph demonstrating guidewire and screw placement for fixation of fifth metatarsal fracture.

Nonoperative Management
- First MT fractures nondisplaced, stable: immobilization (short leg cast or cast boot) for 6 weeks, weight bearing as tolerated.
- Lesser MT fractures nondisplaced or mild displacement (<4 mm translation, ≤10-degree sagittal angulation): hard-sole shoe for 4 to 6 weeks, weight bearing as tolerated.
- Fifth MT fractures:
  - Zone 1: hard-soled shoe or short cast boot for 4 to 6 weeks, weight bearing as tolerated. Consider ORIF for significantly displaced fractures.
  - Zone 2: short leg cast immobilization for 6 to 8 weeks, non–weight bearing.
  - Concern for nonunion with nonoperative treatment exists, especially in noncompliant patients. ORIF is recommended for high-level athletes.
  - Zone 3: high risk of nonunion, most surgeons recommend ORIF. If nonoperative treatment used, short leg cast immobilization with protected weight bearing for up to 3 months.

Operative Management
ICD-10: S92.309A Metatarsal fracture
CPT: 28485 ORIF fifth MT fracture, zone 2 or Jones fracture
Indications
- Significantly displaced fracture or fracture in zone 2 or 3. Treatment of zone 2 fractures is controversial and can be treated operatively or nonoperatively.
- ORIF or percutaneous pinning is recommended for fractures with significant displacement. Approach

and exact procedure depend on location and fracture type.
Informed consent and counseling
- Risks include nonunion, surgical site infection, hardware irritation, and nerve or vascular injury. Nonunions are often associated with early return to weight-bearing activity. Structures at risk during fifth MT ORIF include cutaneous branches of sural nerve and peroneal tendons.
Anesthesia
- General anesthesia, may use peripheral nerve block (ankle)
Patient positioning
- Supine, a bump under the ipsilateral hip can help to internally rotate leg and allow for easier access to lateral foot

Surgical Procedure
ORIF Fifth Metatarsal Fracture: Fig. 8.19
Surgical fixation for a fifth metatarsal fracture/Jones fracture occurs via intramedullary screw fixation of the fifth metatarsal. The patient is placed in the lateral position to facilitate exposure to the lateral aspect of the foot, as well as intraoperative radiographs. A longitudinal incision is made proximal to the base of the metatarsal, just dorsal to the border of the dorsal and plantar skin. Blunt dissection is performed down to bone/base of the fifth metatarsal. A guide wire is used to access the intramedullary canal from the dorsal and medial position, under guidance of an intraoperative radiograph.

Trajectory of the pin, and subsequent screw, is confirmed via radiograph to be within the intramedullary canal. Appropriate screw length is determined. Typically, a 5.5-mm screw is placed across the fracture. When using a partially threaded screw, all threads must cross the fracture site to obtain optimal fixation. The screw is countersunk to decrease the risk of soft tissue irritation postoperatively. Due to the bow of the fifth metatarsal, a screw with excess length can increase varus stress and result in nonunion or secondary fracture. A postoperative short leg splint/Robert Jones dressing is applied before leaving the operating room, and the patient is non–weight bearing for at least 2 weeks.[3]

Estimated Postoperative Course

Postoperative 2 weeks:

- Sutures removed and patient transitioned to a cast boot, bearing weight as tolerated.

Postoperative 6 to 12 weeks:

- Return to athletics depending on clinical and x-ray healing.

Board Review

A Jones fracture of the fifth metatarsal occurs distal to the tuberosity and extends to the fourth/fifth intermetatarsal joint. A fifth metatarsal fracture proximal to that area is considered a tuberosity avulsion fracture. A fracture distal to that area, in the diaphysis of the fifth metatarsal, is sometimes referred to as a Dancer's fracture.

SUGGESTED READINGS

Miller MD, editor: *Review of orthopedics*, ed 7, Philadelphia, PA, 2015, Saunders.

Bettin CC: Fractures and dislocations of the foot, Chapter 89. In Beaty JH, Azar FM, Canale ST, Authors. *Campbell's operative orthopedics*, Elsevier, pp 4407–4494, 2020.

REFERENCES

1. Hatch R, Alsobrook J, Clugston J: Diagnosis and management of metatarsal fractures, *Am Fam Physician* 76:817–827, 2007.
2. Portland G, Kelikian A, Kodros S: Acute surgical management of Jones' fractures, *Foot Ankle Int* 24:829–833, 2003.
3. Schenck RC, Heckman JD: Fractures and dislocations of the forefoot: operative and non-operative treatment, *J Am Acad Orthop Surg* 3:70–78, 1995.

LISFRANC FRACTURE/INJURY (TARSOMETATARSAL JOINT COMPLEX INJURY)

Lisfranc injuries are not particularly common. The Lisfranc ligament is between the medial cuneiform and second metatarsal. Injuries traditionally are associated with high-energy trauma, such as motor vehicle crash (MVC) and industrial accidents. Almost 40% of Lisfranc fracture dislocations are not recognized in polytrauma patients.[1] Recently, greater appreciation of midfoot sprains represents a new spectrum of injury to the Lisfranc ligament complex from low-energy, sport-related injuries.

History

- The Lisfranc ligament is a strong, interosseous attachment between the medial cuneiform and second metatarsal. A Lisfranc fracture describes an injury to the base of the metatarsal(s) at the attachment to the distal tarsal bones and Lisfranc ligament.
- Mechanism is trauma. About two-thirds of injuries result from high-energy trauma (MVC, fall from height), and one-third result from lower-energy mechanisms (e.g., athletics).
- Symptoms include pain, inability to weight bear on affected foot, swelling, and bruising.
- Most injuries are subtle, and many are missed on first evaluation and radiograph.

Physical Examination

- Edema of midfoot and forefoot, tenderness midfoot/tarsometatarsal joints, and plantar ecchymosis are present.
- The neurovascular examination is usually normal, but severe dislocation of the second MT can compromise blood flow, resulting in decreased or absent dorsalis pedis pulse.

Imaging

- Radiograph: weight-bearing AP, lateral, oblique of the foot. Include weight-bearing AP with both feet on same film for comparison.
  - Most common finding in Lisfranc injury is lateral step-off at second tarsometatarsal (TMT) joint.
  - Normal/uninjured foot: Medial border of second MT and medial border of middle cuneiform align on AP view. Oblique view demonstrates alignment

of medial border fourth MT and medial border of cuboid (Fig. 8.20).

Additional Imaging

- If radiographs appear normal, but high suspicion for Lisfranc injury, evaluate with CT scan or MRI.
  - CT scan: can be used to evaluate subtle or occult fractures. CT scans allow for more precise evaluation of fractures including comminution and intraarticular extension (Fig. 8.21).
  - MRI: can be used to evaluate soft tissues including Lisfranc ligament. MRI is used less frequently than CT scan to evaluate Lisfranc injuries.

Initial Management

- When Lisfranc injury is suspected, initialize immobilization in a sugar tong splint or cast boot and instruct patient to not bear weight. Refer to an orthopaedic surgeon.
- **Patient Education.** Unstable fractures that are not appropriately managed lead to posttraumatic arthritis of the midfoot. Posttraumatic arthritis can develop quickly.

Nonoperative Management

Indications

- Nonoperative treatment is recommended for low-demand patients (little ambulation or nonambulatory), preexisting inflammatory arthritis, or insensate foot.

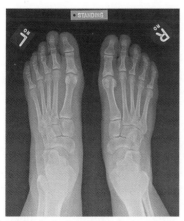

Fig. 8.20 On the right (uninjured foot), there is good alignment of the medial borders of the second metatarsal (MT) and middle cuneiform. On the left, a subtle fracture is noted at the base of the second MT.

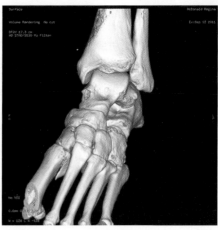

Fig. 8.21 Computed tomography scan three-dimensional reconstruction demonstrating Lisfranc injury with fracture at the base of the first and second metatarsal.

- Consider nonoperative management for stable injuries (no subluxation on radiograph or CT, no ligament tear on MRI, and negative stress examination under anesthesia).
- Immobilize in cast boot for 6 to 10 weeks, and bear weight as tolerated.
- Repeat weight-bearing radiographs 2 weeks postinjury. If there is a change in alignment, consider ORIF.
- After 6 to 10 weeks of immobilization, physical therapy may be indicated for gait training, balance, and functional strengthening. Full recovery occurs approximately 4 months postinjury.
- If pain is persistent in the future, midfoot arthrodesis can be performed.

Operative Management

ICD-10

S93.326A Closed dislocation of tarsometatarsal joint (Lisfranc injury)

S93.316A Open dislocation of tarsometatarsal joint

CPT

28615 Open reduction, internal fixation of tarsometatarsal fracture

Indications

- Unstable injury (subluxation on radiograph or CT scan, ligament tear on MRI, or positive stress radiograph under anesthesia)

Informed consent and counseling

- If unstable injury is left untreated, significant posttraumatic arthritis develops resulting in persistent pain. Major structures at risk include dorsalis pedis artery and sensory branch of deep peroneal nerve. A second procedure is necessary 3 to 4 months after fixation to remove hardware.

Anesthesia

- General anesthesia, with or without ankle block

Patient positioning

- Supine with toes toward ceiling

Surgical Procedure

Open Reduction Internal Fixation

There are many fixation techniques that can be used, as well as multiple devices available for fixation of midfoot fractures. A dorsal incision is made over the involved joints of the mid foot. Fractures are reduced, correcting the alignment of the TMT joints and hardware is placed. Intraoperative radiographs are used to determine correct alignment and the placement of hardware (Fig. 8.22). A postoperative short leg splint/Robert Jones dressing is applied before leaving the operating room and the patient is to be likely non–weight-bearing for 4 to 8 weeks.[2]

Estimated Postoperative Course

Postoperative 2 weeks:

- Sutures are removed at about 2 weeks, and the patient is transitioned to a short leg cast.

Postoperative 4 to 6 weeks:

- Apply walking boot and begin partial weight bearing. K-wires are removed at about 6 weeks postoperative if present.

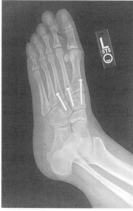

Fig. 8.22 Postoperative oblique view of open reduction, internal fixation first, second, and third tarsometatarsal joints.

Postoperative 8 weeks:

- Progress to full weight bearing in a cast boot. Continue boot for 3 to 4 months postoperative.

Hardware removal is performed about 4 months postoperative. Use walking boot, and bear weight as tolerated for 2 to 4 weeks after hardware removal. Progress to normal shoe full weight bearing.

Board Review

The Lisfranc ligament/ligamentous structures of the midfoot are critical to stabilizing the second metatarsal base—the "keystone" in the maintenance of the midfoot arch. Injury to this ligament, between the medial cuneiform and the second metatarsal, often results in severe pain, inability to bear weight, and marked swelling. Plantar ecchymosis should raise suspicion for a TMT/Lisfranc injury.

SUGGESTED READINGS

Bellabarba C, Barei DP, Sanders RW: Dislocations of the foot. In Coughlin MJ, Mann RA, Saltzman CL, editors: *Coughlin: Mann's surgery of the foot and ankle*, ed 9, Philadelphia, 2014, Mosby.

Coetzee JC: Making sense of Lisfranc injuries, *Foot Ankle Clin* 13:695–704, 2008.

Miller MD, editor: *Review of orthopedics*, ed 7, Philadelphia, PA, 2015, Saunders.

Bettin CC: Fractures and dislocations of the foot, Chapter 89. In Beaty JH, Azar FM, Canale ST, Authors. *Campbell's operative orthopedics*, Elsevier, pp 4407–4494, 2020.

REFERENCES

1. Thompson M, Mormino M: Injury to the tarsometatarsal joint complex, *J Am Acad Orthop Surg* 11:260–268, 2003.
2. Watson T, Shurnas P, Denker J: Treatment of Lisfranc joint injury: current concepts, *J Am Acad Orthop Surg* 18:718–728, 2010.

PHALANGEAL FRACTURES

Phalangeal fractures are commonly occurring fractures of the lower extremity. They are typically caused by a crushing injury or direct axial force. Fractures with associated circulatory compromise, open fractures, significant soft tissue injury, involvement of articular surface, or gross significant displacement may require referral for possible surgical intervention, although rare. Treatment often consists of buddy taping affected toe and use of a rigid soled shoe that extends beyond the toes to prevent repeat injury due to recurrent axial load.

History

- Common mechanisms include stubbing a toe or a direct blow from a falling object.
- Symptoms include pain, swelling, bruising, and difficulty walking or wearing a shoe.
- Sesamoid fractures are caused by overuse or avulsion forces or direct trauma. Patients report pain directly under the first MTP joint with weight bearing. The medial (tibial) sesamoid is more commonly injured than the lateral (fibular).[1]

Physical Examination

- The affected area is edematous, tender to palpation, and ecchymotic.
- Evaluate skin for signs of open fracture.

Imaging

- Radiograph: weight-bearing AP and lateral views, as well as oblique view. If there is concern for sesamoid injury, obtain a tangential view of the sesamoid.

Additional Imaging

- CT/MRI is usually not indicated unless additional injury is noted or there is significant involvement of the first MTP joint.

Initial Management

- Open fractures require immediate irrigation and débridement followed by a course of antibiotics.

Nonoperative Management

- Nearly all phalangeal fractures can be treated non-operatively.
- Displaced fractures of lesser toes can be treated with closed reduction with traction after digital block. After reduction, splint to adjacent toe (buddy taping) for 2 to 4 weeks. Weight bearing as tolerated in hard-soled shoe for 4 to 6 weeks.
- Nondisplaced fractures of the great toe require immobilization in hard-soled shoe or boot for 2 to 3 weeks, weight bearing as tolerated primarily through heel.

- Sesamoid fractures: cast boot with sesamoid orthotic (dancer's pad) for 6 weeks, then transition to shoe with sesamoid orthotic for an additional 6 weeks.

Operative Management

ICD-10

    S92.919A Fracture of one or more phalanges of the foot

CPT

    28525: Open treatment of fracture of phalanx or phalanges other than the great toe

    28496: Open treatment of fracture of the great toe (proximal or distal phalanx)

    Indications

- Rarely indicated. Operative intervention is only recommended for displaced fractures of the great toe.

Surgical Procedure

Surgical interventions for phalanx fractures are rarely indicated. Operative intervention is only recommended for displaced fractures of the first toe. Surgical fixation is obtained via percutaneous pinning with K-wires. Patient will likely be weight-bearing as tolerated in a postoperative shoe after surgery. K-wires are removed 4 to 6 weeks postoperative.

SUGGESTED READINGS

DiGiovanni C, Greisberg J: *Foot and ankle: core knowledge in orthopaedics*, Philadelphia, 2007, Elsevier.

Miller MD, editor: *Review of orthopedics*, ed 7, Philadelphia, PA, 2015, Saunders.

Sander RW, Papp S: Fractures of the midfoot and forefoot. In Coughlin MJ, Mann RA, Saltzman CL, editors: *Coughlin: surgery of the foot and ankle*, ed 8, Philadelphia, 2007, Mosby.

REFERENCE

1. Schenck RC, Heckman JD: Fractures and dislocations of the forefoot: operative and non-operative treatment, *J Am Acad Orthop Surg* 3:70–78, 1995.

TARSAL TUNNEL SYNDROME

Tarsal tunnel syndrome and its symptoms may be vague and misleading, including diffuse burning sensation about the medial ankle and plantar foot. It is a compressive neuropathy of the tibial nerve in the fibroosseous tunnel posterior and inferior to medial malleolus, akin to carpal tunnel syndrome of the wrist. Reported causes of tarsal tunnel are largely in relation to anatomic issues causing mass effect and impingement of the nerve within the restricted tarsal tunnel. Systemic diseases such as diabetes mellitus, rheumatoid arthritis, and ankylosing spondylitis may indirectly cause tarsal tunnel symptoms due to generalized inflammatory edema.

History

- Tarsal tunnel syndrome may present with a history of injury or trauma.
- Patients complain of burning, tingling, and numbness over the plantar aspect of the foot, which may radiate distally or proximally. Symptoms increase with protracted walking or standing and resolve with rest, elevation, and loose shoes. Patients may experience severe pain at night.
- Obtain history related to systemic disorders that can affect nerves (i.e., rheumatologic disorders, diabetes, ankylosing spondylitis, Lyme disease, thyroid disorder).

Physical Examination

- Note valgus or varus heel alignment.
- Palpate course of tibial nerve for thickness, edema, or paresthesias.
- Look for a positive percussion sign (Tinel) or cuff test.
  - **Cuff test:** This tests for tarsal tunnel syndrome secondary to venous insufficiency. A pneumatic cuff is placed above the ankle and inflated to 60 to 80 mm Hg. This occludes venous flow and increases venous pressure around the nerve and is positive if the patient's symptoms are reproduced.

Imaging

- Electromyography (EMG) or nerve conduction study (NCS)
- Radiograph: weight-bearing foot (AP, oblique, lateral) and ankle (AP, mortise, lateral)

Additional Imaging

- MRI to evaluate for space-occupying lesion

Classification of Origin

- Trauma
- Space-occupying lesion
- Foot deformity

Initial Management

- Nonoperative treatment is the first line and mainstay of treatment for tarsal tunnel syndrome, unless acute. Surgical intervention is to be proceeded with much caution and may not alleviate all of the patient's symptoms.
- Primary care providers can initiate ordering diagnostic studies such as MRI or EMG or NCS.
- Refer to orthopaedic surgeon on a nonurgent basis.

Nonoperative Management

- Non-operative management is most effective when the underlying etiology is tenosynovitis or foot deformity.
- Includes use of corticosteroid injection, orthotics, NSAIDs, and immobilization (see Tarsal Tunnel Injection, p. 316).
- Can consider prescribing medications such as tricyclic antidepressants, selective serotonin reuptake inhibitors (SSRIs), antiseizure medication, or other antidepressants. Refer patient to pain management or neurologist if not comfortable prescribing these medications.

Operative Management

ICD-10

    G57.50 Tarsal tunnel syndrome
CPT

    28035 Tarsal tunnel release
    Indications
- Recalcitrant symptoms despite appropriate conservative management
- Evidence of space-occupying lesion on MRI
    Informed consent and counseling
- Risks and complications include continued pain despite release, increased symptoms, numbness dysesthesias, persistent tenderness or paresthesias over the tarsal tunnel, edema, nerve damage, vascular damage, infection, wound complications, difficulty with footwear, and causalgia or complex regional pain syndrome.[1]
    Anesthesia
- Surgeon and patient discretion, likely general anesthesia with regional nerve block

Patient positioning
- Supine or mild Trendelenburg
- Tourniquet optional

Surgical Procedures
Tibial Nerve Release/Tarsal Tunnel Release
Surgical release of the tibial nerve occurs via a curved medial incision extending above, behind, and below the medial malleolus beginning 10 cm proximal to the medial malleolus and 2 cm posterior to the tibia. The incision is deepened to expose the flexor retinaculum. The tibial nerve sheath is identified and opened proximally. The flexor retinaculum is then carefully released. Any anatomic structures causing impingement on the nerve are also subsequently released/excised. Terminal branches of the tibial nerve should be identified and released. The wound is closed in layers, leaving the retinaculum open to prevent recurrence due to scar formation. Patient is placed a well molded postoperative splint and is non–weight bearing for 2 to 4 weeks postoperatively.

Estimated Postoperative Course
Postoperative 10 days to 2 weeks:
- Splint and sutures removed. May continue to protect incision with controlled ankle motion (CAM) boot. Begin gently with ROM exercises to prevent adhesions.

Postoperative 3 to 4 weeks:
- Weight bearing as tolerated, increase activities as tolerated. May begin more aggressive therapy as indicated.

Board Review
Tarsal tunnel syndrome is a compressive neuropathy of the tibial nerve within the fibroosseous tunnel posterior and inferior to the medial malleolus. It is roughly equivalent to carpal tunnel of the wrist. Symptoms are often vague and misleading, and often include burning sensation along the plantar surface of the foot and medial ankle.

SUGGESTED READINGS

Antoniadis G, Scheglmann K: Posterior tarsal tunnel syndrome, *Dtsch Arxtebl Int* 105:776–781, 2008.

Coughlin M, editor: *Mann's Surgery of the foot and ankle*, ed 9, Philadelphia, 2014, Mosby.

Miller MD, editor: *Review of orthopedics*, ed 7, Philadelphia, PA, 2015, Saunders.

Grear BJ: Neurogenic disorders, Chapter 87, e 2. In Beaty JH, Azar FM, Canale ST, Authors. *Campbell's operative orthopedics*, Elsevier, pp 4345–4381, 2020.

REFERENCE

1. Lau J, Daniels T: Tarsal tunnel syndrome: a review of the literature, *Foot Ankle Inter* 20:201–209, 1999.

ACHILLES TENDINOPATHY AND RUPTURE

Achilles tendon injuries are the most common tendon injury of the lower extremity. An increase in acute ruptures is attributed to increased participation in physically demanding activities by the "weekend warrior" patients in the fourth to fifth decade of life. Treatment decisions are often made on an individual basis, with both nonoperative and operative interventions being advocated. Managing the expectations of the patient sustaining an Achilles tendon injury is paramount to achieving a successful outcome. Typical recovery from injury, or any surgical intervention, is routinely 6 months to a year before returning to regular sporting activity.

Achilles Tendon Rupture
History
- Sharp unexpected dorsiflexion force to the ankle in conjunction with a strong contraction of the calf (e.g., tripping on a curb, unexpectedly stepping into a hole), pushing off the weight-bearing foot with the knee in extension (e.g., lunging for a tennis shot), and a strong or violent dorsiflexion force on a plantar-flexed ankle (e.g., jumping from a height).
- Sensation of a snap or audible pop in posterior calf followed by acute pain like "got kicked from behind" or sounds "like a gun being shot," difficulty walking, and weakened plantarflexion.

Physical Examination
- Palpable defect approximately 2 to 6 cm from insertion of Achilles tendon.
- Increased ankle dorsiflexion ROM and decreased plantarflexion strength compared with uninjured extremity.

- **Positive Thompson test:** assesses the continuity of Achilles tendon. Patient is placed in a prone position with both feet extended past end of examination table. The affected calf is squeezed, and reflex plantarflexion is assessed. A positive test is when there is no reflex plantarflexion with a squeeze of the calf, indicating an Achilles injury/tear.
- Be sure to palpate for calcaneal tenderness.

Imaging
- Radiographs only if calcaneal bony tenderness

Additional Imaging
- MRI or ultrasound not necessary to confirm diagnosis with strong history and physical examination findings—may order if considering nonoperative treatment.

Initial Management
- Immobilize affected extremity in plantarflexed position, non–weight bearing.
- Refer immediately to orthopaedic surgeon.
- **Patient Education.** Acute Achilles ruptures may be treated surgically or nonsurgically with similar outcomes with appropriate patient selection. Nonsurgical treatment has lower complication rates; however, surgical repair has a faster recovery time, quicker return to sport activities, and slightly lower re-rupture rates. Missed or improperly treated ruptures can lead to significant weakness and altered gait mechanics.

> **! CLINICAL ALERT**
>
> Quinolone use has been associated with rupture of Achilles tendon most commonly in the elderly and patients using corticosterioids.[1]

Nonoperative Management
- With dynamic ultrasound or MRI, rupture gap must be less than 5 mm with maximum plantarflexion, less than a 10-mm gap with foot in neutral dorsiflexion, or greater than 75% apposition of tendon in 20 degrees of plantarflexion
- Good candidates for nonoperative management include those with systemic disease, medical comorbidities, patient who use tobacco or have diabetes, as well as healthy individuals who meet the previously mentioned criteria and do not want to have surgery
- Treatment protocol (Table 8.5)

Operative Management
ICD-10 S86.019A

727.67 Achilles tendon rupture
CPT

27650 Acute Achilles rupture repair

TABLE 8.5   Nonoperative Treatment Protocol for Achilles Tendon Rupture

Initial evaluation	Ultrasound (U/S) or magnetic resonance imaging (MRI) examination showing <5-mm gap of tendon ends with maximal plantarflexion, <10-mm gap with neutral, or >75% apposition of tendon ends in 20 degrees plantarflexion (PF).
Initial management	Cast in full PF, non–weight bearing.
2-week evaluation	May transition to pneumatic walking boot or bivalved cast with foot in 20 degrees PF with two 1-cm heel wedges, may be weight bearing. Must wear boot 24 hours/day.
4-week evaluation	On examination, palpable continuity of tendon. If concern tendon not apposed, order repeat U/S or MRI. Patient may remove boot 5 minutes per hour to perform active dorsiflexion to neutral with passive plantarflexion.
6-week evaluation	On examination, continue to document continuity of tendon. Patient may remove one 1-cm lift. Continue range-of-motion exercises, may initiate more formal physical therapy protocol.
8-week evaluation	Document continued continuity of tendon. May decrease to zero lifts in boot and discontinue use of boot at night. Continue therapy program.
10-week evaluation	Discontinue use of boot and transition into a shoe with one 1-cm heel lift to be used for 3 additional months. Continue therapy program, and avoid aggressive sport activity until heel lift is discontinued.

Indications

- Greater than 1-cm gap in neutral dorsiflexion
- Patient preference

Informed consent and counseling

- Risks include infection and wound complications, which can be catastrophic, re-rupture, keloid formation, sural nerve injury, and adhesions
- Most people are back to sport activity at 6 months postoperatively
- Full recovery in terms of pain, edema, and strength can take a full year to achieve

Anesthesia

- General anesthesia with regional block such as popliteal block

Patient positioning

- Prone or modified lateral
- Nonsterile tourniquet on upper thigh

Surgical Procedure

Primary Repair of Achilles Tendon Rupture

The patient is placed in the prone position, with the affected extremity elevated to facilitate exposure of the surgical site. A 10-cm incision is made 0.5 cm medial to Achilles tendon and extended proximally to insertion into the calcaneus. Dissection down to peritenon, which is then cut longitudinally to expose ruptured tendon. Care is taken not to undermine the skin or create increased skin tension on wound edges with retractors. The ankle is plantarflexed to approximate tendon ends, and the hematoma débrided. Nonabsorbable suture is used to repair the rupture using a modified Kessler, Bunnell, or Krackow stitch. The peritenon is closed and skin sutured. Place the patient in non–weight bearing, well-padded, molded posterior splint in plantarflexion.

Estimated Postoperative Course

Early protected weight bearing and use of a protective device that allows mobilization is key in successful rehabilitation of Achilles tendon ruptures.

Postoperative 1 to 2 weeks:

- Postoperative splint removed and wound inspected, well-healed sutures removed. If not, patient placed back into short leg cast for 1 week.
- Once sutures removed, patient placed in removable boot with 2 heel wedges and allowed to initiate weight bearing as tolerated.

Postoperative 4 to 5 weeks:

- Heel wedges are gradually decreased over the course of the next 2 to 3 weeks, until the patient is weight bearing in the boot with no lifts.

Postoperative 6 to 8 weeks:

- Boot is discontinued after 2-4 weeks of weight bearing in boot with no lifts.
- Physical therapy program initiated.
- Patient may increase activities as tolerated after discontinuing use of boot, starting with non-impact activities. Most people do not return to sport activity until at least 6 months after surgery.

Board Review

Acute Achilles tendon ruptures are the most common tendon rupture of the lower extremity. Complete rupture is associated with sudden, violent dorsiflexion of the ankle. There is increased risk of rupture with intratendinous degeneration, fluroquinolone usage, previous steroid injections, or history of inflammatory arthritis. A positive Thompson test, with lack of plantarflexion response with calf compression, indicates a complete Achilles rupture.

ACHILLES TENDINOPATHY

Achilles tendinosis/tendinopathy is a spectrum of pathology affecting the Achilles tendon. It often begins with an episode of acute inflammation, and over time experiencing repetitive microtrauma which progresses to degenerative changes within the tendon. The cumulative effect of the degenerative changes leads to an increased risk of subsequent rupture of the tendon.

History

- Due to overuse injuries with primary contributing factors of host susceptibility and mechanical overload.
- Associated with advancing age, usually insidious and chronic in nature.
- Patient complains of pain in Achilles tendon with activities, thickness or edema of tendon, and impaired performance. May be related to training errors and inappropriate footwear.

Physical Examination

- Tender to palpation, thickened and/or edematous Achilles tendon or bony prominence at posterior calcaneus

- Decreased plantarflexion strength, calf atrophy, palpable gap if chronic or missed rupture
- Antalgic gait
- Assess for heel cord tightness

Imaging

- Radiographs: weight-bearing foot (AP/oblique/lateral) and ankle (AP/mortise/lateral)

Additional Imaging

- Ultrasound or MRI to delineate source of pathology or for surgical planning

Classification

- Paratendinopathy—inflammation of the tendon sheath
- Noninsertional—tendinopathy within the substance of the tendon
- Insertional—tendinopathy where the Achilles inserts onto the calcaneus
- Retrocalcaneal bursitis—inflammation of the fluid-filled sac that lies between the Achilles and the calcaneus

Initial Management

- Prescribe heel lifts, NSAIDs, rest, ice, and an eccentric physical therapy program (see Nonoperative Management later).
- Refer to orthopaedic surgeon if you suspect acute rupture or if symptoms are recalcitrant to prescribed treatment program.
- **Patient Education.** This condition is likely chronic and noninflammatory in nature. It responds well to a specific rehabilitation program in which the patient's compliance is crucial in its success. The goal of treatment is symptomatic only. The patient may always have thickened tendon or calcaneal bony prominence unless he or she undergoes surgical intervention. Recovery may follow a prolonged time course, taking 4 to 6 months before noticing improvement and even longer until the patient is back to reasonable activities comfortably.

Nonoperative Management

- Mainstay of treatment, especially for patients with no prior formal treatment.
- Eccentric loading proven to be beneficial in treatment of symptoms but may take up to 12 weeks to notice improvements in symptom.[2]

- Immobilization in walking cast or boot necessary initially if symptoms severe.
- Physical therapy prescription for Alfredson's 12-week Eccentric Loading Protocol.
- Follow-up in 4 to 6 months if no significant improvement to discuss possible need for surgical intervention.[3]

Operative Management
ICD-10
  M76.60 Achilles bursitis or tendonitis
CPT
  27654 Achilles débridement mid-substance w or w/o flexor hallucis longus (FHL) tendon transfer
  27680 Achilles débridement, Haglund excision with FHL tendon transfer
Indications
- Symptoms recalcitrant to appropriate conservative treatment
- Missed or chronic Achilles tendon rupture
Informed consent and counseling
- Risks include infection and wound complications, which can be catastrophic; painful scar; nerve injury; and continued pain.[4]
- In cases where there is a missed Achilles tendon rupture or more than 50% of the tendon is débrided, an FHL tendon transfer is necessary to augment Achilles.
Anesthesia
- General anesthesia with regional nerve block, likely popliteal
Patient positioning
- Prone or modified lateral
- Nonsterile tourniquet on upper thigh

Surgical Procedures
Achilles Tendon Reconstruction Using Flexor Hallicus Longus Transfer
The patient is placed in the prone position with the surgical extremity slightly elevated to facilitate exposure. A longitudinal incision is made medial to Achilles tendon from musculotendinous junction to 2 cm distal to insertion. The peritenon is incised, and the Achilles tendon inspected and débrided. The FHL muscle belly is exposed by retracting the posterior tibial artery, vein, and nerve and incising the deep posterior compartment. The FHL is harvested distally through a second longitudinal incision made along the medial border of the foot; it is pulled through the proximal wound and passed through a calcaneal drill hole made 1 cm distal and 1 cm anterior to the

Achilles tendon insertion. The FHL is secured through the drill hole in the calcaneus or through a suture to the Achilles tendon. The muscle belly of the FHL is often approximated to the affected area of tendon to facilitate increased vascularity and promote healing. The peritenon is repaired, followed by careful wound closure to minimize disruption of wound edges. The patient is placed in a posterior mold splint in slight plantarflexion. The patient will be non–weight bearing for 6 to 8 weeks.[5]

Estimated Postoperative Course

Postoperative course similar to recovery for acute rupture repair; may be delayed only if tendon transfer is used to augment the Achilles tendon
Postoperative 1 to 2 weeks:

- Splint and sutures removed; patient placed into cast or boot in 10 to 20 degrees of plantarflexion.

Postoperative 4 to 6 weeks:

- Place the patient in neutral dorsiflexion boot or cast and initiate weight bearing at 8 weeks postoperatively.
- Initiate rehabilitation program.

Postoperative 12 weeks:

- Transition out of boot into regular shoe with 2.5-cm heel lift for another 3 months.

Board Review

Achilles tendinopathy issues can involve the midsubstance of the Achilles tendon and the retrocalcaneal bursa, as well as an enlarged prominence of the posterosuperior calcaneal tuberosity commonly referred to as a Haglund deformity.

SUGGESTED READINGS

Miller MD, editor: *Review of orthopedics*, ed 7, Philadelphia, PA, 2015, Saunders.

Bettin CC: Fractures and dislocations of the foot, Chapter 89. In Beaty JH, Azar FM, Canale ST, Authors. *Campbell's operative orthopedics*, Elsevier, pp 4407–4494, 2020.

REFERENCES

1. Lewis JR, gums JG, Dickensheets DL: Levofloxacin-induced bilateral Achilles tendonitis, *Ann Pharmacother* 33(7-8):792–795, 1999.
2. Alfredson H, Pietila T, Jonsson P, et al.: Heavy-load eccentric calf muscle training for the treatment of chronic Achilles tendinosis, *Am J Sports Med* 26:360–366, 1998.
3. Tan G, Sabb B, Kadakia A: Non-surgical management of Achilles ruptures, *Foot Ankle Clin N Am* 14:675–684, 2009.
4. Reddy S, Pedowitz D, Parekh S, et al.: Surgical treatment for chronic disease and disorders of the Achilles tendon, *J Am Acad Orthop Surg* 17:3–14, 2009.
5. Wilcox D, Bohay D, Anderson J: Treatment of chronic Achilles tendon disorders with flexor hallucis longus tendon transfer/augmentation, *Foot Ankle Intern* 21:1004–1010, 2000.

ANKLE SPRAIN

Lateral ankle sprains are the most common injury in sports but can occur just as easily from a misstep. The lateral ankle ligaments stabilize the ankle joint both statically and dynamically. A high ankle sprain refers to an injury to the tibiofibular syndesmosis. Syndesmosis refers to the bony articulation between the distal fibula and tibia, as well as ligamentous structures to support the articulation. The majority of ankle sprains are treated successfully with nonsurgical management.

History

- Inversion injury in plantar-flexed position
- Injury to lateral ligamentous complex including the anterior talofibular ligament (ATFL), calcaneofibular ligament (CFL), and posterior talofibular ligament (PTFL)
- External rotation forces in syndesmotic sprains or high ankle sprain
- Patients complain of pain, swelling, bruising, inability to bear weight, and loss of functional ability

Physical Examination

- Inspect for lateral ankle edema and ecchymosis.
- Tenderness to palpation occurs over ATFL and CFL.
- **Anterior drawer test** to assess injury to ATFL (Fig. 8.23): The patient is seated with the leg hanging off the side of the bed or table with the knee bent, the tibia is stabilized with one hand, and the foot is translated anteriorly with the other hand at the level of the heel. With sprain or partial rupture of ligaments, pain may be elicited. With a complete tear, the patient may demonstrate a suction sign.
- Conduct an **inversion stress test** to assess injury to the CFL: With the ankle in neutral or slightly dorsiflexed position, invert the ankle by grasping the

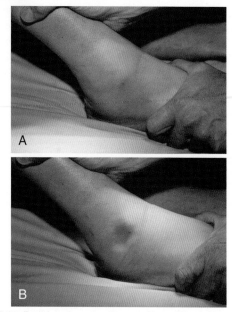

Fig. 8.23 Positive Anterior Drawer Test. (From Clanton TO, McGarvey W: Athletic injuries to the soft tissues of the foot and ankle. In Coughlin MJ, et al., editors: *Surgery of the foot and ankle*, ed 8, St. Louis, 2007, Elsevier.)

lateral calcaneus. This may elicit pain with injury to the CFL.
- Use **squeeze test** or **cross-legged test** to assess syndesmotic injury: A positive result occurs when a squeeze of the proximal calf causes pain in the distal syndesmosis. Squeezing the calf will cause separation of the distal fibula and anterior tibiofibular ligament and therefore, if injured, elicits discomfort.

Imaging
- Radiograph: Weight-bearing foot (AP/oblique/lateral) and ankle (AP/mortise/lateral) if indicated per Ottawa Rules for Ankle radiographs (can be any one of the following):
  - Bone tenderness along distal 6 cm of posterior tibia or medial malleolus
  - Bone tenderness along distal 6 cm of the fibula or lateral malleolus
  - Inability to bear weight for four steps

Additional Imaging
- MRI or CT if ankle sprain symptomatic for more than 6 weeks to assess for osteochondral injury, tendon injury, or missed fracture

Classification System
- Grade 1—ATFL stretched, no frank ligament tear, no laxity on examination
- Grade 2—Moderate injury to ligamentous complex, complete tear of ATFL ± partial tear of CFL; may or may not have increased laxity
- Grade 3—Complete tear of ATFL and CFL ± capsular tear ± PTFL tear

Initial Management
- Engage in RICE therapy (rest, ice, compression, and elevation)
- Functional immobilization in lace-up or semirigid ankle support devices such as CAM walking boot for more severe injuries or ankle stabilizing orthosis (ASO) brace for less severe
- Weight bearing as tolerated unless significant amount of pain
- Referral to orthopaedic surgeon appropriate if concern or evidence of fracture or dislocation, neurovascular compromise, tendon rupture or subluxation, mechanical "locking" of joint, open wound penetrating the joint, and syndesmotic injury[1]
- **Patient Education.** Lateral ligament ankle sprains are the most common musculoskeletal injuries in the United States. Goals of treatment include reduction in pain and edema and prevention of further injury. Inadequate treatment can lead to chronic problems including joint instability, pain, and loss of ROM

Nonoperative Management
- Most patients will recover well from an ankle sprain with nonsurgical management with surgical management reserved for high-performance athletes.
- Functional rehabilitation is superior to prolonged immobilization with protection of injured tissue during postinjury days 1 to 5 and protected stress in a CAM walker boot during days 6 to 32 postinjury.[2]
- If patient is placed in a CAM walker boot, see back in the office 2 to 3 weeks postinjury to reassess ability to transition into semirigid device such as an ASO brace.
- Initiate physical therapy 2 to 3 weeks postinjury.
- If continued or worsening symptoms 6 or more weeks postinjury, consider MRI and/or orthopaedic referral.

Rehabilitation

- An effective rehabilitation program involves resumption of preinjury ROM, strength, proprioception, and motor control.
- Physical therapy prescription should include ankle ROM and strengthening, as well as peroneal strengthening and proprioception one to three times a week for 6 weeks.[3]
- The patient may return to normal activity depending on pain and with guidance of a therapist once rehabilitation goals are met.

Prevention

- Use of an ankle brace with activity has been shown to prevent injury with minimal to no performance decrements.

Board Review

Ankle sprains are one of the most common sports-related injuries. Sprains often involve the lateral ankle ligaments, particularly the anterior talofibular ligament. Patients often report "hearing a pop" with associated swelling and ecchymosis of the lateral ankle. Stability of the ankle is assessed with the anterior drawer test. Treatment is tailored to the severity of the sprain, but should always include "RICE" (rest, ice, compression, and elevation).

SUGGESTED READINGS

Miller MD, editor: *Review of orthopedics*, ed 7, Philadelphia, PA, 2015, Saunders.

Richardson DR: Sports injuries of the ankle, Chapter 90. In Beaty JH, Azar FM, Canale ST, Authors. *Campbell's operative orthopedics*, Elsevier, pp 4495–4536, 2020.

Ivins D: Acute ankle sprain: an update, *Am Fam Physician* 74:1714–1720, 2006.

REFERENCES

1. Lin C-W, Hiller C, de Bie R: Evidence-based treatment for ankle injuries: a clinical perspective, *J Man Manip Ther* 18:22–28, 2010.
2. Maffulli N, Ferran N: Management of acute and chronic ankle instability, *J Am Acad Orthop Surg* 16:608–615, 2008.
3. Mattacola C, Dwyer M: Rehabilitation of the ankle after acute sprain or chronic instability, *J Athl Train* 37:413–429, 2002.

CAVOVARUS FOOT DEFORMITY

Cavovarus foot refers to a foot that is both cavus (high arch) and varus alignment of the heel (a heel that is positioned inward/medially). It is not as common as flatfoot, pes planus deformity. Varus alignment of the hindfoot can occur from calcaneal or talar fracture malunions, as well as sequelae from compartment syndrome. In all cases, it leads to increased load/stress to the lateral aspect/lateral column of the affected foot and ankle. This can lead to issues with ankle instability, peroneal tendon pathology, and even stress reactions/fractures of the lateral bones of the foot and ankle.

History

- Foot deformity characterized by hindfoot varus and forefoot valgus or pronated position
- Increased pain over lateral border of foot, first metatarsal (MT) head or lateral metatarsal heads
- High arch
- Stress fractures of fifth metatarsal
- Lateral ankle instability
- Family history of similar foot shape
- History of Charcot-Marie-Tooth (CMT)

Physical Examination

- "Peek-a-boo heel" sign on standing examination: positive test is when patient's heel pad is visible from the front with feet aligned straight ahead
- May have abnormal callus formation at plantar first MT head and lateral border of foot
- Decreased strength with dorsiflexion and eversion with CMT[1]
- Coleman block testing to assess flexibility of deformity and pronation of forefoot: heel varus is correctable or flexible if hindfoot alignment corrects with use of 2.5- to 4-cm thick Coleman block placed under the lateral border of the foot allowing first, second, and third metatarsal to drop
- May have tenderness over peroneal tendons

Imaging

- Radiographs: weight-bearing ankle (AP/mortise/lateral) and foot (AP/lateral/oblique) (Fig. 8.24)

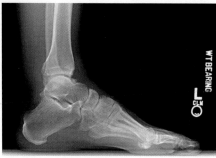

Fig. 8.24 Lateral Radiograph of Cavovarus Foot. Note increased calcaneal pitch.

Classification: Table 8.6

TABLE 8.6   Classification of Cavovarus Foot Deformity
Neurologic
Hereditary sensory & motor neuropathies
Cerebral palsy
Cerebrovascular accident
Spinal root injury
Traumatic
Compartment syndrome
Peroneal nerve injury
Knee dislocation (neurovascular injury)
Talar neck malunion
Residual Clubfoot
Idiopathic

Initial Management

- **Patient Education.** The goal of treatment is to improve gait and prevent overload that may contribute to ankle instability, peroneal tendinitis, stress fractures, and arthritic joints. Surgery is indicated to rebalance tendons and muscle control to prevent deterioration of the foot.
- Initiate neurologic and genetic testing if indicated.
- Initiate orthotic management if flexible deformity.
- Refer to orthopaedic surgeon for recurrent symptoms or injury and for surgical evaluation.

Nonoperative Management

- Orthotics—custom versus modifying OTC inserts
- AFO brace—indicated for patients with muscle imbalance

Operative Management
ICD-10

    Q66.1 Cavovarus deformity of the foot

Surgery may involve tendon transfers and corrective osteotomy for fusion, with the goal to improve function and decrease the risk of injury and progressive foot deterioration.[2]

Indications
- Presence of progressive deformity due to muscular imbalance
- Continued pain or injury despite appropriate conservative management

Informed consent and counseling
- Risks of surgery include nonunion or malunion of bony procedures and the continued need for brace or orthotic management.
- The patient may require extensive physical therapy after surgery.

Anesthesia
- General anesthesia with regional nerve block

Patient positioning
- Supine
- Nonsterile tourniquet on upper thigh

Surgical Procedures

There are multiple surgical procedures considered for the treatment and correction of cavovarus foot alignment. Surgical interventions are often a combination of soft tissue and bony procedures, which are numerous. Patient specific indications and surgeon preference dictate type of procedure(s) used for correction procedures. Surgery entails soft tissue release and tendon lengthening, as well as tendon transfer. Osteotomies of the calcaneus, midfoot, dorsiflexion of first ray, talar neck, and lateral column shortening procedures are often used in conjunction. May also consider fusion/arthrodesis procedures along with clawtoe reconstruction. Postoperative recovery times may vary considerably, depending on patient and surgical procedure.

SUGGESTED READINGS

Manoli A, Graham B: The subtle cavus foot, "The Underpronator," a review, *Foot Ankle Int* 26:256–263, 2005.

Miller MD, editor: *Review of orthopedics*, ed 7, Philadelphia, PA, 2015, Saunders.

Grear BJ: Neurogenic disorders, Chapter 87, e 2. In Beaty JH, Azar FM, Canale ST, Authors. *Campbell's operative orthopedics*, Elsevier, pp 4345–4381, 2020.

REFERENCES

1. Guyton G: Current concepts review: orthopaedic aspects of Charcot-Marie-Tooth disease, *Foot Ankle Int* 27:1003–1010, 2006.
2. Younger A, Hansen S: Adult cavovarus foot, *J Am Acad Orthop Surg* 13:302–315, 2005.

HALLUX RIGIDUS

Hallux rigidus refers to degenerative changes to the articular cartilage of the first MTP joint. The development of this condition can lead to decreased ROM and increased discomfort in the joint that can hinder weight-bearing activities. There are conservative and surgical options available that can improve symptoms and overall function.

History

- Osteoarthritis of the first MTP joint
- Insidious onset of pain and stiffness at the great toe MTP joint
- Presence of dorsal bony prominence can cause pain with shoe wear and impingement with activities
- Patient may complain of lateral foot pain due to compensatory overload

Physical Examination

- Decreased motion, especially dorsiflexion
- Pain with motion, initially with terminal dorsiflexion and plantarflexion progressing to pain and crepitus with midrange motion as disease progresses
- Evidence of dorsal bony prominence at MTP joint
- Antalgic gait
- Note evidence of transfer metatarsalgia, lesser toe deformities, or foot malalignment

Imaging

- Radiographs: weight-bearing foot—AP, lateral, and oblique (Fig. 8.25)

Radiographic Classification

- Grade I: mild to moderate osteophyte formation with preservation of joint space
- Grade II: moderate osteophyte with joint space narrowing and subchondral sclerosis
- Grade III: marked osteophyte with severe loss of joint space and subchondral cyst formation

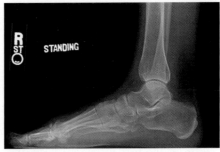

Fig. 8.25 Lateral Foot X-Ray Demonstrating Dorsal Osteophyte Formation.

Initial Management

- **Patient Education.** Hallux rigidus is one of the most common disorders of the great toe and the most common form of arthritis in the foot. The exact etiology is unclear because many biomechanical and structural factors may play a role in its development.[1]
- Engage in shoe modifications, activity modifications, ice, and antiinflammatories.
- Refer to orthopaedic surgeon for surgical consult as needed.

Nonoperative Management

- Use of shoe with adequate width and height to accommodate dorsal bony prominence
- Carbon fiber plate/Morton's extension or rigid soled shoe
- Intermittent corticosteroid injections

Operative Management

ICD-10

    M20.20 Hallux rigidus

CPT

    28289 Cheilectomy—First MTP

    28750 Arthrodesis—First MTP

Indications

- Failed nonoperative treatment

Informed consent and counseling

- Risks of surgery include infection, nerve trapped in scar, progression of arthritis, and need for further surgery, such as arthrodesis, if pain continues.
- It is important to discuss the objectives of surgery with the patient. In case of cheilectomy, the arthritic joint still remains; therefore, pain may still be present when stressed.

Anesthesia

- General anesthesia with regional or local block

Patient positioning

- Supine
- Nonsterile tourniquet on upper thigh

Surgical Procedures

There are two surgical considerations for hallux rigidus/first MTP joint arthritis. Cheilectomy consists of bone spur excision of the first metatarsal head and proximal phalanx, and is indicated for grade I and grade II arthritis. First MTP arthrodesis is indicated for grade III arthritis, arthritis in addition to hallux valgus deformity, failed prior surgical intervention, or underlying rheumatoid arthritis or other neuromuscular conditions. Both procedures occur via a dorsal longitudinal incision made over the first MTP joint. The extensor hood and joint capsule are incised, and deep dissection is done either lateral or medial to the EHL. Thorough synovectomy is performed, and osteophytes are located. The joint is inspected to assess cartilage loss. The metatarsal osteophyte is resected on the dorsal, dorsomedial, and dorsolateral aspects using an osteotome or rongeur. Articular cartilage irregularities including loose bodies are assessed and removed. If adequate articular cartilage remains, cheilectomy is carried out with the goal of achieving 60 degrees of dorsiflexion. If there is significant cartilage loss/eburnation, proceed with first MTP arthrodesis via a cross screw fixation or dorsal plate and screw construct.[2] The joint capsule is sutured, followed by subcutaneous and skin closure. A dry bulky dressing and a postoperative shoe are applied. The patient may be heel weight bearing or full weight bearing depending on the surgeon's preference.

Estimated Postoperative Course

Postoperative 2 weeks:

- Sutures are removed.
- The patient may transition back into a regular shoe and start activities as tolerated. Active ROM is encouraged.

Maximal medical improvement can take up to 3 to 4 months to achieve.

SUGGESTED READINGS

Mann R: Disorders of the first metatarsophalangeal joint, *J Am Acad Ortho Surg* 3:34–43, 1995.

Miller MD, editor: *Review of orthopedics*, ed 7, Philadelphia, PA, 2015, Saunders.

Murphy GA: Disorders of the Hallux, Chapter 82, e 7. In Beaty JH, Azar FM, Canale ST, Authors. *Campbell's operative orthopedics*, Elsevier, pp 4041–4153, 2020.

REFERENCES

1. Yee G, Lau J: Current concepts review: hallux rigidus, *Foot Ankle Int* 29:637–646, 2008.
2. Coughlin M: In *Mann's Surgery of the foot and ankle*, ed 9, Philadelphia, 2014, Mosby.

HALLUX VALGUS

Hallux valgus (bunion) is a common, painful orthopaedic foot and ankle deformity. A hallux valgus deformity occurs when there is medial deviation of the first metatarsal and lateral deviation of the first toe (hallux). With lateral migration of the first toe, there is plantar lateral migration of the abductor hallucis which leads to plantar flexion and pronation of the first toe. The condition can lead to painful motion of the joint and shoe wear difficulty. Most hallux valgus deformities can be treated with shoe-wear modifications, orthotics, and bunion splints. Surgery is indicated for deformities recalcitrant to conservative measures in order to improve the patient's pain and overall function.

History

- Lateral deviation of the great toe with medial deviation of the first metatarsal, commonly known as a "bunion"
- Pain over medial eminence of first metatarsal with shoe wear, especially narrow toe box shoes
- Other locations of pain include within first MTP joint, plantar aspect of second metatarsal head, and with impingement of the first toe onto the second
- May be present since childhood and/or worsening deformity over time
- Cosmetic deformity

Physical Examination

- Note severity of hallux valgus deformity and presence of pes planus while patient is weight bearing.
- Note skin changes (erythema, skin breakdown, callus formation).
- Assess pain over medial eminence, with first MTP joint motion and first TMT joint laxity.

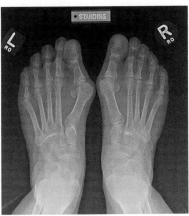

Fig. 8.26 Anteroposterior View of Bilateral Hallux Valgus Deformities.

- Evaluate second MTP joint for synovitis, second toe deformity, and metatarsal head overload.

Imaging

- Weight-bearing foot radiograph (AP, lateral, oblique) (Fig. 8.26)
- Measure hallux valgus angle (HVA)—intersection of longitudinal axes of diaphysis of first metatarsal and proximal phalanx
- Measure intermetatarsal angle (IMA)—angle between diaphysis of first and second metatarsals

Classification

- Mild: HVA less than 30 degrees and IMA less than 10 to 15 degrees
- Moderate: HVA 30 to 40 degrees and IMA 10 to 15 degrees
- Severe: HVA greater than 40 degrees and IMA greater than 15 to 20 degrees

Initial Management

- **Patient Education.** The cause of a bunion is thought to be multifactorial and largely due to shoe/foot size mismatch, some genetic predisposition, and from repetitive forces applied to the first MTP joint. Only surgery can correct the deformity, but patients' symptoms can be significantly relieved with appropriate conservative management.[1]
- Initially advise patient of proper accommodative shoe wear to include wider toe box and use of shoe stretchers.
- Refer to orthopaedic surgeon if patient has failed appropriate conservative treatment.

Nonoperative Management

- The main goal is symptomatic relief only, but it will not permanently correct the deformity.
- Shoe modifications include shoes with a wider toe box and use of shoe stretcher or ball and ring stretcher.
- Use devices such as toe spacers, bunion sleeve, and padding over medial eminence.

Operative Management

ICD-10

    M20.10 Acquired hallux valgus

CPT

    28296 Hallux valgus—distal/proximal osteotomy

    28297 Hallux valgus—Lapidus procedure

    28750 First MTP fusion

    Operative indications

- Pain recalcitrant to appropriate nonoperative treatment

    Informed consent and counseling

- There are more than 100 described bunion surgeries.
- Risks/complications of surgery include reoccurrence of deformity or residual deformity, stiffness at the first MTP joint, and inability to return to level of activity before surgery.
- Surgery should not be done to achieve unlimited shoe wear potential.

    Anesthesia

- Surgeon and patient discretion, likely general anesthesia with regional block

    Patient positioning

- Supine
- Nonsterile tourniquet

Surgical Procedures

Surgical management of hallux valgus deformities can vary. The degree of deformity usually dictates the surgical procedure of choice. Mild to moderate deformity requires distal soft tissue and bony alignment procedure. Severe deformity with increased intermetatarsal deviation requires a proximal procedure (Lapidus) with associated distal soft tissue procedures. If patient has noted concurrent hallux rigidus or underlying rheumatoid arthritis, proceed with MTP joint arthrodesis.

Mild to moderate deformity often requires only distal alignment procedure. A distal Chevron osteotomy (Fig. 8.27) occurs via a longitudinal incision made over the medial eminence with dissection down to the joint

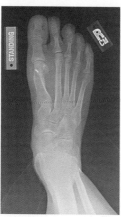

Fig. 8.27 Distal Chevron Osteotomy for Hallux Valgus Correction.

capsule. Full-thickness dorsal and plantar skin flaps are created, being careful to avoid the dorsomedial and plantar medial cutaneous nerve. An L-shaped, distally based capsular flap is made for distal soft tissue release. The type of osteotomy performed varies per surgeon preference. The medial eminence is resected using an oscillating saw parallel to the medial border of the foot. An oscillating saw is used for the horizontal osteotomy in the metaphyseal region with a divergent angle of approximately 60 degrees. Care must be taken to avoid over penetrating the lateral cortex and entering the soft tissues, which may compromise the metatarsal head blood supply. The osteotomy is displaced by approximately 30% of the metatarsal's width. The capital fragment is impacted and fixated on the proximal fragment, with a Kirschner wire or screw fixation, directed from proximal dorsal to distal plantar with care not to penetrate the MTP.[2] Any bony prominence is beveled with a saw. The medial capsule is repaired with interrupted absorbable sutures with the toe in neutral position. Skin closure is per surgeon's preference. Dry, compressive dressing is applied with a postoperative shoe, making sure to provide adequate dressing between the first and second toes to maintain first ray alignment and reduce stress across the surgical site.

Estimated Postoperative Course

Postoperative 1 to 2 weeks:

- Postoperative dressing removed and bunion dressing applied if indicated; change every week for 10 days for 8 weeks.
- Sutures removed 2 to 3 weeks postoperative.

- Immobilization in a postoperative shoe or CAM boot, weight bearing through heel only.

Postoperative 4 weeks:

- Kirschner wire removed.

Postoperative 6 to 8 weeks:

- Discontinue bunion dressing, if indicated.
- Transition into full weight bearing in postoperative shoe or CAM boot.
- Initiate ROM at first MTP joint to prevent stiffness and pain.

Postoperative 10 to 12 weeks:

- Transition into regular shoe as tolerated.
- Increase activities as tolerated.

Board Review

Bunion deformity (hallux valgus) of the first toe is the most common deformity of the MTP joint, with lateral deviation of the proximal phalanx. They are more common in women than men, often caused by wearing tight, pointed-toe footwear. Other causes include congenital deformity and systemic diseases such as rheumatoid arthritis.

SUGGESTED READINGS

Coughlin M, editor: *Mann's surgery of the foot and ankle*, ed 9, Philadelphia, 2014, Mosby.

Miller MD, editor: *Review of orthopedics*, ed 7, Philadelphia, PA, 2015, Saunders.

Murphy GA: Disorders of the Hallux, Chapter 82, e 7. In Beaty JH, Azar FM, Canale ST, Authors. *Campbell's operative orthopedics*, Elsevier, pp 4041–4153, 2020.

REFERENCES

1. Easley M, Trnka H-J: Current concepts review: hallux valgus part I: pathomechanics, clinical assessment, and non-operative treatment, *Foot Ankle Int* 28:654–659, 2007.
2. Easley M, Trnka H-J: Current concepts review: hallux valgus part II: operative treatment, *Foot Ankle Int* 28:748–758, 2007.

POSTERIOR TIBIAL TENDON DYSFUNCTION OR ACQUIRED ADULT FLATFOOT DEFORMITY (AAFD)

Posterior tibial tendon insufficiency is a common pathology affecting more women than men, and can lead to significant disability. It is commonly referred to as flatfoot deformity (pes planus). The posterior tibial tendon is the main dynamic stabilizer of the midfoot and arch. Insufficiency/acquired laxity of the posterior tibial tendon can lead to progressive flatfoot deformity, whereby the hindfoot bones sublux with respect to the talus. Conservative treatment consists largely of orthotic usage. Surgical management can vary significantly and is dictated by whether the flatfoot deformity is fixed versus flexible, if the forefoot is abducted or the medial column is stable or unstable, and the nature of the spring ligament. It is important to realize the deformity occurs in multiple planes and at multiple joint levels.

History

- Gradual-onset medial hindfoot pain and swelling caused by lateral impingement in the subfibular and sinus tarsi region
- Pain increases with activity
- Gait disturbance to include inability to run, push off, and do heel raise
- Also known as "fallen arches"/flatfoot deformity.

Physical Examination

- Flatfoot deformity on affected side to include flattening of medial longitudinal arch, hindfoot valgus, and abduction of midfoot onto hindfoot
- "Too many toes" sign: When examining standing patient from the rear, most of the lesser toes are visible because of midfoot abduction
- Edema, thickness, tenderness to palpation over posterior tibial tendon (PTT), subfibular region, and sinus tarsi
- Inability to do single heel raise
- Assess ROM of hindfoot for flexible or rigid deformity and dorsiflexion ROM for equinus contracture

Imaging

- Radiographs: Weight-bearing foot (AP/oblique/lateral) and ankle (AP/mortise/lateral) (Figs. 8.28 and 8.29).

Additional Imaging

- MRI: not needed to make diagnosis; can be ordered to assess status of soft tissues (i.e., PTT, spring ligament, deltoid ligament)

Classification System

- Stage I—No deformity
- Stage IIa—Mild/moderate flexible deformity

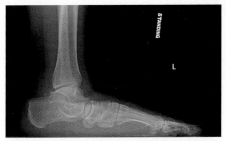

Fig. 8.28 Lateral Radiograph Demonstrating Pes Planus.

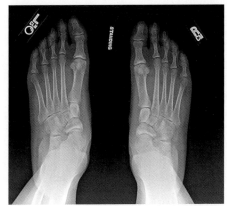

Fig. 8.29 Anteroposterior Radiograph Demonstrating Talar Uncovering.

- Stage IIb—Severe flexible deformity
- Stage III—Fixed deformity
- Stage IV—Includes ankle deformity (lateral talar tilt)
- Stage IVa—Flexible foot deformity
- Stage IVb—Fixed foot deformity

Initial Management

- Acute exacerbation treated in CAM boot, NSAIDs, ice.
- Refer to orthopaedics for orthotic and surgical management.
- **Patient Education.** Deformity can be effectively treated nonoperatively, but surgery may be indicated if deformity and pain progress.[1]

Nonoperative Management

- Custom orthotics with flexible deformity with goal to support the longitudinal arch and decrease hindfoot valgus
- Custom ankle bracing to include Arizona or AFO for rigid deformity[2]
- Physical therapy may be beneficial in the early stages

Operative Management

ICD-10

M21.40 Pes Planus/Flat foot

M66.879/ M76.829 Posterior tibial tendon rupture/ dysfunction

CPT

28300 Medial slide calcaneal osteotomy

27691 Posterior tibial tendon reconstruction with FDL to navicular

27687 Gastrocnemius recession

Indications

- Failed appropriate nonoperative management with continued pain and deformity

Informed consent and counseling

- Risks to include infection, nerve injury, nonunion or malunion, and persistent pain and deformity[3]

Anesthesia

- General anesthesia with regional nerve block, likely popliteal

Patient positioning

- Supine
- Nonsterile tourniquet on upper thigh

Surgical Procedures

Several surgical options are available dependent upon degree of deformity. Posterior tibial tenosynovectomy is indicated for stage I deformity. Flatfoot reconstruction occurs via medial slide calcaneal osteotomy, FHL augmentation of PTT, gastrocnemius recession, ± lateral column lengthening and medial column fusion and is indicated for stage II flexible deformity. A triple arthrodesis (arthrodesis of the subtalar, talonavicular, and calcaneocuboid joints) is indicated for rigid deformity.

Flatfoot reconstruction (Fig. 8.30) is performed via an incision from the posterosuperior to anteroinferior along the lateral aspect calcaneus, dissecting down to the calcaneus with careful consideration of the sural nerve. An osteotomy is performed at a 45-degree angle to its longitudinal axis. Posterior segment is translated medially, and temporarily fixated with Kirschner wire, followed by one to two cannulated screws. A second incision is made from the tip of the medial malleolus extending distally to the navicular. The PTT sheath is incised and the tendon exposed. Tendon is examined and débrided as indicated. Flexor digitorum longus (FDL) is located deep to the PTT by flexing and extending toes; once located, the tendon sheath is incised. The FDL is traced distally into the foot until

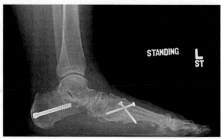

Fig. 8.30 Lateral Weight-Bearing Radiograph Demonstrating Calcaneal Osteotomy.

the fibrous connection between the FDL and FHL is reached, where a side-to-side tenodesis is performed. A Krakow suture technique is used at the distal aspect of the FDL. The dorsomedial aspect of the navicular bone is exposed in anticipation of tendon transfer. The FDL is passed inferior to superior through the navicular and appropriately tensioned using nonabsorbable suture. Gastrocnemius recession is then performed as indicated. All incisions are sutured; a posterior mold/ sugar tong splint is applied.

Estimated Postoperative Course

Postoperative 2 weeks:

- Postoperative dressing is removed, sutures removed.
- Patient placed in non–weight-bearing short leg cast or removable CAM boot.

Postoperative 6 weeks:

- Initiate weight bearing in CAM boot.
- Rehabilitation exercises to include ankle dorsiflexion and plantarflexion.

Postoperative 12 weeks:

- Transition from CAM to tennis shoe with ASO ankle brace as indicated.
- Allowed to initiate non–weight-bearing exercise.
- Evaluate need for custom orthotics.

SUGGESTED READINGS

Coughlin M: In *Mann's surgery of the foot and ankle*, ed 9, Philadelphia, 2014, Mosby.

Miller MD, editor: *Review of orthopedics*, ed 7, Philadelphia, PA, 2015, Saunders.

Grear BJ: Disorders of tendons and fascia and adolescent and adult pes planus, Chapter 83, e 10. In Beaty JH, Azar FM, Canale ST, Authors. *Campbell's operative orthopedics*, Elsevier, pp 4154–4226, 2020.

REFERENCES

1. Deland J: Adult-acquired flatfoot deformity, *J Am Acad Orthop Surg* 16:399–406, 2008.
2. Haddad S, Myerson M, Younger A, et al.: Adult acquired flatfoot deformity, *Foot Ankle Int* 32:95–111, 2011.
3. Pinney S, Lin S: Current concept review: acquired adult flatfoot deformity, *Foot Ankle Int* 27:66–75, 2006.

SUBTALAR JOINT DISLOCATION

Subtalar joint dislocations are relatively rare injuries. They are usually the result of a high-energy trauma; therefore 90% of subtalar dislocations are associated with tarsal bone fractures.[1] Most subtalar dislocations are medial. Reduction of medial dislocations is often obstructed by the extensor digitorum brevis, the extensor retinaculum, and the peroneal tendons. Lateral dislocations are less frequent, but reduction may be obstructed by interposed posterior tibial and FHL tendon. The severity of the original injury closely correlates to subsequent symptomatology, including development of posttraumatic arthritis and associated pain.

History

- Results from high-energy trauma (e.g., MVC, fall from height, sport activity)
- Pain and deformity to affected extremity
- Relatively uncommon injury, less than 1% of all dislocations

Physical Examination

- Inspect for open wounds.
- Determine type of deformity present: medial, lateral, anterior, or posterior.
- Assess neurovascular status to include a dorsalis pedis pulse and sensation to superficial peroneal nerve, deep peroneal nerve, sural, saphenous, and tibial nerves.
- Assess for associated injuries.

Imaging

- Radiographs: initial and postreduction—ankle (AP/mortise/lateral) and foot (AP/lateral/oblique) (Fig. 8.31)

Additional Imaging

- CT scan: evaluation for osteochondral injuries and occult trauma

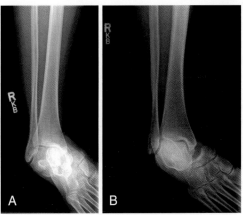

Fig. 8.31 Subtalar dislocation anteroposterior view (**A**) and oblique view. Note dislocation at talonavicular joint (**B**).

Classification

- Dislocation at the talonavicular joint with intact calcaneocuboid and tibiotalar joints
- Medial: inversion force, most common
- Lateral: eversion force, usually associated with concomitant fractures
- Anterior
- Posterior

Initial Management

- Immediate referral to emergency department for prompt evaluation and reduction.
- Postreduction follow-up with orthopaedic surgeon.

Nonoperative Management

- Closed reduction under sedation: Traction is placed on the foot and heel in line with the deformity. Countertraction is applied with the knee in flexion to relax the gastrocnemius. For medial dislocations, the foot is abducted and ankle is dorsiflexed. For lateral dislocations, the foot is adducted and the ankle is dorsiflexed.
- Immobilize patient in non–weight-bearing short leg cast for 4 to 6 weeks, followed by protected mobilization and weight bearing.

Operative Management

ICD-10

    S93.316A Closed dislocation of subtalar/tarsal joint

CPT

    27846 Open treatment of ankle dislocation, w or w/o percutaneous skeletal fixation, w or w/o repair or internal fixation

27848 Open treatment of ankle dislocation, w or w/o percutaneous skeletal fixation; with repair or internal or external fixation

Indications

- If unsuccessful closed reduction and/or open dislocation

Informed consent and counseling

- Associated foot and ankle injuries are common and can lead to future pain and morbidity.
- Restriction of subtalar joint motion and progression of posttraumatic arthritis are common.[2]

Anesthesia

- General anesthesia

Patient positioning

- Supine

Surgical Procedures

Subtalar dislocations may be difficult to reduce. If unable to reduce medial subtalar dislocation, often reduction is obstructed by extensor digitorum brevis, the extensor retinaculum, and peroneal tendons.[3] If unable to reduce lateral subtalar dislocation, reduction is obstructed by the interposed posterior tibial tendon and FHL tendon. Surgical intervention is warranted if closed reduction cannot be obtained or maintained. Surgery entails irrigation and débridement with rigid fixation such as ORIF and/or external fixator, if needed.

Estimated Postoperative Course

- Immobilization in non–weight-bearing short leg cast for 4 to 6 weeks followed by protected immobilization and weight bearing
- Physical therapy as needed after cast removal to improve ROM of subtalar joint

SUGGESTED READINGS

Jones CB, Wenke JC: *Skeletal trauma: basic science, management, and reconstruction,* Elsevier, 2015.
Miller MD, editor: *Review of orthopedics,* ed 7, Philadelphia, PA, 2015, Saunders.

REFERENCES

1. Bibbo C, Anderson B, Davis WH: Injury characteristics and clinical outcomes of subtalar dislocations: a clinical and radiographic analysis of 25 cases, *Foot Ankle Int* 24:158–163, 2003.
2. DeLee J, Curtis R: Subtalar dislocation of the foot, *J Bone Joint Surg Am* 64:433–437, 1982.
3. Heppenstall R, Farahvar H, Balderston R, et al.: Evaluation and management of subtalar dislocations, *J Trauma* 20:494–497, 1980.

CALCANEAL FRACTURES

The calcaneus is the largest of the tarsal bones of the foot. It articulates with the talus through the posterior, middle, and anterior facets. The largest and most important of these is the posterior facet. Calcaneal fractures are typically the result of a significant axial load, impacting the talus into the calcaneus. This mechanism often leads to articular incongruity, a widened heel with varus angulation, and loss of calcaneal height. Calcaneal fractures are challenging injuries with significant impact on long-term morbidity. Patient education is one of the keys to optimizing management/care of the patient with a calcaneal fracture.

History

- High-energy, axial load such as fall from height or MVC
- Pain in heel, inability to bear weight
- Most common tarsal bone fracture, approximately 2% of all fractures[1]

Physical Examination

- Edema and hematoma of hindfoot and ankle, possible deformity
- Tenderness to palpation in heel
- Associated injuries possible (e.g., low back pain/injury)

Imaging

- Radiographs: ankle (AP/mortise/lateral) and foot (AP/oblique/lateral) and Harris view (Fig. 8.32)

Additional Imaging

- CT: used to evaluate fracture for preoperative planning

Classification
Sanders Classification

- Type I: extraarticular, nondisplaced
- Type II: one displaced fracture line
- Type III: two displaced fracture lines
- Type IV: three or more displaced fracture lines

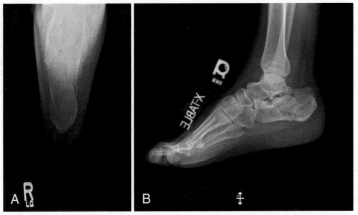

Fig. 8.32 Harris view (**A**) and lateral radiograph of calcaneus fracture (**B**).

Initial Management

- Immobilize affected extremity in non–weight-bearing posterior and stirrup splint.
- Refer to orthopaedic surgeon for management.
- **Patient Education.** Calcaneus fractures are notoriously bad injuries with a high probability of developing posttraumatic arthritis. The goal of operative intervention is to restore anatomy and prevent severity of arthritis in the future.

Nonoperative Management

Indications

- Nondisplaced or minimally displaced fractures; local or systemic contraindications to surgery
  - Non–weight-bearing splint, cast, or CAM boot for 6 weeks, followed by weight bearing in boot for additional 4 to 6 weeks
  - Subtalar joint ROM initiated after 2 to 6 weeks of treatment

Operative Management

ICD-10
  S92.009A Closed fracture of calcaneus
CPT
  28415 ORIF calcaneus fracture

Indications

- Displaced intraarticular fracture with joint displacement greater than 1 mm
- Extraarticular fractures with significant hindfoot valgus/varus or considerable flattening, broadening, or shortening of the heel

- Primary subtalar fusion in case of highly comminuted fractures where restoration of joint is impossible

Informed consent and counseling

- Risks of surgery include but are not limited to surgical wound infection, malunion/nonunion, and nerve injury.
- The patient may need subtalar fusion in the future if he or she has persistent pain and evidence of posttraumatic osteoarthritis of subtalar joint.
- Maximal medical improvement can take up to 1 year to achieve.

Anesthesia

- General anesthesia with ankle or popliteal block

Patient positioning

- Lateral decubitus on noninjured side
- Nonsterile tourniquet on upper thigh

Surgical Procedure

ORIF of the calcaneus options vary with extent/fracture pattern and degree of soft tissue involvement. ORIF calcaneus through a minimally invasive sinus tarsi approach[2] is ideally performed shortly after injury (within 1 week) as fracture fragments are more mobile. ORIF calcaneus via an extended lateral approach occurs once the soft tissue envelope has stabilized, typically in the 2- to 3-week postinjury timeframe. If the patient's calcaneal fracture is severe with additional soft tissue involvement, a delayed surgical intervention of the primary subtalar arthrodesis with or without bone block distraction may be considered, as described earlier in the chapter.

ORIF of the calcaneus via the minimally invasive sinus tarsi approach occurs via an incision similar to that of subtalar arthrodesis. Fixation options vary per surgeon preference, but often include specially designed wave plate construct. Percutaneous leverage is used to reduce the main tuberosity fracture fragment. A 6.5-mm Schanz screw with a handle is placed into the main portion of tuberosity fragment parallel to its upper aspect. The handle is used to manipulate the fracture fragments to achieve fluoroscopic-guided anatomic reduction. Fracture fragments are fixed with three to six cortical screws introduced independently via stab incisions, or through guide block for wave plate construct. One or two screws are placed into the thalamic portion toward sustenaculum tali to achieve maximum stability. Wound closure is followed by splinting in a well-molded posterior non–weight-bearing splint.

Estimated Postoperative Course

Postoperative 1 to 2 weeks:
- First office visit and wound check. Sutures removed 10 to 14 days postoperatively.
- Placed into immoveable device such as CAM walker boot or bivalve cast.
- Strictly non–weight bearing, may initiate gentle ROM of ankle.

Postoperative 6 weeks:
- Initiate weight bearing in a CAM boot.
- Initiate non–weight bearing ROM subtalar joint out of boot.

Postoperative 12 weeks:
- Transition from boot to tennis shoe.
- Increase therapy to include weight-bearing ROM and strengthening and gait training.
- The patient may initiate non–weight-bearing exercise; no impact for additional 4 to 6 weeks

TALUS FRACTURE

The talus is a unique bone in that 60% of it is covered in cartilage and there are no muscular attachments. The talus is divided into distinct anatomic regions, mainly the body, neck, and head. The vascular supply to the talus is tenuous and often disrupted in case of talar neck fractures. The most common mechanism of injury is high impact axial load causing forceful dorsiflexion of the foot, leading to impaction of the narrow talar neck on the anterior tibia.[3] A thorough understanding of the relationship of fracture pattern and talar vascularity is important when considering operative approaches and planned fixation.

History
- Axial load on plantarflexed foot—talar head fracture
- High-velocity trauma—talar neck fracture
- Ankle inversion, dorsiflexion—lateral process fracture, "snowboarder's fracture"
- Ankle pain, swelling, inability to bear weight

Physical Examination
- Note edema or tenderness over affected area (e.g., talonavicular joint, proximal dorsal foot).
- Assess for deformity or change in normal ankle contours.
- Assess for associated injuries.

Imaging: (Fig. 8.33)
- Radiographs: Foot (AP/lateral/oblique) and ankle (AP/lateral/mortise). May consider Canale's view (foot in maximum equinus, pronated 15 degrees, beam directed at 75-degree angle from horizontal plane) and Broden's view (foot in neutral flexion with leg internally rotated 30 to 40 degrees. The beam is centered over the lateral malleolus; radiographs are taken at 40, 30, 20, and 10 degrees toward patient's head) for further evaluation.

Additional Imaging
- CT: A scan provides better fracture detail, which is useful in assessing comminution, success of reduction, and congruency of subtalar joint.

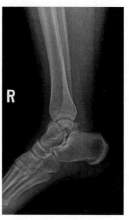

Fig. 8.33 Lateral View, Talar Body Fracture.

TABLE 8.7 **Hawkins Classification of Talar Neck Fractures**
Type I: Nondisplaced
Type II: Displaced with subtalar joint subluxation
Type III: Displaced with dislocation of ankle and subtalar joint
Type IV: Displaced with dislocation at talonavicular joint

Classification

- Talar head
- Talar neck: Hawkins classification (Table 8.7)
- Talar body

Initial Management

- Immobilization in non–weight-bearing posterior/stirrup lower leg splint.
- Referral to orthopaedic surgery for further management.
- **Patient Education.** Treatment of talus fractures provides a difficult challenge because of the large amount of articular surface present, vulnerable blood supply, and crucial biomechanical role in function of the foot and ankle. Injury to the talus puts patients at high risk for osteoarthrosis and osteonecrosis.

Nonoperative Management

Indications

- Talar neck fracture Hawkins type I; stable talar head fracture; talar osteochondral fractures less than 10 mm; nondisplaced talar body fractures less than 2 mm fracture gaping; types I and III lateral process fracture[4]
  - Immobilization in non–weight-bearing short leg cast for 6 to 8 weeks

Operative Management

ICD-10

  S92.109A Closed fracture of talus

CPT

  28445 ORIF talus

Indications

- Unstable talar fracture or risk of significant morbidity with nonoperative treatment

Informed consent and counseling

- Talar fractures can be difficult to treat and can lead to disability despite the appropriate treatment.

- Recovery may require prolonged course of immobilization and non–weight bearing.

Anesthesia

- General anesthesia with regional nerve block

Patient positioning

- Supine
- Nonsterile tourniquet on upper thigh

Surgical Procedures

- ORIF talar neck fracture
- ORIF talar head fracture
- ORIF talar body fracture
- ORIF versus excision of lateral process fracture

Estimated Postoperative Course

Postoperative 1 to 2 weeks:
  - Wound check and suture removal.
  - Placed into non–weight-bearing CAM boot or cast.

Postoperative 6 to 8 weeks:
  - Transition into weight bearing in CAM boot.

Postoperative 12 weeks:
  - Transition from CAM boot to tennis shoe, likely with ASO ankle brace for additional 4 to 6 weeks.
  - Patient can gradually increase activities.
  - Therapy if indicated for ankle and subtalar joint ROM and strengthening.

SUGGESTED READINGS

Jones CB, Wenke JC: *Skeletal trauma: basic science, management, and reconstruction*, Elsevier, 2015.

Kitaoka Harold B: In *Master techniques in orthopaedic surgery: the foot and ankle*, ed 3, Lippincott Williams and Wilkins, 2013.

Levine David: *Hospital for Special Surgery's illustrated tips and tricks in foot and ankle surgery*, Lippincott Williams and Wilkins, 2019.

Miller MD, editor: *Review of orthopedics*, ed 7, Philadelphia, PA, 2015, Saunders.

Rudloff MI: Fractures of the lower extremity, Chapter 54, e 17. In Beaty JH, Azar FM, Canale ST, Authors. *Campbell's operative orthopedics*, Elsevier, pp 2812–2908, 2020.

REFERENCES

1. Rammelt S, Zwipp H: Calcaneus fractures, *Trauma* 8:197–212, 2006.
2. Zhang T, Su Y, Chen W, Zhang Q, Wu Z, Zhang Y: Displaced intra-articular calcaneal fractures treated in a minimally

invasive fashion: longitudinal approach versus sinus tarsi approach, *J Bone Joint Surg Am* 96(4):302–309, 2014.

3. Ahmad J, Raikin S: Current concepts review: talar fractures, *Foot Ankle Int* 27:475–482, 2006.

4. Higgins T, Baumgaertner M: Diagnosis and treatment of fractures of the talus: a comprehensive review of the literature, *Foot Ankle Int* 20:595–605, 1999.

ORTHOPAEDIC PROCEDURES

Ankle Injection/Aspiration

CPT code
20605

Indications
- Arthritis, synovitis, crystal arthropathies

Contraindications
- Infection
- Local skin rash

Equipment Needed
- Sterile gloves
- Topical bactericidal solution
- 18-gauge needle for aspiration, 25-gauge needle for injection
- 5- to 10-mL syringe
- Injectate: 1% lidocaine without epinephrine (4 to 8 mL) and corticosteroid (Celestone or Solumedrol) (1 mL)
- Sterile bandage

Procedure: Fig. 8.34
1. Place patient in supine position with the ankle relaxed.
2. Palpate the anterior joint line between anterior tibial tendon and anterior border of medial malleolus.

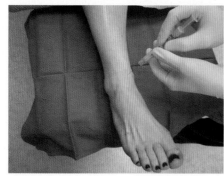

Fig. 8.34 See text for the ankle injection/aspiration procedure.

3. Prepare the skin with a bactericidal agent at the injection site.
4. Using sterile technique, insert needle into identified joint space, aiming posterolateral. Once the needle is in the joint space, there will be reduced resistance, allowing aspiration and/or easy injection of medication.
5. Apply sterile dressing.

Aftercare Instructions
1. Monitor for local erythema, edema, increased pain, or systemic symptoms. Notify clinician.
2. Local anesthetic effect will wear off within a few hours, and corticosteroid will take effect within 3 to 5 days. Patients may experience steroid flare where symptoms may be worse for the first 24 to 48 hours. This can be treated with NSAIDs and ice.
3. The patient should remain in the office for 30 minutes after injection to monitor for adverse effects.
4. He or she should avoid strenuous activity for 48 hours after injection.

Plantar Fasciitis Injection

CPT code
20550

Indications
- Plantar fasciitis not resolved with stretching and inserts

Contraindications
- Foot infection
- Local skin rash
- Allergy to any injection material
- Multiple previous injections to the same area

Equipment Needed
- Sterile gloves
- Bactericidal solution
- 25-gauge needle
- 5- to 10-mL syringe
- Injectate: 1% lidocaine without epinephrine (2 to 3 mL), corticosteroid (1 mL of Celestone or Solumedrol)
- Sterile bandage

Procedure: Fig. 8.35
1. Place the patient in supine or lateral recumbent position on the examination table.

2. Palpate insertion of plantar fascia on the medial, plantar calcaneus.
3. Prepare the medial aspect of the plantar heel with bactericidal solution.
4. Using sterile technique, insert a 25-gauge needle perpendicular to the skin from the medial aspect directly down to midline of the foot. Aspirate to ensure needle is not in a vessel and then slowly inject medication evenly as the needle is slowly withdrawn. Use caution to avoid injecting the calcaneal fat pad.
5. Apply sterile dressing.

Aftercare Instructions
1. Monitor for local erythema, edema, increased pain, or systemic symptoms and notify clinician of any symptoms.
2. Local anesthesia will wear off within a few hours, and the corticosteroid will take effect within 3 to 5 days. Patients may experience steroid flare where symptoms may be worse for the first 24 to 48 hours. This can be treated with NSAIDs and ice.
3. The patient should remain in the office for 30 minutes after injection to monitor for adverse effects.
4. Avoid strenuous activity for at least 48 hours after injection.

Morton's Neuroma Injection
CPT code:
    64455, 64632

Indications
• Pain, paresthesias, and/or burning sensation into toes of affected interdigital nerve
• Positive Mulder click or pain with squeeze of the metatarsal heads

• Continued pain despite other appropriate treatment to include NSAIDs, ice, and orthotics

Contraindications
• Local skin irritation or infection
• Allergy to anesthetic or steroid

Equipment Needed
• Topical cleansing agent (e.g., Betadine)
• Sterile gloves
• Syringe, 3- to 5-mL
• 25-gauge needle, 1.5-inch
• Injectate:1 mL Lidocaine (1%) or Bupivacaine (0.25% or 0.5%) and 1 mL steroid (e.g., Celestone, Solumedrol)
• Clean dressing (gauze and tape)

Procedure: Fig. 8.36
1. Place patient in supine position with foot in relaxed neutral position.
2. Palpate area of tenderness and mark location.
3. Apply Betadine.
4. Insert needle on dorsal surface, pointed distal to proximal, at 45-degree angle to skin at marked site until reaching area of fullness. Be careful not to puncture through plantar skin.
5. Aspirate and then inject steroid/anesthetic medication.
6. Withdraw needle, and apply clean dressing.

Aftercare Instructions
1. Patients should remain in the office for 30 minutes after injection to monitor for adverse effects.
2. Patients should avoid any strenuous activity for at least 48 hours after injection.

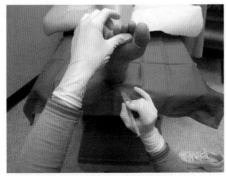

Fig. 8.35 See text for the plantar/fasciitis injection procedure.

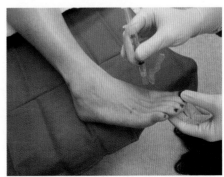

Fig. 8.36 See text for the Morton's neuroma injection procedure.

3. Caution patients on possible steroid flare where symptoms may be worse for the first 24 to 48 hours. This can be treated with NSAIDs and ice.
4. Call the office with any complaints of local erythema or systemic reaction.

Tarsal Tunnel Injection
CPT code
64450

Indications
- Pain, paresthesias, and/or burning sensation over the tibial nerve distribution
- Positive Tinel sign over tibial nerve
- Continued pain despite other appropriate treatment to include NSAIDs, ice, and orthotics

Contraindications
- Local skin irritation or infection
- Allergy to anesthetic or steroid

Equipment Needed
- Topical cleansing agent (e.g., Betadine)
- Sterile gloves
- Syringe, 3- to 5-mL
- 25-gauge needle, 1- to 1.5-inch
- Injectate: 1 to 2 mL Lidocaine (1%) or Bupivacaine (0.25% or 0.5%) and 1 mL steroid (e.g., Celestone or Solumedrol)
- Clean dressing (gauze and tape)

Procedure: Fig. 8.37
1. Place patient in lateral recombinant position.
2. Percuss posterior to medial malleolus to locate area of pain; mark. Also identify PTT.
3. Apply Betadine.

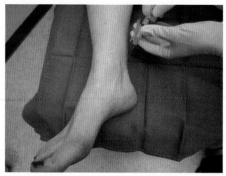

Fig. 8.37 See text for the tarsal tunnel injection procedure.

4. Insert needle, pointed distally, approximately 2 cm proximal to marked location with needle at 30-degree angle to the skin.
5. Aspirate and then inject steroid/anesthetic medication.
6. Withdraw needle, and apply clean dressing.

Aftercare Instructions
1. Patients should remain in the office for 30 minutes after injection to monitor for adverse effects.
2. Patients should avoid any strenuous activity for at least 48 hours after injection.
3. Caution patients on possible steroid flare where symptoms may be worse for the first 24 to 48 hours. This can be treated with NSAIDs and ice.
4. Call the office with any complaints of local erythema or systemic reaction.

ACKNOWLEDGMENTS

The authors would like to acknowledge the contribution of the previous edition authors, Suzanne Eiss and Margaret Schick.

9

Pediatrics

Michelle Post

INTRODUCTION

Development and Growth

- Developmental milestones (Table 9.1)

Lower Extremity Rotational and Coronal Alignment During Growth

- Children progress through development with predictable changes in the rotational and coronal alignment. This is a common cause of parental concern and it is necessary to have a systematic approach to discern normal from abnormal.
- Parental concerns can be addressed with a thorough exam, validation of the presenting complaint, concise explanation of exam findings, and appropriate follow up.
- Take a thorough history to include birth history, family history, developmental milestones, trauma, and serious infection. Take particular notice of an asymmetry in rotational or coronal alignment, which is more likely to be pathologic.

- Rotational profile: The rotation of a child's lower limb changes during the first decade of life with both the tibia and femur rotating externally over time. Intoeing tends to improve over time whereas outtoeing tends to get worse as a child grows.
  - Assess the child's gait first, noticing the **foot progression angle**, which is the angle subtended by the axis of the foot versus the line created by the direction of walking (in-toeing, out-toeing, or neutral), and then evaluate each segment of the lower extremity independently to determine the etiology.
  - Assess **femoral rotation** (version) by determining internal and external hip rotation with the patient prone and the knees flexed to 90 degrees. Increased internal hip rotation may cause the knees to point towards each other during gait and/or the child to in-toe. This also explains a child's ability to "W" sit and "egg beater" run. Increased external rotation

TABLE 9.1 **Developmental Milestones**		
Milestone	**Age (Months)**	**Consider Further Evaluation if:**
Rolls from back to stomach	3.6 ± 1.4	Not rolling by 6 months
Sits unsupported	6.3 ± 1.2	Not sitting by 8 months
Pull to stand	8.1 ± 1.6	
Walk	11.7 ± 2	Not walking by 18 months
Run	15 ± 3	

Modified from Palmer F: Keys to developmental assessment. In McMillan J, editor: *Oski's pediatrics*, ed 3, Philadelphia, 2006, Lippincott Williams & Wilkins, p 789.

may cause the child to out-toe. Normal internal hip rotation is less than 70 degrees.

- Next assess the **thigh-foot angle**, which is the angle created between the axis of the thigh and the axis of the foot when the child is prone and the knees are flexed to 90 degrees. Thigh-foot angle is used to determine internal or external rotation (version) of the tibia.
- Observe the **foot shape** to assess for forefoot adductus as a cause for in-toeing or calcaneovalgus deformity as a cause for out-toeing. The lateral border of the foot should be straight.
- Coronal alignment: During early childhood, the alignment of the lower extremities follows a predictable pattern. When children start walking, the legs are in varus alignment. By age 2, the alignment changes into valgus alignment. Persistent genu varum beyond age 18 months that is unilateral and progressive is concerning for Blount's disease or Ricket's disease and warrants a full length x-ray of both lower extremities to assess the proximal tibial physis and overall alignment. Usually by age 8, the legs are neutral. Order a bilateral lower extremity standing x-ray if the distance between the knees (intracondylar distance) or the distance between the ankles (intramalleolar distance) is greater than 9 cm with the patient standing and the ankles or knees, respectively, barely touching.
- Treatment of coronal and rotational problems is rarely necessary with less than 1% of femoral and tibial deformities that do not resolve with observation alone. Twister cables, braces, shoe wedges, and night splints have all been shown to be ineffective. Operative treatment, if needed, includes guided growth procedures for persistent coronal plane deformity and rotational osteotomy for persistent rotational deformity.

Structure and Function of Bone

- Basic bone anatomy—children's bones are more porous than adults, which creates different fracture patterns than those seen in adults.
  - Epiphysis—This region of bone is closest to a joint and lined with articular cartilage.
    - Ossification of the child's epiphysis depends on age and location: Distal femoral, proximal tibial, and proximal humeral epiphysis are ossified at birth.

- Ossification of the elbow epiphysis follows a sequence in pneumonic. Remember CRITOE and 1,3,5,7,9,11 for a rough age guideline for evaluating elbow radiographs:
  - **C**—capitellum: ossifies around 1 year
  - **R**—radial head: ossifies around 3 years
  - **I**—internal (medial) epicondyle: ossifies around 5 years
  - **T**—trochlea: ossifies around 7 years
  - **O**—olecranon: ossifies around 9 years
  - **E**—external (lateral) epicondyle: ossifies around 11 years
- Fractures through the epiphysis cannot be seen by plain radiograph until they are ossified.
- Physis—also called the "growth plate" is the stripe of cartilage that separates the epiphysis from the metaphysis and is responsible for longitudinal growth of bones. The epiphysis narrows over time and is obliterated normally at skeletal maturity when the epiphysis fuses with the metaphysis.
- Metaphysis—the region of most porous bone that is the transition zone to the shaft of the long bone.
- Diaphysis—the shaft of a long bone.
- Periosteum—the layer of connective tissue that covers the bone. The periosteum is thick and strong in children which helps decrease the risk of fracture displacement and also quickly produces early fracture healing, called callus.

Skeletal Growth

- Skeletal growth over the lifetime is not constant—the rate of growth is highest in the first 4 years and levels off until adolescence.
- Growth proportion varies by anatomic region (i.e., proximal tibial physis contributes more to tibial length than distal tibial physis). Familiarity with the contributions of growth from a particular physis is relevant because it impacts the remodeling potential of displaced fractures as well as the effect of physeal injury on future growth. For instance, the proximal humerus is a very active physis and contributes 80% of the longitudinal growth of the humerus. Angular deformity up to 70 degrees in young children (under 5 years old) and up to 40 degrees in older children (over 12 years old) is acceptable in part because the proximity to an active physis allows for considerable remodeling.

- Longitudinal growth of limbs occurs via endochondral ossification.
  - Endochondral ossification occurs when cartilage cells mature → hypertrophy → calcify → and are replaced by mature bone.
  - Endochondral ossification occurs at the physis, or growth plate, of each bone pushing new bone towards the diaphysis.

- Physeal anatomy:
  - In long bones, the physis is located near a joint, lying in between the epiphysis and metaphysis.
  - Physis contains four continuous zones starting adjacent to the epiphysis to the metaphysis: resting zone (near epiphysis), proliferating zone, hypertrophic zone, and provisional calcification zone (near metaphysis) (Table 9.2).

TABLE 9.2 Physeal Zones

Zone	Resting Zone	Proliferating Zone	Hypertrophic Zone	Provisional Calcification Zone
Actions in the zone	Resting immature chondrocytes supply necessary cells for growth	Chondrocytes grow and divide, and arrange into columns, develop extracellular matrix	Chondrocytes hypertrophy, produce type X collagen, which is important for extracellular matrix calcification	Chondrocytes die, cartilage matrix becomes calcified, which leads to vascular invasion and invasion of osteoblasts and osteoclasts for bone formation
Clinical Pearls	Injury to this zone causes growth arrest	Achondroplastic dwarves have a genetic mutation that prevents cartilage growth in this zone	• Weakest part of physis, fractures tend to propagate through this region • Slipped capital femoral epiphysis occurs in this weak zone • Rickets (vitamin D deficiency) prevents calcification of cells past this zone	Scurvy (severe vitamin C deficiency) causes failure of collagen cross-linking in the transition between this zone and the metaphysis leading to brittleness of this region

TABLE 9.3 Salter-Harris Classification for Growth Plate Injuries

Type	Fig.	Description	Significance
I		Fracture line through the physis only (zone of hypertrophy)	• Low chance of growth disturbance if nondisplaced • Occurs most commonly in hypertrophic zone of physis
II		Fracture line through the physis and extending to include a portion of the metaphysis	• Most common • Variable growth disturbance—depends on location (i.e., rarer in wrist but high in distal femur)
III		Fracture line through the physis and exiting through the epiphysis into a joint	• Variable growth disturbance • Anatomic reduction important as fracture involves joint
IV		Vertical fracture line through the epiphysis, physis, and metaphysis	• Physeal bar formation possible as fracture line traverses cartilage reserve zone of physis • Anatomic reduction important as fracture involves joint
V		Crush injury to the physis	• Rare, hard to distinguish from nondisplaced Salter-Harris type I • High chance of growth disturbance

- Fractures in children require special consideration due to the potential for physeal fractures to cause growth disturbances such as limb length inequality from physeal arrest and deformity from asymmetric growth from development of a physeal bar in one portion of the physis.
- The Salter-Harris classification is for growth plate injuries (Table 9.3).

Fracture Care Principles

- Examine the whole extremity for tenderness, deformity, and limitations in range of motion.
- X-rays need to include the joint above and below the point of tenderness.
- Tenderness at the physis despite normal x-rays warrants immobilization.
- Computed tomography (CT) is used to characterize fractures that are difficult to evaluate with x-ray.
- Articular displacement greater than 2 mm is an indication for surgical consultation.
- For unstable fractures or fractures requiring reduction, x-rays are repeated at 1 and 2 weeks to assess fracture alignment and early callus formation.
- Fracture remodeling is the process whereby a fracture deformity can improve over time in children with open physes.
- Remodeling potential is determined by a patient's age, the proximity of the fracture to the physis, and the percentage of growth that a particular physis contributes to bone growth. For instance, a proximal humerus metaphysis fracture in a 4-year-old will have higher remodeling potential than a mid-shaft diaphyseal humerus fracture in a 12-year-old.
- Re-check x-rays 6 months after fracture healing for fractures that involve the physis to assess for growth arrest and angular deformity. Look for a Park Harris growth arrest line to be parallel to the physis.

SUGGESTED READINGS

Rang M, Stearns P, Chambers H: Radius and ulna. In Wenger DE, Pring ME, editors: *Rang's children's fractures*, Philadelphia, 2005, Lippincott, Williams & Wilkins, pp 135–150.

Staheli L: Spine and pelvis. In *International pediatric orthopedic pocketbook*, Staheli, 2005, Seattle, pp 131–142.

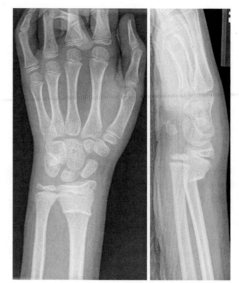

Fig. 9.1 Distal radius fracture in an 8-year-old boy.

PEDIATRIC WRIST FRACTURES

History

- Background: Pediatric distal radius and ulna fractures are common injuries. Younger children generally sustain metaphyseal buckle fractures, whereas older children can sustain distal radius and ulna physeal fractures.
- A fall onto an outstretched hand is the most common mechanism. Most fractures occur with a hyperextended wrist leading to dorsal displacement of the distal fracture fragment.
- The patient may report pain and may have a wrist deformity or swelling.

Physical Examination

- Inspect for significant edema and deformity of the wrist.
- Palpate for significant tenderness at fracture site.
- Perform a careful neurovascular examination.
  - High-energy injuries can be associated with carpal tunnel syndrome.
- Assess the extremity proximal and distal to the injury site to rule out other associated injuries.

Imaging: Fig. 9.1

- Take posteroanterior (PA) and lateral radiographs of the wrist.
- Consider radiographs of the hand, forearm, and elbow to rule out adjacent injuries.

Classification System

- Salter-Harris classification for physeal injuries
- Nondisplaced versus displaced metaphyseal fractures
  - Nondisplaced fractures can be treated in a splint or cast without reduction.
  - Displaced fractures require closed reduction.

Initial Management

- Low-energy trauma and nondisplaced: splint or casting in the outpatient setting
- Higher-energy trauma + displaced injury: closed reduction and splinting under conscious sedation in the emergency department
- **Patient Education.** Physeal arrest is a risk. It can occur in up to 10% of physeal distal radius and ulna fractures. Repeat x-rays 6 months after healing if the physis is involved and look for asymmetric Park Harris growth arrest line, physeal bridge, and ulnar overgrowth.
- For nondisplaced fractures, apply a sugar tong splint without manipulation of the fracture. Provide the patient with an appropriately fitting sling.
- Displaced fractures: Apply a temporary volar splint in a position of comfort. Arrange for the patient to be seen in an acute care setting that will allow for reduction and sedation.

Nonoperative Management

Codes

ICD-10 S52.5 Closed fracture of the distal radius
CPT: 25606 Closed reduction of distal radius fracture

- Closed manipulation and reduction of dorsally displaced distal radius and ulna fracture.
  - After adequate anesthesia is established, the displaced fracture is reduced with slight traction (excessive traction may be counterproductive due to tightening of thick periosteum in children), recreation of the injury force by wrist dorsiflexion, and then volar pressure of the distal fragment. The reduction is held in place manually and confirmed with fluoroscopy. A sugar tong splint or long-arm cast with a three-point mold is then applied to hold the reduction in place.
  - Displacement of the fracture in the splint/cast can occur, and hence repeat radiographs are recommended 1 week after injury and subsequent weeks per discretion of the clinician.
  - Mild residual dorsal angulation (<30 degrees) in children after reduction can remodel with time.

- The splint or cast should be held in place for 4 to 6 weeks. Radiographs should be obtained within 1 week after reduction to confirm that displacement has not occurred. Cast can be discontinued around 1 month when the fracture has healed and the patient is nontender at the injury site. Transition to a removable wrist splint to help prevent re-fracture.

Operative Management

Indications

- Surgical intervention is rare for this injury and is reserved for open fractures, fractures with significant neurovascular compromise, or irreducible fractures

SUGGESTED READINGS

Bae DS: Pediatric distal radius and forearm fractures, *J Hand Surg Am* 33(10):1911–1923, 2008.

Beatty E, Light TR, Belsole RJ, Ogden JA, et al.: Wrist and hand skeletal injuries in children, *Hand Clin* 6(4):723–738, 1990.

Campbell Jr RM: Operative treatment of fractures and dislocations of the hand and wrist region in children, *Orthop Clin North Am* 21(2):217–243, 1990.

de Putter CE, van Beeck EF, Looman CW, et al.: Trends in wrist fractures in children and adolescents, *J Hand Surg Am* 36(11):1810–1815, 2011.

Dolan M, Waters PM: Fractures and dislocations of the forearm, wrist, and hand. In Green NE, Swiontkowski MF, editors: *Skeletal trauma in children*, Philadelphia, 2009, Saunders, pp 159–205.

Rang M, Stearns P, Chambers H: Radius and ulna. In Wenger DE, Pring ME, editors: *Rang's children's fractures*, Philadelphia, 2005, Lippincott Williams & Wilkins, pp 135–150.

Webb GR, Galpin RD, Armstrong DG: Comparison of long and short arm plaster casts for displaced fractures in the distal third of the forearm in children, *J Bone & Joint Surg Am.* 88(1):9–17, 2006.

PEDIATRIC FOREARM FRACTURES

History

- Background: Pediatric forearm fractures include fractures of the diaphysis of the radius and/or ulna. Forearm bony anatomy is unforgiving of significant displacement or malrotation with regard to subsequent range of motion and function.
- Common mechanisms include a fall onto an outstretched hand or direct blow to the forearm.

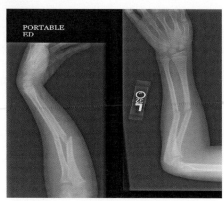

Fig. 9.2 Both bone forearm fracture in a 9-year-old boy.

- Severe pain or neurovascular problems should prompt suspicion for compartment syndrome of the forearm.
- The patient may report forearm pain, swelling, or deformity.

Physical Examination

- Inspect for edema and rotational deformity (a key component to the injury).
  - Inspect for the apex of the deformity, which serves as a clue for malrotation: An apex dorsal deformity suggests a pronation deformity of the distal fragment, whereas an apex volar deformity suggests a supination deformity of the distal fragment.
- Palpate for significant tenderness at the fracture site.
- Perform a careful neurovascular examination.

Imaging: Fig. 9.2

- Anteroposterior (AP) and lateral radiographs of forearm (full length)
- Wrist and elbow radiographs to rule out associated injuries (injuries to the wrist, disruption of the distal radioulnar joint—Galeazzi fracture, radial head dislocation–Monteggia fracture)
- Evaluate images for the apex of the deformity and clues to malrotation including the relationship between the bicipital tuberosity and radial styloid (which should be facing opposite to each other in the normal forearm)

Initial Management

- Forearm fractures are common injuries in children. These injuries must be reduced in near anatomic alignment, or limited range of motion and deformity may develop. Most preadolescents can be treated with casting. Children approaching maturity may be considered for operative open reduction and internal fixation (ORIF).
- Refracture rate is 1.4%, with the highest rate of refracture in patients with mid-shaft forearm fractures with residual fracture angulation of greater than 10 degrees.
- The patient's forearm should be immobilized with a temporary splint until transport to a facility that can offer adequate anesthesia (conscious sedation or general anesthesia) can be arranged.
- All patients with displaced radius and ulna fractures should undergo manipulative reduction or fixation.

Nonoperative Management

- Nonoperative management with closed manipulation under sedation/anesthesia is the mainstay of treatment. Monteggia fractures with plastic deformation or greenstick fracture of the ulna may be treated with closed reduction and immobilization.
- The deformity should be reduced, paying particular attention to the fact that forearm injuries often require reduction of a rotational deformity.
- Acceptable alignment: For age less than 8, up to 20 degrees. For age over 10, less than 10 degrees. Complete translation will remodel in younger children. Bayonet apposition is acceptable.
- A long-arm cast or sugar tong splint with the elbow at 90 degrees with a flat ulna and interosseous mold can be used to hold the reduction. The cast should look more like a rectangle than a cylinder through the forearm segment.
- The patient should be followed up weekly for repeat radiographs for 2 to 3 weeks with cast immobilization for a total of 6 weeks.
- Educate the family that there will be a palpable bump at the fracture site when the cast is removed.

Operative Management

Codes

ICD-10: S52.90XA Closed fracture of radius and ulna
CPT: 25575 ORIF both bone forearm fracture, flexible intramedullary (IM) nailing of both bone forearm fracture

Indications

- Adolescents approaching skeletal maturity should be treated with rigid internal fixation.
- Younger children with displaced fractures for which closed treatment fails to hold acceptable alignment can be treated with flexible IM nailing.
- Monteggia fractures with a complete, length stable ulna fracture should be treated with an IM nail. Complete, length unstable ulna fractures should be treated with open reduction and rigid internal fixation

Informed consent and counseling

- Decreased forearm rotation can occur with non-anatomic reductions.
- Risk of infection and nerve damage can occur with surgical approaches for ORIF.

Anesthesia

- General

Patient positioning

- Supine with operative extremity placed on a hand table. A tourniquet is applied to the operative extremity.

Surgical Procedures

Intramedullary Nailing of Forearm Fracture

- Using C-arm guidance, an appropriate start point is determined for insertion of elastic nail. A nail of 2 to 2.5 mm in diameter is usually used. In the radius, the entry point is 2 cm proximal to the distal physis along the radial border. A small incision is made and bluntly spread down to bone to prevent injury to the superficial branch of the radial nerve. The nail is inserted and passed down the shaft of the radius with the bone held reduced. In the ulna the entry point is 2 cm distal to the apophyseal plate (proximal, along the dorsoradial side). The nails are cut within 6 mm from the bone. A bivalved long-arm cast is placed.

ORIF of Forearm Fracture

- See Chapter 3, page 98, the section on Forearm (Radius and Ulna) Fractures and Dislocations

Estimated Postoperative Course

- Postoperative week 1 and 2: Repeat radiographs.
- Postoperative 6 weeks: Repeat radiographs, discontinue cast; if healing, gradual progression to activities.

SUGGESTED READINGS

Dolan M, Waters PM: Fractures and dislocations of the forearm, wrist, and hand. In Green NE, Swiontkowski MF, editors: *Skeletal trauma in children*, Philadelphia, 2009, Saunders, pp 159–205.

Flynn JM, Jones KJ, Garner MR, Goebel J: Eleven years' experience in the operative management of pediatric forearm fractures, *J Pediatr Orthop* 30(4):313–319, 2010.

Garg NK, Ballal MS, Malek IA, et al.: Use of elastic stable intramedullary nailing for treating unstable forearm fractures in children, *J Trauma* 65(1):109–115, 2008.

Herman MJ, Marshall ST: Forearm fractures in children and adolescents: a practical approach, *Hand Clin* 22(1):55–67, 2006.

Ramski DE, Hennrikus WP, Bae DS, et al.: Pediatric Monteggia fractures: a multicenter examination of treatment strategy and early clinic and radiographic results, *J Pediatr Orthop* 35(2):115–120, 2015.

Rang M, Stearns P, Chambers H: Radius and ulna. In Wenger DE, Pring ME, editors: *Rang's children's fractures*, Philadelphia, 2005, Lippincott Williams & Wilkins, pp 135–150.

Rodriguez-Merchan EC: Pediatric fractures of the forearm, *Clin Orthop Relat Res* 342:65–72, 2005.

Tisosky AJ, Werger NM, McPartland TG, et al.: The factors influencing the refracture of pediatric forearms, *J Pediatr Orthop* 35(7):677–681, 2015.

RADIAL HEAD SUBLUXATION (NURSEMAID'S ELBOW)

History

- Background: Nursemaid's elbow is radial head subluxation with an annular ligament tear and interposition of annular ligament between the radial head and capitellum.
- This is a common injury in young children, where a longitudinal traction force is placed on the child's extended and pronated forearm (i.e., child being helped up onto a sidewalk). The mechanism of injury is key. This is not an injury that happens from a fall on an outstretched hand (FOOSH) mechanism.
- Children affected are usually younger than 5 years old.
- Initially the condition is painful, but it eventually subsides, although the child will guard the extremity with activities.
- The patient or parents may report that the arm is not being used.

Physical Examination

- Inspect for how the child holds the arm, which is usually flexed and pronated.
- Inspect for use of the arm. Pseudoparalysis is possible in very young children due to pain.
- Palpate for tenderness along the radial head. Also palpate throughout the upper extremity to rule out other injuries.
- Perform neurovascular examination and document.

Imaging

- AP and lateral radiographs of elbow to rule out other injuries

Differential Diagnosis

- Fracture
- Shoulder or wrist injury (young children often have difficulty localizing the pain)

Initial Management

- **Patient Education.** Nursemaid's elbow is a common elbow injury in young children. The vast majority of patients improve with closed reduction without future problems.
- If the patient is uncomfortable, immobilize him or her in a posterior splint with the arm in a position of comfort until reduction can be performed.

Nonoperative Management

Codes

ICD-10: S53.03 Nursemaid's elbow
CPT: 24605 Closed reduction of elbow dislocation

Closed Reduction of Radial Head Subluxation: Fig. 9.3

- Under adequate anesthesia, child's forearm is supinated and maximally flexed with the clinician's thumb placed over the radial head.
- A palpable click is often felt on reduction.
- There is no need to immobilize after reduction if this is a first-time reduction. If this is a repeat injury, consider cast immobilization.

Board Review

Radial head subluxation (nursemaid's elbow) should be on the top of the differential diagnoses list for any complaint of elbow pain in a young child especially in the setting of a traction injury.

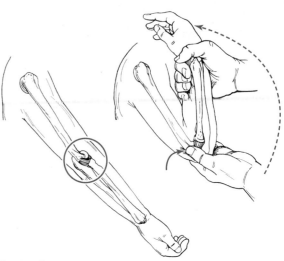

Fig. 9.3 Closed reduction of Nursemaid's elbow. (From Flynn JM, Kolze EA: Upper extremity injuries. In Dormans JP, editor: *Core knowledge in orthopaedics: pediatric orthopaedics*, Philadelphia, 2005, Mosby, p 76.)

SUGGESTED READINGS

Chuong W, Heinrich SD: Acute annular ligament interposition into the radiocapitellar joint in children (nursemaid's elbow), *J Pediatr Orthop* 15(4):454–456, 1995.

Dolan M, Waters PM: Fractures and dislocations of the forearm, wrist, and hand. In Green NE, Swiontkowski MF, editors: *Skeletal trauma in children*, Philadelphia, 2009, Saunders, pp 159–205.

Lewis D, Argall J: Reduction of pulled elbows, *Emerg Med J* 20(1):61–62, 2003.

PEDIATRIC SUPRACONDYLAR HUMERUS FRACTURES

History

- Background: Common elbow injury in children, with location of fracture site above the condyles of the elbow
- Common mechanism of injury is fall onto an outstretched hand or direct blow to the elbow
- Patient may report elbow pain, deformity, or swelling

Physical Examination

- Inspect for deformity and edema, refusal to use the injured arm

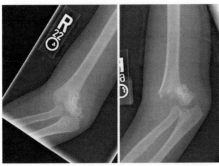

Fig. 9.4 Type III supracondylar humerus fracture in a 5-year-old girl.

- Palpate forearm and evaluate for additional fracture and compartment syndrome. 10% of elbow fractures have a concomitant forearm fracture
- Perform and document a neurovascular examination (critical as major vessels and nerves cross the elbow)

Imaging: Fig. 9.4

- AP, lateral, and oblique radiographs of elbow
  - For nondisplaced or occult fractures, evaluate for the presence of elevated posterior fat pads on the lateral radiograph. Treat for fracture even if x-rays are negative as 76% of children with a history of trauma and elevated posterior fat pad sign have an elbow fracture.
  - The radial head should be opposite the capitellum in all views and the anterior humeral line should intersect the capitellum on the lateral radiograph in a normal elbow.

Classification System

- Flexion- and extension-type injuries depending on whether the arm was flexed or extended at the time of injury; majority of injuries are of the extension type
- Gartland classification (extension-type injuries)—type I: nondisplaced, type II: angulated with an intact posterior cortex, type III: displaced with no intact cortex, type IV: multidirectional instability (determined intraoperatively)

Differential Diagnoses

- Other bony fracture
- Nursemaid's elbow

Initial Management

- **Patient Education.** Supracondylar humerus fractures are the most common elbow injuries in young children, with a 10% to 15% neurovascular injury rate in displaced fractures. These injuries should be evaluated and treated urgently in an emergency department where a pediatric orthopedist is available. The standard of care is to pin displaced fractures.
- Place in a temporary posterior long-arm splint in a position of comfort and send to the emergency department for evaluation.

Nonoperative Management

- Type I injuries: Immobilize initially in a posterior long arm splint and then transition to a long arm cast with the elbow at 70 to 80 degrees. Avoid hyperflexion.
- Type II injuries without significant angulation, intact medial cortex, and in which the anterior humeral line intersects the capitellum: Immobilize initially in a splint and then transition to a cast as indicated earlier.

Operative Management

Codes

ICD-10: S42.413A Closed fracture of supracondylar humerus

CPT: 24538 Closed reduction and percutaneous pinning of supracondylar humerus fracture

Indications

- Any fracture with significant displacement should be treated with closed reduction and percutaneous pinning.
- A patient with a pulseless hand and a supracondylar humerus fracture requires emergent reduction and pinning with reevaluation of vascular status. Persistent pulseless hand with capillary refill greater than 2 seconds warrants open antecubital fossa exploration.

Informed consent and counseling

- Risks of neurovascular injury from pinning can occur, especially to the ulnar nerve with medial-based pins. Most nerve injuries from the initial trauma are neuropraxia and resolve with time. Despite accurate reduction, risk of malunion and elbow deformity can occur.

Anesthesia

- General anesthesia

Patient positioning

- Supine with the patient's arm resting on a draped fluoroscopy machine

Surgical Procedures
Closed Reduction and Percutaneous Pinning of Displaced Supracondylar Humerus Fracture

- The patient's arm is prepped and draped as proximally as possible. The fluoroscopy machine is then draped, and the patient's arm is placed on the base of the fluoroscopy machine.
- Gentle traction is applied to the arm, and varus/valgus angulation is corrected with fluoroscopic guidance. The elbow is then flexed to reduce the extended fracture. The reduction is held in place until pinned.
- Two to three lateral 0.062-inch diverging pins are placed from the lateral condyle engaging the medial diaphyseal cortex to hold the fracture in place.
- The arm is splinted in a long arm posterior splint in approximately 70 degrees of elbow flexion.

Estimated Postoperative Course
- Postoperative days 7 to 10: Repeat radiographs of elbow in splint and transition to long arm cast.
- Postoperative week 3: Repeat radiographs of elbow, cast removal, and pin removal in clinic if radiographs demonstrate acceptable alignment. Anesthesia (local or sedation) is not necessary for pin removal, although it can be anxiety provoking for children and parents.
- Start range of motion at 3 weeks with activity restriction, with gradual progression based on healing.
- Postoperative month 3: Repeat radiographs if necessary and clinical evaluation of range of motion.

Board Review
Supracondylar humerus fractures are the most common elbow injury in children.

SUGGESTED READINGS

Abzug JM, Herman MJ: Management of supracondylar humerus fractures in children: current concepts, *J Am Acad Orthop Surg* 20(2):69–77, 2012.

Brauer CA, Lee BM, Bae DS, et al.: A systematic review of medial and lateral entry pinning versus lateral entry pinning for supracondylar fractures of the humerus, *J Pediatr Orthop* 27(2):181–186, 2007.

Green NE, Van Zeeland NL, et al.: Fractures and dislocations about the elbow. In Green NE, Swiontkowski MF, editors: *Skeletal trauma in children*, Philadelphia, 2009, Saunders, pp 207–282.

Omid R, Choi, PD, Skaggs DL: Supracondylar humeral fractures in children, *J Bone Joint Surg Am* 90(5):1121–1132, 2008.

Rang M, Stearns P, Chambers H: Radius and ulna. In Wenger DE, Pring ME, editors: *Rang's children's fractures*, Philadelphia, 2005, Lippincott Williams & Wilkins, pp 135–150.

Skaggs DL, Mirzayan R: The posterior fat pad sign in association with occult fracture of the elbow in children, *J of Bone & Joint Surg Am*. 81(10):1429–1433, 1999.

Woratanarat P, Angsanuntsukh C, Rattanasirri S, et al.: Meta-analysis of pinning in supracondylar fracture of the humerus in children, *J Orthop Trauma* 26(1):48–53, 2012.

PEDIATRIC FEMUR FRACTURES

Age Range
- Age 0 to 6 months
- Age 6 months to 5 years
- Age 6 years to 11 years
- Age older than 12 years

History
- Background: Femur fractures in children can be related to both low-energy and high-energy mechanisms, including torsional-type injuries and motor vehicle accidents. Child abuse is not an uncommon mechanism of fracture in younger children (16% to 35% in children younger than 1, 1.5% to 6% in children older than 12 months). Be particularly suspicious for nonaccidental trauma in children less than 12 months old, nonambulatory, inconsistent history, or other concomitant injuries.
- Patient characteristics (age and patient size); fracture characteristics (spiral, transverse, comminuted); and mechanism of injury are all important in determining appropriate treatment.
- Patients present with pain and deformity and an impaired ability to bear weight on the affected lower extremity.

Physical Examination
- If a high-energy mechanism occurred, a thorough trauma evaluation is necessary.
- Inspect for evidence of open injury and identify abrasions, edema, and deformity.
- Palpate throughout the lower extremity to evaluate for other injuries.
- Perform and document a neurovascular examination.

Imaging: Fig. 9.5
(Note differences in age and severity of mechanism.)
- AP and lateral radiographs of the femur

Initial Management

- **Patient Education.** The appropriate treatment of pediatric femur fractures includes many variables. Most low-energy mechanism injuries can be treated in a closed fashion in young children. Internal fixation options in older children include intramedullary stabilization options. Common complications can include leg length inequality, malrotation, and angular malunion.
- Initiate a pediatric trauma evaluation for high-energy injuries.
- Immobilize the extremity in a temporary posterior long leg splint.
- Depending on fracture location, the muscles that attach to the fracture fragments may cause varus, valgus, extension, or rotation of the fracture
- Consider pain management and treatment of muscle spasm in the first few weeks until early fracture healing occurs.

Nonoperative Management

- **0 to 6 months**: Apply a Pavlik harness and immobilize the patient for 2 to 3 weeks. Rapid healing with exuberant callous formation is expected. Up to 2 cm of shortening is acceptable in anticipation of femoral overgrowth with fracture healing
- **6 months to 5 years**: Apply a Spica cast under anesthesia **(CPT Code 29325).** Reduce the fracture with fluoroscopic guidance. Acceptable reduction includes up to 15 degrees of varus-valgus angulation, up to 20 degrees of sagittal angulation, and 1 to 2 cm of shortening. Apply a Spica cast positioning the injured extremity in approximately 45 degrees hip flexion and 45- to 60-degree knee flexion. Repeat radiographs within 2 weeks, and continue Spica cast for approximately 6 weeks until healing.
  - Treatment in a Spica cast requires extensive teaching about cast care, diapering, and modifications to the child's car seat

Operative Management

Codes

ICD-10: S72.309 Closed fracture of shaft of femur
CPT: 27506 Intramedullary stabilization of femoral shaft fracture

Indications

- Surgical treatment should be considered in all displaced femoral shaft fractures in the appropriate age group (older than 5 years). For age greater than 10, the acceptable reduction parameters include 5 to 10 degrees of varus-valgus, 10 degrees of angulation in the sagittal plane, and less than 1 cm of shortening.

Informed consent and counseling

- The risk of malunion, leg length discrepancy, and malrotation exists for any treatment type. Decreased tolerance for shortening due to decreased anticipated femoral overgrowth as compared to younger children.

Anesthesia

- General anesthesia

Patient positioning

- Supine positioning on a fracture table

Surgical Procedures

- **5 to 11 years**
  - *Flexible intramedullary nailing (for patients <50 kg, length stable fracture patterns)*
  - The appropriate-sized nail is planned on the basis of radiographs and should be selected to be less than 40% of the narrowest portion of the femoral canal. The patient is placed supine on the fracture

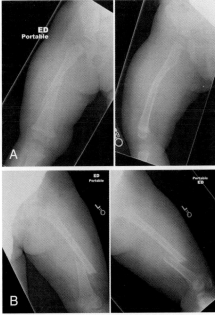

Fig. 9.5 A, Spiral femur fracture in a toddler from a fall. **B,** Transverse femur fracture in a 10-year-old from a motor vehicle accident.

table, and closed reduction is obtained with gentle traction under C-arm guidance. The nails are manually contoured such that the apex of the bow is at the fracture site. A fluoroscope is used to identify the nail entry point on the lateral femur approximately 3 cm above the physis. A small stab incision is made along the lateral aspect of the distal femur, and a drill is used to open the femoral cortex. The nail is inserted to the level of the fracture. The opposite medial cortex is drilled at the same level and opened analogous to the lateral side, and a second nail is passed up to the level of the fracture. Each nail is then inserted in diverging directions past the fracture site sequentially while the fracture is held reduced. The nails are advanced until they just pass the proximal femoral physis. The nails are then cut (within 1 cm off the cortex of insertion site) and bent. Wounds are then closed.

- **Over 12 years**
  - *Lateral entry with intramedullary nailing (weight >50 kg, length unstable fracture patterns)*
  - The patient is placed supine on a fracture table. C-arm images are obtained of the proximal femur before prepping to ensure adequate images are obtained. The fracture is reduced using traction on the fracture table. A small incision is made proximal to the greater trochanter, and a guidewire is used to determine the appropriate start point just lateral to the tip of the greater trochanter. Avoid piriformis fossa entry. The guidewire is drilled into the greater trochanter under C-arm guidance in the AP and lateral planes to verify accurate placement. An entry reamer is used to open the proximal femoral canal over the guidewire. A reaming guidewire is then placed down the intramedullary canal past the fracture site ending proximal to the physis. The appropriate length nail is then measured with the measuring guide. The femur is then reamed to the appropriate width. An IM nail is then placed down the reaming guidewire with the fracture held reduced in place. The reaming guidewire is removed. Using C-arm guidance, proximal and distal nail interlocking screws are placed through stab incisions. Wounds are then irrigated and closed.

Estimated Postoperative Course

- Postoperative day 0: Ensure hemodynamic stability and monitor in the hospital. Patients generally may start partial weight bearing unless there is concern for fracture stability postoperatively.
- Postoperative days 10 to 14: Check the wound and take radiographs.
- Postoperative weeks 6 to 8: Repeat radiographs and clinical evaluation, and progress activities gradually if healing. Educate the family that the child will be reluctant to walk at first and then limp for several months.
- Postoperative months 3 to 6: Gradual progression to normal activities follows.
- Postoperative months 6 to 12: Consider removal of flexible nails at 6 to 12 months as the nail ends can become prominent and alter the shape of the femoral metaphysis. Up to a 1 cm discrepancy is acceptable.

SUGGESTED READINGS

Anglen JO, Choi L: Treatment options in pediatric femoral shaft fractures, *J Orthop Trauma* 19(10):724–733, 2005.

Bopst L, Reinberg O, Lutz N, et al.: Femur fracture in preschool children: experience with flexible intramedullary nailing in 72 children, *J Orthop* 27(3):299–303, 2007.

Flynn JM, Curatolo E: Pediatric femoral shaft fractures: a system for decision making, *Instr Course Lect* 64:453–460, 2015.

Hosalkar HS, Pandya NK, Cho RH, et al.: Intramedullary nailing of pediatric femoral shaft fracture, *J Am Acad Orthop Surg* 19(8):472–481, 2011.

Kocher MS, Sink EL, Blasier RD, et al.: Treatment of pediatric diaphyseal femur fractures, *J Am Acad Orthop Surg* 17(11):718–725, 2009.

Pring M, Newton P, Rang M: Femoral shaft. In Wenger DE, Pring ME, editors: *Rang's children's fractures*, Philadelphia, 2005, Lippincott Williams & Wilkins, pp 181–200.

Shilt J: Fractures of the femoral shaft. In Green NE, Swiontkowski MF, editors: *Skeletal trauma in children*, Philadelphia, 2009, Saunders, pp 397–423.

Wood JN, Fockeye O, Mondestin V, et al.: Prevalence of abuse among young children with femur fractures: a systemic review, *BMC Pediatr* 2(14):169, 2014.

PEDIATRIC TIBIA/FIBULA FRACTURES

Types of Fractures

- Fractures of the proximal tibial metaphysis

- Fractures of the tibial and fibular shafts
- Isolated fractures of the tibial shaft
- Fractures of the distal tibial metaphysis

History

- The mechanism of injury commonly includes motor vehicle accidents, falls, and sports.
- Pain is the most reliable clinical history.
- In young children, inability to walk may be the clue, especially in nondisplaced toddler spiral fractures of the tibia.
- Incidence peaks at 3 to 4 years (mostly torus fractures of the proximal metaphysis and spiral fractures) and 15 to 16 years (mostly transverse fractures).
- Direct and indirect forces can contribute to tibia fractures in which direct injuries cause transverse or segmental fractures, whereas indirect forces can cause oblique fractures.

Physical Examination

- Inspect for deformity and open fracture.
- Palpate throughout the tibia if the deformity is not obvious (nondisplaced fractures are common in young children with a low-energy mechanism).
- Palpate compartments because of risk of compartment syndrome, especially in a high-energy mechanism.
- Perform and document a neurovascular examination.

Imaging

- Obtain AP and lateral radiographs of the tibia/fibula (Fig. 9.6).
- Image the joints above and below (ankle, knee).

Classification System

- Fractures of the proximal tibial metaphysis (common in children 3 to 6 years; most fractures are nondisplaced or greenstick with tendency to develop posttraumatic valgus)
- Fractures of the tibial and fibular shafts (complete both bone fractures are associated with higher energy mechanisms and direct blows)
- Isolated fractures of the tibial shaft or fibular shaft (tibial shaft—torsional injuries without significant displacement or shortening due to intact fibula; fibular shaft—direct-impact injuries)
- Fractures of the distal tibial metaphysis (rare injuries that generally heal without significant malalignment)

Initial Management

- **Patient Education.** Tibia/fibula fractures represent a wide spectrum of injury severity and are common fractures in children. In general, most low-energy mechanism injuries are expected to heal well with closed treatment. Higher-energy mechanism injuries can be associated with open fractures and a higher rate of subsequent disability as well as compartment syndrome.
- Pediatric trauma evaluation is necessary for high-energy injuries.
- Apply a long leg posterior splint to prevent further damage to soft tissues.
- Open fractures need to be débrided in the operating room.

Nonoperative Management
Fractures of the proximal tibial metaphysis

- Closed manipulation to correct valgus angulation under anesthesia and application of a long leg cast with knee flexed to 10 to 15 degrees is the treatment of choice.
- Immobilize for 4 to 6 weeks in a cast.
- Monitor weekly radiographs for first 3 weeks and then at 6 weeks.
- Remove cast when fracture is healed. Progress knee range of motion and activities as tolerated.
- Valgus deformity of less than 15 degrees generally remodels and improves with time. Follow with long standing x-rays for 2 years. Persistent deformity can be corrected with a hemiepiphysiodesis guided growth procedure prior to physeal closure.

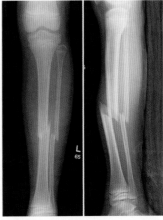

Fig. 9.6 Tibial and fibular shaft fracture in a 12-year-old boy.

Fractures of the tibial and fibular shafts, isolated fractures of the tibial shaft, fractures of the distal tibial metaphysis

- Closed fractures should be treated with immobilization in a cast.
- Obtain closed reduction and long leg casting with approximately 30 degrees of knee flexion if you anticipate allowing the child to weight bear. To prevent weight bearing, flex the knee to 80 degrees in the cast for unstable fractures.
- Acceptable alignment is 5 degrees varus/valgus in children older than 8 years old (10 degrees if less than 8 years old), 5 degrees flexion/extension, less than 1 cm shortening, and less than 50% translation.
- Immobilize for 4 to 6 weeks in long leg cast. For low energy mechanism of injury injuries, earlier weight bearing is acceptable without increased malalignment or time to healing.
- Monitor weekly radiographs for first 3 weeks, and then spread out future radiographs.
- Transition to short leg cast or boot with healing fracture for 4 to 6 more weeks. Longer immobilization times are required for older children and more significant fracture patterns.

Operative Management

Codes
ICD-10:

S82.10 Proximal tibial metaphysis fracture

S82.20 Fracture of tibial shaft

S82.40 Fracture of fibular shaft

CPT:

27752 Closed reduction of tibia/fibula fracture

27759 Intramedullary fixation of tibia fracture

Indications
- Any open fracture or compartment syndrome should undergo débridement and fasciotomy, respectively.
- Failure to adequately maintain closed reduction in pediatric tibia fracture should be considered for operative stabilization (rare). Consider cast wedging to improve alignment.

Informed consent and counseling
- Tibia fractures can develop rotational or angular malunion, as well as length discrepancy to the contralateral leg. Proximal metaphyseal fractures tend to angulate toward valgus, whereas isolated tibial fractures tend to angulate in varus after initial casting.

Repeat manipulations may be necessary to maintain some reductions, and if these fail, operative management is indicated.

Anesthesia
- General anesthesia

Patient positioning
- Supine on a regular table, tourniquet applied to proximal thigh

Surgical Procedures

Closed Reduction and Flexible Intramedullary Nailing of Tibia Fracture: Fig. 9.7

- The appropriate-sized nail is planned on the basis of radiographs, and should be selected to be less than 40% of the narrowest portion of the tibial canal. The patient is placed supine on a regular table and closed reduction is obtained under C-arm guidance. The nails are manually contoured such that the apex of the bow is at the fracture site. A fluoroscope is used to identify the nail entry point on the anteromedial proximal tibia approximately 2 cm distal to the proximal physis. A small stab incision is made along the anteromedial proximal tibia, and a drill used to open the tibial cortex. The nail is inserted to the level of the fracture. The opposite anterolateral cortex is drilled at the same level and opened analogous to the medial side, and a second nail is inserted up to the level of the fracture. Each nail is then inserted in diverging directions past the fracture site sequentially while the fracture is held reduced. The nails are advanced until they are several centimeters proximal to the distal tibial physis. The nails are then cut (within 1 cm off the

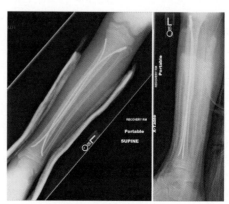

Fig. 9.7 Tibial and fibular shaft fracture in a 12-year-old boy treated with flexible intramedullary nails.

cortex of insertion site) and bent. Wounds are then closed. A long leg cast is placed to protect the fixation, and the patient remains non–weight bearing.

Estimated Postoperative Course

- Postoperative days 10 to 14: Return for clinical evaluation and radiographs in the cast.
- Postoperative weeks 6 to 8: Cast removed; radiographs should show signs of healing.
- Postoperative months 3 to 6: Gradual progression to normal activities.

SUGGESTED READINGS

Mashru RP, Herman MJ, Pizzutillo PD: Tibial shaft fractures in children and adolescents, *J Am Acad Orthop Surg* 13(5):345–352, 2005.

Sankar WN, Jones KJ, David Horn B, Wells L: Titanium elastic nails for pediatric tibial shaft fractures, *J Child Orthop* 1(5):281–286, 2007.

Shannak AO: Tibial fractures in children: follow-up study, *J Pediatr Orthop* 8(3):306–310, 2007.

Silva M, Eagan MJ, Wong MA, et al.: A comparison of two approaches for the closed treatment of low energy tibial fractures in children, *J Bone Joint Surg Am* 94(20):1853–1860, 2012.

Thompson GH, Son-Hing J: Fractures and dislocations of the tibia and fibula. In Green NE, Swiontkowski MF, editors: *Skeletal trauma in children*, Philadelphia, 2009, Saunders, pp 471–506.

ADOLESCENT IDIOPATHIC SCOLIOSIS

History

- Adolescent idiopathic scoliosis is abnormal curvature of the adolescent spine, with greater than 10 degrees coronal plane deformity and rotational deformity not associated with other conditions.
- Back pain may or may not be present.
- Patients may complain of rib hump and shoulder asymmetry.
- Menarche status (to assess remaining growth) and family history (positive in 30%) should be assessed.

Physical Examination

- Inspect the body for cutaneous lesions (café au lait spots, dimples, hemangiomas or hairy patches) or congenital malformations to rule out non-idiopathic scoliosis.
- Inspect for shoulder asymmetry, forward-bending rib hump, direction and level of curve, pelvic obliquity, and kyphosis/lordosis (Fig. 9.8). A Scoliometer is an instrument that measures truncal rotation and a reading greater than 7 degrees is an indication for x-rays.
- Perform thorough neurologic examination including abdominal reflexes.
- Assess body for general assessment of maturity (breast appearance, axillary hair, facial hair).

Imaging: Fig. 9.9

- Full-length standing PA and lateral scoliosis radiographs. Look for wedged or hemi vertebrae.
  - Assess location, apex and magnitude of curvature. Classic idiopathic scoliosis exhibits an apex to the right thoracic curve.
  - Assess Risser grade on iliac apophysis (grade 1: 25% ossified, 2: 50% ossified, 3: 75% ossified,

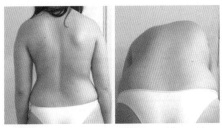

Fig. 9.8 Common deformity in adolescent idiopathic scoliosis. Note shoulder asymmetry and rib hump.

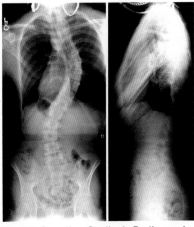

Fig. 9.9 Standing Scoliosis Radiographs.

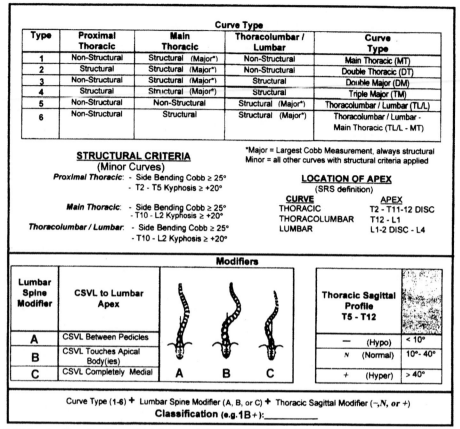

Fig. 9.10 Lenke Classification of Adolescent Idiopathic Scoliosis. (From Pierz, K, Dormans JP: Spinal disorders. In Dormans JP, editor: *Core knowledge in orthopaedics: pediatric orthopaedics*, Philadelphia, 2005, Mosby, p 277.)

4: 100% ossified, 5: 100% ossified and fused). Ossification progresses from lateral to medial, with higher grades indicating progression to skeletal maturity.

- Magnetic resonance imaging (MRI) is indicated if there are neurological findings or if there is an apex to the left thoracic curve to assess for cord abnormalities

Classification System

- Lenke classification (Fig. 9.10)

Initial Management

- **Patient Education.** Adolescent idiopathic scoliosis is an abnormal curvature in the spine with the age of onset after 10 years. There is an equal female to male prevalence in the general population. Risk of progression is associated with female gender, curve magnitude, younger age (less than 12 years old), and time remaining until skeletal maturity.

Nonoperative Management

- Observation is indicated for skeletally immature patients with curves less than 25 degrees or patients with nonprogressive curves near maturity.
  - Patients should be observed serially with radiographs every 6 months to 1 year.
- Schroth method: intensive physical therapy program developed in Germany and gaining traction in the United States. The goals of the program are to improve muscle symmetry, rotation, and posture. This is an alternative and sometimes an adjunct to

bracing, but requires diligent adherence and is not effective for severe curves.

- Bracing is indicated for skeletally immature patients (Risser 0–1) with curves of 25 to 40 degrees. Goal is to reduce the magnitude of the curve by 50% when the patient is wearing the brace.
  - Full-time bracing with a thoracolumbar orthosis is recommended until the patient reaches Risser grade 4. Outcomes with bracing are dependent on the number of hours the brace is worn during the day (13 hour/day minimum wear time according to the BRAIST trial).
  - Follow with serial x-rays out of the brace every 6 months

Operative Management
Codes
ICD-10: M41.20 Idiopathic scoliosis
CPT:
  - 22842 Posterior spinal instrumentation 3 to 6 vertebral segments
  - 22843 Posterior spinal instrumentation 7 to 12 vertebral segments
  - 22844 Posterior spinal instrumentation 13 or more vertebral segments
  - 26610 Arthrodesis, posterior or posterolateral technique, single level (thoracic)
  - 26612 Arthrodesis, posterior or posterolateral technique, single level (lumbar)
  - 26614 Arthrodesis, posterior or posterolateral technique, each additional level
Indications
- Curves greater than 50 degrees or greater than 40 degrees in skeletally immature patients
Informed consent and counseling
- Surgery for adolescent idiopathic scoliosis is major surgery, with high blood loss and possible observational monitoring in the intensive care unit postoperatively. Complications of spine surgery include infection, nerve damage/cord injury (rare), pseudoarthrosis, and hardware-related complications.
Anesthesia
- General anesthesia
Patient positioning
- Prone positioning on a Jackson table with neuromonitoring setup

Surgical Procedures
Posterior Spinal Instrumentation and Fusion
- This is the most common procedure for adolescent idiopathic scoliosis. The patient is positioned prone, and posterior exposure of the spine is carried out with a midline incision, carefully exposing the spinous processes and lamina of the instrumented levels by sub-periosteal dissection and cautery of paraspinal musculature. For pedicle screw instrumentation, the vertebrae are exposed to show the transverse process and superior articular facet. Pedicle screws are inserted on the basis of a thorough understanding of vertebral anatomy because screw trajectories differ on the basis of both location in the spine and intrinsic patient anatomy. Osteotomies and facetectomies are performed to allow for correction of deformity. Segmental instrumentation is performed, and rods are contoured and affixed to reduce the spinal deformity. The wound is irrigated thoroughly and closed.

Estimated Postoperative Course
- Postoperative days 0 to 1: Close hemodynamic monitoring in the intensive care unit (ICU) due to possibility of large-volume blood loss.
- Postoperative days 2 to 5: Normalization in the hospital, work on improving mobility until safe discharge from the hospital.
- Postoperative days 14 to 21: Wound evaluation, remove stitches, standing scoliosis radiographs.
- Postoperative week 6: Routine follow-up, standing scoliosis radiographs. Progress activities as tolerated; follow-up visits spaced out.

SUGGESTED READINGS

Cuartas E, Rasouli A, O'Brien M, Shufflebarger HL: Use of all-pedicle screw constructs in the treatment of adolescent idiopathic scoliosis, *J Am Acad Orthop Surg* 17(9):550–561, 2009.

Kim HJ, Blanco JS, Ridman RF: Update on the management of idiopathic scoliosis, *Curr Opin Pediatr* 21(1):55–64, 2009.

Kuru T, Yelden I, Dereli EE, et al.: The efficacy of three-dimensional Schroth exercises in adolescent idiopathic scoliosis: a randomized controlled clinical trial, *Clin Rehabil* 30(2):181–190, 2016.

Lenke LG, Betz RR, Harms J, et al.: Adolescent idiopathic scoliosis: a new classification to determine extent of spinal arthrodesis, *J Bone Joint Surg Am* 83:1169–1181, 2001.

Sponseller PD: Bracing for adolescent idiopathic scoliosis in practice today, *J Pediatr Orthop* 31(1 Suppl):S53–60, 2011.

Staheli L: Spine and pelvis. In *International pediatric orthopedic pocketbook*, Staheli, 2005, Seattle, pp 291–320.

DEVELOPMENTAL DYSPLASIA OF THE HIP

History

- Definition: Developmental dysplasia of the hip (DDH) is a spectrum that includes acetabulum and/or femoral head anatomic or hip stability abnormalities (dislocation or subluxation) that occurs in utero, infancy, or early childhood.
- Dysplasia is generally caused by abnormal forces acting on the hip in utero leading to abnormal development of the acetabulum, and in severe cases it leads to eventual hip dislocation because of insufficient bony coverage for the femoral head.
- Risk factors include family history of DDH, breech positioning before birth, female, and large gestational weight.
- Early diagnosis and treatment is critical to improving or, at minimum, optimizing long-term outcomes

Physical Examination
Newborn

- Every infant needs to be screened at every well baby visit. Examine one hip at a time.
- **Barlow test** is performed by flexing (90 degrees), then applying posteriorly directed force. Test is positive if the hip dislocates.
- **Ortolani test** is performed by flexing (90 degrees) and adducting the thigh to subluxate the hip, then abducting the hip while simultaneously applying an anteriorly directed pressure along the greater trochanter. Test is positive if a clunk is felt to indicate reduction of the dislocated hip.

Infant/Toddler

- Asymmetric or limitation of abduction (less than 45 degrees) could indicate hip dysplasia.
- Evaluate for asymmetric thigh folds and the Galeazzi sign. Asymmetric thigh folds can also be a normal finding.
  - **Galeazzi sign:** The child's hips and knees are flexed to 90 degrees and adducted to midline. The

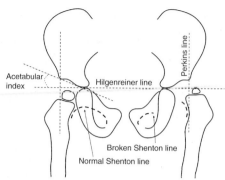

Fig. 9.11 Radiographic assessment of hip dysplasia. (From Erol B, Dormans JP: Hip disorders. In Dormans JP, editor: *Core knowledge in orthopaedics: pediatric orthopaedics*, Philadelphia, 2005, Mosby, p 232.)

test is positive if one knee appears shorter than the other knee, indicating possible DDH on the shorter side. Asymmetric femur lengths is another cause for a positive Galeazzi sign. In addition, the Galeazzi test may be negative in a patient with bilateral DDH.
- Walking children can have leg length discrepancy, Trendelenburg gait, and excessive lumbar lordosis.

Imaging: Fig. 9.11

Newborn to 6 months: The acetabulum and femoral head do not readily appear on radiographs until 4 to 6 months. Hence, ultrasound is the preferred modality for evaluation at this age.

- Ultrasound is indicated at 6 to 8 weeks old when screening for patients with risk factors for DDH, when the diagnosis is in question, or to evaluate the efficacy of Pavlik harness treatment in children younger than 6 months old.

6 months and older: Radiographic evaluation is appropriate in this age group. An AP view of the pelvis is reviewed for several criteria illustrated in Table 9.4 and Fig. 9.11.

Initial Management

- **Patient Education.** Hip dysplasia describes a spectrum of hip anatomic and/or instability problems that are congenital or develop in early childhood. If left untreated, abnormal forces and contact from developmental dysplasia can lead to a progressive problem that impairs normal development of the

TABLE 9.4 Radiographic Assessment of Hip Dysplasia

Radiographic Landmark	Abnormal if:
Intersection of Hilgenreiner line and Perkin line	Femoral head not located in the medial lower quadrant
Shenton line	Break in the continuity of the line
Acetabular index	>24 degrees at 24 months old (age dependent—can be higher in newborn, but >40 is always abnormal)

acetabulum and femoral head. It is important to develop a treatment plan once a diagnosis has been established.

- The goal of non-operative treatment is to achieve a concentric reduction of the femoral head in the acetabulum in order to promote optimal development of the hip joint and avoid long-term sequelae, such as chronic hip dislocation, early onset degenerative disease, chronic limp, and early hip arthroplasty.

Newborn to 6 Months

- A Pavlik harness is the initial treatment, which is worn 23 hours/day, and has a success rate of 85% to 95%. Reassess ultrasound in 2 weeks for reduction. If the hip is not reduced on ultrasound, the patient may need a closed reduction under anesthesia. If reduced, continue using the Pavlik harness full time (6 weeks), then night time (6 weeks) or until x-rays normalize.
  - Risks of femoral nerve palsy exist from excessive hip flexion, avascular necrosis with excessive hip abduction, and brachial plexus palsy from shoulder straps.

6 Months to 18 months

- Closed reduction and Spica casting under anesthesia.
  - Risks of avascular necrosis exist with excessive hip abduction and cast-related complications including skin breakdown and irritation.
  - Technique for closed reduction of the hip:
  - Gentle traction is applied manually to the leg, and the hip is brought into approximately 120 degrees flexion and then abduction. After a reduction is felt,

the hip is considered stable if it remains reduced with adduction greater than 30 degrees past maximal abduction and less than 90 degrees of flexion. An arthrogram of the hip is performed to confirm adequate reduction. Percutaneous adductor tenotomy is considered to relieve pressure on the reduction if the adductors are tight in the reduced position. A hip Spica cast is then applied and maintained for approximately 3 months.

- Skin traction may be considered before closed reduction to relieve muscular contraction.
- Confirm reduction with radiograph or single-cut CT.
- If hip does not remain reduced in a cast, open reduction should be performed.
- AP pelvis x-ray quarterly until 12 months old and then yearly for 3 years, then every 3 years.

18 Months and Older

- Open reduction is the initial treatment. By this point, chronic dislocation is difficult to reduce due to significant acetabular dysplasia.
- Consideration of femoral shortening osteotomy should be made to avoid excessive pressure on the proximal femur after reduction.
- Acetabular coverage is often deficient, and remodeling potential is lower at this age; hence pelvic osteotomy (Pemberton or Salter) should be considered to provide adequate femoral head coverage.
- Postoperative CT scan to confirm reduction.
- Spica cast for 6 to 12 weeks.

Operative Management

Codes

ICD-10: Q65.2 Congenital dislocation of hip
ICD-10: Q65.89 Congenital hip dysplasia
CPT: 27257 Closed reduction of congenital hip dislocation
27258 Open reduction of congenital hip dislocation
29325 Application of hip Spica cast

Indications

- Open reduction under anesthesia for dysplasia diagnosed in children older than 18 months or those with failed attempts at closed reduction.

Informed consent and counseling

- Open reduction and spica cast are associated with risks depending on the approach. If using a medial approach to the hip, there is a risk of medial femoral circumflex artery disruption. If using an anterior approach to the hip, there is a risk of damage to iliac crest apophysis and lateral femoral cutaneous nerve. There is always a risk of avascular necrosis with reduction and application of a Spica cast.

Anesthesia

- General anesthesia

Patient positioning

- Supine positioning on standard operating room table

Surgical Procedures

Open Reduction of the Hip via a Medial Approach

- Prepare the skin for the entire operative leg and hemipelvis. Create an oblique skin incision approximately 5 cm long, 1 cm distal and parallel to the inguinal crease, and centered over the adductor longus. The deep fascia is incised, and the saphenous vein is avoided if possible or ligated. The pectineus muscle is identified and retracted inferomedially. The femoral neurovascular structures are retracted laterally. The femoral circumflex vessels are also then retracted laterally. The psoas tendon is divided and allowed to retract proximally. The capsule is opened in line to the acetabular margin. The transverse acetabular ligament is identified and released. Next, the ligamentum teres/pulvinar is removed allowing for reduction of the femoral head. The limbus, which will develop into the acetabular labrum, is left intact. The hip is held reduced, and the wound is closed. A hip Spica is then applied with the hip in 90 to 100 degrees of flexion, 30 to 40 degrees of abduction, and neutral rotation.

Open Reduction of the Hip via an Anterior Approach

- Prepare the skin for the entire operative leg and hemipelvis. Place a bump under the operative hip. An incision is made in a curvilinear fashion starting at a point two-thirds above the greater trochanter and the iliac crest and immediately crossing the anterior inferior iliac spine. The apophysis of the iliac crest is exposed. The interval between the tensor fascia lata and sartorius is bluntly developed, being careful to avoid the lateral femoral cutaneous nerve. The iliac apophysis is split sharply down to bone and exposed subperiosteally, allowing for retraction of the sartorius medially and the tensor fascia lata laterally. The rectus femoris is identified deep to this interval,

reflected from its origin, and tagged. The hip capsule is then dissected with a periosteal elevator and then opened sharply with a knife (T-shaped incision). The ligamentum teres is then cut with scissors. The hip is then reduced under direct visualization. Additional procedures such as pelvic osteotomies can be added at this point if the femoral head coverage is inadequate. The wound is closed, and a hip Spica cast is applied as previously described.

Estimated Postoperative Course

- Postoperative days 10 to 14: First clinical visit, evaluate cast hygiene, patient, and parent education.
- Postoperative week 6: Radiographs to evaluate hip reduction, removal or change of Spica cast.
- Postoperative months 2 to 3: Radiographs to evaluate hip reduction, mobilize gradually.
- Continue to follow clinically and/or radiographically until skeletal maturity.

Board Review

Barlow and Ortolani tests are routinely the most commonly used way to evaluate for hip dysplasia in an infant.

SUGGESTED READINGS

Bohm P, Brzuske A: Salter innominate osteotomy for the treatment of development dysplasia of the hip in children: results of seventy-three consecutive osteotomies after twenty-six to thirty-five years of follow-up, *J Bone Joint Surg Am.* 2002;84(A)-2:178–186.

Erol B, Dormans J: Hip disorders. In Dormans JP, editor: *Core knowledge in orthopaedics: pediatric orthopaedics*, Philadelphia, 2005, Mosby.

Herring JA, Sucato DJ: Developmental dysplasia of the hip. In Herring JA, editor: *Tachdjian's pediatric orthopaedics*, ed 4, Philadelphia, 2008, Saunders.

Ramsey P, Lasser S, MacEwen GD: Congenital dislocation of the hip, *J Bone Joint Surg Am* 58(7):1000–1004, 1976.

Staheli L: Spine and pelvis. In *International pediatric orthopedic pocketbook*, Staheli, 2005, Seattle, pp 250–261.

LEGG-CALVE-PERTHES DISEASE

History

- Background: Legg-Calve-Perthes disease (LCPD) is avascular necrosis of the femoral head without a known etiology, possibly from a temporary interruption to the blood supply to the capital femoral epiphysis. There are four stages. Initially, there is *synovitis of the hip capsule and necrosis* of the femoral head, which may last for weeks to months. The capital femoral epiphysis undergoes necrosis leading to relative decreased size compared with the unaffected side and radiographic physeal irregularity. The femoral epiphysis then undergoes *collapse and fragmentation*. In this second stage, the epiphysis appears fragmented and begins to resorb and collapse. This stage lasts for months to years. With collapse, the femoral head can migrate proximally and laterally to uncover the lateral portion of the head. The third stage is *reossification,* with necrotic bone being replaced by new bone. The femoral head then *remodels* until maturity.

- Younger children (age <6) have a better prognosis in part due to a greater number of remaining years of growth and therefore remodeling potential.
- The age of a child affected is usually between 4 and 10, with a 4:1 male: female ratio. Perthes is bilateral in 10% to 15% of patients, usually with asynchronous presentation of symptoms.
- The limping child has mild or no pain. Pain is usually activity related and can be located from hip/groin all the way to the knee.

Physical Examination

- Inspect child's gait—are they limping?
- Inspect for leg length discrepancy (from contractures or femoral head collapse).
- Assess hip range of motion: loss of internal rotation and abduction.

Imaging

- Obtain AP and frog leg lateral views of the hip (Fig. 9.12).

- Radiographs are normal initially and then follow a predictable progression as the patient moves through the four stages of the disease (Table 9.5).

Classification System

- Herring lateral pillar classification is the most commonly used, most prognostic radiographic classification system that also guides treatment algorithms. Radiographs are taken in the early fragmentation stage and evaluated for lucencies in the lateral pillar of the femoral head (Table 9.6).
  - The lateral pillar is the lateral 15% to 30% of the femoral head width.
  - Preserved height of the lateral pillar is associated with a better prognosis.

Differential Diagnoses

- Hip dysplasia
- Slipped capital femoral epiphysis
- Epiphyseal dysplasia (especially if seen bilaterally)

Initial Management

- **Patient Education.** LCPD is caused by a disruption to blood flow to the femoral head. The mechanism is still not completely understood. The femoral head undergoes a process of remodeling over time. The younger the child is when the disease first presents, the better the remodeling prognosis. Prognosis also depends on the severity of the lateral pillar femoral head collapse (Herring classification). The patient may experience loss of range of motion and early hip degenerative changes with an aspherical femoral head at maturity.

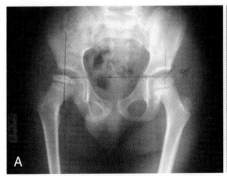
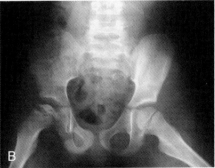

Fig. 9.12 A and **B,** Anteroposterior and frog-leg lateral radiographs of Legg-Calve-Perthes disease of the right hip (initial stage). (From Erol B, Dormans JP: Hip disorders. In Dormans JP, editor: *Core knowledge in orthopaedics: pediatric orthopaedics*, Philadelphia, 2005, Mosby, p 239.)

TABLE 9.5	**Radiographic Findings in Legg-Calve-Perthes Disease**
Stage	**Findings**
Initial (synovitis and avascular necrosis)	• Smaller ossific nucleus of femoral head, lateralization of the femoral head relative to the acetabulum • Later, subchondral fractures and increased density of the femoral head
Fragmentation	Areas of radiolucency in the femoral head (resorbed areas)
Reossification	Radiolucent areas replaced by new bone
Remodeling	Gradual remodeling of the reossified femoral head and acetabulum

TABLE 9.6	**Lateral Pillar Classification**	
Lateral Pillar Group	**Characteristics**	**Prognosis**
A	Lateral pillar not involved	Good; spherical femoral head at maturity
B	>50% of the lateral pillar height maintained	Mixed; improved outcomes when children affected with disease at earlier age
C	<50% of the lateral pillar height maintained	Poor; aspherical femoral head at maturity

• Goal of treatment: maintain range of motion and containment of femoral head in the acetabulum. Avoid femoral head extrusion as it leads to coxa plana and an aspherical incongruent joint.

Nonoperative Management

• Children younger than age 6 at the onset of disease with all Herring lateral pillar grades can be treated with nonoperative management.
  • Pain control with nonsteroidal antiinflammatory drugs (NSAIDs) and observation is the mainstay of treatment.
  • Use of an abduction orthosis (Atlanta Scottish Rite brace) is controversial and poorly tolerated. An orthosis can be used in mild disease part time during the day until reossification is verified on radiographs (>9 months).
  • Physical therapy is helpful to maintain hip range of motion.

Operative Management

Codes
ICD-10:M91.10 Juvenile osteochondrosis of the femur
CPT: 27145 Osteotomy, iliac, acetabular or innominate bone

27151 Osteotomy, iliac, or innominate bone; with femoral osteotomy
27165 Osteotomy, intertrochanteric or subtrochanteric including Internet fixation and/or cast
Indications
• Age older than 6 to 8 years at onset of disease with Herring lateral pillar grade B or B/C border, without severe motion loss
• Femoral varus osteotomy and Salter innominate acetabular osteotomy can be considered for realignment and containment.
  • The concept is that the femoral head spherical congruity can be restored if the femoral head can be contained in the acetabulum to allow for subsequent remodeling.
Informed consent and counseling
• Complications with femoral osteotomy: abductor limp, failure of remodeling leading to persistent varus angulation, leg length discrepancy
• Complications with Salter innominate osteotomy: hip stiffness
Anesthesia
• General anesthesia
Patient positioning
• Supine positioning on a radiolucent table with a bump under the hip

Surgical Procedures
Proximal Femoral Varus Osteotomy

- An incision is made longitudinally centered just distal to the greater trochanter, and the fascia lata is split. The vastus lateralis fascia is incised using an L-shaped incision along the vastus ridge. The vastus lateralis is retracted anteriorly, and the proximal femur is exposed subperiosteally under this. A degree of desired varus correction is planned, and a transverse osteotomy cut is made just proximal to the lesser trochanter. Then the chisel for the blade plate is introduced into the proximal fragment, and the proximal fragment is tipped into the desired amount of varus correction. A wedge of medial bone is then removed to allow for the desired amount of varus. The blade plate is then inserted into the chiseled portion and affixed to the distal fragment.

Salter Innominate Pelvic Osteotomy

- Several pelvic osteotomies exist and are beyond the scope of this text. The Salter osteotomy is a rotational osteotomy of the acetabulum aimed to gain anterior and lateral coverage for the femoral head by rotating through the pubic symphysis. The entire extremity to inferior rib cage is prepped. An anterior approach to the hip as previously described in developmental dysplasia of the hip section is used. The inner and outer tables are subperiosteally dissected using periosteal elevators to the sciatic notch, and retractors are placed into the sciatic notch from the inner and outer tables overlapping each other. Subperiosteal dissection into the notch is crucial to avoid neurovascular injury to the gluteal vessels/nerves and the sciatic nerve. A gigli saw is passed on top of the retractors using a right-angle clamp and pulled to create a cut from the sciatic notch to the anterior inferior iliac spine (AIIS). This cut creates a proximal and distal pelvic fragment. A bone graft from the iliac wing is removed with a saw laterally, along a path just above the AIIS to the iliac tubercle. The graft is shaped to a 30-degree triangular wedge. The distal pelvic fragment is then hinged anterolaterally with towel clamps. The graft wedge is then placed in the osteotomy gap and affixed with two threaded pins from proximal to distal, stopping short of the triradiate cartilage. The iliac apophysis is then closed, and threaded pins are cut above the apophysis. The exposure is then closed in the usual fashion. A hip Spica cast is applied.

Estimated Postoperative Course

- Postoperative days 10 to 14: Evaluate cast hygiene, and educate the patient and parent.
- Postoperative week 6: Obtain radiographs to evaluate healing osteotomy, and remove Spica cast. If the osteotomy has healed, remove the pins (for pelvic osteotomy). A physical therapist should gradually mobilize the hips.
- Postoperative months 2 to 3: Obtain radiographs to evaluate healing osteotomy, and mobilize as tolerated.

Board Review

Legg-Calve-Perthes disease is most commonly seen in males between the ages of 4 to 10 and results in progressive bony remodeling of the femoral head due to disruption of blood supply.

SUGGESTED READINGS

Herring JA, Neustadt JB, Williams JA, et al. The lateral pillar classification of Legg-Calvé-Perthes disease, *J Pediatr Orthop.* 12(2):143–150.

Herring JA: Legg-Calvé-Perthes disease. In Herring JA, editor: *Tachdjian's pediatric orthopaedics,* 4. Philadelphia, 2008, Saunders.

Stulberg SD, Cooperman DR, Wallenstein R, et al.: The natural history of Legg-Calvé-Perthes disease, *J Bone Joint Surg Am* 63(7):1095–1108, 1981.

Thompson GH, Price CT, Roy D, et al.: Legg-Calvé-Perthes disease, *Instr Course Lect* 51:367–384, 2002.

Thompson GH: Salter osteotomy in Legg-Calve-Perthes disease, *J Pediatr Orthop* 31(2 Suppl):S192–197, 2011.

SLIPPED CAPITAL FEMORAL EPIPHYSIS

History

- Definition: Slipped capital femoral epiphysis (SCFE) is the displacement of the femoral neck and shaft from the femoral epiphysis, in which the femoral neck moves anterior-superior relative to the epiphysis.
- It usually occurs during a period of rapid growth in adolescence (ages 12 to 15).
- Obesity, mechanical (i.e., femoral neck retroversion), and endocrine factors (i.e., hypothyroidism, hypogonadism) are all proposed risk factors.
- Patients present with either acute onset of severe pain to the hip region (acute SCFE) or more commonly several months' duration of insidious vague groin and thigh pain (chronic SCFE).

- Minimal to no trauma before significant pain distinguishes acute SCFE from Salter-Harris type I injury to the proximal femoral epiphysis.
- It is essential to do a hip examination for every patient who complains of knee pain. Due to the innervation of the obturator nerve, patients with a SCFE may present with isolated thigh or knee pain.

Physical Examination

- Generally obese child
- Chronic SCFE:
  - Inspect for antalgic gait with limp, limb externally rotated at rest
  - Assess obligatory external rotation with hip flexion due to anatomic distortion of proximal femur (Drehmann sign)
- Acute SCFE:
  - Inspect for refusal to bear weight, limb shortened and externally rotated

Imaging: Fig. 9.13

- Obtain AP and frog pelvis radiographs with a single lateral hip radiograph.
- Widening of the proximal femoral physis can be seen in early SCFE. Grading of a SCFE is based on the amount of epiphyseal displacement as compared to the femoral neck with mild (less than 1/3 displacement), moderate (greater than 1/3, less than 2/3), and severe (greater than 2/3).
- Slip angle can also be calculated on the lateral hip radiograph to help determine the severity of the SCFE with mild (less than 30 degrees, moderate 30 to 50 degrees, and severe greater than 50 degrees.
- Klein's line—A line drawn along the superior femoral neck on the AP radiograph intersects the lateral epiphysis normally and does not intersect in SCFE.
- MRI can help evaluate for early SCFE if radiographic findings are inconclusive.

Classification System

- Onset of symptoms:
  - Acute—prodromal symptoms less than 3 weeks before sudden acute severe pain without significant trauma. No remodeling of the proximal femur on radiographs
  - Chronic—prodromal symptoms more than several months of vague groin and thigh pain. Remodeling of the femoral neck on radiographs

- Acute on chronic—prodromal symptoms more than 3 weeks, although sudden acute severe pain and radiographic evidence of minor prior femoral neck remodeling
- Clinical function:
  - Stable—pain tolerable enough for patient to bear weight
  - Unstable—pain intolerable, patient unable to bear weight; risk of avascular necrosis up to 24%

Differential Diagnoses

- Salter-Harris fracture
- Legg-Calve-Perthes disease

Initial Management

- **Patient Education.** SCFE is a separation of the proximal femur from the proximal femoral growth plate. It can occur on both hips. The cause is unknown, although obesity is a risk factor. The most devastating result is the risk of avascular necrosis, especially in acute, unstable, or significantly displaced slips, as well as risk of early osteoarthritis from proximal femoral deformity in significantly displaced slip.
- Evaluate other hip because up to 20% to 40% of slips are bilateral at the time of presentation.
- Rule out fracture/dislocation of affected hip.
- Once a diagnosis of SCFE has been confirmed by radiographs, the patient must be strictly non–weight bearing and a pediatric orthopedist should be involved in formulating a definitive management plan. The patient should be admitted to the hospital for bed rest and pain control until fixation.

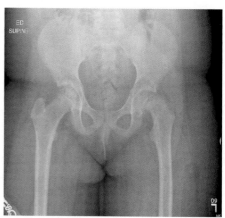

Fig. 9.13 Acute-on-chronic slipped capital femoral epiphysis in a 12-year-old girl.

Nonoperative Management

- Spica casting for patients with chronic SCFE has fallen out of favor due to associated risks including recurrent slip and chondrolysis.

Operative Management

Codes

ICD-10: M93.003 Slipped upper femoral epiphysis
CPT: 27176 In-situ pinning of SCFE

Indications

- Operative management is the standard of care to stabilize the epiphysis and prevent further displacement.

Informed consent and counseling

- Consider prophylactic contralateral pinning
- Technical risk of screw penetration into the hip joint and risk of avascular necrosis postoperative

Anesthesia

- General anesthesia

Patient positioning

- Patient is positioned supine on a fracture table, with the operative leg in neutral position. The other leg can be positioned flexed and abducted in a leg holder to clear it from fluoroscopic view. Reduction prior to in situ screw fixation is controversial.

Surgical Procedures

In Situ Screw Fixation of the Hip: Fig. 9.14

- Before prepping the operative leg, it is important to be able to obtain adequate fluoroscopic AP and lateral views of the hip.
- Ideal screw placement is perpendicular to the physis and in the center of the epiphysis.

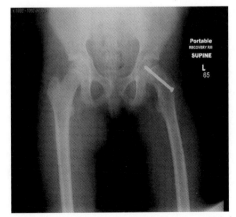

Fig. 9.14 In situ screw fixation of slipped capital femoral epiphysis.

- A guidewire is placed on the skin to estimate the trajectory of the screw in the AP and lateral planes. The trajectories are marked on the skin with a marking pen.
- The guidewire is inserted through a small stab incision and placed through the femoral neck, physis, and epiphysis using fluoroscopic guidance, being careful not to penetrate the hip joint. The guidewire length is measured using a depth gauge to estimate the screw length.
- A drill and tap are used over the guidewire to prepare for screw insertion.
- A cannulated partially threaded screw is then inserted over the guidewire, with at least three screw threads passing into the epiphysis.
- The skin is closed in the usual fashion. The patient may be discharged on toe-touch weight bearing on crutches.

Estimated Postoperative Course

- For stable slips, patients can bear weight as tolerated.
- For unstable slips, patients remain partial weight bearing for up to 6 weeks.
- Postoperative days 10 to 14: Perform clinical evaluation, check wounds, and obtain radiographs.
- Postoperative week 6: Perform clinical evaluation, obtain radiographs, and progress with weight bearing as tolerated.
- Continue radiographs every 3 months until physeal closure monitoring for chondrolysis (decreased joint space), avascular necrosis, hardware penetration into the joint, and contralateral SCFE. Complications usually occur within 6 to 12 months.

Board Review

Slipped capital femoral epiphysis is most commonly seen in obese patients between the ages of 12 to 15 during periods of growth spurts. Obesity is a risk factor for SCFE.

SUGGESTED READINGS

Goodman WW, Johnson JT, Robertson Jr WW, et al.: Single screw fixation for acute and acute-on-chronic slipped capital femoral epiphysis, *Clin Orthop Related Res* 322:86–90, 1996.

Larson AN, Sierra RJ, Yu EM, et al.: Outcomes of slipped capital femoral epiphysis treated with in situ pinning, *J Pediatr Orthop* 32(2):125–130, 2012.

Loder RT, Aronsson DD, Dobbs MB, Weinstein SL: Slipped capital femoral epiphysis, *Instr Course Lect* 50:1141–1147, 2001.

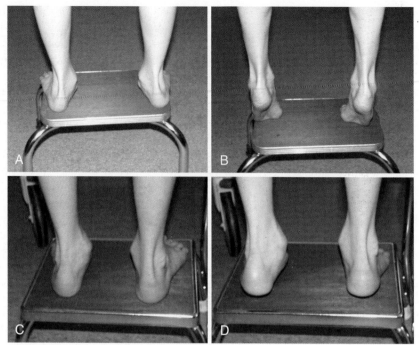

Fig. 9.15 Flexible Flat Foot and Rigid Flat Foot. **A** and **B**, Flexible flat foot. Note inversion of hind foot with plantarflexion. **C** and **D**, Rigid flat foot. Note hind foot does not invert with plantarflexion. ((From Wallach D, Davidson RS: Pediatric lower limb disorders. In Dormans JP, editor: *Core knowledge in orthopaedics: pediatric orthopaedics*, Philadelphia, 2005, Mosby, pp 212.))

Loder RT, Richards BS, Shapiro BS, et al.: Acute slipped capital femoral epiphysis: the importance of physeal stability, *J Bone Joint Surg Am* 75(8):1134–1140, 1993.

Staheli L: Hip. In *International pediatric orthopedic pocketbook*, Staheli, 2005, Seattle, pp 278–284.

Zaltz I, Baca G, Clohisy JC: Unstable SCFE: review of treatment modalities and prevalence of osteonecrosis, *Clin Orthop Relat Res* 471(7):2192–2198, 2013.

PES PLANOVALGUS (FLAT FEET)

History

- Definition: loss of medial foot arch
- Commonly presents as painless flexible deformity in early childhood
- Flexible flat foot is common in toddlers, and prevalence decreases by preschool years
- Foot arch develops around 5 to 6 years of age
- Parents often concerned about appearance of deformity, asymmetric shoe wear, and potential future disability

- Important to rule out other conditions including tarsal coalition, equinus, and congenital vertical talus before diagnosis of flat feet
- Higher prevalence in children with ligamentous laxity and obesity

Physical Examination

- Inspect patient's feet for an abnormal callus pattern.
- Assess if flat foot is rigid or mobile (Fig. 9.15):
  - If arch is restored by the patient standing on tiptoe, deformity is flexible.
  - Observe the patient standing flat and then rising to tip toes. Normally, the heels will be in valgus while standing flat and swing into varus when patient stands on tip toes indicating intact subtalar motion.
  - Rigid flat foot is always pathologic and can indicate other conditions such as tarsal coalition.
- Assess the flexibility of the subtalar joint by inverting and everting the heel with a hand cupped on the calcaneus.

- Assess for contracture of the heel cord, which can also predispose to flat feet. This is often associated with callous formation along the head of the talus.
- Perform a **Silfverskiöld test** for tight heel cord: Check ankle dorsiflexion with knee in flexion (normally 20 degrees of dorsiflexion above neutral) and extension (normally 10 degrees above neutral). If improved ankle dorsiflexion with knee flexion exists, then gastrocnemius is tight. If equivalent ankle dorsiflexion with knee flexion and extension exists, then the gastrocnemius and soleus muscles are tight.

Imaging

- Radiographs are not routinely necessary for the evaluation of flat feet unless they are associated with pain or rigid deformity exists. Order standing radiographs when indicated to assess for calcaneal pitch, talus-first metatarsal angle, and C sign of Latour or anteater sign as seen in tarsal coalition.
- In rigid deformity, consider a CT scan to evaluate for tarsal coalition of the midfoot or hind foot.

Classification System

- Mild flat foot: arch depressed on standing but visible
- Moderate flat foot: arch obliterated on standing though present when non–weight bearing
- Severe flat foot: arch not present when non–weight bearing, with convex medial border of the foot

Initial Management

- Flat foot has two characteristic components to the deformity in which the hind foot is in valgus and the forefoot is in supination, leading to loss of the medial foot arch.
- **Patient Education.** Most cases of mobile flat feet do not require specific treatment, and no future adverse sequelae is the norm in asymptomatic flexible flat foot.
- First, rule out rigid and significantly painful flat foot. Reassure patient and parents that no significant future disability is substantiated by the presence of the asymptomatic flat foot.
- If mild or moderate flat foot and mostly asymptomatic or with mild symptoms of foot strain, consider arch support or heel cups.

Nonoperative Management

- Nonoperative management with reassurance and consideration of arch supports is the mainstay of treatment of mild to moderate flat foot.

Operative Management

Codes

ICD-10: M21.40 Flat foot

CPT: 28300 Lateral column lengthening via calcaneal osteotomy

    27685 Lengthening or shortening of tendon, leg or ankle

Indications

- Operative management is indicated for older children with severe or painful flat feet.
- If the patient has severe flat feet without significant pain and appearance is bothersome for child and parents, consider medial calcaneal displacement osteotomy or lateral column lengthening.
- If patient has severe flat feet with significant pain, consider subtalar fusion.

Informed consent and counseling

- Long-term results of arch reconstruction are lacking, and treatment should be aimed toward joint-sparing procedures if possible.
- There is a risk of graft failure or nonunion (for lateral column lengthening), and infection and continued pain should be discussed.

Anesthesia

- General anesthesia

Patient positioning

- The patient is positioned supine on a regular table, with a bump under the ipsilateral hip. A tourniquet is applied to the operative extremity.

Surgical Procedures

Lateral Column Lengthening

- An oblique incision is made along the lateral ankle anterior and parallel to the peroneus brevis. The peroneal tendons are released from their sheaths to allow for retraction.
- The sinus tarsi is exposed, and the calcaneocuboid joint is visualized.
- An oblique osteotomy of the calcaneus is made using an oscillating saw starting at the inferior aspect of the calcaneus 2 cm proximal to the calcaneocuboid joint

and exiting the junction between the anterior and middle facets.

- An osteotome is used to open the osteotomy, and a tricortical iliac crest graft is impacted in the osteotomy. A Steinman pin can be used to affix the graft for additional fixation.
- The peroneal brevis tendon is lengthened and repaired, and the wound irrigated and closed.
- A padded short leg cast is placed and bivalved.

Achilles Tendon Lengthening

- If the Silfverskiöld test shows tight Achilles tendon, lengthening is indicated as an adjunct to lateral column lengthening procedure.
- A longitudinal skin incision anteromedial to the Achilles tendon is made along the tendon to just proximal to the tendon insertion.
- The paratenon sheath is incised along the tendon.
- Two incisions are made along the tendon: (1) distally just proximal to the tendon insertion, an incision directed from anterior to posterior (two-thirds the width of the tendon); and (2) proximally along the medial two-thirds from medial to lateral (two-thirds the width of the tendon).
- The ankle is dorsiflexed (being careful not to be too aggressive) to the desired position.
- A short leg cast is applied.

Estimated Postoperative Course

- Non–weight bearing for 6 to 8 weeks.
- Postoperative days 10 to 14: Routine follow-up, patient and parent education.
- Postoperative 6 to 8 weeks: Cast and pin removal, with standing radiographs at that time. Use arch supports to supplement walking out of cast.

SUGGESTED READINGS

Bordelon RL: Hypermobile flatfoot in children. Comprehension, evaluation, and treatment, *Clin Orthop Relat Res* 181:7–14, 1983.

Koutsogiannis E: Treatment of mobile flat foot by displacement osteotomy of the calcaneus, *J Bone Joint Surg Br* 53:96–100, 1971.

Mosca VS: Calcaneal lengthening for valgus deformity of the hind foot. Results in children who had severe, symptomatic flatfoot and skewfoot, *J Bone Joint Surg Am* 77:500–512, 1995.

Staheli LT, Chew DE, Corbett M, et al.: The longitudinal arch: a survey of eight hundred and eighty-two feet in normal children and adults, *J Bone Joint Surg Am* 69(3):426–428, 1987.

CLUBFOOT (TALIPES EQUINOVARUS DEFORMITY)

History

- Background: Congenital deformity of the foot, in which foot is shaped like a "club" and includes equinus, varus, forefoot adductus, and medial rotation
- Deformity present at birth and hypothesized to be caused by several factors including intrauterine restriction, genetics, and neuromuscular conditions
- Can be unilateral or bilateral

Physical Examination

- Assess position and flexibility of foot:
  - The hind foot is in equinus and the subtalar joint is in varus (inversion and adduction). The posterior tibial tendon and Achilles tendon are tight. Look for a single posterior heel crease.
  - The midfoot is adducted and plantar flexed. Look for a single medial midfoot crease.
  - Previously, infants with idiopathic clubfoot were thought to be at increased risk for developmental dysplasia of the hips, but this is no longer supported by recent research.

Imaging

- Imaging is not required in the diagnosis or management of clubfoot.

Initial Management

- **Patient Education.** Clubfoot occurs in approximately 1 in 1000 births, and although many theories on etiology exist, there is no definitive answer regarding etiology. Nonoperative treatment with Ponseti casting is the initial treatment of choice, although Achilles tendon releases are necessary in 90% of cases to help with contracture. Ponseti casting can be initiated in the first week of life. Parental patience and diligence is key because patients post-casting will require long-term foot bracing to prevent recurrence of deformity. With adherence to the Ponseti casting and bracing recommendations, there is a 90%+ success rate.

Nonoperative Management

Serial Ponseti casting

- In children younger than 2 years old, the majority of the deformity can be corrected with four to six long leg casts in a sequence described by Ponseti.
- Sequence: C.A.V.E.:
  - C—Cavus: The first cast is used to elevate the first ray into alignment with other rays.
  - A—Adductus: A second to third cast is used to decrease the adduction deformity of the forefoot. Counter-pressure should be applied to the head of the talus to ensure abduction around the talus.
  - V—Varus: A second to third cast is also used to gradually decrease varus of the hind foot.
  - E—Equinus: A fourth cast is used to correct any equinus of the calcaneus.
  - Each cast should be left on for 5 to 7 days before the next cast change. Once appropriate cavus, adductus, and varus are achieved, it is often necessary to perform percutaneous Achilles tenotomy, which is done in the office, to correct hind foot equinus, after which point the final cast can be applied for 3 weeks.
  - Check perfusion of toes after each cast change to ensure that the cast has not been applied too tightly.

Operative Management

Codes

ICD-10: Q66.1 Congenital talipes equinovarus
CPT: 27605 Tenotomy, percutaneous, Achilles tendon
  28262 Capsulotomy, midfoot; extensive

Indications

- Hind foot equinus after Ponseti casting → percutaneous Achilles tenotomy
- Recalcitrant clubfoot or long-standing clubfoot not amenable to Ponseti technique → surgical release of clubfoot

Informed consent and counseling

- Surgical release of clubfoot can be associated with wound problems, damage to nerves and vessels, overcorrection or undercorrection of deformity, recurrence of deformity, stiffness, and weakness.

Anesthesia

- Local anesthesia for percutaneous Achilles tenotomy
- General anesthesia for open release of resistant clubfoot

Patient positioning

- Supine position with knee flexed and ankle maximally dorsiflexed for percutaneous Achilles tenotomy
- Prone position with knee extended for surgical release of clubfoot, with tourniquet applied to the upper thigh

Surgical Procedures

Percutaneous Achilles Tenotomy

- The patient is placed supine, and 1% lidocaine is applied topically or injected into a region approximately 2 cm proximal to the calcaneal insertion of the Achilles tendon.
- An assistant holds the foot in dorsiflexion, which accentuates the Achilles tendon.
- A #11 blade is inserted from the medial side, anterior to the Achilles tendon. The blade is oriented such that on insertion the sharp portion of the blade does not touch the Achilles tendon (parallel to the tendon).
- Once the blade is passed gently past the entire width of the tendon, the blade is gently twisted 90 degrees such that it is perpendicular to and facing the tendon.
- Gentle pressure is placed with a thumb over the tendon until release is complete, which should allow for approximately 15 degrees more dorsiflexion.
- Pressure over the small stab wound is applied until bleeding is stopped, and a long leg cast is applied with increased dorsiflexion. This cast is the final cast in the Ponseti method that addresses equinus.

Surgical Release of Clubfoot

- Soft tissue release of multiple contracted structures may be necessary in older children where Ponseti method will not work due to secondary adaptive changes from long-term clubfoot.
- Intraoperative assessment of tight structures determines which soft tissues need to be released.
- A Cincinnati incision is made. This large incision starts medially along the talonavicular joint, courses posteriorly above the calcaneal tuberosity, and progresses laterally at the level of the talonavicular joint. Parts of the incision can be used if selective releases are being carried out.
- Posterior structures are assessed first, and the Achilles tendon is lengthened with a Z-plasty. If the ankle is still tight in equinus, release the posterior ankle joint capsule

by simple incision, being careful to protect peroneal tendons and posteromedial neurovascular structures.

- Medial structures are assessed next if further correction is necessary. The posterior tibial neurovascular bundle lies between the flexor digitorum longus and flexor hallucis longus and should be protected throughout the case. Identifying tight structures, the posterior tibial tendon, abductor hallucis muscle, flexor digitorum, and flexor hallucis longus can be lengthened. If this does not provide adequate correction of hind foot varus and forefoot adduction, then release the talonavicular joint capsule and subtalar joint capsule.
- Lateral structures are assessed next and, rarely, if anatomic alignment cannot be achieved, a completion of the talonavicular and subtalar joint capsule release can be performed on the lateral side.
- The subtalar joint is reduced to create a straight lateral border of the foot and held in place with a 0.062–K-wire passing from the posteromedial talus, navicular, medial cuneiform, and the first web space.
- Wound closure is performed, and a bulky soft dressing is applied.

Estimated Postoperative Course
- Percutaneous Achilles tenotomy
  - The final Ponseti cast after tenotomy should be left on for 3 weeks, after which it can be removed.
  - A Denis-Browne boot with derotation bar is used continuously for 3 months and then gradually changed to nighttime only wear until the child is school age.
  - Compliance with bracing can be challenging as a child grows, but it is important to counteract the tendency for the deformity to recur.
- Surgical release of clubfoot
  - Postoperative week 1: dressing removed, wound evaluated, long leg cast applied.
  - Postoperative week 4: pins removed, cast changed.
  - Postoperative week 12: cast removed.

SUGGESTED READINGS

Cooper DM, Dietz FR: Treatment of idiopathic clubfoot: a thirty-year follow-up noted, *J Bone Joint Surg Am* 77A:1477–1489, 1995.

Davidson R: Posteromedial and posterolateral release for the treatment of resistant clubfoot. In Wiese SW, editor: *Operative techniques in orthopaedic surgery*, Philadelphia, 2010, Lippincott Williams & Wilkins.

Mahan ST, Yazdy MM, Kasser JR, Werler MM: Is it worthwhile to routinely ultrasound screen children with idiopathic clubfoot for hip dysplasia? *J Pediatr Orthop* 33(8):847–851, 2013.

Ponseti IV, Zhivkov M, Davis N, et al.: Treatment of the complex idiopathic clubfoot, *Clin Orthop Relat Res* 251:171–176, 2006.

Roye Jr DP, Roye BD: Idiopathic congenital talipes equinovarus, *J Am Acad Orthop Surg* 10(4):239–248, 2002.

PEDIATRIC SPORTS MEDICINE

OSTEOCHONDROSIS

History
- History of repetitive activity and year-round sports that causes traction at a tendon origin/insertion to bone which can occur in several classic locations. The name of the condition is specific to the location:
  - Sinding-Larsen-Johansson: inferior pole of the patella
  - Osgood-Schlatter: tibial tubercle
  - Sever: calcaneus
  - Iselin apophysitis: fifth metatarsal at the insertion of the peroneus brevis
- Typically, patients are between 8 and 14 years old and frequently with current or recent growth spurt during which bones elongate quickly, soft tissue flexibility decreases, and biomechanics change.
- Recent change in sports or activity schedule/frequency often precedes symptoms.
- Pain and swelling at the effected site that is worse with increased activity and better with rest.
- Limping as symptoms become more severe.

Physical Examination
- Inspect for swelling.
- Palpate for tenderness and overgrowth.
- Stress the tendinous attachment with resisted knee extension or heel/toe walking depending on the site of concern.
- Assess flexibility using popliteal angle (hamstring), Ely's test (quad/hip flexor), and Silfverskiöld (gastrocnemius/soleus).
- Observe a double leg and single leg squat looking for proper mechanics (hips pushing back, knees staying in line with the toes, avoiding valgus at the knees).

Imaging

- X-rays are indicated for pain greater than 6 weeks which is not responding to conservative treatment
  - Knee: AP, lateral, sunrise radiographs. Heel: lateral weight-bearing foot radiographs
  - A spectrum of findings of the apophysis: irregular ossification (early disease), enlargement, or fragmentation (late disease)
- MRI is rarely needed and only helpful if the diagnosis is in question

Initial Management

- **Patient Education.** Osteochondrosis is a result of repetitive microtrauma to the tendinous attachment to bone, leading to inflammation, pain, and bony overgrowth, if chronic. Most patients improve with rest (up to 3 months) and activity modification. A sport specific rehabilitation and evaluation may be helpful.

Nonoperative Management

- Antiinflammatories and ice for pain control
- Bracing can be helpful
  - Chopat strap for Sinding-Larsen-Johansson and Osgood-Schlatter disease
  - Heel cups for Sever disease
- 4 to 6 weeks of relative rest
- Structured rehabilitation program with a focus on stretching and proper mechanics. Gradual progression of activity if pain free
- Recalcitrant symptoms indicative of inadequate rest
- Symptoms can flare intermittently and generally resolve completely when the physes close
  Codes

ICD-10:M92.40 Juvenile osteochondrosis of the patella (Osgood-Schlatter or Sinding-Larsen-Johansson)
ICD-10:M92.80 Other specified juvenile osteochondrosis (Sever disease or Iselin apophysitis)

SUGGESTED READINGS

Milewski MD, Wylie J, Nissen CW, Prokop PR: Knee injuries in skeletally immature athletes. In DeLee Drez, Miller 's, editors: *orthopaedic sports medicine*, ed 5, Philadelphia, 2020, Elsevier, pp 1697–1724.
Sullivan JA, Gregory JR: Foot and ankle injuries in the adolescent athlete. In DeLee Drez, Miller 's, editors: *orthopaedic sports medicine*, ed 5, Philadelphia, 2020, Elsevier, pp 1725–1740.

LITTLE LEAGUER'S ELBOW

History

- History of repetitive throwing/pitching, which places valgus stress along the flexor-pronator origin (medial epicondyle) and the medial epicondylar apophysis with compression stress to the lateral elbow.
- Medial elbow pain and swelling, decreased throwing distance and accuracy. Complaints of constant elbow pain that is worse with throwing is more concerning than soreness just after activity.
- Previously, curve balls were perceived to increase the risk of elbow pain but more recent studies have shown that fastballs and sliders cause increased torque on the elbow.
- The same mechanism can also cause osteochondritis of the capitellum or osteochondral injury to the radial head.

Physical Examination

- Inspect for medial elbow swelling.
- Palpate for medial elbow tenderness and overgrowth.
- Valgus stress on the elbow reproduces pain.

Imaging

- Elbow AP, lateral, oblique radiographs
  - A spectrum of findings of the medial epicondyle apophysis: irregular ossification, enlargement, or partial avulsion
- MRI helpful if the diagnosis is in question or the patient/family needs further convincing to comply with treatment

Initial Management

- **Patient Education.** Little Leaguer's elbow is a result of repetitive microtrauma to the flexor-pronator mass, leading to inflammation along the medial epicondyle and at the medial epicondylar apophysis. Most patients improve with rest (up to 3 months) and activity modification. A throwing rehabilitation and evaluation of pitching mechanics may be helpful. To prevent injury, the recommended per-game pitch counts are 7 to 8 years, 50 pitches; 9 to 10 years, 75 pitches; 11 to 12 years, 85 pitches, 13 to 16 years, 95 pitches; and 17 to 18 years, 105 pitches allowing for appropriate rest between pitching days.

Nonoperative Management

- Antiinflammatories for pain control
- 4 to 6 weeks of complete rest from throwing
- Structured throwing program starting at 6 to 8 weeks with gradual progression if pain free
- Return to throwing at around 12 weeks
- Recalcitrant symptoms indicative of inadequate rest
  Codes

ICD-10:M77.00 Medial epicondylitis, unspecified elbow

SUGGESTED READINGS

Chen FS, Diaz VA, Loebenberg M, et al.: Shoulder and elbow injuries in the skeletally immature athlete, *J Am Acad Orthop Surg* 13:172–185, 2005.

Fleisig GS, Andrews JR, Cutter GR, et al.: Risk of serious injury for young baseball pitchers: a 10-year prospective study, *Am J Sports Med* 39(2):253–257, 2011.

Klingele KE, Kocher MS: Little League elbow: valgus overload injury in the paediatric athlete, *Sports Med* 32(15): 1005–1015, 2002.

Kocher MS, Waters PM, Micheli LJ: Upper extremity injuries in the paediatric athlete, *Sports Med* 30(2): 117–135, 2000.

Wei AS, Khana S, Limpisvasti O, et al.: Clinical and magnetic resonance imaging findings associated with Little League elbow, *J Pediatr Orthop* 30(7):715–719, 2010.

LITTLE LEAGUER'S SHOULDER (PROXIMAL HUMERUS EPIPHYSIOLYSIS)

History

- Definition: chondral injury to the proximal humerus physis
- Repetitive microtrauma to the proximal humeral physis causes the injury and it is most common in patients 11 to 14 years old
- Recent increase in throwing regimen or transition to a year-round team precedes pain
- Shoulder pain that is activity related, worse with throwing activities
- Decreased ball control and velocity with fatigue

Physical Examination

- Pain and tenderness along the shoulder near the physis
- Weakness with resisted abduction and internal rotation
- Glenohumeral internal rotation deficit (GIRD)

Imaging: Fig. 9.16

- AP and axillary radiographic views of the shoulder
  - Radiographs may show physeal widening of the proximal humeral epiphysis, metaphyseal demineralization, sclerosis, and/or fragmentation.
  - Comparison views are helpful because the proximal humeral physis is normally irregular.
- MRI of shoulder may be helpful to rule out other pathology if diagnosis unclear; may show edema around physis.

Initial Management

- **Patient Education.** Little Leaguer's shoulder is an overuse type injury to the pediatric shoulder. Most patients get better with rest and activity modification for several months with gradual progression to a throwing program. Physeal injury, which is rare, can lead to growth arrest. Abnormal pitching mechanics may contribute, and supervised throwing mechanics evaluation may be helpful. To prevent injury, the recommended per-game pitch counts are 7 to 8 years, 50 pitches; 9 to 10 years, 75 pitches; 11 to 12 years, 85 pitches, 13 to 16 years, 95 pitches; and 17 to 18 years, 105 pitches allowing for appropriate rest between pitching days.

Nonoperative Management

- Rest and activity modification for 6 weeks.
- Antiinflammatory medications for pain control.
- Start physical therapy after 6 weeks with evaluation of pitching mechanics and prevent excessive

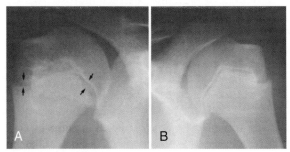

Fig. 9.16 Little Leaguer's shoulder. (**A**) Widening of the proximal humeral physis compared with (**B**) unaffected side. (From Wilkins K: Shoulder, section J: injuries of the proximal humerus in the skeletally immature athlete. In DeLee JC, Drez D, Miller MD, et al, editors: *DeLee and Drez's orthopaedic sports medicine*, Philadelphia, 2010, Saunders, p 1093.)

pitch count. Return to full activity usually at 8 to 12 weeks.

- Radiographic abnormalities may persist after clinical improvement.

    Codes. ICD-10: M89.12 Partial physeal arrest proximal humerus

SUGGESTED READINGS

Chen FS, Diaz VA, Loebenberg M, Rosen JE, et al.: Shoulder and elbow injuries in the skeletally immature athlete, *J Am Acad Orthop Surg* 13:172–185, 2005.

Fleisig GS, Andrews JR, Cutter GR, et al.: Risk of serious injury for young baseball pitchers: a 10-year prospective study, *Am J Sports Med* 39(2):253–257, 2011.

Keeley DW, Hackett T, Keirns M, et al.: A biomechanical analysis of youth pitching mechanics, *J Pediatr Orthop* 28(4):452–459, 2008.

Kocher MS, Waters PM, Micheli LJ: Upper extremity injuries in the paediatric athlete, *Sports Med* 30(2):117–135, 2000.

McFarland EG, Ireland ML: Rehabilitation programs and prevention strategies in adolescent throwing athletes, *Instr Course Lect* 52:37–42, 2003.

OSTEOCHONDRITIS DISSECANS LESIONS

History

- Definition: lesion of subchondral bone that may be associated with overlying chondral fissuring or delamination without a known etiology. Spontaneous avascular necrosis and microtrauma are proposed etiologies.
- Classic locations include the knee (lateral aspect of the medial femoral condyle), talus, and distal humerus in descending order, although osteochondritis dissecans (OCD) lesions can occur in other locations also.
- Symptoms include activity dependent pain, swelling, and mechanical symptoms such as catching or locking if the OCD fragment dislodges.
- Patients with open physes are more likely to be treated successfully with nonoperative intervention.

Physical Examination

- Joint swelling, tenderness over the lesion

Imaging

- Lesions are frequently visualized on x-rays
  - Knee: AP, lateral, sunrise, and tunnel views
  - Ankle: AP, lateral, and mortise views
  - Elbow: AP, lateral, internal and external oblique views
- MRI is used to assess the integrity of the overlying articular cartilage, presence of synovial fluid deep to the lesion, and help predict lesion stability as well as prognosis for healing. Disruption in the articular cartilage, presence of synovial fluid deep to the lesion, loose body, or impending loose body are indicative of unstable lesions.

Initial Management

- As articular cartilage is avascular, healing capacity is extremely limited. Treatment is guided by physeal status, size of the lesion, stability of the lesion, and displacement of the OCD fragment.
- Initially, rest from impact activity for 6 to 8 weeks is the mainstay of treatment for stable lesions. If walking is painful, crutches and partial or non–weight bearing are indicated.

Nonoperative Management

- Rest and activity modification for 6 to 8 weeks.
- Antiinflammatory medications for pain control.
- Radiographic abnormalities may persist after clinical improvement. Repeat x-rays at 3 and 6 months.

Operative Management

Codes

ICD-10: M93.20 Osteochondritis dissecans lesion of unspecified site

CPT: 29885 Knee arthroscopy drilling of OCD lesion with or without fixation

   29879 Knee arthroscopy, microfracture of OCD lesion

Knee autograft (29866) or allograft (29867) osteochondral transfer procedure (OATS)

   29892 Ankle arthroscopy, drilling or microfracture of OCD lesion

Ankle autograft (28446) or allograft (28899) osteochondral transfer procedure (OATS)

Indications

- Failure of nonoperative treatment
- Patient nearing skeletal maturity
- Intact Drilling of Osteochondritis Dissecans Lesion fragment with fluid tracking under the fragment
- Displaced Drilling of Osteochondritis Dissecans Lesion fragment

Informed consent and counseling

- Joint stiffness, risk of recurrent symptoms or failure of OCD lesion to heal, need for additional procedures

  Anesthesia

- General anesthesia

  Patient positioning

- Supine position with a lateral thigh post and tourniquet to the thigh

Surgical Procedures

Surgical technique is based on the size of the lesion, integrity of the overlying articular cartilage, remaining skeletal growth, and stability of the lesion. **Antegrade or retrograde drilling** is utilized for stable lesions that are small with intact articular cartilage and especially in skeletally immature patients. OCD lesion **elevation, bone grafting and screw fixation** is utilized for small unstable lesions if bone is present on the OCD fragment, indicating a potential for healing. **Microfracture** is utilized in lesions less than 2 cm that are not amenable to drilling because the cartilage is no longer intact and also not amenable to fixation because there is no bone on the OCD lesion. Microfracture involves débriding the lesion to establish stable borders and using an awl to cause bleeding of the subchondral bone and stimulate formation of a blood clot and then fibrocartilage in the base of the lesion. Type I fibrocartilage is inferior to type II articular cartilage, but superior to exposed subchondral bone with regard to symptom resolution and delaying the onset of osteoarthritis. Unstable lesions without bone on the OCD fragment or lesions that have failed prior operative treatment are indicated for **osteochondral autograft or allograft transfer** (OAT) procedure. Allograft is utilized for lesions greater than 3 cm. A study published in 2012 demonstrated superiority of OAT procedure as compared to microfracture with regard to return to play in young athletes with 10-year follow up.

Knee Arthroscopy, Drilling of Osteochondritis Dissecans Lesion

- The patient is positioned supine on a regular table with a lateral post along the thigh. A tourniquet is placed along the proximal thigh. The leg is exsanguinated and the tourniquet pressure is elevated. A small stab incision directed toward the notch is made along the lateral joint line just lateral to the inferior aspect of the patellar tendon and used as a viewing

portal. The arthroscope is inserted into this portal, and inflow is established. An inferomedial portal is established for the working portal.

- A diagnostic arthroscopy is performed, and the osteochondral lesion is assessed with careful attention to the integrity of the overlying cartilage. A probe is used to detect softening and/or fissuring of the articular cartilage and the lesion is measured.
- A Steinman pin is used to drill antegrade as directed by fluoroscopy or retrograde into the area of cartilage softening with several passes made a few millimeters apart in a stellate pattern. Stimulating the subchondral bone to bleed promotes healing of the lesion.
- The arthroscopic inflow is paused to assess for bleeding from the Steinman pin holes.
- Portal sites are closed with a single nylon suture.

Estimated Postoperative Course

- 50% weight bearing for 6 weeks.
- Postoperative day 0: Start knee range of motion and isometric quadriceps and hamstring exercises.
- Postoperative days 10 to 14: Wound check.
- Postoperative weeks 6: Clinical examination for range of motion and tenderness over the OCD lesion; progress activities as tolerated.

Knee Arthroscopy, Open Osteochondral Allograft Transfer

- The patient is positioned supine on a regular table with a lateral post along the thigh. A tourniquet is placed along the proximal thigh. The leg is exsanguinated and the tourniquet pressure is elevated. A small stab incision directed toward the notch is made along the lateral joint line just lateral to the inferior aspect of the patellar tendon and used as a viewing portal. The arthroscope is inserted into this portal, and inflow is established. An inferomedial portal is established for the working portal.
- A diagnostic arthroscopy is performed, and the osteochondral lesion is assessed with careful attention to the integrity of the overlying cartilage. A probe is used to assess the articular cartilage and the lesion is measured. The knee is then drained of arthroscopic fluid.
- A medial para-patellar incision is made with extension proximally and distally as necessary to expose the OCD lesion. Subcutaneous dissection is carried out followed by a longitudinal incision through the

retinaculum, leaving a cuff of soft tissue on the patella to close at the conclusion of the procedure.

- The patella is displaced laterally and a bent Homann is placed in the intracondylar notch. The knee is flexed to bring the OCD lesion into the field of view. Hoffa's fat pad is excised to aid in visualization. The lesion is circumscribed and an appropriate size is determined. A guidewire is placed in the center of the lesion and an appropriate-sized reamer is used to core out the lesion in entirety to a depth of 6 to 8 mm.
- Allograft femoral hemicondyle is secured on the back table and the donor site is selected on the hemicondyle to match the contour of the patient's condyle. A coring device that corresponds with the lesion size is used to harvest the donor osteochondral graft. The graft is trimmed to match the depth of the recipient site and washed with irrigation.
- Attention is turned back to the patient's OCD lesion site. The wound is irrigated and the allograft plug is delivered into the prepared site with care not to leave the graft either proud or recessed.
- Retinaculum is closed with interrupted figure-of-eight sutures, followed by subcutaneous layers and finally, a running subcuticular layer. The lateral portal site is closed with a single nylon suture.

Estimated Postoperative Course

- 50% weight bearing for 6 weeks to protect the graft.
- Postoperative day 0: Start knee range of motion and isometric quadriceps and hamstring exercises.
- Postoperative days 10 to 14: Wound check.
- Postoperative weeks 6: Clinical examination for range of motion and tenderness over the OCD lesion; progress therapy to include full weight bearing and progressive strengthening.
- Postoperative months 3 to 6: Progress therapy to include sport specific drills.

SUGGESTED READINGS

Gudas R, Gudaite A, Pocius A, et al.: Ten-year follow-up of a prospective, randomized clinical study of mosaic osteochondral autologous transplantation versus microfracture for the treatment of osteochondral defects in the knee joint of athletes, *Am J Sports Med* 40:2499–2508, 2012.

Gunton MJ, Carey JL, Shaw CR, Murnaghan ML: Drilling juvenile osteochondritis dissecans: retro- or transarticular? *Clin Orthop Relat Res* 471(4):1144–1151, 2013.

Laidlaw MS: Articular cartilage lesions. In *DeLee, Drez, & Miller's orthopaedic sports medicine*, ed 5, Philadelphia, 2020, Elsevier, pp 1161–1177.

Perumal V, Wall E, Babekir N: Juvenile osteochondritis dissecans of the talus, *J Pediatr Orthop* 27(7):821–825, 2007.

DISCOID MENISCUS

History

- Definition: abnormal development of meniscus leading to enlarged and discoid-shaped meniscus
- Majority of cases involve lateral meniscus
- Frequently an incidental finding because most cases are asymptomatic
- Young child can present with lateral knee catching or popping, with or without pain

Physical Examination

- Inspect for any blocks to knee range of motion.
- Palpate the lateral joint line for tenderness.
- Perform the **McMurray test** to evaluate for painful pop/click along the joint line:
  - One hand stabilizes the medial knee at the joint line while the other hand holds the sole of the foot. The knee is in full flexion, then simultaneously extended and internally rotated. If click or pain occurs, the test suggests a lateral meniscus tear.
- Perform a varus stress test to evaluate for lateral collateral ligament laxity because the lateral knee joint line may be widened to accommodate a larger lateral meniscus.

Imaging

- AP and lateral radiographs of the knee
  - May show widening of lateral compartment compared with medial or a flattened lateral femoral condyle
  - Assess for OCD of the lateral femoral condyle
- MRI of the knee
  - Best study to evaluate discoid meniscus
  - A discoid meniscus appears as three consecutive sagittal 3-mm cuts without a bow-tie appearance of the anterior and posterior horns

Classification System

- Stable—posterior meniscofemoral ligament is intact securing the discoid meniscus

- Unstable (Wrisberg type)—posterior meniscofemoral ligament is lacking, leading to hypermobile discoid meniscus

Differential Diagnoses

- Other patterns of meniscus tears
- OCD
- Patellofemoral pain

Initial Management

- **Patient Education.** Discoid meniscus is present in 3% to 5% of the population, and in most cases is asymptomatic and does not require treatment. However, discoid menisci may have a propensity to develop intrasubstance tears or, if unstable, cause pain and mechanical symptoms such as knee locking and popping.

Nonoperative Management

- Establish diagnosis on the basis of an examination and MRI of stable or unstable type.
- Rest and antiinflammatory medications with observation is the mainstay of nonoperative treatment.

Operative Management

Codes

ICD-10: Q68.6 Discoid meniscus
CPT: 29881 Knee arthroscopy and partial meniscectomy (medial or lateral)
29882   Knee arthroscopy with meniscus repair (medial or lateral)

Indications

- Persistent loss of range of motion/locking or pain

Informed consent and counseling

- Knee stiffness, risk of recurrent tear, failure of meniscal stabilization after surgery can occur postoperatively

Anesthesia

- General anesthesia

Patient positioning

- Supine position with a lateral thigh post and tourniquet to the thigh

Surgical Procedures

Arthroscopic Partial Lateral Meniscectomy and Saucerization: Fig. 9.17

- The patient is positioned supine on a regular table with a lateral post along the thigh. A tourniquet is placed along the proximal thigh. The leg is exsanguinated by elevation only, and the tourniquet pressure is elevated. A small stab incision directed toward the notch is made along the lateral joint line just lateral to the inferior aspect of the patellar tendon and used as a viewing portal. The arthroscope is inserted into this portal, and inflow is established. An inferomedial portal is established for the working portal.
- A diagnostic arthroscopy is performed, and if the discoid meniscus is unstable, a posterolateral approach to the knee is made in preparation for an inside-out suture repair of the meniscus. All inside meniscus repair devices can also be utilized.
  - A 3-cm lateral joint line incision is made in line with the posterior aspect of the fibular head.
  - The interval between the biceps femoris and iliotibial band is found, and a retractor is placed into this interval. The peroneal nerve lies posterior to the biceps femoris.
- Using a combination of biters and shavers, the lateral meniscus is saucerized to leave an approximately 15-mm rim of meniscus. The discoid meniscus is stabilized as needed with an inside-out suture fixation, passing suture through the meniscus and out the open lateral wound and tying knots superficial to the joint capsule. A minimum of 3 sutures are used to repair an unstable meniscus.

Estimated Postoperative Course

- 50% weight bearing and hinged knee brace with range of motion limited to 0 to 90 degrees for 6 weeks if meniscal stabilization was performed. No squatting beyond 90 degrees for 6–12 weeks.
- Postoperative day 0: Start knee range of motion.
- Postoperative days 10 to 14: Wound check.
- Postoperative weeks 6: Clinical examination for range of motion; progress activities as tolerated.

SUGGESTED READINGS

Atay OA, Doral MN, Leblebicioglu G, et al.: Management of discoid lateral meniscus tears: observations in 34 knees, *Arthroscopy* 19(4):346–352, 2003.

Carter CW, Hoellwarth J, Weiss JM: Clinical outcomes as a function of meniscal stability in the discoid meniscus: a preliminary report, *J Pediatr Orthop* 32(1):9–14, 2012.

Good CR, Green DW, Griffith MH, et al.: Arthroscopic treatment of symptomatic discoid meniscus in children: classification, technique, and results, *Arthroscopy* 23(2):157–163, 2007.

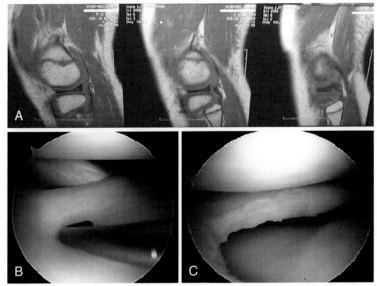

Fig. 9.17 Discoid Lateral Meniscus. **A**, Magnetic resonance imaging showing lack of bow-tie appearance of lateral meniscus. **B**, Arthroscopy: complete discoid lateral meniscus. **C**, Arthroscopy: saucerization of discoid lateral meniscus. (From Brockmeier S, Rodeo S. Knee, Section B: Meniscal injuries. In DeLee JC, Drez D, Miller MD et al, editors: *DeLee and Drez's orthopaedic sports medicine*, Philadelphia, 2010, Saunders, pp 1615.)

Kramer DE, Micheli LJ: Meniscal tears and discoid meniscus in children: diagnosis and treatment, *J Am Acad Orthop Surg* 17:698–707, 2009.

PEDIATRIC MUSCULOSKELETAL INFECTION

Introduction

- Musculoskeletal infection in the child has a wide spectrum of severity, and a systematic approach to each patient is essential. Musculoskeletal infection is most common in children younger than 5 who are otherwise healthy.
- Osteomyelitis (infection of the bone) and septic arthritis (infection of the joint) are the focus of this topic discussion.
- Infants younger than 18 months have contiguous metaphyseal and epiphyseal circulation, making simultaneous osteomyelitis and septic arthritis common in this group.
- The metaphyseal outflow circulation is turbulent in children, predisposing this region to osteomyelitis. The femur, tibia, and humerus are most commonly involved.
  - The hip, ankle, and shoulder are common sites where septic arthritis can occur adjacent to bone infection due to the intracapsular location of the metaphysis.

OSTEOMYELITIS

History

- Definition: Osteomyelitis is infection of the bone.
- Timing and severity of symptoms include the following:
  - Acute hematogenous osteomyelitis (AHO)—Child often presents with sudden illness and localized symptoms within a matter of a few days
  - Subacute osteomyelitis (SO)—Child presents with more than 2 weeks of vague or moderate symptoms
  - Chronic osteomyelitis (CO)—Child presents with months to years of mild symptoms, likely as a result of inadequately treated acute infection
- Evaluate for constitutional symptoms such as fevers, chills, and malaise. Children often appear obviously sick in acute severe cases.
- The patient is unable to bear weight and has worsening pain in the affected extremity.
- Patients and family should be queried about recent systemic and respiratory infections and recent travel history.

- Most common organisms include *Staphylococcus, Streptococci, and Pseudomonas* (in the foot).

Physical Examination

- Fever is higher than 38.5°C.
- Inspect for inability to bear weight or use the affected extremity or pseudoparalysis of the affected extremity.
- Palpate for swelling, warmth, and significant tenderness in affected extremity.
- It may be difficult to localize, so always consider referred pain from a more distant site in children.

Imaging

- Obtain AP and lateral radiographs of the affected extremity.
  - Soft tissue swelling is seen early, and cortical erosion and destruction is seen late (10 to 14 days later).
- Ultrasound is useful to determine deep soft tissue swelling and subperiosteal fluid collections.
- Bone scan is useful when osteomyelitis is suspected, although location is in question.
- MRI allows clear visualization of osteomyelitis and associated abscesses but frequently requires sedation for children (Fig. 9.18).

Laboratory Evaluation

- Peripheral complete blood cell count (CBC) with differential, erythrocyte sedimentation rate (ESR), C-reactive protein (CRP), and blood cultures × 2 sets. White blood cell count (WBC) is often normal. CRP elevates first, then ESR. Blood cultures are positive in only 30% to 50% of patients with osteomyelitis.

Classification System

- Timing and severity classify osteomyelitis into three major categories: AHO, SO, and CO.
- Age is important in addition to the classification as common causative organisms differ per age group: neonatal (0 to 8 weeks), infant and early child (younger than 3 years), child (greater than 3 years), and adolescent (greater than 12 years) (Table 9.7).

Initial Management

- **Patient Education.** Osteomyelitis is an infection to the bone. Adequate treatment of osteomyelitis may take considerable time and effort, including

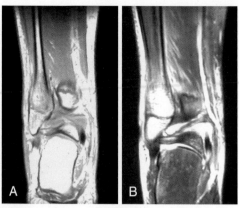

Fig. 9.18 A and B, Magnetic resonance imaging of osteomyelitis of the fibula. (From Copley LA, Dormans JP: Musculoskeletal infections. In Dormans JP, editor: *Core knowledge in orthopaedics: pediatric orthopaedics*, Philadelphia, 2005, Mosby, p 337.)

long-term antibiotics, surgical débridement, and reconstructive procedures.

- In all cases of AHO, the patient should be admitted to the hospital for a thorough workup, empiric antibiotics, medical management, and possible surgical débridement.
- For cases of SO, completion of a thorough workup to confirm the diagnosis should be made. Consideration of a bone biopsy should also be made to confirm the diagnosis, and then the patient should be treated with appropriate antibiotics.
- For cases of CO, a thorough workup including possible MRI and bone biopsy should be obtained. A plan for surgical débridement and reconstruction should be made after confirmation of diagnosis.

Nonoperative Management

- All types of osteomyelitis have a component of antibiotic therapy with or without adjunctive surgical débridement.
- Some cases of AHO (if identified early without abscess formation) and most cases of SO can possibly be treated with antibiotics alone.
- Antibiotic selection based on organism, age, and concurrent illness. Initial therapy is IV, then transition to oral antibiotics. Duration of antibiotic therapy is generally 4 to 6 weeks and guided by the extent of infection, presence of abscess, inflammatory labs, and clinical symptoms. Inflammatory markers and

TABLE 9.7 Common Pathogens by Age

Age	Organism (Top 3)
Neonatal (0–8 week)	*Staphylococcus aureus*, Group B *Streptococcus*, *Staphylococcus epidermidis*
Infant and early child (<3 year)	*Staphylococcus aureus*, *Kingella kingae*, *Streptococcus pneumonia*
Child (>3 year)	*Staphylococcus aureus*, Group A *streptococcus*
Adolescent (>12 year)	*Staphylococcus aureus*, *Neisseria gonorrhoeae*

clinical symptoms should continue to improve or should prompt repeat imaging.

- Patients are frequently comanaged with the infectious disease service.
- If no improvement in 24 to 48 hours, there is increased suspicion for abscess.

Operative Management

Codes
ICD-10: M86.10 Acute osteomyelitis
M86.60 Chronic osteomyelitis
CPT: 11044 Débridement of skin, subcutaneous tissue, muscle, and bone

Indications
- Limited response to antibiotics alone, presence of subperiosteal or intraosseous abscess

Informed consent and counseling
- Risk of chronic osteomyelitis, pathologic fracture, growth disturbance, and avascular necrosis
- The need for more than a single procedure for adequate débridement of the infection
- Multisystem involvement of infection and side effects of long-term antibiotics

Anesthesia
- General anesthesia

Patient positioning
- Supine positioning is the norm in most extremity cases.

Surgical Procedures

Surgical Débridement of Osteomyelitis
- Operative débridement is the goal in complex cases of AHO and almost all cases of CO, and approaches vary by anatomic location of the infection. Drilling, decompression, and cortical windowing are among the available techniques for débridement.

- Serial débridement may be necessary, as well as the placement of local antibiotic cement beads.
- Common themes regardless of location and approach are drainage of pus and abscess and débridement of necrotic tissue.
- Surgical treatment of chronic osteomyelitis includes débridement of sequestrum (dead bone), involucrum (reactive new bone) and any existing sinus tracts.
- It is important to perform a careful biopsy if diagnosis is unclear before aggressive débridement to rule out aggressive malignancies.

Estimated Postoperative Course
- Approximately 6 weeks of antibiotics is the norm, at the discretion of the pediatric infectious disease specialist. Protected weight-bearing may be necessary depending on the surgical location to decrease the risk of pathologic fracture
- Postoperative days 0 to 7: Continued clinical and laboratory evaluation (serial WBC, CRP, and ESR). Clinical and laboratory value improvement is expected within 72 to 96 hours.
- Postoperative days 10 to 14: Wound evaluation, repeat laboratory tests.
- Postoperative week 6 onwards: Gradual increase in time between follow-up visits as improvement is seen.

SUGGESTED READINGS

Copley LA, Dormans JP: Musculoskeletal infections. In Dormans JP, editor: *Core knowledge in orthopaedics: pediatric orthopaedics*, Philadelphia, 2005, Mosby.

Song KM, Sloboda JF: Acute hematogenous osteomyelitis in children, *J Am Acad Orthop Surg* 9:166–175, 2001.

Staheli L: Infection. In *International pediatric orthopedic pocketbook*, Staheli, 2005, Seattle, pp 373–392.

Stanitski CL: Changes in pediatric acute hematogenous osteomyelitis management, *J Pediatr Orthop* 24(4):444–445, 2004.

SEPTIC ARTHRITIS

History

- Definition: Septic arthritis is infection of a joint space.
- Most cases of septic arthritis occur in children younger than 5 years.
- Most cases are monoarticular with the hip, knee, ankle, elbow, wrist, and shoulder the most commonly affected sites. Expeditious diagnosis and treatment is vital as joint destruction occurs quickly.
- Hematogenous seeding of the joint is the most common mechanism.
- As in osteomyelitis, historical features include sudden inability to use or bear weight on the affected extremity. Recent sick contacts and illnesses should be assessed.
- *Staphylococcus, Streptococcus, and Kingella* are the most common organisms. *Enterococcus* and Group B *Streptococcus* are more prevalent in neonates.

Physical Examination

- Fever is higher than 38.5°C. Fever is frequently not present in neonates.
- Inspect for inability to bear weight or use the affected extremity (pseudoparalysis).
- Palpate for edema, warmth, and significant tenderness in the joint.
- Assess passive range of motion of the joint, which is painful in septic arthritis.

Imaging

- AP and lateral radiographs for the affected joint, which are frequently normal.
  - Effusion will be present in acute cases.
  - Joint space widening may be present.
  - Rule out trauma.
- Ultrasound—helpful to identify effusion, especially in the hip.

Laboratory Evaluation

- As in osteomyelitis, all patients should have CBC with differential, ESR, CRP, and blood cultures × 2

sets drawn. Joint aspiration should be performed and the aspirate sent for culture.
- Kocher criteria: Fever greater than 38.5°C, inability to bear weight on the affected limb, ESR greater than 40 mm/hour, WBC greater than 12,000/ml. If three of these criteria are met, there is a 93.1% probability of septic arthritis. If four of these criteria are met, there is a 99.6% probability of septic arthritis.

Initial Management

- **Patient Education.** Septic arthritis is an infection of the joint space that can lead to damage from severe inflammation. Cartilage and joint destruction can occur if treatment is not initiated expeditiously. Parents should expect at least 4 weeks of antibiotic therapy.
- The patient should be evaluated in the emergency department and receive no food or drink (kept non per os [NPO]) in case urgent joint decompression is necessary.
- An aspiration of the joint should be performed and sent for synovial profile (cell count), and a Gram stain with culture should be obtained. Joint aspirate is typically cloudy or frank pus with greater than 50,000 WBC. Due to the bacteriostatic properties of synovial fluid, culture is only positive in approximately 35% of joint aspirate cultures.
- Empiric intravenous antibiotics should be started to include gram-positive coverage for the most common pathologies (*Staphylococcus aureus*). Joint decompression should start as soon as possible to prevent joint damage.

Nonoperative Management

- There is little role for nonoperative management of septic arthritis once a diagnosis has been made.

Operative Management

Codes

- ICD-10:M00.9 Pyogenic arthritis, unspecified site
- CPT: 29871 Arthroscopic lavage of knee for infection

Indications

- Consideration of formal irrigation and débridement should be given for all septic joints.

Informed consent and counseling

- Risk of joint damage without decompression of the affected joint

- Possible need for serial procedures to adequately eradicate infection
  Anesthesia
- General anesthesia
  Patient positioning
- Supine positioning is the norm in most extremity cases.

Surgical Procedures

Arthroscopic Joint Lavage and Débridement of the Knee

- The patient is positioned supine on a regular table with a lateral post along the thigh. A tourniquet is placed along the proximal thigh. The leg is exsanguinated by elevation only, and the tourniquet pressure is elevated. A small stab incision directed toward the notch is made along the lateral joint line just lateral to the patellar tendon inferolateral and used as a viewing portal. The arthroscope is inserted into this portal, and inflow is established. An outflow portal is made along the medial joint line just medial to the patellar tendon using a small stab incision directed toward the notch. This portal can also be used to débride inflamed synovium using an arthroscopic shaver. Copious irrigation is allowed through the knee to lavage the infection.

Open Joint Arthrotomy and Lavage

- The approach to the particular site of infection varies by the type of joint infected and is beyond the scope of this text. In general, the joint is opened and copious saline is used to lavage the joint to decrease the bacterial burden and reduce the effects of proteolytic enzymes from inflammation, which cause proteoglycan and collagen degradation.

Estimated Postoperative Course

- At least 4 weeks of antibiotics is the norm, at the discretion of the pediatric infectious disease specialist.

- Postoperative days 0 to 7: Immediately post surgically, a temporary splint may be applied to immobilize the joint and allow for rest. After the patient's comfort improves, therapy should be started to initiate motion of the joint to prevent stiffness. Follow serial inflammatory laboratory tests to help guide transition to oral antibiotics.
- Postoperative days 10 to 14: Check the wound, remove sutures, perform clinical assessment of joint, and continue to work on range of motion.
- Postoperative weeks 2 to 6: There should be a gradual increase in time between follow-up visits as improvement is seen.

SUGGESTED READINGS

Copley LA, Dormans JP: Musculoskeletal infections. In Dormans JP, editor: *Core knowledge in orthopaedics: Pediatric orthopaedics*, Philadelphia, 2005, Mosby.

Copley LA: Infections of the musculoskeletal system. In Herring JA, editor: *Tachdjian's pediatric orthopaedics*, ed 4, Philadelphia, 2008, Saunders.

Kocher MS, Zurakowski D, Kasser JR, et al.: Differentiating between septic arthritis and transient synovitis of the hip in children: an evidence-based clinical prediction algorithm, *J Bone Joint Surg Am* 81:1662–1670, 1999.

Perlman MH, Patzakis MJ, Kumar PJ, Holtom P: The incidence of joint involvement with adjacent osteomyelitis in pediatric patients, *J Pediatr Orthop* 20:40–43, 2000.

Section J, Gibbons SD, Barton T, et al.: Microbiological culture methods for pediatric musculoskeletal infection: A guideline for optimal use, *J Bone Joint Surg Am* 97(6):441–449, 2015.

ACKNOWLEDGMENTS

The authors would like to acknowledge the contribution of the previous edition author, Scott Yang.

10

Orthopaedic Tumors and Masses

Deana Bhamidipati

INTRODUCTION

- Orthopaedic oncology is a field of orthopaedic surgery that specializes in the diagnosis and treatment of both benign and malignant tumors of the bones and soft tissues of the extremities, pelvis, and spine. Although definitions vary, a tumor can be thought of simply as any mass in the soft tissues or bone that otherwise should not be there. For example, a tumor may be a neoplasm, which is an abnormal proliferation of abnormal cells; a hamartoma, which is an abnormal proliferation of normal cells; or simply an infection causing a masslike effect. The focus of this chapter will be the common neoplasms encountered by the musculoskeletal oncologist.
- Musculoskeletal neoplasms can first be divided into benign and malignant entities. Benign neoplasms are proliferations of abnormal cells that have no potential to metastasize to other areas of the body. Locally, some benign neoplasms can be aggressive and cause significant problems. However, despite its local activity, if a neoplasm has the ability to travel to a distant organ (such as the lungs or lymph nodes) it is considered malignant.

MALIGNANT BONE DISEASE

- There are many categories of malignant neoplasms. Some of these include carcinomas (from epithelial origin), adenocarcinomas (from epithelial cells with secretory properties), lymphomas (arising from lymphocytes), leukemia (from bone marrow cells), and melanomas (from transformed melanocytes). A sarcoma is a malignant neoplasm that arises from cells of mesenchymal origin. Mesenchymal tissues include those found in the limbs and pelvis: bone, cartilage, muscle, fat, vessels, and nerves. Sarcomas are exceedingly rare. Every year in the United States there are fewer than 10,000 new cases of bone sarcoma and fewer than 15,000 new soft tissue sarcomas.
- Malignant bone disease often causes bone destruction or lysis. A permeative or moth-eaten pattern of lysis (Fig. 10.1), in which the bone is aggressively destroyed with indistinct margins, is usually displayed. A more geographic pattern, in which there is a clear margin between normal and abnormal bone, is seen with benign tumors (Fig. 10.2).

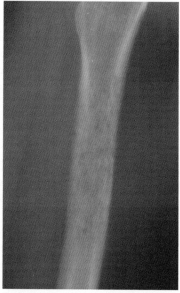

Fig. 10.1 A Permeative Pattern of Destruction from a Metastatic Lesion in the Diaphysis of a Femur.

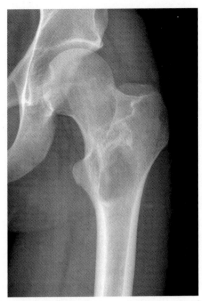

Fig. 10.2 A Geographic Pattern of Bone Lysis Seen in a Simple Bone Cyst of the Femur.

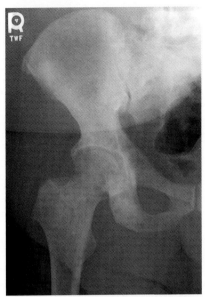

Fig. 10.3 A Mixed Lytic and Blastic Pattern of Metastasis Seen with Widespread Breast Cancer.

Metastatic Disease

- Metastatic carcinoma to bone is 25 times more likely to occur than primary bone sarcoma. The five primary carcinomas that most commonly metastasize to bone are breast, prostate, lung, kidney, and thyroid. In contrast to the small numbers of primary bone sarcoma, there are roughly 800,000 new cases of these five carcinomas in the United States every year. Metastatic carcinoma most commonly occurs in the thoracic and lumbar spine (theoretically because of the valveless Batson's venous system there) but can occur in virtually any bone. It commonly presents as pain and can lead to weakened bone and pathologic fractures (fractures that occur at normal physiologic loads).

- Metastatic breast cancer is common in women with advanced disease. Radiographically, it is classically a mixed lytic and blastic lesion; that is, it causes lysis of bone and formation of bone (Fig. 10.3). It typically responds to radiation therapy but commonly requires surgical stabilization. Metastatic prostate cancer is also radiosensitive but typically is a purely blastic process (Fig. 10.4). Lung, kidney, and thyroid disease usually cause purely lytic and destructive lesions (Fig. 10.5). Renal cell carcinoma and thyroid disease are extremely vascular lesions that often require embolization before open surgical treatment.

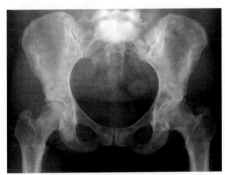

Fig. 10.4 Widespread Blastic Metastases Throughout the Pelvis, Lumbar Spine, and Femurs.

- Because of the overwhelming preponderance of potentially metastatic carcinoma, any lytic bone lesion in a patient older than 40 years of age should be considered metastatic disease until proven otherwise. Work-up for these patients should include radiographs of the entire affected bone, magnetic resonance imaging (MRI) of the area to assess soft tissue extent, a bone scan to assess other skeletal disease, and a computed tomography (CT) scan of the chest, abdomen, and pelvis in an attempt to identify the primary site (Fig. 10.6). Often a biopsy will still be necessary to secure a definitive tissue diagnosis.

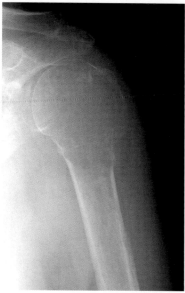

Fig. 10.5 Purely Lytic Lung Metastasis to the Proximal Humerus.

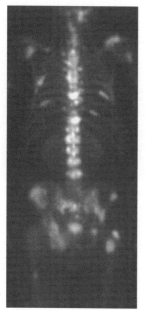

Fig. 10.6 A Bone Scan Demonstrating Widespread Adenocarcinoma Metastases.

• Surgical treatment of metastatic disease can be challenging. Painful lesions in weight-bearing bones should be aggressively stabilized, but many lesions may not have definite surgical indications, especially in patients with limited life spans. A team approach with medical oncology, radiation oncology, orthopaedic oncology, and the patient should be used to optimize treatment and outcomes. Unfortunately, bone metastasis is an ominous finding with little chance of cure.

• Although much rarer, other malignancies such as melanoma, colon, bladder, and cervical cancer can all metastasize to bone and should be suspected in patients with a positive medical history. Metastatic bone disease in children is not common but can be seen with neuroblastoma and Wilms tumor.

Multiple Myeloma

• Multiple myeloma, a malignant disease of monoclonal plasma cells, is the second most common cause of lytic lesions in adults. It is more common in men in their 60s and in African Americans. The bone lesions are well-defined, punched-out lytic areas that can be seen in any bone (Fig. 10.7) and are often seen in the skull. Patients will often have anemia (from bone marrow replacement by tumor), hypercalcemia (from the bone lysis), a monoclonal protein spike on urine and serum protein electrophoresis, and impaired renal function (from the increased protein secretion by the malignant cells). Treatment is multimodal, requiring medical oncology, radiation oncology, and orthopaedics.

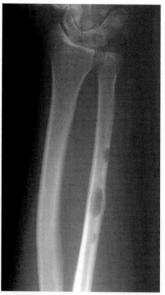

Fig. 10.7 Multiple, Well-Defined, "Punched Out" Lesions Seen in Multiple Myeloma.

Lymphoma

- Metastatic disease and multiple myeloma account for the vast majority of malignant lesions of bone in adults and should be the first and second entities on any differential diagnosis. Lymphoma that arises primarily in bone, although rare, can also be seen. It is often in younger and middle-age adults and classically has a large soft tissue mass with little bony change or destruction. Surgery for lymphoma of bone is for biopsy and bone stabilization only; definitive treatment with high cure rates is a combination of chemotherapy and radiation.

Primary Sarcoma of Bone

- Except for chondrosarcoma (which is seen almost exclusively in adults) the primary sarcomas of bone occur more commonly in the pediatric population. Therefore, entities like osteosarcoma and chondrosarcoma should be considered at the bottom of the differential diagnosis of malignant bone lesions in adults (behind metastatic disease, multiple myeloma, and lymphoma). Primary sarcoma should be at the top of the differential diagnosis of aggressive lesions in children. The primary sarcomas in the following sections account for the most common entities.
- Secondary sarcomas of bone are rarely seen but should be considered when there is a lytic lesion or a mass in a bone with preexisting Paget's disease or previous radiation therapy (osteosarcoma is the most common variant). Enchondromas and osteochondromas can transform into chondrosarcomas less than 1% of the time. Rarely, secondary sarcomas can arise from bone infarcts or fibrous dysplasia.

Osteosarcoma

- Osteosarcoma is the most common primary sarcoma of bone. It is a high-grade disease that has a bimodal age distribution; it arises mostly in children but also in the elderly (often secondary to a preexisting condition like Paget's disease). It can occur in any bone but is most common around the knee. Radiographically, it is classically a mixed lytic and blastic lesion with a soft tissue mass characterized by a "sunburst," radial pattern of osteoid formation (Fig. 10.8). Pathologically, the tumor is required to have malignant cells producing osteoid (Fig. 10.9).
- The work-up for osteosarcoma should include an MRI of the entire bone to assess tumor extent (Fig. 10.10),

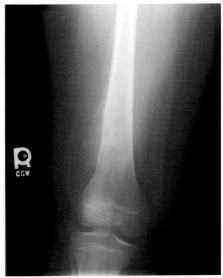

Fig. 10.8 Osteosarcoma of the Distal Femur. Note the blastic soft tissue mass.

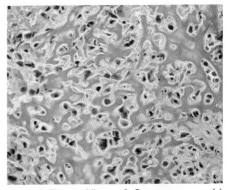

Fig. 10.9 High-Power View of Osteosarcoma. Malignant cells are evident among the pink bands of osteoid.

assist with preoperative planning, and rule out any skip metastases (anatomically separate areas of tumor in the same bone); a CT scan of the chest to evaluate the lungs for metastatic disease (the most common site); and a bone scan to evaluate the skeleton (the second most common site of metastatic disease). A biopsy performed by the treating physician is the next step to secure the diagnosis.

- Treatment for osteosarcoma is typically multidrug chemotherapy, followed by wide excision of the lesion (80% to 90% of cases are limb salvage; see Fig. 10.11), followed by more chemotherapy. Radiation is rarely used as adjuvant therapy, but may be included in cases that are unresectable. Five-year survival rates

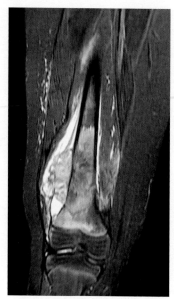

Fig. 10.10 Coronal Magnetic Resonance Imaging of the Osteosarcoma Seen in Fig. 10.8.

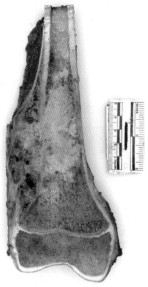

Fig. 10.11 The Gross Specimen From Fig. 10.8 After Chemotherapy and Limb Salvage Surgery.

are currently approaching 80%. Chemotherapy can have ototoxic and cardiotoxic side effects.

Ewing's Sarcoma

- Ewing's sarcoma is the second most common primary sarcoma in children. Pathologically, it is a

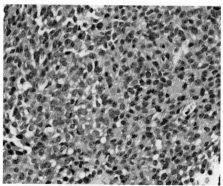

Fig. 10.12 High-Powered View of Ewing Sarcoma Showing the Uniform, Small, Round, Blue Cells.

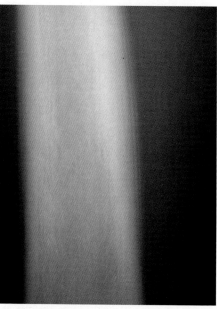

Fig. 10.13 Plain Radiograph Showing the Layered, Periosteal Reaction Known as "Onion Skinning."

high-grade tumor composed of monotonous, small round blue cells (Fig. 10.12). The majority of Ewing's sarcomas have a characteristic t(11,22) translocation that results in the formation of the EWS-FLI1 oncogene.

- Ewing's sarcoma is often seen in flat bones and the metaphyseal-diaphyseal regions of long bones. Classically, it has an "onion skin" appearance (multiple thin layers of periosteal reaction at the site of the tumor; see Fig. 10.13). The work-up for Ewing sarcoma is the same as for osteosarcoma, but the prognosis is slightly worse. Treatment involves chemotherapy and local treatment. Most tumors are surgically excised, but because Ewing sarcoma is sensitive to radiation, it can be used to treat tumors that are otherwise unresectable.

Chondrosarcoma

- Chondrosarcoma is a primary bone tumor of chondroid origin. Except for clear cell chondrosarcoma (a rare variant seen in the epiphysis of younger patients), chondrosarcomas are seen almost exclusively in adults. They can range from low-grade (grades 1 and 2) to aggressive, high-grade (3) tumors. On radiographs (especially with lower-grade lesions) they often display the punctate calcifications and rings and whorls classic for cartilaginous tissue. They sometimes arise from preexisting benign cartilaginous tumors like enchondromas (Figs. 10.14 and 10.15) and osteochondromas.
- Chondrosarcomas can arise in any bone and are often seen in the pelvis, where they carry a worse prognosis. The work-up for a chondrosarcoma includes an MRI of the affected area, a bone scan, and a chest CT. Chondrosarcomas are not responsive to chemotherapy or radiation, so wide surgical excision is the treatment of choice.

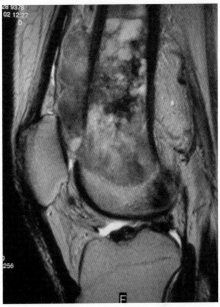

Fig. 10.15 Sagittal Magnetic Resonance Image Showing the Anterior Soft Tissue Mass of the Chondrosarcoma from Fig. 10.14.

BENIGN BONE TUMORS

- Benign tumors are much more common than malignant bony disease. Benign tumors are characterized by a geographic pattern of bone destruction and often have a well-defined rim of reactive bone around the lesion, "walling it off." According to the Enneking/Musculoskeletal Tumor Society staging system, they can be stage 1 or latent lesions, which are asymptomatic and often found incidentally; they can be stage 2 or active lesions, which are symptomatic and usually require treatment; or they can be stage 3 or aggressive lesions, which can mimic a malignant tumor with local destruction and activity.
- Benign tumors can be classified into bone forming, cartilage forming, and others. Careful examination of plain radiography can reveal clues to the lesion's histology and help in subclassifying and diagnosing the tumor. An MRI is then used to define the anatomic extent of disease and aid in preoperative planning.

Benign Bone-Forming Tumors
Bone Island

- A bone island, or enostosis, is a benign formation of histologically normal cortical bone that is usually

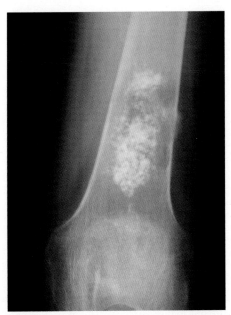

Fig. 10.14 Plain Radiograph of a Chondrosarcoma Arising from an Enchondroma. Note the lucency and periosteal reaction around the stippled calcification of the enchondroma.

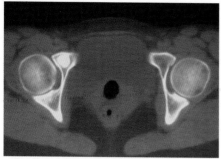

Fig. 10.16 Computed Tomography Scan of the Pelvis Showing the Dense Cortical Bone of a Bone Island.

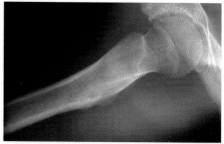

Fig. 10.17 Plain Radiograph of an Osteoid Osteoma of the Femur. Note the lucent nidus.

seen as an incidental finding on radiography done for other reasons. Enostoses are commonly seen in the pelvis bones on CT scans (Fig. 10.16). Typically, they are small punctate areas of dense bone. They may have mild activity on bone scan. Rarely, they can become large or symptomatic. Treatment is benign neglect. An autosomal dominant disorder in which multiple bone islands can be seen is called osteopoikolosis or spotted bone disease.

Osteoid Osteoma

- Osteoid osteoma is a benign bone tumor seen in young people (usually teenagers) presenting as pain, worse at night, that responds to nonsteroidal antiinflammatory drugs. The actual tumor is a small nidus composed of osteoblasts and osteoid that creates a reactive area of dense cortical bone easily identified on plain films and CT scan (Figs. 10.17 and 10.18). They often occur around the proximal femur and acetabulum but can occur in any bone. They often arise in the posterior elements of the spine, where they are the most common cause of painful scoliosis (found on the concave side at the apex of the curve). The natural history is to gradually burn out, so long-term treatment with NSAIDs is an option, but most patients choose a radiofrequency ablation of the nidus with good results.

Osteoblastoma

- Osteoblastomas (Fig. 10.19) are also known as giant osteoid osteomas. Pathologically, they are virtually identical. Osteoblastomas are more aggressive than osteoid osteomas and cause a geographic pattern of destruction with expansile remodeling. Stage 3 lesions can mimic malignant disease. They can be found in any bone (like osteoid osteomas, they too are seen in the posterior elements of the spine). The

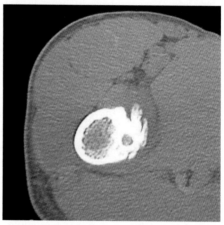

Fig. 10.18 A Computed Tomography Scan of the Osteoid Osteoma in Fig. 10.17 Shows the Reactive Bone Formation Around the Nidus.

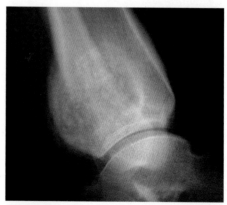

Fig. 10.19 A Benign, Bone-Forming Osteoblastoma of the Distal Tibia.

work-up should include plain films, an MRI of the area, and possibly a biopsy in the aggressive lesions to rule out malignancy. Treatment is curettage of the lesion and reconstruction of the defect, often with bone graft.

Benign Cartilage-Forming Tumors
Enchondroma

- Enchondromas are extremely common benign areas of mature hyaline cartilage that occur in the metaphyseal and diaphyseal areas of virtually any bone (Fig. 10.20). It is theorized that they arise from persistent rests of cartilage from the physis. They are usually incidental and can be treated with serial radiographs to follow for the rare instance of malignant degeneration. Sometimes, they can occupy large portions of the intramedullary canal and raise the possibility of a low-grade chondrosarcoma. The most reliable indicator of malignancy is pain at the site of the lesion, but this can be clinically difficult to distinguish from other musculoskeletal conditions. In cases of possibly painful enchondromas, it is advisable to refer the patient to a musculoskeletal oncologist for treatment. Enchondromas in the hand are often more aggressive clinically (although it is extremely uncommon for malignant degeneration) and can be treated with curettage and bone graft.
- Ollier disease, also known as *enchondromatosis*, is an autosomal dominant condition characterized by multiple enchondromas throughout the skeleton (Fig. 10.21). The patients often have growth disturbances and are of short stature. Because of the sheer number of lesions, there is a significant chance one of them will become malignant over the course of the patient's lifetime.

Osteochondroma

- Osteochondromas, otherwise known as *exostoses*, are common benign bone tumors that present as exophytic boney masses (Fig. 10.22). They are thought to be aberrations of the growth plate and can be pedunculated (with a well-defined stalk) or sessile (having a more broad-based attachment to the underlying bone). All osteochondromas have

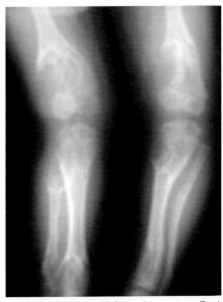

Fig. 10.21 A Severe Case of Ollier Disease, or Enchondromatosis, of Bilateral Lower Extremities.

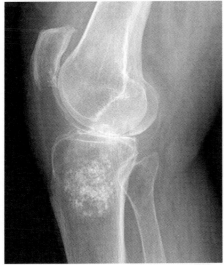

Fig. 10.20 The Enchondroma in the Proximal Tibia Shows the Classic, Stippled, or "Rings and Arcs" Calcification.

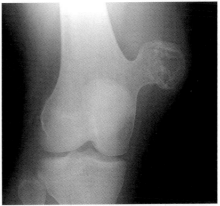

Fig. 10.22 A Large Pedunculated Osteochondroma of the Distal Femur.

corticomedullary continuity; that is, the medullary canal of the bone flows into the osteochondroma without interruption. The surface of osteochondromas is made up of a cartilage cap that is subject to the same growth regulation as any physis. Therefore, osteochondromas will grow until skeletal maturity, and then the cap tends to become thin and growth ceases. There is a small chance that the cartilage cap can degenerate into a (usually low-grade) chondrosarcoma. Treatment is excision for symptomatic lesions.

- Multiple hereditary exostosis (MHE), also known as osteochondromatosis, is an autosomal dominant disorder with many exostoses. Patients have growth disturbances (especially around the elbows, forearms, and ankles) and are of short stature. Like with Ollier disease, the chance of malignant transformation is much higher due to the numerous lesions.

Periosteal Chondroma

- A periosteal chondroma is a benign cartilaginous tumor on the surface of a bone that is often painful. On plain radiography it appears as a "scalloped-out" lesion on the surface of cortical bone with a thin rim of reactive bone around the actual cartilaginous tissue (Fig. 10.23). Microscopically it is benign lobules of cartilage. Treatment is curettage of the lesion and bone grafting of the defect if necessary.

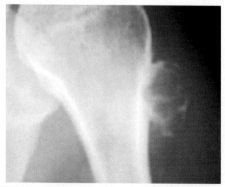

Fig. 10.23 A Periosteal Chondroma of the Proximal Humerus. Note the surface lesion and the thin periosteal rim of bone.

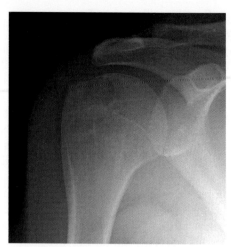

Fig. 10.24 A Chondroblastoma of the Proximal Humerus. Note the well-defined lucency in the epiphysis and the reactive bone laterally.

Chondroblastoma

- Chondroblastoma is a rare, benign proliferation of chondroblasts seen almost exclusively as a well-defined lytic lesion (occasionally with stippled calcifications) in the epiphyseal region of bone (Fig. 10.24). Benign fetal chondroblasts with characteristic "chicken wire" calcification are seen under the microscope. It is most commonly seen in patients between the ages of 15 and 25. In patients with open physes the other entity to consider is a Brodie's abscess. Treatment is curettage and bone grafting. Occasionally chondroblastoma can metastasize to the lungs in a "benign fashion." These lesions are usually treated successfully with wedge resection.

Chondromyxoid Fibroma

- Chondromyxoid fibroma is a rare, benign cartilaginous tumor characteristically seen in the metaphysis of the proximal tibia (although it can be seen in any bone) as a multiloculated lesion with a sclerotic rim that resembles a "soap bubble" (Fig. 10.25). These fibromas have a trimodal appearance under the microscope (hence the name) with characteristic spindle cells that have cytoplasmic projections resembling boat propellers. They can be locally aggressive and should be treated with curettage and bone grafting.

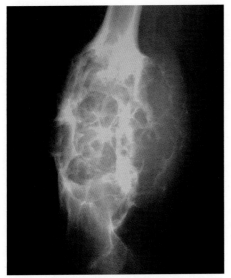

Fig. 10.25 An Extremely Large and Aggressive Chondromyxoid Fibroma of the Femur Displaying the Classic "Soap Bubble" Appearance.

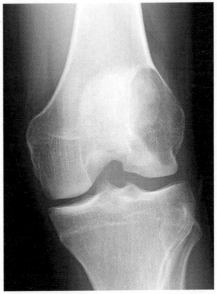

Fig. 10.26 A Giant Cell Tumor of the Distal Femur. Note the involvement of the epiphysis and metaphysis.

Giant Cell Tumor of Bone

- Giant cell tumor of bone is a benign bone tumor that arises in the metaphyseal-epiphyseal region of bone (and almost always extends to the subchondral region) in patients in their third through fifth decades of life. It is a lytic lesion usually without any sclerotic rim that can be aggressive and is often associated with a soft tissue mass (Figs. 10.26 and 10.27). Microscopically, there are large osteoclast-like giant cells with many nuclei in a stroma of mononuclear cells (Fig. 10.28). Rarely giant cell tumors of the bone undergo spontaneous malignant transformation. Like with chondroblastoma, "benign metastases" to the lung can occur and a chest radiograph to evaluate these patients is advisable (especially with lesions of the distal radius, which tend to be more aggressive).
- Because of their epiphyseal location, giant cell tumors can be challenging to treat. Curettage, high-speed burring, and some adjuvants (e.g., argon beam, cryotherapy, phenol) can reduce the rate of local recurrence and the defect can be filled with cement and/or bone graft. However, some aggressive disease requires wide excision and more complex reconstructions like joint replacement or fusion depending on the location and extent of disease. Denosumab, a monoclonal antibody preventing osteoclast formation, can be

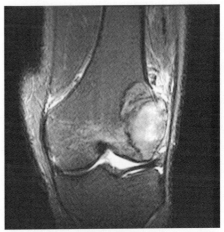

Fig. 10.27 A T2-Weighted Magnetic Resonance Image of the Giant Cell Tumor from Fig. 10.26.

used for tumors that are unresectable or patients who are not surgical candidates.

Fibrous Lesions
Nonossifying Fibroma

- Nonossifying fibroma, or NOF, is a benign, eccentric, metaphyseal lesion often seen as an incidental finding on radiographs done for another reason. The lesion presents as a well-defined area of radiolucency

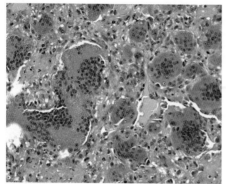

Fig. 10.28 A High-Power Micrograph of a Giant Cell Tumor Demonstrating the Large, Multinucleated Giant Cells.

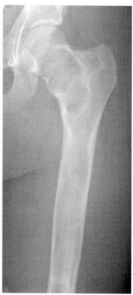

Fig. 10.30 The "Ground Glass" Appearance of Fibrous Dysplasia. Note the involvement of the entire bone.

with a sclerotic border found on the endosteal surface of bone in children and teenagers (Fig. 10.29). The natural history is to fill in with bone over time, and NOFs can usually be treated expectantly. However, some lesions are large and can cause pain and even pathologic fracture. In these instances, curettage, bone grafting, and fixation are often necessary.

Fibrous Dysplasia
- Fibrous dysplasia is a benign fibro-osseous proliferation during skeletal maturation that can occur in any bone but is most commonly seen in the femur and tibia. Eighty percent of cases are isolated to a single bone (monostotic). Severe polyostotic cases are often associated with pigmented skin lesion and endocrine abnormalities (often precocious puberty), a syndrome called *McCune Albright disease.*

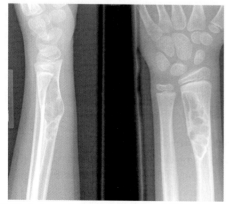

Fig. 10.29 Anteroposterior and Lateral Views of a Large Nonossifying Fibroma of the Radius.

- Radiographically, fibrous dysplasia displays symmetric cortical thinning and expansile remodeling down the long axis of the bone leading to the "long lesion in a long bone" description of the disease (Fig. 10.30). The matrix of the tumor on radiographs is classically described as "ground glass" and represents the microscopic areas of dysplastic bone (in an "alphabet soup" or "Chinese letters" configuration) in a benign fibrous stroma.
- Fibrous dysplasia can weaken the bone, cause pain, and lead to fractures. Multiple fractures of the proximal femur over time lead to deformity and the classic "shepherd's crook" appearance. Asymptomatic lesions can be observed. Symptomatic lesions can be curetted and bone grafted. Unfortunately, the disease often returns and destroys the bone graft, so instrumentation or bulk allograft is usually employed. Bisphosphonates have been shown to reduce pain associated with the disease.

Adamantinoma
- Adamantinoma is an exceedingly rare low-grade malignant fibrous tumor that almost always arises in the anterior cortex of the tibia in younger patients with closed growth plates. Radiographically, it is a bubbly, multiloculated lesion with sclerotic borders

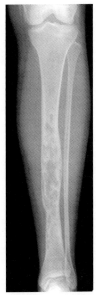

Fig. 10.31 An Adamantinoma Showing the Expansile Remodeling of the Tibial Cortex.

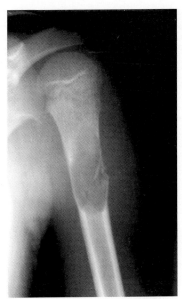

Fig. 10.32 A Pathologic Fracture Through a Simple Bone Cyst of the Humerus. The wafer of cortical bone laterally is a "fallen leaf" sign.

(Fig. 10.31). It has several different pathologic patterns, but cytokeratin is always expressed. It is a malignancy, so the patients have to be worked up for metastatic disease. Treatment is wide surgical excision only. A bulk allograft is often used for reconstruction.

Osteofibrous Dysplasia

- Osteofibrous dysplasia, also known as OFD or Campanacci disease, is a benign condition with a similar appearance to adamantinoma seen in the anterior cortex of the tibia in patients with open physes. Some experts believe it could represent a precursor lesion to adamantinoma. It resembles fibrous dysplasia under the microscope, except the areas of dysplastic bone are rimmed by osteoblasts. Most cases are self-limited and stop growing at skeletal maturity, so watchful waiting is the treatment of choice.

Bone Cysts

- Bone cysts are benign, fluid-filled cavities that appear as radiolucent lesions on radiograph. MRI confirms the fluid nature and rules out a solid tumor.

Simple Bone Cyst

- A simple or unicameral bone cyst is a single-chambered, symmetric, and central lytic lesion seen

in children and adolescents most commonly in the metaphysis of the proximal humerus just below the growth plate (although lesions in the proximal femur and about the knee occur). The lesion thins and expands the cortical bone, presenting with pain or a pathologic fracture (Fig. 10.32). A thin wafer of cortical bone that fractures and floats to the bottom of the cyst is called a "fallen leaf" sign. In the proximal humerus, these fractures will heal with the cyst often recurring. Multiple fractures can lead to deformity. Treatment of proximal humerus lesions should begin with allowing fractures to heal followed by aspiration and injection of bone graft into the cyst. Sometimes, when the cyst has migrated away from the physis, intramedullary rods can be used to correct deformity or prevent further fractures. Because of the high stresses around the proximal femur, simple cysts in that area should be treated more aggressively with instrumentation.

Aneurysmal Bone Cyst

- An aneurysmal bone cyst, or ABC, is a benign, eccentric, expansile, lytic lesion made up of multiple cavities filled with blood (Fig. 10.33). On MRI, the blood settles out and characteristic fluid-fluid levels are seen on T2-weighted images (Fig. 10.34).

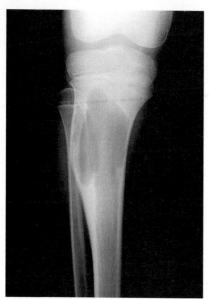

Fig. 10.33 The Eccentric, Benign Lucency of an Aneurysmal Bone Cyst.

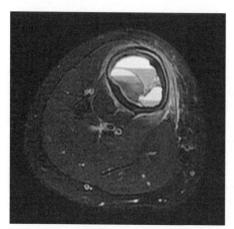

Fig. 10.34 An Axial Magnetic Resonance Image of the Cyst in Fig. 10.33 Shows the Multiple Septations and Fluid-Fluid Levels.

They most commonly occur around the knee but can also be seen in the posterior elements of the spine. ABCs can be locally aggressive and mimic a telangiectatic osteosarcoma. Pathology should be carefully examined to rule out malignancy and a precursor lesion (such as chondroblastoma or chondromyxoid fibroma). Standard treatment is curettage and bone graft, but large lesions may need to be embolized as well.

Subchondral Cysts
- Subchondral cysts are radiographically lucent lesions just below the joint surface that represent the collection of simple fluid through defects in the articular cartilage. The most common causes are osteoarthritis and posttraumatic. Treatment of large cysts may require curettage and bone grafting.

Epidermal Inclusion Cyst
- An epidermal inclusion cyst can be seen in bone as a lytic lesion in the distal phalanges of the fingers and toes. There is normally a history of trauma, and theoretically epidermal tissue is introduced into the periosteum, where it proliferates into a cyst. These may present with pain or a fracture and can require curettage and bone grafting.

Intraarticular Tumors
Synovial Chondromatosis
- Synovial chondromatosis is an intraarticular metaplastic disease in which the synovial tissue forms multiple nodules of otherwise normal hyaline cartilage. These can be seen as a sea of calcified masses around a joint, with the knee being the most commonly affected (Fig. 10.35). The many loose bodies can damage the normal cartilage, so removal and synovectomy are the treatments of choice.

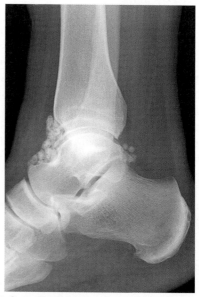

Fig. 10.35 Synovial Chondromatosis of the Tibiotalar Joint.

Pigmented Villonodular Synovitis

- Pigmented villonodular synovitis, or PVNS, is a benign, proliferative disease of the synovium. It can affect almost any joint, but it is most common in the knee of patients in their third or fourth decade of life. On MRI, due to the hemosiderin deposition in the tissue, the lesions have a characteristic low intensity on both T1- and T2-weighted images (Fig. 10.36). It can present as a focal, nodular mass or as a more diffuse, villous involvement of the entire joint. The nodular form is easily treated with excision, but the diffuse form can damage the joint and be challenging to treat (recurrence is common even after attempted total synovectomy).

Eosinophilic Granuloma

- Eosinophilic granuloma (EG) is a benign, lytic bone lesion seen in children and adolescents, most commonly in flat bones and the diaphysis of long bones. It is often called the great imitator because of its varied appearance radiographically, but classically it is a well-defined "hole in bone" (Fig. 10.37). Histologically, eosinophils are usually seen along with larger histiocytic cells called Langerhans cells. EG can manifest as a systemic disease (Langerhans cell granulomatosis) and be seen in multiple bones and other organs. Treatment for bone disease can simply be steroid injection. Larger or unstable lesions may need curettage and fixation.

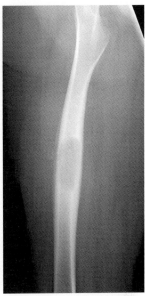

Fig. 10.37 The "Hole-in-Bone" appearance of an eosinophilic granuloma of the femoral diaphysis with abundant periosteal reaction.

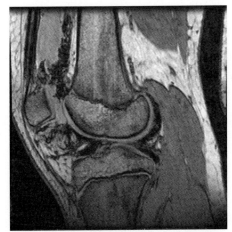

Fig. 10.36 A sagittal magnetic resonance image of the knee joint demonstrating diffuse pigmented villonodular synovitis. The low-intensity areas represent the hemosiderin-rich tumor.

Soft Tissue Lesions

- The orthopaedic oncologist also treats soft tissue masses of the extremities and joints. There are many different benign and malignant soft tissue masses that may present in children and adults. These should be worked up with an MRI to gain as much knowledge about the actual tissue in addition to the anatomic location.
- Classically, a soft tissue sarcoma presents as an enlarging, painless mass in an older patient. The classic MRI findings of a soft tissue sarcoma (no matter what the histologic subtype) are intermediate intensity on T1-weighted images and bright and heterogeneous on T2-weighted images (Fig. 10.38). After being staged for metastatic disease with CT scans, these masses should be biopsied by or under the direction of the treating surgeon. Standard treatment is surgery and radiation therapy (it may be preoperative or postoperative depending on the tumor and surgeon preference). Chemotherapy is being used as adjuvant treatment for medium to large high-grade soft tissue sarcomas. Local recurrence rates for soft tissue sarcomas are low, but 5-year survival rates are poor, especially in patients with metastatic disease.

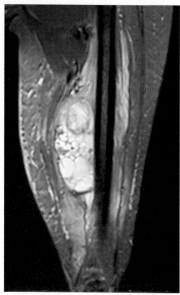

Fig. 10.38 A T2-Weighted Magnetic Resonance Image of the Thigh Demonstrating the Heterogenous, High-Signal Intensity of a Soft Tissue Sarcoma.

- Soft tissue masses in the extremities are most commonly benign, and there are many possible diagnoses. Lipomas, or benign fatty tumors, are exceedingly common and can be diagnosed from MRI alone before surgical resection. However, many benign soft tissue masses can have indeterminate MRI findings or even mimic a sarcoma. These masses should be referred to a treating surgeon for further treatment.

Board Review

- The five primary carcinomas that most commonly metastasize to bone are breast, lung, prostate, kidney, and thyroid.
- Multiple myeloma is most common in older patients, African Americans, and males, and often presents with fatigue, generalized pain, anemia, hypercalcemia, and renal failure. X-rays may show punched-out lytic bony lesions. The mnemonic CRAB (C= elevated calcium, R= renal failure, A= anemia, B= bone lesions) is used to remember some of the common presenting symptoms. Elevated calcium comes from bone lysis, renal failure from increased protein secretion by malignant cells, anemia second to bone marrow replacement by tumor, and boney lesions are typically seen in the ribs and vertebrae.

- An osteosarcoma should be suspected in a pediatric patient presenting with knee pain and x-rays showing a mixed lytic and blastic lesion with a soft tissue mass characterized by a "starburst" radial pattern of osteoid formation. Work-up to confirm should include an MRI of the entire bone, CT of the chest, bone scan, and referral to an orthopedic oncologist for biopsy.
- Ewing's sarcoma should be suspected in a pediatric patient with a bone biopsy of a tumor at the metaphyseal-diaphyseal region of the femur which shows uniform, small, round, blue cells under high-power microscope.
- Osteosarcoma most commonly metastasizes to the lung.
- A sarcoma is a malignant neoplasm that arises from cells of mesenchymal origin.
- Metastatic carcinomas most often occur in the thoracic and lumbar spine.
- Metastatic bone disease is not common in children, but can be seen with Wilms tumors.
- An osteoid osteoma is best treated with NSAID use and radiofrequency ablation.

SUGGESTED READINGS

Attar S, Peabody T: *Orthopaedic oncology: primary and metastatic tumors of the skeletal system*, Switzerland, 2014, Springer.

Collins MT: *Fibrous dysplasia overview*, . https://www.bones.nih.gov/sites/bones/files/pdfs/fibrousdysplasia-508-12-18.pdf, 2018.

Delaney TF, Park L, Goldberg SI, et al.: Radiotherapy for local control of osteosarcoma, *Int J Rad Oncol Biol Physics* 61(2):492, 2005.

Goldschmidt H, Moehler T: *Multiple myeloma*, Heidelberg, Germany, 2011, Springer.

Jamshidi K, Gharehdaghi M, Hajialiloo SS, Mirkazemi M, Ghaffarzadehgan K, Izanloo A: Denosumab in Patients with giant cell tumor and its recurrence: a systematic review, *Arch Bone Joint Surg* 6(4):260–268, 2018.

Jemal A, Miller K, Siegel R: Cancer facts & figures, *American Cancer Society Journal, CA: A Cancer Journal for Clinicians* 67(1):7–30, 2017.

ACKNOWLEDGMENTS

The authors would like to acknowledge the contribution of the previous edition author, Gregory Domson.

11

Splinting and Casting

Damond A. Cromer

INTRODUCTION

Splints and casts share a common purpose, which is to immobilize, protect, and/or counter a given musculoskeletal injury. The most notable difference between a splint and a cast, however, is that splints are designed to immobilize along three or fewer margins of an injured extremity, where casts immobilize circumferentially. Thus, splints are noncircumferential by design which is often essential for the acute care of an injury; the aim being to adequately constrain an injury while still providing for any edema inherent to the resulting acute inflammatory response. Subsequently, casts are best used for the managed care of an injury, where edema has either resolved or is considered negligible to firmly immobilizing the injury.

PEARLS OF SPLINTING AND CASTING

The following are some guidelines, tips, and recommendations for applying some of the more common extremity splints and casts. Bear in mind that these recommendations, although intended to suit most patients, should be adjusted accordingly. Children and smaller individuals will often be better fit in more narrow-width materials than described later, and likewise, larger individuals may be better suited in wider-width materials. Common terms and considerations follow:

- Stockinette should fit the extremity without being too loose or tight.
- Cast/undercast padding should be appropriate to the diameter and length of the extremity.
- Plaster or synthetic (prefabricated) splint material must not overlap circumferentially but be large enough to adequately maintain reduction of the injury.
- An elastic bandage or wrap should be appropriate to the diameter and length of the extremity.
- When wrapping an elastic bandage, do not pull too much tension or it could compromise circulation.
- When rolling the cast/undercast padding or synthetic cast tape, respectively, a 50% overlay technique is commonly employed (i.e., each new layer overlaps half the prior).
- When rolling the cast/undercast padding:
  - Pull just enough tension so that it is taut, but not so much that the material thins or tears away.
  - The padding should be predominantly rolled from distal toward proximal.
  - Commonly, roll just enough padding to eliminate any residual shadow-effect (i.e., the padding should be relatively opaque versus the layers below, typically three layers thick).
- When ready to apply the splint:
  - Thoroughly wet the selected material with clean room-temperature water and squeeze out the excess liquid. A dry towel may be used to help absorb or damp dry the material as needed.
  - The warmer the water, the quicker the set time of the material; however, the heat released by the material also increases and this may potentially cause skin burns or irritation.
  - If using plaster, keep in mind while measuring to fit the splint, the material will contract a bit when wet.
  - For the typical adult, a plaster splint will need to be between 10 and 15 layers thick for adequate stability.

- When ready to apply the cast:
  - Thoroughly wet the selected cast tape with clean room-temperature water and leave the material wet or lightly wring depending on time projected for end application.
  - It is best to leave the material a bit saturated because any wringing will quicken the set time of the material, and care must be taken that the material does not cure before the cast has finished being rolled in its entirety.
  - The warmer the water, the quicker the set time of the material also, so follow the same guidelines.
  - Pay great care not to pull significant tension on the tape when wrapping the cast; simply unroll it onto the extremity to avoid compromising circulation.

SPLINTS

Upper Extremity Sugar Tong (Reverse) Splint:
Fig. 11.1A
Common Indications
- Nondisplaced or minimally displaced fractures of the distal radius and ulna
- Maintaining reduced fractures of the distal radius
- Forearm fractures (radius or ulna shaft fractures)

Recommended Materials
- Stockinette: 2-inch width (1-inch width optional)
- Cast padding/undercast padding: 3- and 4-inch width
- Plaster or synthetic (prefabricated) splint material: 3- or 4-inch width
- Elastic bandage/wrap: 2-, 3-, and 4-inch width

Application
1. With the patient's arm flexed to approximately 90 degrees and their wrist at neutral, fit the 2-inch width stockinette in length from just beyond the fingertips up to midway of the humerus. Cut a hole in the stockinette to adequately accommodate the thumb (Fig. 11.1B).
   - The 1-inch width stockinette may be used specifically for the thumb to create a protective sleeve of padding by folding suitable length over on itself three times.
2. At the antecubital fossa, cut a slit in the stockinette (epicondyle to epicondyle), and pull the proximal portion of the stockinette to overlap the distal portion (or vice versa) (Fig. 11.1C and D).
3. Begin wrapping the padding at the metacarpal heads (MCHs) and proceed proximally with a 50% overlay. Figure-of-eight wrap around the elbow and apply ample padding around the bony prominences of the epicondyles. Continue wrap up to the midhumerus, but keep about two fingerbreadths distal to the stockinette edge (Fig. 11.1E).
   - The 3-inch width padding works for wrapping the hand, wrist, and forearm, whereas the 4-inch width is suitable for wrapping from the forearm, elbow, and arm.
4. Measure so that the selected splint material fits as a "U" around the elbow and along the dorsal and volar sides of the arm all the way to the MCHs, respectively (Fig. 11.1F).
5. Apply the splint material beginning on the volar side at the palmar crease of the hand, proximally toward the elbow, around the elbow, and back to just distal to the MCHs on the dorsal side of the hand. Any excess material can be trimmed away or folded back on itself.
   - Pay particular care to any material obstructing the thumb.
   - At the elbow, you may cut slits (ulnar toward radial) partway through the splint on both the volar and dorsal aspects, and overlap the wings of the splint material on itself to allow for a better mold around the elbow (Fig. 11.1G and H).
6. Pull the underlying stockinette and padding back over the splint at the distal and proximal ends, respectively (Fig. 11.1I). This will protect and pad the patient from the edge of the splint at those areas.
7. Wrap the elastic bandage over the wet splint to just secure it in place. Wrap distal toward proximal; use a figure-of-eight wrap to cover around the elbow (Fig. 11.1J).
8. Mold the splint to maintain given reduction or with the wrist at neutral (functional) unless otherwise indicated.

Upper Extremity Long Arm Posterior Splint:
Fig. 11.2A
Common Indications
- Distal humerus fractures
- Radial head/neck fractures

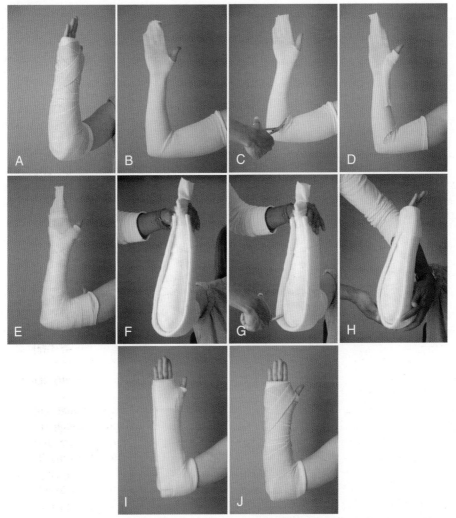

Fig. 11.1 A, Upper extremity sugar tong (reverse) splint. B, Apply stockinette. C, Cut the stockinette and overlap at the antecubital fossa. D, Create a protective sleeve of padding over the thumb with the stockinette and fold over on itself. E, Apply cast padding. F, Apply splint and trim to fit. G, Cut slits in the splint at the elbow to create wings that overlap. H, Mold the wings around the elbow. I, Fold the ends of the stockinette back over the splint. J, Wrap elastic bandage over splint to secure in place.

- Proximal ulna fractures
- Reduced elbow dislocations
- Elbow sprains/strains

Recommended Materials
- Stockinette: 3-inch width (1-inch width optional)
- Cast padding/undercast padding: 3- and 4-inch width
- Plaster or fiberglass (prefabricated) splint material: 4- or 5-inch width
- Elastic bandage/wrap: 2-, 3-, and 4-inch width

Application
1. With the patient's arm flexed to approximately 90 degrees and their wrist at neutral, fit the 3-inch width stockinette in length from just beyond the fingertips up to (and with some gather at) the axilla. Cut a hole in the stockinette to adequately accommodate the thumb (Fig. 11.2B).
   - The 1-inch width stockinette may be used specifically for the thumb to create a protective sleeve of padding by folding suitable length over on itself three times.

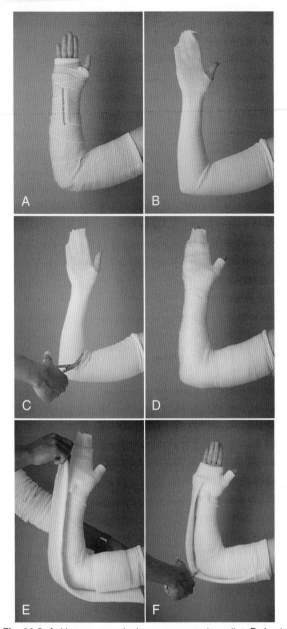

Fig. 11.2 A, Upper extremity long arm posterior splint. **B,** Apply stockinette. **C,** Cut the stockinette and overlap at the antecubital fossa. **D,** Apply cast padding. **E,** Apply splint and trim to fit. **F,** Fold the ends of the stockinette back over the splint. Cut slits in the splint at the elbow to create wings that overlap to mold around the elbow.

2. At the antecubital fossa, cut a slit in the stockinette (epicondyle to epicondyle) and pull the proximal portion of the stockinette to overlap the distal portion (or vice versa) (Fig. 11.2C).

3. Begin wrapping the padding at the MCHs and proceed proximally with a 50% overlay. Figure-of-eight wrap at the elbow, and apply ample padding around the bony prominences of the epicondyles. Continue wrapping up to the axilla (Fig. 11.2D).
   - The 3-inch width padding works for wrapping the hand, wrist, and forearm, whereas the 4-inch width is suitable for wrapping from the forearm, elbow, and arm.
4. Measure so that the selected splint material fits from the fifth MCH to the axilla.
5. Apply the splint material beginning on the ulnar side at the palmar crease along the fifth metacarpal of the hand, along the ulna, posteriorly along the elbow up just distal to the axilla. Any excess material can be trimmed away or folded back on itself (Fig. 11.2E).
   - Pay particular care to any material obstructing the axilla.
   - At the elbow, you may cut partway through the splint on both the volar and dorsal aspects, and then overlap the wings of the splint material on itself to allow for a better mold around the elbow (Fig. 11.2F).
6. Pull the underlying stockinette and padding back over the splint at the distal and proximal ends, respectively. This will protect and pad the patient from the edge of the splint at those areas.
7. Wrap the elastic bandage over the wet splint to just secure it in place. Wrap distal toward proximal; use a figure-of-eight wrap to cover around the elbow.
8. Mold the splint to maintain given reduction and with the wrist in a functional position unless otherwise indicated.

Upper Extremity Volar Short Arm Splint: Fig. 11.3A
Common Indications
- Finger injuries
- Metacarpal injuries
- Carpal injuries (excluding occult scaphoid or trapezium fractures)
- Protection of lacerations of the hand/wrist/forearm
- Wrist sprains/strains

Recommended Materials
- Stockinette: 2-inch width (1-inch width optional)
- Cast padding/undercast padding: 3-inch width

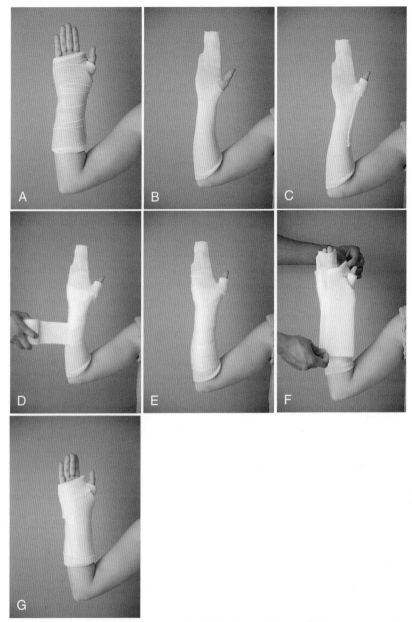

Fig. 11.3 **A**, Upper extremity volar short arm splint. **B**, Apply stockinette. **C**, Create a protective sleeve of padding over the thumb with the stockinette and fold over on itself. **D**, Apply cast padding. **E**, Cast padding applied. **F**, Apply splint and trim to fit. **G**, Fold the ends of the stockinette back over the splint.

- Plaster or synthetic (prefabricated) splint material: 3- or 4-inch width
- Elastic bandage/wrap: 2-inch and 3-inch width

Application

1. With the patient's wrist at neutral, fit the 2-inch width stockinette in length from just beyond the fingertips up to the antecubital fossa. Cut a hole in the stockinette to adequately accommodate the thumb (Fig. 11.3B).

- If enclosing the fingers in the splint, place padding between each finger, respectively, to protect against skin maceration.
- The 1-inch width stockinette may be used specifically for the thumb to create a protective sleeve of

padding by folding suitable length over on itself three times (Fig. 11.3C).

2. Begin wrapping the padding at the MCHs and proceed proximally with a 50% overlay. Continue wrapping up to the antecubital fossa (Fig. 11.3D and E).
   - If enclosing the fingers in the splint, alternatively begin wrapping the padding at the distal phalanges.
3. Measure so that the selected splint material fits in length from the MCHs to within about two to three fingerbreadths (about 2 inches) of the antecubital fossa.
   - Start measuring from the distal phalanges if protecting for finger or metacarpal injuries.
4. Apply the splint material beginning on the volar side at the palmar crease of the hand, proximally toward the antecubital fossa. Any excess material can be trimmed away or folded back on itself (Fig. 11.3F).
   - Pay particular care to any material obstructing the thumb or antecubital fossa.
5. Pull the underlying stockinette and padding back over the splint at the distal and proximal ends, respectively. This will protect and pad the patient from the edge of the splint at those areas (Fig. 11.3G).
6. Wrap the elastic bandage over the wet splint to secure it in place. Wrap distal toward proximal.
7. Mold the splint as to counter the given injury or with the wrist at neutral unless otherwise indicated.

Upper Extremity Thumb Spica Splint: Fig. 11.4A
Common Indications
- Thumb injuries
- Wrist injuries (occult/suspected scaphoid or trapezium fractures)
- Wrist sprains/strains

Recommended Materials
- Stockinette: 2-inch width (1-inch width optional but shown)
- Cast padding/undercast padding: 3-inch width
- Plaster or synthetic (prefabricated) splint material: 3- or 4-inch width
- Elastic bandage/wrap: 2- and 3-inch width

Application
1. With the patient's wrist at neutral, fit the 2-inch width stockinette in length from just beyond the fingertips up to the antecubital fossa. Cut a hole in the stockinette to adequately accommodate the thumb (Fig. 11.4B).
   - The 1-inch width stockinette may be used specifically for the thumb to create a protective sleeve of padding by folding suitable length over on itself three times (Fig. 11.4C):
   - Interphalangeal joint (IP) free: If leaving the distal phalanx free, the collar should be just proximal to the distal interphalangeal joint (DIP).
   - IP joint included: If enclosing the distal phalanx, the collar should approach the thumb tip.
   - Alternative to 1-inch width stockinette, about three layers of 3-inch width cast/undercast padding may be wrapped circumferentially around the thumb (same considerations as earlier).
2. Begin wrapping the padding at the MCHs and proceed proximally with a 50% overlay. Continue wrapping up to just distal to the antecubital fossa (Fig. 11.4D and E).
3. Measure so that the selected splint material fits in length from the MCHs to within about two to three fingerbreadths (about 2 inches) of the antecubital fossa.
4. Apply the splint material centered over the radial border of the thumb and forearm, beginning just proximal to the padded edge of stockinette (or cast/undercast padding) protecting the thumb proximally toward the antecubital fossa. Any excess material can be trimmed away or folded back on itself (Fig. 11.4F).
   - Pay particular care to any material that would otherwise make the splint circumferential about the thumb.
5. Pull the underlying stockinette back just over the padding at the distal and proximal ends, respectively. This will protect and pad the patient from the edge of the cast at those areas (Fig. 11.4G).
6. Wrap the elastic bandage over the wet splint to secure it in place. Wrap distal toward proximal.
7. Position the thumb as to reduce the given injury and with the wrist at neutral unless otherwise indicated.

Upper Extremity Ulnar Gutter Splint: Fig. 11.5A
Common Indications
- Ring and small finger injuries
- Ring and small finger metacarpal injuries

Recommended Materials
- Stockinette: 2-inch width (1-inch width optional)
- Cast/undercast padding: 3-inch width

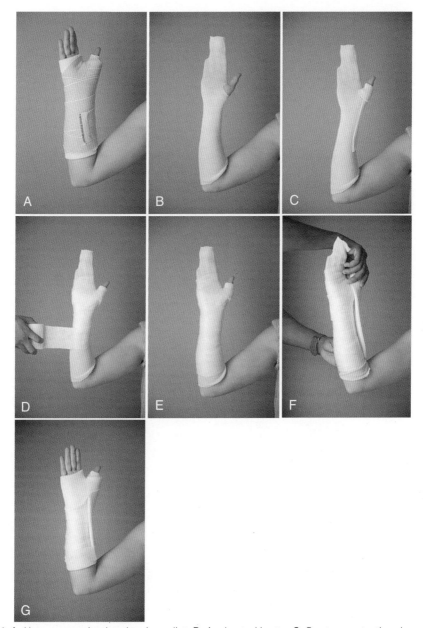

Fig. 11.4 A, Upper extremity thumb spica splint. **B**, Apply stockinette. **C**, Create a protective sleeve of padding over the thumb with the stockinette and fold over on itself. **D**, Apply cast padding. **E**, Cast padding applied. **F**, Apply splint and trim to fit. **G**, Fold the ends of the stockinette back over the splint.

- Plaster or synthetic (prefabricated) splint material: 4- or 5-inch width
- Elastic bandage/wrap: 2- and 3-inch width

Application

1. With the patient's wrist at neutral, fit the 2-inch width stockinette in length from about 1 inch beyond the fingertips up to the antecubital fossa. Cut a hole in the stockinette to adequately accommodate the thumb (Fig. 11.5B).

- The 1-inch width stockinette may be used specifically for the thumb to create a protective sleeve of padding by folding suitable length over on itself three times (Fig. 11.5C).

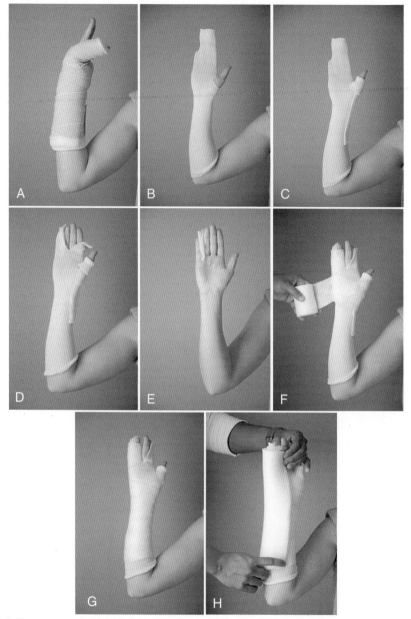

Fig. 11.5 A, Upper extremity ulnar gutter splint. **B,** Apply stockinette. **C,** Create a protective sleeve of padding over the thumb with the stockinette and fold over on itself. **D,** Cut a slit in the stockinette between the long and ring fingers. **E,** Place some cast padding between the fingers to prevent skin maceration. **F,** Apply cast padding starting around the wrist and fingers. **G,** Continue cast padding proximally. **H,** Apply splint and trim to fit.

- The 1-inch width stockinette may also be used specifically for the ring and small fingers (instead of cast/undercast padding as described later) to create a similar sleeve of padding to capture both digits. In this case, fit the stockinette and roll the cast/undercast padding in the same manner as for the volar short arm splint, omitting the relevant steps that follow.

2. At the distal end of the stockinette, cut a slit in the stockinette longitudinally toward the web space between the long and ring fingers (Fig. 11.5D).

3. Trim or fold a few layers of cast/undercast padding to place between the length of the ring and small fingers to prevent skin maceration (Fig. 11.5E).
4. Begin wrapping the padding just at the tips of the ring and small fingers and proceed proximally with a 50% overlay. Continue wrapping up to just distal to the antecubital fossa (Fig. 11.5F and G).
5. Measure so that the selected splint material fits from the tip of the ring finger to the antecubital fossa.
6. Apply the splint material beginning on the ulnar side of the small finger (distally equal to the ring ginger) forming a "gutter" along the fifth metacarpal and the ulna proceeding toward the antecubital fossa. Any excess material can be trimmed away or folded back on itself (Fig. 11.5H).
   - Pay particular care to any material obstructing the antecubital fossa.
7. Pull the underlying stockinette and padding back over the splint at the distal and proximal ends, respectively. This will protect and pad the patient from the edge of the splint at those areas.
8. Wrap the elastic bandage over the wet splint to just secure it in place. Wrap distal toward proximal.
9. Mold the splint at the fingers, hand, and wrist to maintain a given reduction or counter the given injury as indicated.
   - Commonly the ring and small fingers are molded fully extended in the intrinsic plus position (metacarpal phalangeal joints in 70 degrees of flexion, IP joints extended).

Lower Extremity Sugar Tong (Ankle-Stirrup/U) Splint: Fig. 11.6A

Common Indications
- Ankle sprains/strains
- Medial and lateral malleolus injuries

Recommended Materials
- Stockinette: 3-inch width
- Cast/undercast padding: 4- and/or 6-inch width
- Plaster or synthetic (prefabricated) splint material: 3-inch width
- Elastic bandage/wrap: 4- and 6-inch width

Application
1. With the patient's ankle at neutral (ankle dorsiflexed to approximately 90 degrees), fit the 3-inch width stockinette in length distally from the metatarsal heads (MTHs) up to the patella and popliteal fossa.

2. At the ankle joint, cut a slit in the stockinette (malleolus to malleolus) and pull the proximal portion of the stockinette to overlap the distal portion (or vice versa) (Fig. 11.6B).
3. Begin wrapping the padding just proximal to the MTHs and proceed proximally with a 50% overlay. Figure-of-eight wrap at the ankle/heel and apply ample padding around the bony prominences of the malleoli. Continue wrapping up to the tibial tuberosity (Fig. 11.6C).
   - The 4-inch width padding works for wrapping the midfoot and ankle, whereas the 6-inch width is suitable for wrapping from the ankle up to the tibial tuberosity.
4. Measure so that the selected splint material fits as a "U" under the heel of the foot and up the ankle along the lateral and medial sides of the leg all the way to even with the level of the fibular head (Fig. 11.6D).
5. Apply the splint material in the same manner used to measure above. Any excess material can be trimmed away or folded back on itself.
   - Pay particular care to any material obstructing the motion of the knee.
   - Center the splint on the lateral and medial sides of the leg and take care not to overlap the proximal ends (Fig. 11.6E).
6. Pull the underlying stockinette and padding back over the splint at the distal and proximal ends, respectively. This will protect and pad the patient from the edge of the splint at those areas.
7. Wrap the elastic bandage over the wet splint to just secure it in place. Wrap distal toward proximal; use a figure-of-eight wrap to cover around the ankle and heel.
8. Mold the splint with the ankle at neutral unless otherwise indicated.

Lower Extremity Posterior Leg Splint: Fig. 11.7A

Common Indications
- Ankle sprains/strains
- Ankle dislocations
- Achilles tendon ruptures
- Distal tibia and fibula fractures
- Tarsal injuries
- Metatarsal injuries

Recommended Materials
- Stockinette: 3-inch width
- Cast/undercast padding: 4- and 6-inch width

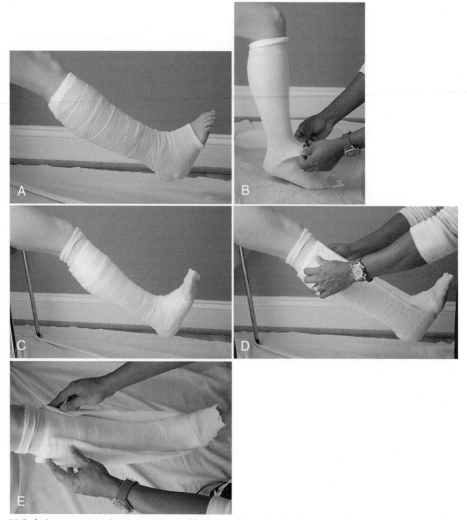

Fig. 11.6 **A,** Lower extremity sugar tong (ankle stirrup/U) splint. **B,** Apply stockinette and create a fold over the anterior ankle. **C,** Apply cast padding. **D,** Apply splint and trim to fit. **E,** Center the splint on the lateral and medial sides of the leg and take care not to overlap the proximal ends.

- Plaster or synthetic (prefabricated) splint material: 4-inch width
- Elastic bandage/wrap: 4- and 6-inch width

Application

1. With the patient's ankle at neutral (ankle dorsiflexed ≈ 90 degrees), fit the 3-inch width stockinette in length about 1 inch distal to the hallux up to the patella and popliteal fossa.
    - In the case of an Achilles tendon injury, particularly, the foot should be kept in slight equinus (plantar flexion).

2. At the ankle joint, cut a slit in the stockinette (malleolus to malleolus) and pull the proximal portion of the stockinette to overlap the distal portion (or vice versa) (Fig. 11.7B).

3. Begin wrapping the padding just distal to the MTHs and proceed proximally with a 50% overlay. Figure-of-eight wrap at the ankle and heel and apply ample padding around the bony prominences of the malleoli. Continue wrapping up to the tibial tuberosity (Fig. 11.7C and D).
    - The 4-inch width padding works for wrapping the foot and ankle, whereas the 6-inch width is suitable for wrapping the leg.

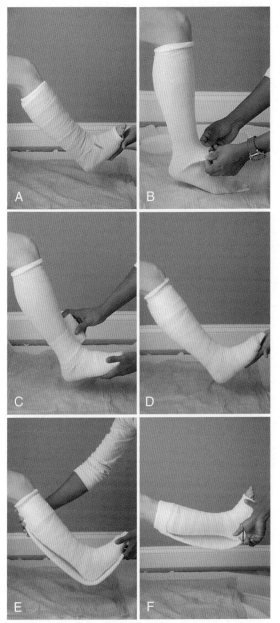

Fig. 11.7 **A,** Lower extremity posterior leg splint. **B,** Apply stockinette and create a fold over the anterior ankle. **C,** Apply cast padding. **D,** Apply cast padding with ankle in neutral. **E,** Apply splint and trim to fit. **F,** Fold the ends of the stockinette back over the splint and cut splint to create wings that mold around the ankle.

4. Measure so that the selected splint material fits in length posteriorly from the MTHs to the popliteal fossa.

5. Apply the splint material in the same manner used to measure above. Any excess material can be trimmed away or folded back on itself (Fig. 11.7E).
   - Pay particular care to any material obstructing the motion of the knee or encroaching the popliteal fossa.
   - At the heel, you may cut partway through the splint on both the lateral and medial aspects and then overlap the wings of the splint material on itself to allow for a better mold around calcaneus (Fig. 11.7F).
6. Pull the underlying stockinette and padding back over the splint at the distal and proximal ends, respectively. This will protect and pad the patient from the edge of the splint at those areas.
7. Wrap the elastic bandage over the wet splint to just secure it in place. Wrap distal toward proximal; use a figure-of-eight wrap to cover around the ankle and heel.
8. Mold the splint to maintain the patient's ankle at neutral unless otherwise indicated.

Lower Extremity Long Leg Splint: Fig. 11.8A
Common Indications
- Knee injuries
- Unstable tibia and fibula fractures

Recommended Materials
- Stockinette: 4-inch width
- Cast/undercast padding: 4- and 6-inch width
- Plaster or synthetic (prefabricated) splint material: 4- or 5-inch width
- Elastic bandage/wrap: 4- and 6-inch width

Application
1. With the patient's ankle at neutral (ankle dorsiflexed ≈90 degrees) and the knee just slightly flexed (≈15 degrees), fit the 4-inch width stockinette in length about 1 inch distal to the hallux up to (and with some gather at) the groin (Fig. 11.8B).
2. At the ankle joint, cut a slit in the stockinette (malleolus to malleolus) and pull the proximal portion of the stockinette to overlap the distal portion (or vice versa).
3. Begin wrapping the padding just distal to the MTHs and proceed proximally with a 50% overlay. Figure-of-eight wrap about the ankle and heel and apply

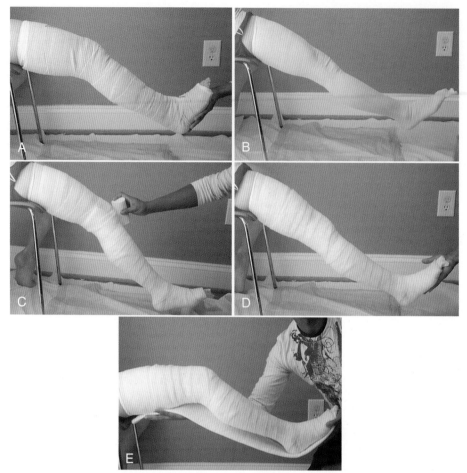

Fig. 11.8 **A**, Lower extremity long leg splint. **B**, Apply stockinette. **C**, Apply cast padding. **D**, Apply cast padding with ankle in neutral. **E**, Apply splint and trim to fit.

ample padding around the bony prominences of the malleoli. Likewise, use ample padding on the bony prominences of the knee. Continue wrapping up to the groin (Fig. 11.8C and D).

- The 4-inch width padding works for wrapping the distal portion, whereas the 6-inch width is suitable for the proximal portion.

4. Measure so that the selected splint material fits in length posteriorly from the MTHs to the gluteal sulcus.

5. Apply the splint material in the same manner used to measure above. Any excess material can be trimmed away or folded back on itself (Fig. 11.8E).

- Pay particular care to any material obstructing the motion of the leg or intruding the groin or buttock.

- At the heel, you may cut partway through the splint on both the lateral and medial aspects and then overlap the wings of the splint material on itself to allow for a better mold around the calcaneus.

6. Pull the underlying stockinette and padding back over the splint at the distal and proximal ends, respectively. This will protect and pad the patient from the edge of the splint at those areas.

7. Wrap the elastic bandage over the wet splint to just secure it in place. Wrap distal toward proximal; use a figure-of-eight wrap to cover around the ankle and heel.

8. Mold the splint to maintain the patient's ankle at neutral and knee slightly bent unless otherwise indicated.

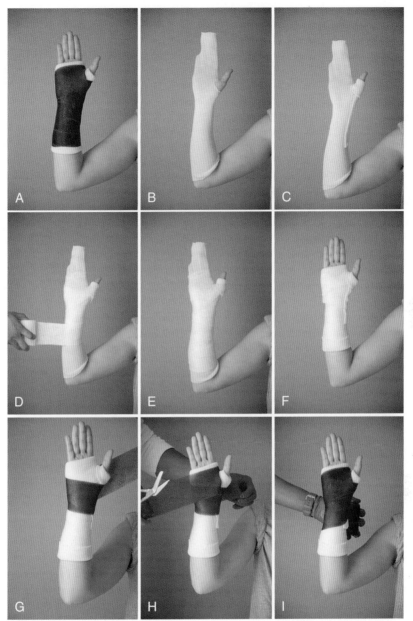

Fig. 11.9 A, Short arm cast. B, Apply stockinette. C, Create a protective sleeve of padding over the thumb with the stockinette and fold over on itself. D, Apply cast padding. E, Cast padding applied. F, Fold the ends of the stockinette back over the cast padding. G, Begin wrapping the cast tape at the wrist. H, Partially cut the cast tape from proximal to distal and place between the first web space and repeat two additional times. I, Continue wrapping cast tape proximally.

CASTS

Short Arm Cast: Fig. 11.9A
Common Indications
- Metacarpal fractures
- Carpal fractures (*excluding* scaphoid or trapezium fractures)
- Distal radius and ulna fractures
- Management of soft tissue injuries affecting the hand or wrist

Recommended Materials

- Stockinette: 2-inch width (1-inch width optional but shown)
- Cast padding/undercast padding: 3-inch width
- Synthetic (fiberglass, polyester) cast tape: 3-inch width

Application

1. With the patient's wrist at neutral, fit the 2-inch width stockinette in length from just beyond the fingertips up to the antecubital fossa. Cut a hole in the stockinette to adequately accommodate the thumb (Fig. 11.9B).
   - The 1-inch width stockinette may be used specifically for the thumb to create a protective sleeve of padding by folding suitable length over on itself three times (Fig. 11.9C).
2. Begin wrapping the padding at the MCHs and proceed proximally with a 50% overlay. Continue wrapping up to just distal to the antecubital fossa (Fig. 11.9D and E).
3. Pull the underlying stockinette back just over the padding at the distal and proximal ends, respectively. This will protect and pad the patient from the edge of the cast at those areas (Fig. 11.9F).
4. Begin wrapping the cast tape at the wrist joint (Fig. 11.9G). One wrap circumferentially around to anchor is suitable before proceeding distally to fit the tape proper about the hand/palm. At the first web space, cut proportionately through the width of the tape proximal toward distal, laying the remaining width through web space and the newly cut ends dorsal and volar about the base of the thumb, respectively (Fig. 11.9H). Roll the tape circumferentially en route just proximal to the base of the thumb to overlay both of the cut ends. Fit the tape through the web space in this manner two additional times (for three layers total).
   - Keep the tape proximal to the padded edge of stockinette (i.e., proximal to the distal palmar crease and proximal to the MCHs dorsally).
5. Continue wrap proceeding proximally with a 50% overlay up toward the antecubital fossa, but keep about one fingerbreadth distal to the padded edge of stockinette (Fig. 11.9I).
6. Roll the tape three times around the proximal end before proceeding back distally with a 50% overlay toward the wrist.
   - Roll the tape to its completion or cut the roll free when enough tape has been applied to eliminate

any shadow effect or noticeable weak points (typically three layers of tape is ideal).
7. Mold the cast to counter the given injury or with the wrist at neutral unless otherwise indicated.
   - Continually rub the cast with open hands to help laminate and smooth the layers until the cast has set firm with care not to create any undue indentations or pressure points.
   - Avoid using fingertips while molding.
   - Be sure to apply a careful interosseous mold about the distal radius/ulna by sandwiching the palms dorsally and volarly, respectively, with adequate pressure.
   - This is particularly important when casting fractures in children.

Long Arm Cast: Fig. 11.10A
Common Indications
- Distal humerus fractures
- Radius and ulna shaft fractures
- Proximal radius and ulna fractures
- Distal radius and ulna fractures in children

Recommended Materials
- Stockinette: 2-inch width (1-inch width optional but shown)
- Cast padding/undercast padding: 3- and 4-inch width
- Synthetic (fiberglass, polyester) cast tape: 3- and 4-inch width

Application
1. With the patient's elbow flexed to approximately 90 degrees and his or her wrist at neutral, fit the 2-inch width stockinette in length from just beyond the fingertips up to (and with some gather at) the axilla. Cut a hole in the stockinette to adequately accommodate the thumb (Fig. 11.10B).
   - The 1-inch width stockinette may be used specifically for the thumb to create a protective sleeve of padding by folding suitable length over on itself three times.
2. At the antecubital fossa, cut a slit in the stockinette (epicondyle to epicondyle) and pull the proximal portion of the stockinette to overlap the distal portion (or vice versa) (Fig. 11.10C).
3. Begin wrapping the padding at the MCHs and proceed proximally with a 50% overlay. Figure-of-eight

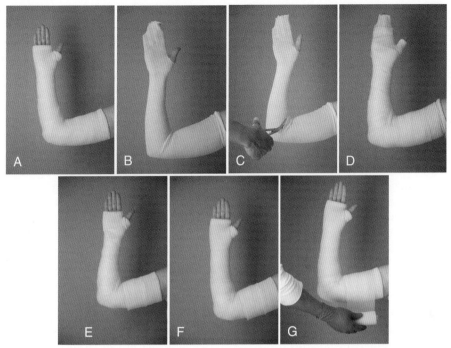

Fig. 11.10 A, Long arm cast. **B,** Apply stockinette. **C,** Cut the stockinette and overlap at the antecubital fossa. **D,** Apply cast padding. **E,** Fold the ends of the stockinette back over the cast padding. **F,** Apply cast tape from distal to proximal. Partially cut the cast tape from proximal to distal and place between the first web space and repeat two additional times. **G,** Apply the cast tape proximally and use a figure-of-eight around the elbow.

wrap at the elbow, and apply ample padding around the bony prominences of the epicondyles. Continue wrapping up to the axilla (Fig. 11.10D).

- The 3-inch width padding works for wrapping the hand, wrist, and forearm, whereas the 4-inch width is suitable for wrapping from the forearm, elbow, and arm.

4. Pull the underlying stockinette back just over the padding at the distal and proximal ends, respectively. This will protect and pad the patient from the edge of the cast at those areas (Fig. 11.10E).

5. Begin wrapping the 3-inch width cast tape at the wrist joint. One wrap circumferentially around to anchor is suitable before proceeding distally to fit the tape properly about the hand and palm. At the first web space, cut proportionately through the width of the tape proximal toward distal, laying the remaining width through web space and the newly cut ends dorsal and volar about the base of the thumb, respectively. Roll the tape circumferentially en route just proximal to the base of the thumb to overlay both of the cut ends. Fit the tape through

the web space in this manner two additional times (for three layers total).

- Keep the tape proximal to the padded edge of stockinette (i.e., proximal to the distal palmar crease and proximal to the MCH dorsally).

6. Continue wrap proceeding proximally with a 50% overlay up toward the antecubital fossa, but keep about one fingerbreadth distal to the antecubital fossa.

7. Roll the tape three layers thick around the proximal forearm before proceeding back distally with a 50% overlay toward the wrist (Fig. 11.10F).

- Roll the tape to its completion or cut the roll free when enough tape has been applied to eliminate any shadow effect or noticeable weak points (typically ≥ three layers of coverage ideal).
- The cast should resemble a short arm cast at this point.

8. Begin wrapping the 4-inch width cast tape about two fingerbreadths distal to the padded edge of stockinette at the axilla. Roll circumferentially three layers thick around before proceeding distally with a 50% overlay toward the elbow.

9. Figure-of-eight wrap the elbow three times, and overlap at least half width the still wet end of the cast at the proximal forearm (Fig. 11.10G). Ensure adequate coverage at the elbow (three or more layers) before proceeding proximally with a 50% overlay toward the axilla.
   - Roll the tape to its completion or cut the roll free when enough tape has been applied to eliminate any shadow effect or noticeable weak points (typically three or more layers of coverage is ideal).
10. To further unify the distal and proximal portions of the cast, wrap another 3-inch width cast tape beginning at the distal end capturing the hand (one layer as earlier) before proceeding proximally with a 50% overlay to the proximal end at the axilla (one layer).
    - Cut the roll free or optionally roll the tape to its completion with a 50% overlay proceeding distally again toward the hand and wrist.
11. Mold the cast to counter the given injury or with the wrist at neutral unless otherwise indicated.
    - Continually rub the cast with open hands to help laminate and smooth the layers until the cast has set firm with care not to create any undue indentations or pressure points.
    - Avoid using fingertips while molding.
    - Be sure to apply a careful interosseous mold about the distal radius/ulna by sandwiching the palms dorsally and volarly, respectively, with adequate pressure.
    - This is particularly important when casting fractures in children.

Thumb Spica Cast: Fig. 11.11A
Common Indications
- Thumb fractures
- Thumb sprains/strains
- Scaphoid or trapezium fractures (*including* occult or suspected fractures)
- Management of some wrist sprains/strains

Recommended Materials
- Stockinette: 2-inch width (1-inch width optional but shown)
- Cast padding/undercast padding: 3-inch width
- Synthetic (fiberglass, polyester) cast tape: 3-inch width

Application
1. With the patient's wrist at neutral, fit the 2-inch width stockinette in length from just beyond the fingertips up to the antecubital fossa. Cut a hole in the stockinette to adequately accommodate the thumb (Fig. 11.11B).
   - The 1-inch width stockinette may be used specifically for the thumb to create a protective sleeve of padding by folding suitable length over on itself three times (Fig. 11.11C):
   - IP free: If leaving the distal phalanx free, the collar should be just proximal to the DIP.
   - IP joint included: If enclosing the distal phalanx, the collar should approach the thumb tip.
   - Alternative to 1-inch width stockinette, about three layers of 3-inch width cast/undercast padding may be wrapped circumferentially around the thumb (same considerations as mentioned earlier).
2. Begin wrapping the padding at the MCHs and proceed proximally with a 50% overlay. Continue wrapping up to just distal to the antecubital fossa (Fig. 11.11D and E).
3. Pull the underlying stockinette back just over the padding at the distal and proximal ends, respectively. This will protect and pad the patient from the edge of the cast at those areas (Fig. 11.11F).
4. Begin wrapping the 3-inch width cast tape at the wrist joint. One wrap circumferentially around to anchor is suitable before proceeding distally to fit the tape proper about the thumb, hand, and palm.
5. To fit the tape around the thumb, roll the tape to the dorsal-radial border of the thumb and approaching the first web space, cut partially through the width (proximal toward distal) to just fit the tape around the proximal phalanx segment of the thumb (or distal phalanx segment additionally if IP joint is included). Continue through and around the respective phalanx segment(s) circumferentially back to the dorsal-radial border of the thumb again. Fit the tape around the thumb in this manner two additional times (for three layers total) (Fig. 11.11G and H).
   - Keep the tape just proximal to the padded edge of stockinette (or cast/undercast padding) protecting the thumb.
6. To fit the tape about the hand and palm, from the thumb roll toward the first web space, cut proportionately through the width of the tape proximal toward distal,

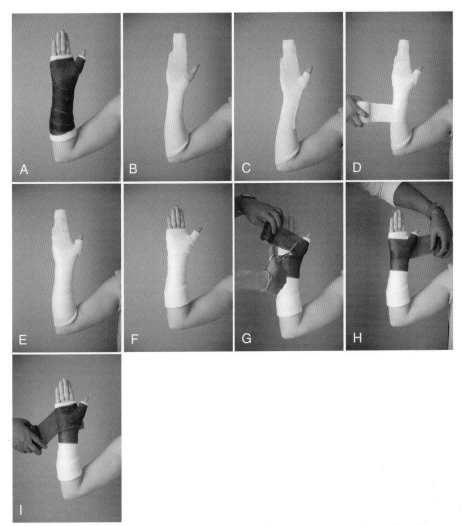

Fig. 11.11 A, Thumb spica cast. **B,** Apply stockinette. **C,** Create a protective sleeve of padding over the thumb with the stockinette and fold over on itself. **D,** Apply cast padding. **E,** Cast padding applied. **F,** Fold the ends of the stockinette back over the cast padding. **G,** Apply the cast tape starting at the wrist. Wrap from the dorsal-radial thumb toward the first web space. Cut the cast tape from proximal to distal in order to cover the proximal phalanx when placed into the first web space. **H,** Repeat two additional times around the thumb. **I,** To fit the tape over the hand and palm, cut the tape from proximal to distal and lay into the first web space so that the newly cut ends surround the thumb.

laying the remaining width through the web space and the newly cut ends dorsal and volar about the base of the thumb, respectively (Fig. 11.11I). Roll the tape circumferentially en route just proximal to the base of the thumb to overlay both of the cut ends. Fit the tape through the web space in this manner two additional times (for three layers total).

- Keep the tape proximal to the padded edge of the stockinette (i.e., proximal to the distal palmar crease and proximal to the MCH dorsally).
- When fitting the tape through the web space and about the thumb as described earlier, be sure to overlay the proximal-most portion of tape of the thumb spica.

7. Continue wrap proceeding proximally with a 50% overlay up toward the antecubital fossa, but keep about one fingerbreadth distal to the padded edge of the stockinette.
8. Roll the tape three times around the proximal end before proceeding back distally with a 50% overlay toward the wrist.
   - Roll the tape to its completion or cut the roll free when enough tape has been applied to eliminate any shadow effect or noticeable weak points (typically three layers of tape is ideal).
9. Mold the cast to counter the given injury or with the wrist and thumb at neutral unless otherwise indicated.
   - Continually rub the cast with open hands to help laminate and smooth the layers until the cast has set firm, taking care to not create any undue indentations or pressure points.
     - Avoid using fingertips while molding.
   - Be sure to apply a careful interosseous mold about the distal radius/ulna by sandwiching the palms dorsally and volarly, respectively, with adequate pressure.
     - This is particularly important when casting fractures in children.

Outrigger (Routinely Ulnar Gutter) Cast:
Fig. 11.12A
Common Indications
- Ring and small finger fractures
- Ring and small finger metacarpal fractures

Recommended Materials
- Stockinette: 2-inch width (1-inch width optional but shown)
- Cast padding/undercast padding: 3-inch width
- Synthetic (fiberglass, polyester) cast tape: 3-inch width

Application
1. With the patient's wrist at neutral, fit the 2-inch width stockinette in length from about 1 inch beyond the fingertips up to the antecubital fossa. Cut a hole in the stockinette to adequately accommodate the thumb (Fig. 11.12B).
   - The 1-inch width stockinette may be used specifically for the thumb to create a protective sleeve of padding by folding suitable length over on itself three times (Fig. 11.12C).

2. At the distal end of the stockinette, cut a slit in the stockinette longitudinally toward the web space between the long and ring fingers (Fig. 11.12D).
3. Trim and fold a few layers of cast/undercast padding to place between the length of the ring and small fingers to prevent skin maceration (Fig. 11.12E).
   - These fingers can (optionally) be secured to one another via buddy-tape to further stabilize the injury.
4. Begin wrapping the padding just at the tips of the ring and small fingers and proceed proximally with a 50% overlay (Fig. 11.12F and G). Continue wrapping up to just distal to the antecubital fossa.
5. Pull the underlying stockinette back just over the padding at the distal and proximal ends, respectively. This will protect and pad the patient from the edge of the cast at those areas (Fig. 11.12H).
6. Begin wrapping the 3-inch width cast tape at the wrist joint (preferably starting on the volar surface rolling radial toward ulnar). One wrap circumferentially around to anchor is suitable before proceeding distally.
7. To fit the tape about the respective phalanges, angle and roll the tape to the dorsal aspect of the phalanges, even with the radial border of the ring finger cut at a slight angle partially through the width (proximal toward distal) to just fit the tape through the long and ring finger web space and around the ring and small finger phalanx segment(s) (Fig. 11.12I). Continue through and around the respective phalanx segment(s) circumferentially back to the dorsal-radial border of the ring finger again. Fit the tape around the phalanges in this manner two additional times (for three layers total).
   - Keep the tape just proximal to the padded edge of stockinette (or cast/undercast padding), protecting the phalanges.
   - Tuck or trim any tape that would intrude the long and ring finger web space or distal palm, respectively.
8. To fit the tape about the hand, from the phalanges roll toward the first web space, cut proportionately through the width of the tape proximal toward distal, laying the remaining width through web space and the newly cut ends dorsal and volar about the base of the thumb, respectively. Roll the tape circumferentially en route just proximal to the base of the thumb to overlay both of the cut ends. Fit

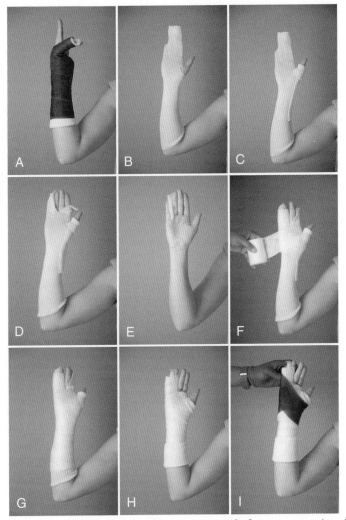

Fig. 11.12 A, Outrigger (ulnar gutter) cast. B, Apply stockinette. C, Create a protective sleeve of padding over the thumb with the stockinette and fold over on itself. D, Cut a slit in the stockinette between the long and ring fingers. E, Place some cast padding between the fingers to prevent skin maceration. F, Apply cast padding starting around the wrist and fingers. G, Continue the cast padding proximally. H, Fold the ends of the stockinette back over the cast padding. I, Begin wrapping the cast tape at the wrist and angle toward the fingers. Wrap around the fingers, cutting the cast tape from proximal to distal to fit between the long and ring finger web space.

the tape through the web space in this manner two additional times (for three layers total).

9. Continue wrap proceeding proximally with a 50% overlay up toward the antecubital fossa, but keep about one fingerbreadth distal to the padded edge of stockinette.

10. Roll the tape three times around the proximal end before proceeding back distally with a 50% overlay toward the wrist.

- Roll the tape to its completion or cut the roll free when enough tape has been applied to eliminate any shadow effect or noticeable weak points (typically three layers of tape is ideal).

11. Mold the cast to counter the given injury, commonly with the wrist in moderate extension and the ring and small fingers molded fully extended in the intrinsic plus position (metacarpal phalangeal joints in about 70 degrees of flexion) unless otherwise indicated.

- Continually rub the cast with open hands to help laminate and smooth the layers until the cast has set firm, taking care to not create any undue indentations or pressure points.
- Avoid using fingertips while molding.
- Be sure to apply a careful interosseous mold around the distal radius/ulna by sandwiching the palms dorsally and volarly, respectively, with adequate pressure.
- This is particularly important when casting fractures in children.

Muenster Cast: Fig. 11.13A
Common Indications
- Distal radius and ulna fractures
- Radius and ulna shaft fractures

Recommended Materials
- Stockinette: 2-inch width (1-inch width optional but shown)
- Cast padding/undercast padding: 3- and 4-inch width
- Synthetic (fiberglass, polyester) cast tape: 3- and 4-inch width

Application
1. With the patient's elbow flexed to approximately 90 degrees and the wrist at neutral, fit the 2-inch width stockinette in length from just beyond the fingertips up to midway of the humerus. Cut a hole in the stockinette to adequately accommodate the thumb (Fig. 11.13B).
   - The 1-inch width stockinette may be used specifically for the thumb to create a protective sleeve of padding by folding suitable length over on itself three times (Fig. 11.13C).
2. At the antecubital fossa, pull the proximal portion of the stockinette to overlap the distal portion to create a measurable fold (tongue) to be used subsequently.
   - The tongue should resemble a crescent that extends from epicondyle to epicondyle (as shown in preceding Fig.).
3. Begin wrapping the padding at MCHs and proceed proximally with a 50% overlay. Figure-of-eight wrap at the elbow and apply ample padding around the bony prominences of the epicondyles. Continue wrapping up to the midhumerus, but keep about two fingerbreadths distal to the stockinette edge (Fig. 11.13D).
   - The 3-inch width padding works for wrapping the hand, wrist, and forearm, whereas the 4-inch width is suitable for wrapping from the forearm, elbow, and arm.
4. Pull the underlying stockinette back just over the padding at the distal end. This will protect and pad the patient from the edge of the cast at that area (Fig. 11.13E).
   - The underlying stockinette at the proximal end will be pulled back over for padding at that end subsequently.
5. Begin wrapping the 3-inch width cast tape at the wrist joint. One wrap circumferentially around to anchor is suitable before proceeding distally to fit the tape proper about the hand. At the first web space, cut proportionately through the width of the tape proximal toward distal, laying the remaining width through the web space and the newly cut ends dorsal and volar about the base of the thumb, respectively. Roll the tape circumferentially en route just proximal to the base of the thumb to overlay both of the cut ends. Fit the tape through the web space in this manner two additional times (for three layers total) (Fig. 11.13F).
   - Keep the tape proximal to the padded edge of the stockinette (i.e., proximal to the distal palmar crease and proximal to the MCHs dorsally).
6. Continue wrapping, proceeding proximally with a 50% overlay up toward the antecubital fossa but keeping about one fingerbreadth distal to the antecubital fossa.
7. Roll the tape three layers thick around the proximal forearm before proceeding back distally with a 50% overlay toward the wrist.
   - Roll the tape to its completion or cut the roll free when enough tape has been applied to eliminate any shadow effect or noticeable weak points (typically ≥ 3 layers of coverage ideal)
   - The cast should resemble a short arm cast at this point.
8. Begin wrapping the 4-inch width cast tape just distal to the cast/undercast padding at the mid-humerus. Roll circumferentially three layers total around before proceeding distally with a 50% overlay toward the elbow.
9. Figure-of-eight wrap about the elbow three times, and overlap at least one-half width (2 inches) the

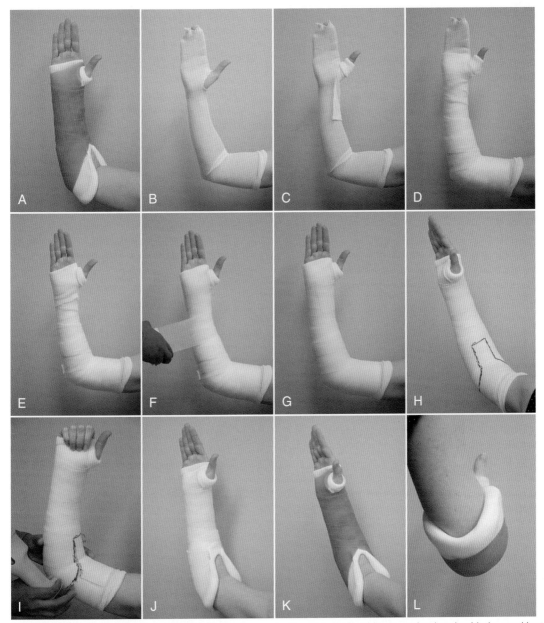

Fig. 11.13 **A,** Muenster cast. **B,** Apply stockinette. **C,** Create a protective sleeve of padding over the thumb with the stockinette and fold over on itself. **D,** Apply cast padding. **E,** Fold the ends of the stockinette back over the cast padding. **F,** Apply cast tape from distal to proximal. Partially cut the cast tape from proximal to distal and place between the first web space and repeat two additional times. **G,** Continue wrapping the cast tape proximally up the arm and use a figure-of-eight around the elbow. Allow to set with the elbow in the desired position. **H,** Draw lines around the elbow to guide cutting. **I,** Cut the splint using an oscillating cast saw. **J,** Fold the ends of the stockinette back over the cut end of the cast. **K,** Apply another layer of cast tape from distal to proximal and lay over the ends of the stockinette. **L,** Posterior view of completed cast.

still wet end of the cast at the proximal forearm. Ensure adequate coverage about the elbow (three or more layers) before proceeding proximally with a 50% overlay toward the midhumerus (Fig. 11.13G).

- Roll the tape to its completion or cut the roll free when enough tape has been applied to eliminate any shadow effect or noticeable weak points (typically three or more layers of coverage is ideal).
- The cast should resemble a shortened long arm cast at this point.

10. Mold the cast to counter the given injury or with the wrist at neutral unless otherwise indicated.
    - Continually rub the cast with open hands to help laminate and smooth the layers until the cast has set firm, taking care to not create any undue indentations or pressure points.
    - Avoid using fingertips while molding.
    - Be sure to apply a careful interosseous mold around the distal radius/ulna by sandwiching the palms dorsally and volarly, respectively, with adequate pressure.
    - This is particularly important when casting fractures in children.

11. Once the cast has set firm, tailor the proximal portion using an oscillating cast saw (Fig. 11.13H and I). Remove the areas otherwise obstructing the extension and flexion of the elbow while still leaving the portions that reduce the pronation and supination of the wrist.
    - Ergo, the cast should ultimately curve around two to three fingerbreadths proximal to the lateral and medial epicondyles, respectively, scoop down (distal) just proximal to the olecranon posteriorly, with an appropriate two to three fingerbreadths' notch extending along the length of the proximal radius anteriorly.
    - Remove the overlying cast with care to remove as little of the underlying cast/undercast padding as possible.

12. Cut a slit through the middle of the anterior cast/undercast padding proximal to distal extending to the notch at the proximal forearm. Fold the padding proximal to distal to rim the proximal margins of the cast, and pull the underlying stockinette taut back over the padding and the cast at the proximal end. This will protect and pad the patient from the edge of the cast at those areas (Fig. 11.13J).

- The tongue of stockinette (created in step 2 earlier) can be accessed once the cast/undercast padding has been slit and the proximal stockinette pulled back over the cast as described. Use this tongue to further tailor the stockinette/padding about the notch by pulling it taut distally, the ends of which will be fixed in place subsequently when overlaid by cast tape.

13. To complete the cast, wet another 3-inch width of cast tape and begin wrap at the distal end capturing the hand (one layer thick as earlier) before proceeding proximally with a 50% overlay to the proximal end to just capture the unsecured stockinette (one layer thick) (Fig. 11.13K and L).
    - Cut the roll free or optionally roll the tape to its completion with a 50% overlay proceeding distally again toward the wrist and hand.

14. Continually rub the cast with open hands to help laminate and smooth the layers until they have set firm.

Short Leg Non–Weight-Bearing Cast:
Fig. 11.14A
Common Indications
- Ankle sprains/strains
- Ankle dislocations
- Achilles tendon ruptures
- Distal tibia and fibula fractures
- Tarsal fractures
- Metatarsal fractures

Recommended Materials
- Stockinette: 3-inch width
- Cast/undercast padding: 4- and/or 6-inch width
- Synthetic (fiberglass, polyester) cast tape: 3- and 4-inch width
- Self-adhering orthopaedic foam: 4-inch width
  - If self-adhering foam is unavailable, about five layers of 4-inch width cast/undercast padding may be substituted.

Application
1. With the patient's ankle at neutral (ankle dorsiflexed to approximately 90 degrees) fit the 3-inch width stockinette in length about 1 inch distal to the hallux up to the patella and popliteal fossa.
   - In the case of an Achilles tendon injury, particularly, the foot should be kept in moderate equinus (plantar flexion).

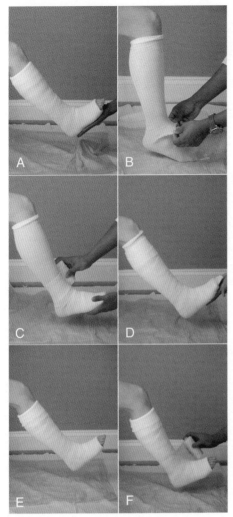

Fig. 11.14 A, Short leg non–weight-bearing cast. **B,** Apply stockinette and create a fold over the anterior ankle. **C,** Apply cast padding. **D,** Apply cast padding with the ankle in neutral. **E,** Fold the ends of the stockinette back over the cast padding. **F,** Apply cast tape from distal to proximal and use a figure-of-eight around the ankle.

4. Fit and apply the self-adhering orthopaedic foam (or cast/undercast padding) to extend anteriorly from just distal to the MTHs up to the tibial tuberosity (centered directly over the foot/shin). Additionally, apply a section of foam just even with the tibial tuberosity yet extending laterally from fibular head to proximal-medial tibia. Lastly, apply a section of foam posteriorly at the heel with length and width adequate to protect the Achilles tendon insertion.

5. Pull the underlying stockinette back just over the padding at the distal and proximal ends, respectively. This will protect and pad the patient from the edge of the cast at those areas (Fig. 11.14E).

6. Begin wrapping the 4-inch width cast tape just proximal to the ankle joint. One wrap circumferentially around to anchor is suitable before proceeding distally to fit the tape properly around the foot and ankle. Figure-of-eight wrap the ankle three times, and ensure adequate coverage around the heel (three or more layers) before proceeding distally with a 50% overlay toward the MTHs (Fig. 11.14F).

7. Roll the tape three layers thick around the MTHs before proceeding back proximally with a 50% overlay toward and/or beyond the ankle joint. Roll the tape to its completion.

8. Begin wrapping another 4-inch width cast tape about two fingerbreadths distal to the padded edge of stockinette at the tibial tuberosity/popliteal fossa. Roll circumferentially three layers total around before proceeding distally with a 50% overlay toward the ankle.

9. Figure-of-eight wrap the ankle and further overlap at least the midfoot. Ensure adequate overlay around the heel and ankle before proceeding proximally with a 50% overlay back toward the tibial tuberosity and popliteal fossa.
   • Roll the tape to its completion or cut the roll free when enough tape has been applied to eliminate any shadow effect or noticeable weak points (typically three or more layers of coverage is ideal).

10. Mold the cast to maintain the patient's ankle at neutral unless otherwise indicated.
    • Continually rub the cast with open hands to help laminate and smooth the layers until the cast has just set firm, taking care to not create any undue indentations or pressure points.
    • Avoid using fingertips while molding.

2. At the ankle joint, cut a slit in the stockinette (malleolus to malleolus) and pull the proximal portion of the stockinette to overlap the distal portion (or vice versa) (Fig. 11.14B).

3. Begin wrapping the padding just distal to the MTHs and proceed proximally with a 50% overlay. Use a figure-of-eight wrap about the ankle and heel and apply ample padding around the bony prominences of the malleoli. Continue wrapping up to the tibial tuberosity (Fig. 11.14C and D).

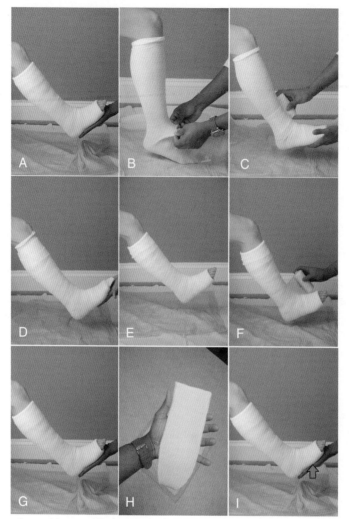

Fig. 11.15 **A,** Short leg walking cast. **B,** Apply stockinette and create a fold over the anterior ankle. **C,** Apply cast padding. **D,** Apply cast padding with the ankle in neutral. **E,** Fold the ends of the stockinette back over the cast padding. **F,** Apply cast tape from distal to proximal and use a figure-of-eight around the ankle. **G,** Allow to set with the ankle in neutral. **H,** Splint material, doubled over and trimmed. **I,** Apply splint material to dorsum of foot and secure with another layer of cast tape around the foot and ankle.

- Shape and mold to accommodate the malleoli and Achilles tendon insertion.
11. To further unify the distal and proximal portions of the cast, wrap another 4-inch width of cast tape (or 3-inch width, alternatively) beginning at the distal end (one layer) before proceeding proximally with a 50% overlay to the proximal end at the tibial tuberosity and popliteal fossa (one layer).
    - Cut the roll free or optionally roll the tape to its completion with a 50% overlay proceeding distally again toward the foot and ankle.

12. Continually rub the cast with open hands to help laminate and smooth the layers until the cast has set firm.

Short Leg Walking Cast: Fig. 11.15A
Common Indications
- Ankle sprains/strains
- Ankle dislocations
- Distal tibia and fibula fractures
- Tarsal fractures
- Metatarsal fractures

Recommended Materials

- Stockinette: 3-inch width
- Cast/undercast padding: 4- and 6-inch width
- Synthetic (fiberglass, polyester) cast tape: 3- and 4-inch width
- Synthetic (prefabricated) splint material: 3- or 4-inch width
- Self-adhering orthopaedic foam: 4-inch width
  - If self-adhering foam is unavailable, about five layers of 4-inch width cast/undercast padding may be substituted.

Application

1. With the patient's ankle at neutral (ankle dorsiflexed ≈ 90 degrees), fit the 3-inch width stockinette in length about 1 inch distal to the hallux up to the patella and popliteal fossa.
   - Casting the ankle at neutral (even minute dorsal flexion) is essential for the walking cast to allow proper balance and toe-off.
2. At the ankle joint, cut a slit in the stockinette (malleolus to malleolus) and pull the proximal portion of the stockinette to overlap the distal portion (or vice versa) (Fig. 11.15B).
3. Begin wrapping the padding just distal to the MTHs and proceed proximally with a 50% overlay. Figure-of-eight wrap the ankle and heel and apply ample padding around the bony prominences of the malleoli. Continue wrapping up to the tibial tuberosity (Fig. 11.15C and D).
4. Fit and apply the self-adhering orthopaedic foam (or cast/undercast padding) to extend anteriorly from just distal to the MTHs up to the tibial tuberosity (centered directly over the foot and anterior tibia). Additionally, apply a section of foam just even with the tibial tuberosity yet extending laterally from fibular head to proximal-medial tibia. Lastly, apply a section of foam posteriorly at the heel with length and width adequate to protect the Achilles tendon insertion.
5. Pull the underlying stockinette back just over the padding at the distal and proximal ends, respectively. This will protect and pad the patient from the edge of the cast at those areas (Fig. 11.15E).
6. Begin wrapping the 4-inch width cast tape just proximal to the ankle joint. One wrap circumferentially around to anchor is suitable before proceeding distally to fit the tape properly around the foot/ankle. Figure-of-eight wrap the ankle three times,

and ensure adequate coverage about the heel (three or more layers) before proceeding distally with a 50% overlay toward the MTHs (Fig. 11.15F).
7. Roll the tape three layers thick around the MTHs before proceeding back proximally with a 50% overlay toward and/or beyond the ankle joint. Roll the tape to its completion.
8. Begin wrapping another 4-inch width cast tape about two fingerbreadths distal to the padded edge of stockinette at the tibial tuberosity and popliteal fossa. Roll circumferentially three layers total around before proceeding distally with a 50% overlay toward the ankle.
9. Figure-of-eight wrap the ankle and further overlap at least the midfoot. Ensure adequate overlay around the heel and ankle before proceeding proximally with a 50% overlay back toward the tibial tuberosity and popliteal fossa.
   - Roll the tape to its completion or cut the roll free when enough tape has been applied to eliminate any shadow effect or noticeable weak points (typically three or more layers of coverage is ideal.)
10. Mold the cast to maintain the patient's ankle at neutral as indicated (Fig. 11.15G).
    - Continually rub the cast with open hands to help laminate and smooth the layers until the cast has set firm, taking care to not create any undue indentations or pressure points.
    - Avoid using fingertips while molding.
11. Measure so that the selected splint material fits double the length of the patient's foot from the MTHs to the heel. Remove the splint material from any protective sleeve it may be contained in, fold the splint over on itself, and subsequently trim it to roughly proportion the sole of the patient's foot. Hold this in place (Fig. 11.15H).
12. To further unify the distal and proximal portions of the cast and to tie in the newly made cast sole, wrap another 4-inch width of cast tape (or 3-inch width alternatively) beginning at the distal end (one layer) before proceeding proximally with a 50% overlay to the proximal end at the tibial tuberosity and popliteal fossa (one layer) (Fig. 11.15I).
    - Cut the roll free or optionally roll the tape to its completion with a 50% overlay proceeding distally again toward the foot/ankle.
13. Continually rub the cast with open hands to help laminate and smooth the layers until the cast has set firm.

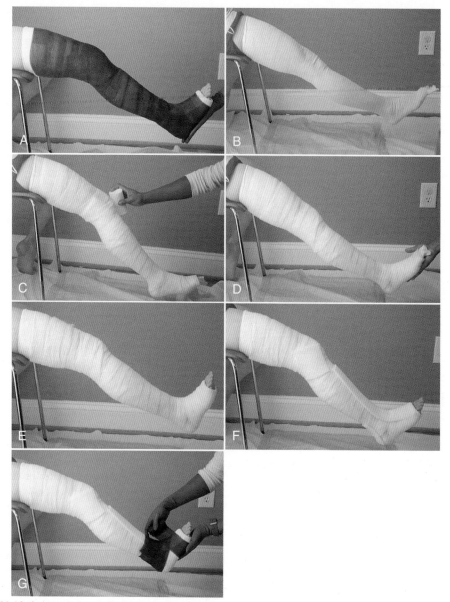

Fig. 11.16 **A**, Long leg cast. **B**, Apply stockinette. **C**, Apply cast padding. **D**, Keep the ankle in neutral. **E**, Fold the ends of the stockinette back over the cast padding. **F**, Apply self-adhering orthopaedic foam padding to the anterior foot, ankle, and tibia, bilateral knee condyles, and the posterior heel. **G**, Apply cast tape from distal to proximal and use a figure-of-eight around the ankle.

Long Leg Cast: Fig. 11.16A
Common Indications
- Unstable tibia/fibula fractures

Recommended Materials
- Stockinette: 4-inch width
- Cast/undercast padding: 4- and/or 6-inch width

- Synthetic (fiberglass, polyester) cast tape: 3- and 4-inch width
- Self-adhering orthopaedic foam: 4-inch width is commonly suitable
  - If self-adhering foam is unavailable, about five layers of 4-inch width cast/undercast padding may be substituted.

Application

1. With the patient's ankle at neutral (ankle dorsiflexed to approximately ≈90 degrees) and the knee just slightly flexed (≈15 degrees), fit the 4-inch width stockinette in length about 1 inch distal to the hallux up to (and with some gather at) the groin (Fig. 11.16B).

2. At the ankle joint, cut a slit in the stockinette (malleolus to malleolus) and pull the proximal portion of the stockinette to overlap the distal portion (or vice versa).

3. Begin wrapping the padding just distal to the MTHs and proceed proximally with a 50% overlay. Figure-of-eight wrap the ankle and heel and apply ample padding around the bony prominences of the malleoli. Likewise, amply pad the bony prominences of the knee. Continue wrapping up to the groin (Fig. 11.16C and D).

4. Pull the underlying stockinette back just over the padding at the distal and proximal ends, respectively. This will protect and pad the patient from the edge of the cast at those areas (Fig. 11.16E).

5. Fit and apply the self-adhering orthopaedic foam (or cast/undercast padding) to extend anteriorly from just distal to the MTHs up to the tibial tuberosity (centered directly overtop the foot and anterior tibia). Additionally, apply a square section of foam over each condyle. Lastly, apply a section of foam posteriorly at the heel with length and width adequate to protect the Achilles tendon insertion (Fig. 11.16F).

6. Begin wrapping the 4-inch width cast tape just proximal to the ankle joint. One wrap circumferentially around to anchor is suitable before proceeding distally to fit the tape properly around the foot and ankle. Figure-of-eight wrap the ankle three times, and ensure adequate coverage around the heel (three or more layers) before proceeding distally with a 50% overlay toward the MTHs (Fig. 11.16G).

7. Roll the tape three layers thick around the MTHs before proceeding back proximally with a 50% overlay toward and/or beyond the ankle joint. Roll the tape to its completion.

8. Begin wrapping another 4-inch width cast tape about two to three fingerbreadths distal to the padded edge of stockinette at the groin and gluteal sulcus. Roll circumferentially three layers thick around before proceeding distally with a 50% overlay toward the knee.

9. Figure-of-eight wrap the knee three times and ensure adequate overlay around the knee and popliteal fossa before proceeding proximally with a 50% overlay back toward the groin and gluteal sulcus. Roll the tape to its completion.

10. Begin wrapping another 4-inch width cast tape to quickly capture the ankle joint before proceeding proximally with a 50% overlay capture the knee.
    - Roll the tape to its completion or cut the roll free when enough tape has been applied to eliminate any shadow effect or noticeable weak points along the length of the entire cast (typically three or more layers of coverage is ideal).

11. Mold the cast to maintain the patient's ankle at neutral and knee slightly bent unless otherwise indicated.
    - Continually rub the cast with open hands to help laminate and smooth the layers until the cast has just set firm, taking care to not create any undue indentations or pressure points.
    - Avoid using fingertips while molding.

12. To further unify the distal and proximal portions of the cast, wrap another 4-inch width of cast tape (or 3-inch width alternatively) beginning at the distal end (one layer) before proceeding proximally with a 50% overlay to the proximal end at the groin and gluteal sulcus (one layer). Use a subsequent roll if necessary.
    - Cut the roll free or optionally roll the tape to its completion with a 50% overlay proceeding distally again toward the foot and ankle.

13. Continually rub the cast with open hands to help laminate and smooth the layers until the cast has set firm.

CRUX OF SPLINTING AND CASTING

The effect of the splint or cast is ultimately as dependent on the compliance of the patient as its proper application. Essential to complete application of the splint or cast, the patient's care instructions on discharge should include the following:

- Keep the splint or cast and the skin around the edges clean and dry:
  - When showering or bathing: Roll up a small towel and wrap it around your arm or leg, just about the splint or cast (do not tuck the towel into the splint or cast) and tape the towel into place. Place an arm or leg into a bag. Tape the bag into place.

- Protect the splint or cast from getting wet during rain.
  - A wet splint or cast must be changed within 24 hours to prevent skin breakdown.
- Do not put anything down inside of your splint or cast:
  - No powder, spray, lotion, water or liquids, or foreign objects to scratch under the splint or cast.
- Do not pull out the padding.
- Do not remove the splint or cast!
- Regular activities should include upper/lower extremity range of motion and edema control:
  - Move all joints/appendages not immobilized by the splint/cast.
  - Massage fingers/toes from the tips toward extremity several times daily as needed.
  - Elevate the extremity above the level of your heart (20 to 30 minutes, several times daily), especially whenever any of the following symptoms occur:
  - Increased swelling
  - Increased pressure
  - Increased tightness of cast
- Increased thumping or throbbing
- Increased pain, tingling, or numbness
- Decreased circulation at the end of the extremity (fingers/toes)
- Use a marker to circle any drainage from wounds on the outside of splint or cast. Report any changes in the amount of drainage.
- A splint or cast is meant to be snug and immobilize the involved joint; however, it should not cut off or decrease circulation to the extremity.
- Report or seek medical assistance for any of the following symptoms within 24 hours of cast or splint application:
  - Increase in pain, pressure, swelling, tingling, or numbness that cannot be controlled with elevation and movement (range of motion)
  - An increase in drainage, foul odor, fever, nausea, or vomiting
  - Any splint or cast that gets wet, cracked, broken, or too loose
  - Any pain related to rubbing or sores caused by rubbing

12

Wound Care and Suturing

Christine Seeger and Sara D. Rynders

WOUNDS

Fundamentals of Wound Healing

- The phases of wound healing are hemostasis, inflammatory, proliferative, and remodeling or maturation phase.
- The wound healing process begins with hemostasis. Within seconds of being injured, the blood vessel constricts and platelets are activated to form a platelet plug. This clot subsequently releases cytokines and growth factors to initiate the first phase of healing, the inflammatory phase.
- I. Inflammatory Phase
  - Occurs from injury through day 4.
  - Inflammatory cells and plasma proteins congregate and neutrophils are activated that secrete enzymes to clear the injury of cellular debris and neutralize bacteria.
  - Monocytes become macrophages, are activated, and secrete cytokines and growth factors to stimulate fibroblasts.
- II. Proliferative Phase
  - Days 4–14.
  - Characterized by epithelization, angiogenesis, and provisional matrix formation.
  - Fibroblasts and endothelial cells are the predominant cells of the proliferative phase.
  - Fibroblasts will synthesize collagen and form ground substance made of fibrin and fibronectin.
- III. Remodeling or Maturation Phase
  - Day 8 through 1 year, can overlap with Phase II.
  - Collagen is deposited and remodeled in an organized manner and reepithelization occurs.
  - Fibroblasts differentiate into myofibroblasts to promote wound contraction.

- The arrest of a wound in one of these phases, as well as prevention of progress to the next phase, may result in a nonhealing wound. As part of a surgical team, it is helpful to recognize potential challenges to normal wound healing and prepare patients for delayed wound healing or refer them promptly when indicated.
- Healing Intention Definitions:
  - Healing by First Intention (def.) when a wound heals with routine closure with minimal manipulation in a minimum amount of time.
  - Healing by Secondary Intention (def.) caused by infection, trauma, tissue loss, or poor wound approximation, secondary intention wound healing usually occurs when a wound is left open to allow granulation and maturation. Slower than first intention healing.
  - Healing by Third Intention (aka delayed primary closure) (def.) a typically traumatic wound that is initially débrided and left open, permitting the development of granulation tissue, and further débrided and closed at a later setting.

Principles of Wound Care
History
- Identify any comorbid medical conditions or medications that could delay normal wound healing:
  - Autoimmune disorders
  - Diabetes
  - Obesity
  - Malnutrition
  - Radiation history (at location of wound)
  - Smoking
  - Vascular disease

401

- Obtain a history of taking anticoagulants (aspirin, clopidogrel, coumadin) and the reason for taking them.
- Medications
  - Immunosuppression (for transplant recipients, autoimmune diseases)
  - Prednisone (steroids)
  - Chemotherapy
- Clarify the wound etiology or mechanism of injury
1. Is it acute or chronic?
   - If chronic, how long has the wound been there, and what has been tried before?
2. Was the offending agent contaminated or relatively clean? Infection risks increase with bite wounds, jagged wound margins with edges, devitalized edges, presence of a foreign body, and lacerations greater than 5 cm.

Physical Examination

- Inspect the wound for injury to neurovascular or tendinous structures
- Inspect the wound for hemostasis, exposed bone, or hardware if postsurgical
- Additional: Anatomic location, length, width and depth, wound classification (trauma, surgical, pressure ulcer), wound color (red, yellow, black or mixed), wound drainage (Table 12.1), presence of infection, patient's pain level

Acute Wounds

- Inspect the wound for the degree of contamination (e.g., road rash, grass, dirt).

TABLE 12.1   Description of Wound Drainage

Drainage	Definition
Serous	Clear, watery plasma
Sanguinous	Bloody (fresh bleeding)
Serosanguinous	Plasma and red blood cells
Purulent	Thick, white blood cells and living or dead organisms , possibly with a yellow, green, or brown color that can suggest the type of infecting organism

- Determine if there is actual tissue loss versus the appearance of a "gaping wound" that is caused by the wound margins being pulled in opposite directions.
  - This helps distinguish between wounds with sharply cut margins that can be reapproximated with suture from ones with skin and soft tissue loss that can be treated with local wound care.
- Determine if there is a skin avulsion, defined as a flap of skin detached from underlying structures but attached to intact skin along one margin.
  - If a skin flap is present, assess the viability of the skin by checking for capillary refill in the flap or seeing if it bleeds after a pinprick from an 18-gauge needle.

Chronic Wounds

- Is the wound clean or does it have necrotic debris? Is there evidence of infection?
- Is the patient sensate in the anatomic location of the wound (i.e., plantar ulcer with lack of plantar sensation)?
- Does the patient have palpable pulses in the extremity with the wound?
- Is there exposed bone (or tendon)? If so, osteomyelitis must be considered.

Principles of Wound Care: Treatment
Acute Wounds

Irrigation and débridement

1. Irrigate the wound with sterile normal saline with a device producing 7 to 15 pounds per square inch (psi) of pressure. Examples include commercially available pulse lavage devices and a 30-mL syringe attached to an 18-gauge angiocatheter.
2. Débride the wound of any contaminants such as grass and gravel. Minimize actual excision of tissue in the acute setting, and only débride obviously nonviable tissues.

Closure

- To minimize scarring, close acute wounds on extremities (excluding the hand, fingers, and foot) in layers.
  - Use monofilament suture for contaminated wounds to minimize bacterial seeding of braided suture (see later section on Sutures).
  - Avoid tension-creating techniques (vertical and horizontal mattress suture repair) because these are more likely to cause necrosis of the skin edges.

- Approximate muscle with strong absorbable monofilament suture that will last around 90 days (e.g., PDS suture).
- Approximate dermis with absorbable monofilament suture that will last around 40 days (e.g., Monocryl).
- Approximate skin with permanent monofilament suture that will be removed in 1 to 2 weeks (e.g., Prolene, Nylon).
- Wounds on the hand, fingers, and plantar foot should be closed in one layer only, with permanent monofilament suture taking bites through the epidermis and dermis.

Chronic Wounds

- Treatment is based on the etiology of the chronicity of the wound. Identify (on the basis of the history) the main etiology for the delayed wound healing.
  - Treat contaminated wounds with mechanical débridement in the office or enzymatic débridement or dressings that will débride the wound (normal saline wet-to-dry dressing changes twice daily). Chemicals such as Dakin solution should not be used for more than 48 hours because they can be toxic to healthy tissues.
  - Treat pressure ulcers with appropriate orthotics for pressure offloading or total contact casts if the patient is a candidate.
  - Treat arterial ulcers with referrals to vascular surgery for evaluation of inflow.
  - Treat diabetic ulcers with education (inspecting footwear and regular extremity examinations) and adequate glucose control.
  - Treat venous ulcers with graduated compression and edema control with an Unna boot, compression stockings, and elevation.
  - Infected wounds need operative débridement and appropriate antibiotic therapy.
- Many commercially available products are available for wound care, which is as much an art as it is a science. Fundamentally the provider must determine if the wound needs débridement or if it needs a moist environment with adjuncts to allow proper healing.
  - The ideal wound healing environment is slightly moist to encourage epithelialization. Topical antimicrobials (e.g., polysporin, bacitracin) or hydrogels are helpful when applied with a gauze dressing changed once a day. Topical antimicrobials can be associated with contact dermatitis.[1] In addition, research has shown that there is no difference in infection rates when comparing treatment of topical antimicrobials and petrolatum.[1]
  - Maceration of tissue indicates a high level of moisture; this may be caused by high drainage, infrequent dressing changes, or the incorrect dressing. Treatment plans should be adjusted.
  - More frequent dressing changes are helpful when trying to débride the wound with dressing changes (as in normal saline wet-to-dry dressing changes).
  - Refer your patient to a dedicated wound care specialist if you are not seeing improvement in the wound.

Negative Pressure Therapy for Wounds

- Wound vac therapy effectively decreases wound surface area and increases blood flow to promote healing in clean wounds.
- Wounds should be clean, without exposed vital structures, before placement of this dressing. Often this is best accomplished in the operating room, and the dressing is then changed every other day.

Hyperbaric Oxygen for Wounds

- This can be a useful adjunct to healing certain chronic wounds. Consider a referral to your local hyperbaric medicine specialist for chronic wounds with a history of radiation or for wounds that you suspect are associated with impaired oxygen delivery.

SUGGESTED READINGS

Broughton II G, Janis JE, Attinger CE: Wound healing: an overview, *Plast Reconstr Surg* 117:1e–S, 2006.

Fan K, Tang J, Escandon J, Kirsner RS: State of the art in topical wound-healing products, *Plast Reconstr Surg* 127:44S, 2011.

REFERENCE

1. Keim A, Marinucci J: Making better wound management decisions, *JAPAA* 32(4):15–22, 2019.

SUTURES

Suture Material
Absorbable or Permanent
- Use absorbable suture for wounds under less tension and permanent suture for wounds under greater tension.
- If using absorbable suture, pick one that will lose strength at the same time the wound is expected to heal and recover that strength.

Monofilament or Braided
- Monofilament suture slides easily through tissues and has fewer potential small spaces for serving as a nidus for opportunistic microorganisms; thus, it is more appropriate for closure of the contaminated wound.

Size
- The numeric designation is based on breaking strength, not diameter.
- Use the smallest possible size that is strong enough to close the wound.

Needle
Taper or Cutting Needle
- A taper needle is more appropriate for tendons, muscles, and deep tissues.
- A reverse cutting needle is more appropriate for skin closure.

Commonly Used Absorbable Suture
Vicryl
- Braided
- Loses all of its strength by 2 weeks
- Good for closing deeper tissues
Monocryl
- Monofilament
- Loses all of its strength by 3 weeks
- Good for closing deeper tissues, especially in contaminated wounds
PDS
- Monofilament
- At 6 weeks, 25% still remains
- Good for closing fascia, muscle, and other deep tissues

Commonly Used Permanent Suture
Nylon
- Monofilament

Prolene
- Monofilament
- Both nylon and Prolene have similar applications: skin closure and tendon repairs. It is often a matter of personal preference as to the choice of one over another.
- Permanent skin suture should be removed as soon as the wound is ready to prevent unsightly cross-hatched scars (7 to 14 days depending on the patient and anatomic site).

Suture Technique
General Principles
- For percutaneous suturing:
  1. Always enter the skin with the needle perpendicular to the skin.
  2. The distance from the entry of the needle to the wound on one side of the wound should equal the distance of the needle entry to exit on the other side of the wound.
  3. The depth of the needle penetration should be equivalent on both sides of the wound to prevent the creation of a shelf, or mismatched wound margins.
  4. Maximize eversion of the wound margins to facilitate optimal appearance of the ultimate scar.
- Strength layers include dermis and fascia. Sutures in subcutaneous fat will not hold tension and will not minimize scarring, but careful placement of buried approximating sutures in the fascia and dermis will result in finer scars.
- Regardless of the technique, if percutaneous sutures remain in place for too long, they will result in a scar with crosshatching or have a so-called "railroad track" appearance. Prevent this with timely removal of sutures. Placement of a deep, buried layer of dermal approximating suture allows expedient removal of percutaneous epidermal sutures.
- Practice atraumatic tissue handling (e.g., avoid pinching skin with forceps) to optimize the appearance of the scar and minimize damage to tissues being repaired.
  Simple interrupted. Fig. 12.1
- *Technique*: With wrist pronated, enter the skin with the needle perpendicular to the skin and wound. Then supinate and travel across the wound, taking equal bites on either side of the wound edge, and grasp the needle. When viewed in cross section the bite should look like a pear, wider in the dermis

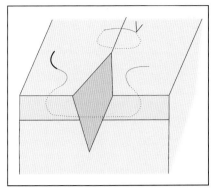

Fig. 12.1 Simple Interrupted Suture.

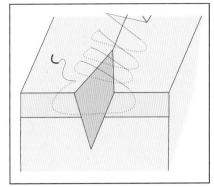

Fig. 12.2 Simple Running Suture.

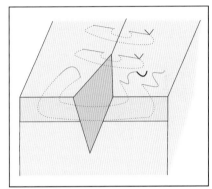

Fig. 12.3 Vertical Mattress Suture.

and narrower in the epidermis to optimize the final appearance of the scar. The knot is secured after the needle passes through both sides of the wound.

- *Common Uses*
  - Percutaneous skin closure
  - Fascial reapproximation

Simple running. *Fig. 12.2*

- *Technique*: See earlier description for a simple interrupted suture. The difference is that after the first bite, the needle is left attached to the suture end and continuously used from one wound margin to the other with a knot secured at the beginning and one secured at the end of the area to be approximated.
- *Common Uses*
  - Percutaneous skin closure, not recommended for wounds under great tension.

Vertical mattress. *Fig. 12.3*

- *Technique*: Also called "far-far-near-near stitch." See earlier description for a simple interrupted suture. After taking the first bite in the deeper layer, the needle is reversed and the "near-near" bite is taken. This is a smaller bite (both in depth and distance to the wound), taken in the opposite direction to the first bite. The knot is secured on the side of the wound. The knot should be secured away from any potentially compromised tissue (e.g., the knot is not secured on the same side as a flap of skin).
- *Common Uses*
  - A vertical mattress suture should not be commonly used in the acute setting because this technique can strangulate tissue if the wound is under great tension.
  - This is an effective technique for eversion of skin edges when the wound is under minimal tension.

Horizontal mattress. *Fig. 12.4*

- *Technique*: See earlier technique for a simple interrupted suture. Before tying the knot, the needle is brought back in the reverse direction across the wound. The second entry point is made after traveling parallel to the wound the same distance as the previous exit point was from the wound edge. The needle is then passed as a simple interrupted suture in the reverse direction and secured on the side of the wound. The knot should be secured away from any potentially compromised tissue (e.g., the knot is not secured on the same side as a flap of skin).
- *Common Uses*
  - Should not be commonly used in the acute setting because this technique can strangulate tissue if the wound is under great tension.
  - This is an effective technique for eversion of skin edges when the wound is under minimal tension.

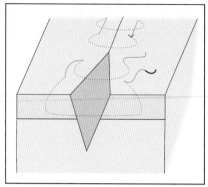

Fig. 12.4 Horizontal Mattress Suture.

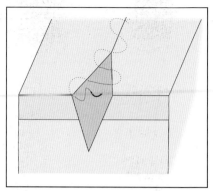

Fig. 12.6 Subcuticular Suture.

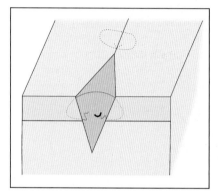

Fig. 12.5 Deep Dermal Buried Suture.

Buried deep dermal. *Fig. 12.5*
- *Technique*: Enter the wound from a deep aspect, not the epidermis. With the needle perpendicular to the dermis, the dermis is entered and the wrist is supinated. The needle should exit just deep to the dermal-epidermal junction and travel across the wound. Enter the other side of the wound at the same level as the exit on the opposite side (just below the dermal-epidermal junction). Supinate and then exit in the deep dermis across from the entry point on the other side. The knot is secured deep in the wound, and the tails of the knot are cut flush with the knot.
- *Common Uses*
  - Deep layer before percutaneous skin closure
  - Effective technique to take tension off of the epidermal closure to optimize ultimate scar outcome

Subcuticular. *Fig. 12.6*
- *Technique*: A buried deep dermal stitch is secured deep in the wound at the apex. Then the needle is passed from deep to superficial at the wound apex, and horizontal bites are taken (in contrast to all the previous bites described in this chapter). The bite is taken at the dermal-epidermal junction. The needle enters perpendicular to the dermis with the needle held parallel to the epidermal surface. The needle then enters the contralateral edge of the wound at the same vertical depth and longitudinal wound distance or mirror image of where it exited on the previous wound margin. This is repeated until closure of the wound, and a buried knot is secured at the end with the tails of the knot cut flush with the knot.
- *Common Uses*
  - Skin closure in areas of minimal tension, in combination with buried deep dermal stitches.

SUGGESTED READINGS

Ethicon: *Knot tying manual*, 2010. Available online. Ethicon.

Ethicon: *Wound closure manual*, 2012. Available online. Ethicon.

Vasconez HC, Habash A: Plastic and reconstructive surgery. In Doherty GM, editor: *Current diagnosis & treatment: surgery*, ed 13, New York, 2010, McGraw-Hill.

Weitzul S, Taylor RS: Suturing technique and other closure materials. In Robinson JK, editor: *Surgery of the skin*, ed 2, Saint Louis, 2010, Elsevier.

ACKNOWLEDGMENTS

The authors would like to acknowledge the contribution of the previous edition authors, Shruti Tannan and Adam Katz.

Page numbers followed by *f* indicate figures, *t* indicate tables, and *b* indicate boxes.